ORTHOPEDIC SECRETS

Third Edition

ORTHOPEDIC SECRETS

Third Edition

David E. Brown, M.D.
Clinical Associate Professor
Department of Orthopedic Surgery and Rehabilitation
University of Nebraska Medical Center
Omaha, Nebraska

Randall D. Neumann, M.D.
Orthopedic Surgeon
Ortho West, P.C.
Omaha, Nebraska

HANLEY & BELFUS
An Affiliate of Elsevier

HANLEY & BELFUS
An Affiliate of Elsevier

The Curtis Center
Independence Square West
Philadelphia, Pennsylvania 19106

DISCLAIMER

Library of Congress Control Number: 2003107383

ORTHOPEDIC SECRETS, 3rd edition   ISBN 1-56053-541-5

Last digit is the print number: 9 8 7 6 5 4 3 2 1

CONTENTS

CONTRIBUTORS

David P. Adkison, M.D.
Orthopedic Surgeon, St. Vincent's Hospital, Birmingham, Alabama

Marc Bouchard, MD
Fellow in Foot and Ankle Surgery, Department of Orthopedic Surgery, Mayo Clinic, Scottsdale, Arizona

Katherine K. Brady, B.A.
Medical Student, Stanford University School of Medicine, Stanford, California

Kristoffer M. Breien, M.D.
Chief Resident, Department of Orthopedic Surgery, University of Nebraska Medical Center, Omaha, Nebraska

Brian E. Brigman, M.D.
Assistant Professor, Department of Orthopedic Surgery, Duke University, Durham, North Carolina

Marcia E. Bromley, M.D.
University of Nebraska College of Medicine, Omaha, Nebraska

Jason A. Browdy, M.D.
Resident, Department of Orthopedic Surgery, University of Nebraska Medical Center, Omaha, Nebraska

David E. Brown, M.D.
Clinical Associate Professor, Department of Orthopedic Surgery and Rehabilitation, University of Nebraska Medical Center, Omaha, Nebraska

Peter K. Buchert, MD
Department of Orthopedic Surgery, University of Missouri Medical School, Columbia, Missouri

Deepak V. Chavda, MD
Medical Director and Orthopedic Surgeon, Texas Bone and Joint Center, North Richland Hills, Texas

Kim J. Chillag, M.D.
Assistant Clinical Professor, Department of Orthopedics, University of South Carolina School of Medicine, Columbia; The Moore Orthopedic Clinic, P.A., Columbia, South Carolina

Michael P. Clare, M.D.
Assistant Professor, Department of Orthopedic Surgery, University of Nebraska Medical Center, Omaha, Nebraska

Christian Clark, M.D.
Resident, Department of Orthopedics, National Naval Medical Center, Bethesda, Maryland

Ian D. Crabb, MD
Orthopedic Surgeon, Ortho West P.C., Omaha, Nebraska

Jeffrey P. Davick, M.D.
Private Practice, Des Moines Orthopaedic Surgeons, P.C., West Des Moines, Iowa

Stephen E. Doran, MD
Section of Neurosurgery, University of Nebraska Medical Center, Omaha, Nebraska

Paul W. Esposito, M.D., FAAP, FAAOS
Associate Professor, Department of Orthopedic Surgery, University of Nebraska Medical Center, Omaha, Nebraska

Edward Vincent Fehringer, M.D.
Assistant Professor, Department of Orthopedics, University of Nebraska College of Medicine, Omaha; Staff Physician, Department of Orthopedic Surgery and Rehabilitation, University of Nebraska Medical Center, Omaha, Nebraska

Brett W. Fischer, M.D.
Medical Director, Department of Rehabilitation, Fremont Area Medical Center, Fremont, Nebraska

Timothy C. Fitzgibbons, M.D.
Private Practice, Gross, Iwersen, Kratchovil and Klein, P.C., Omaha, Nebraska

Jonathan E. Fuller, M.D.
Staff Surgeon, Nebraska Methodist Hospital, Omaha; Staff Surgeon, Immanuel Medical Center, Omaha; Staff Surgeon, Bergan-Mercy Medical Center, Omaha, Nebraska

John P. Furia, M.D.
Director, Department of Sports Medicine, Evangelical Community Hospital, Lewisburg; Department of Orthopedics, Sunbury Community Hospital, Sunbury; Department of Orthopedics, Division of Surgery, Shamukin Area Community Hospital, Coal Township, Pennsylvania

Keith Robert Gabriel, M.D.
Associate Professor, Department of Surgery, Division of Orthopedics and Rehabilitation, Southern Illinois University School of Medicine, Springfield, Illinois

Glen M. Ginsburg, M.D.
Associate Professor, Department of Orthopedics, University of Nebraska Medical Center, Omaha, Nebraska

Stephen Hansen, M.D., MBA
Department of Orthopedic Surgery and Rehabilitation, University of Nebraska Medical Center, Omaha, Nebraska

Brian P. Hasley, M.D.
House Officer, Department of Orthopedic Surgery, University of Nebraska Medical Center, Omaha, Nebraska

Daniel P. Hoeffel, MD
Summit Orthopedics, LTD, St. Paul, Minnesota

Walter W. Huurman, MD
Department of Orthopedics and Rehabilitation, University of Nebraska Medical Center, Omaha, Nebraska

Kirk S. Hutton, M.D.
Clinical Assistant Professor, Department of Orthopedic Surgery, University of Nebraska Medical Center, Omaha, Nebraska

David John Inda, M.D.
Private Practice, Gross, Iwersen, Kratchovi, and Klein, P.C., Omaha, Nebraska

Zubin Gian Khubchandani, M.D.
Private Practice, Texas Bone and Joint Center, North Richland Hills, Texas

Todd A. Kile, M.D.
Assistant Professor, Department of Orthopedic Surgery, Mayo Clini, Scottsdale, Arizona

Brian Konowalchuk, MD
Department of Orthopedic Surgery, University of Minnesota, Minneapolis, Minnesota

Steven G. Kumagai, M.D.
West Omaha Sports Medicine and Orthopedic Surgery, Omaha, Nebraska

Richard A. Kutilek, M.D.
Radiologist, Nebraska Methodist Hospital, Omaha; Assistant Clinical Professor, Department of Radiology, Creighton University Medical Center, Omaha, Nebraska

David M. Lichtman, M.D.
Professor, Department of Surgery, Uniformed Services University of the Health Sciences, Bethesda, Maryland; Chair and Director, Department of Orthopedic Surgery, John Peter Smith Network, Fort Worth; Clinical Professor, University of Texas Southwestern, Dallas, Texas

Adolph V. Lombardi, Jr., M.D., FACS
Clinical Assistant Professor of Orthopedic Surgery, Ohio State University Hospitals, Columbus; Clinical Assistant Professor, Department of Biomedical Engineering, Ohio State University, Columbus, Ohio

Craig R. Mahoney, M.D.
Attending Orthopedic Surgeon, Iowa Orthopedic Center, Des Moines, Iowa

Edward R. McDevitt, M.D.
Department of Orthopedic Surgery, Anne Arundel Medical Center, Annapolis, Maryland

Matthew T. McLeay, M.D.
Clinical Staff, Department of Internal Medicine, University of Nebraska Medical Center, Omaha, Nebraska

Scott T. McMullen, M.D.
Adjunct Assistant Professor, Department of Orthopedic Surgery, University of Nebraska Medical Center, Omaha, Nebraska

John A. Miyano, M.D.
Private Practice, Seattle Hand Surgery Group, P.C., Seattle; Clinical Assistant Professor, Department of Orthopedics, University of Washington, Seattle, Washington

Matthew A. Mormino, M.D.
Assistant Professor, Department of Orthopedic Surgery, University of Nebraska Medical Center, Omaha, Nebraska

Kevin L. Nelson, M.D.
Director of MRI Division, Department of Radiology, Methodist Hospital, Omaha, Nebraska

Randall D. Neumann, M.D.
Orthopedic Surgeon, Ortho West, P.C., Omaha, Nebraska

Peter Norman Ove, M.D.
Anne Arundel Medical Center, Annapolis, Maryland

William R. Palmer, MD
Department of Internal Medicine, University of Nebraska College of Medicine, Omaha, Nebraska

David A. Peterson, M.D.
Orthopaedic Clinic of Salina, Salina, Kansas

Stephen R. Pledger, MD
Staff Physician, Orthopaedic and Sports Medicine Consultants, Inc., Springfield, Ohio

Samar K. Ray, M.D., FRCS
Clinical Assistant Professor, Department of Orthopedic Surgery and Rehabilitation, University of Nebraska Medical Center, Omaha; Active Staff, Methodist Hospital and Children's Hospital, Omaha, Nebraska

Jeffrey A. Rodgers, M.D.
Clinical Teaching Faculty, Division of Hand Surgery, Methodist Hospital, Des Moines, Iowa

Scott G. Rose, M.D.
Chairman, Department of Surgery, Methodist Hospital, Omaha; Faculty, Department of Surgery, University of Nebraska Medical Center, Omaha, Nebraska

Michael J. Schmidt, MD
Orthopaedic and Sports Medicine Clinic, Topeka, Kansas

John A. Schneider, MD
Sports Medicine and Orthopedic Center, Milwaukee, Wisconsin

Jeffrey A. Senall, MD
Fellow in Foot and Ankle Surgery, Department of Orthopedic Surgery, Mayo Clinic, Scottsdale, Arizona

Jeffrey Joseph Tiedeman, M.D.
Clinical Instructor, Department of Orthopedic Surgery, University of Nebraska Medical Center, Omaha, Nebraska

Joshua A. Urban, M.D.
Chief Resident, Department of Orthopedic Surgery and Rehabilitation, University of Nebraska Medical Center, Omaha, Nebraska

Jeremy J. Vanicek, PA-C
Ortho West, P.C., Omaha, Nebraska

Donald J. Walla, MD
Nebraska Orthopedic Associates, Lincoln, Nebraska

W. Michael Walsh, MD
Orthopedic Surgeon, Ortho West, P.C., Omaha; Clinical Associate Professor, Department of Orthopedic Surgery and Rehabilitation, University of Nebraska Medical Center, Omaha, Nebraska

Scott P. Wattenhofer, M.D., FACS
Associate Professor, Department of Surgery, University of Nebraska Medical Center, Omaha, Nebraska

Steven J. Wees, MD
Department of Internal Medicine, University of Nebraska Medical Center, Omaha, Nebraska

Joseph Yao, M.D.
Private Practice, Advanced Orthopaedics of Blytheville, Blytheville, Arkansas

PREFACE TO THE THIRD EDITION

We are gratified by the popularity of the first two editions of *Orthopedic Secrets* and present the third edition as a continuation of that same tradition and purpose: to provide an overview of orthopedics in question-and-answer format covering the common conditions encountered in an orthopedic practice. We have attempted to present a vast amount of information in a concise format that is both informative and thought-provoking without being overly simplistic.

Each chapter in the new edition has been revised and updated, and several new chapters on emerging technologies have been included; most notable are the new chapters on hip arthroscopy and cartilage transplantation, which provide the reader with concise coverage of these new techniques.

As Randy and I have undergone significant practice changes, the third edition has been more challenging than the first two. We have to thank our editor, Jacqueline Mahon, and Linda Belfus for their encouragement, dedication, and support. We could not have completed this without them.

We would also like to thank all of the chapter authors for their contributions to the text. Many are orthopedic residents, graduates, and faculty at the Creighton-Nebraska Orthopaedic Residency Program who also have contributed in the past.

David E. Brown, MD
Randall D. Neumann, MD
EDITORS

I. General

1. OSTEOARTHRITIS

Randall D. Neumann, M.D.

1. What is osteoarthritis?

Osteoarthritis is a noninflammatory disorder of movable joints characterized by deterioration of articular cartilage and formation of new bone at the joint surfaces and margins. This disorder is also known as degenerative joint disease.

2. Describe the pathologic findings in osteoarthritis.

Early degeneration or disruption of the articular cartilage surface, which can be described as flaking or fibrillation, occurs most commonly on the weight-bearing surfaces of the joint. This early finding gradually proceeds to complete loss of articular cartilage and eburnation of the bone, which becomes highly polished and has a sclerotic surface, suggesting ivory. Cyst areas may occur in the subarticular bone, usually on the weight-bearing surface, and are thought to be related to microfractures that degenerate. New bone formation is usually found at the base of the articular cartilage and surrounding the cyst, creating an area of sclerosis.

3. What factors are important in the etiology of degenerative joint disease?

- Obesity
- Genetics and heredity
- Occupation (e.g., interphalangeal joint degeneration in the fingers of cotton mill workers)
- Multiple endocrine disorders, such as diabetes mellitus and acromegaly
- Multiple metabolic disorders, including Paget's disease, gout, and calcium pyrophosphate deposition (CPPD) disease

4. Discuss the epidemiologic features of osteoarthritis.

By age 40 years, 90% of all persons have some degenerative changes in the weight-bearing joints, even though clinical symptoms are generally absent. Roentgenographic manifestations of the disease commonly occur in the third decade. When minimal disease is excluded, the prevalence of osteoarthritis is approximately 20%. In one study 85% of patients aged 55–64 years had some degree of osteoarthritis in one or more joints. Men and women are equally affected by osteoarthritis. Under age 45 years the prevalence was greater among men, whereas prevalence was greater in women after age 55 years. Some studies show that patients with obesity have an increased frequency of osteoarthritis in the weight-bearing joints.

5. What are osteophytes? Why do they form?

Osteophytes, one of the main characteristics of osteoarthritis, are outgrowths, usually marginal, of ossified cartilage. Because of the vascularization in the subchondral bone, proliferation of adjacent cartilage and enchondral ossification occur. Outgrowths extend from the free articular space along the path of least resistance.

6. Describe the pathologic abnormalities of osteoarthritis in correlation with the radiographic abnormalities.

- Cartilage erosion—loss of joint space
- Increased cellularity and bone deposition of subchondral bone—bone eburnation

- Synovial fluid intrusion into bone—subchondral cysts
- Revascularization of the remaining cartilage and capsular traction—osteophytes
- Synovial membrane stimulation—osteophytes
- Compression of weakened bone—bony collapse
- Fragmentation of osteochondral surface—loose bodies
- Destruction and distortion of capsular ligaments—deformity and malalignment

7. Describe the symptoms in patients with osteoarthritis.

The cardinal symptom of osteoarthritis is pain, which first occurs only with joint use and motion but later is relieved only by rest. The pain is usually aching in character and poorly localized. In the severe stages of the disease, pain may awaken the patient from sleep because of loss of protective muscular joint splinting that during the waking hours limits painful motion. Pain may occur with minimal motion and even at rest. Muscle spasms around the joint, often described as sharp, may add to the pain. Most affected patients take nonsteroidal antiinflammatory drugs (NSAIDs) or pain pills for relief of the symptoms.

Stiffness on awakening in the morning and after periods of inactivity during the day is common. As the joint is "limbered up," patients feel better. If the patient sits down for any length of time, pain may develop after commencement of activity. The patient must "loosen" the joint. If loose bodies or meniscal tears are present, patients may complain of giving way or locking episodes. Typically there is some limitation of motion, often involving loss of extension and flexion. In the hip, patients usually maintain 90° of flexion but lose most abduction as well as internal and external rotation. In the knee, most patients develop a flexion contracture, usually mild. Loss of dorsiflexion in the ankle may occur, along with flexion contractures in the proximal and distal interphalangeal joints. Patients may describe crepitation, which generally occurs with any range of motion of the joint. The crepitation may be associated with pain and generally signifies the bone-on-bone quality of degenerative arthritis.

8. What are the clinical signs of patients with osteoarthritis?

Most patients have localized tenderness, generally along the area of the most significant degenerative changes. Patients may have palpable osteophytes. Crepitation may occur with attempts at range of motion. Generally range of motion is diminished compared with the normal extremity. Boggy synovitis, if present, is not as severe as with rheumatoid arthritis. Usually effusion is minimal. Increased effusion is common after slight twisting or giving way episodes.

9. What laboratory abnormalities are seen in primary osteoarthritis?

Erythrocyte sedimentation rate, complete blood count, rheumatoid factor, serum calcium, alkaline phosphates, and electrophoresis are usually within normal limits. Patients may have laboratory abnormalities in secondary osteoarthritis, such as the high levels of uric acid in gout or the high levels of alkaline phosphates in Paget's disease.

10. Describe the synovial fluid analysis in a patient with osteoarthritis.

Synovial fluid in osteoarthritis is generally noninflammatory. The increase in white blood cells is minimal. Viscosity is good. Uric acid or CPPD crystals are not found. Glucose is generally normal. No bacteria are seen on Gram stain.

11. What other radiographic abnormalities are seen with osteoarthritis?

Scanning with ^{99m}technetium shows increased uptake around osteoarthritic joints. Magnetic resonance imaging reveals areas of degenerative changes, subchondral cysts, and osteophyte formation. Such abnormalities are also commonly seen with computed tomography.

12. What is the differential diagnosis of osteoarthritis?

Differential diagnosis includes osteoarthritis, rheumatoid arthritis, gouty arthritis, calcium pyrophosphate arthropathy, osteonecrosis, and a neuropathic joint related to endocrine disease.

13. **List the major complications of degenerative joint disease.**
   - With loss of joint space, angulation in the affected extremity may occur. With complete collapse on the inner or outer side of one of the joints, such as the knee, deformity occurs.
   - Subluxation, as seen in the carpometacarpal joint of the thumb.
   - Ankylosis or complete bony fusion of a joint, such as the great toe metatarsophalangeal joint.
   - Interarticular loose bodies or joint mice related to subchondral fractures.

14. **Name the most common disease processes in which secondary osteoarthritis may develop.**

Acute trauma	Hyperparathyroidism
Chronic trauma	Overuse of interarticular corticosteroid therapy
Alcaptonuria	Neurologic diseases, including diabetes
Wilson's disease	Syringomyelia
Hemochromatosis	Frostbite
Acromegaly	Hemophilia

15. **What is a Heberden's node?**
   Heberden's nodes are the detectable bony enlargements about the distal interphalangeal joints of the hands.

16. **What is Bouchard's node?**
   Bouchard's nodes are bony enlargements in the proximal interphalangeal joints.

17. **What is a mucinous cyst?**
   Mucinous cysts arise from the joint capsule in the distal or proximal interphalangeal joints. They generally contain degenerative myxomatous fibrous tissue from the degenerative arthritis.

18. **Describe osteoarthritis of the first carpometacarpal joint of the thumb.**
   Osteoarthritis of the trapezoimetacarpal articulation is commonly seen in women. Patients have significant pain at the base of the thumb with loss of grip strength and range of motion. This syndrome typically occurs in women > 50 years of age.

19. **List causes of degenerative arthritis in the wrist joint.**
   - Kienbsck's disease (osteonecrosis of the lunate)
   - Trauma
   - Nonunion of the scaphoid
   - Gout
   - CCPD disease
   - Carpal instability from ligamentous disruption of the scapholunate ligament

20. **Describe the clinical presentation of a patient with osteoarthritis of the elbow.**
   Osteoarthritis is four times more common in males than females. The dominant extremity is affected in 80–90% of cases, and a finding of occupational repetitive trauma is common. Loss of extension of the elbow is the most common complaint, along with stiffness. Pain occurs with terminal extension.

21. **Which area of the shoulder has the highest incidence of degenerative arthritis?**
   The acromioclavicular joint has the highest incidence of degenerative arthritis.

22. **What is a bunion?**
   A bunion is a combination of degenerative joint disease at the first metatarsal phalangeal joint and angulation or valgus at the same joint. Symptoms include progression of swelling and pain, difficulty with shoe wear and walking, and inflammation of the bursa of the medial aspect of the joint.

23. Describe the arthritis that occurs in the spine.

Formation is located both anteriorly and posteriorly adjacent to the intervertebral disk. Narrowing of the intervertebral disk is common with actual fusion of the adjacent vertebrae. Subluxation of one vertebral body on another may occur, especially in the lumbar spine. The facet joints with osteophyte formation may cause narrowing of the foraminal space, which may cause nerve root irritation.

24. Discuss the findings of osteoarthritis in the hip.

Osteoarthritis in the hip causes joint space narrowing, which is best seen on an anteroposterior view of the pelvis. Osteophytes occur inferiorly and superiorly on the acetabulum. Osteophytes may be found on the superior and inferior surface of the femoral head. Loose bodies are commonly seen. Sclerosis of the underlying bone with adjacent cystic areas may be seen in the head, neck, and acetabular area of the joint.

25. Describe the clinical and radiographic findings of osteoarthritis in the knee.

Any of the three compartments of the knee—medial, lateral, or patellofemoral—may be involved. Complete collapse of the lateral joint space causes the patient to be "knock-kneed" or in a valgus position. Complete joint space collapse in the medial compartment causes the patient to be bow-legged or in a varus position. Osteophytes may occur medially and laterally or along the patellofemoral joint. Often loose bodies are identified in the intercondylar notch region and in the posterior portions of the medial and lateral joint spaces. Subchondral cysts and sclerosis are common in the affected joint.

26. What is erosive osteoarthritis?

Erosive osteoarthritis involves primarily the distal and proximal interphalangeal joints. The disease may be hereditary. Severe inflammatory episodes lead to joint deformities and sometimes to ankylosis. Cysts may be painful and tender. Postmenopausal women are most frequently affected. Radiographs reveal severe bony erosions and subchondral bony sclerosis. Severe joint destruction is noted.

27. What is DISH?

DISH is the acronym for **d**iffuse **i**diopathic **s**keletal **h**yperostosis, a type of osteoarthritis with a significant amount of osteophyte formation. The spine shows calcification on the anterior longitudinal ligament and the peripheral disk margins. Calcification along the length of the ligaments has been described as following ossification along the vertebral bodies. The disk space height is generally preserved; calcification may be seen in the sacrotuberous, iliolumbar, and patellar ligaments. The main complaint is spinal stiffness, with surprisingly little pain. Patients generally have heel pain related to calcaneal spurs. Marginal osteophytes may be seen in all of the peripheral joints.

28. What new and experimental treatments for osteoarthritis and cartilage defects are available?

- **Soft tissue grafts.** Periosteal or perichondral grafts are sewn over defects (e.g., a small piece of rib perichondrium is transplanted into a metacarpophalangeal joint).
- **Chondrocyte transplantation.** Articular cartilage is harvested from the knee via arthroscopy. The chondrocytes are cultured and then placed in the defect. A periosteal flap is then sutured over the defect with the cells present. Medial femoral condyle defects are being treated this way.
- **Mosaic grafts.** A mosaic graft is an autograft. Osteochondral plugs are taken from the peripheral area of the anteromedial or anterolateral femoral condyle. Corresponding holes are drilled to match the size and depth of the plugs in the chondral defect, which are then inserted into the defect. Differing plug sizes create a "mosaic" look.

- **Artificial matrix.** Caron fiber, collagen, bone matrix, and polylactic acid are used to try to achieve a matrix upon which cartilage can grow.
- **Fresh osteochondral grafts**

BIBLIOGRAPHY

1. Buckwalter JA, Mankin HJ: Articular cartilage: Degeneration and osteoarthritis, repair, regeneration, and transplantation. J Am Acad Orthop Surg Instructional Course Lectures 47:487–504, 1998.
2. Hough AJ, McCarty DJ, Koopman WJ (eds): Pathology of osteoarthritis. In Arthritis and Allied Conditions: A Textbook of Rheumatology, 12th ed. Philadelphia, Lea & Febiger, 1993, pp 1699–1723.
3. Resnick D: Diagnosis of Bone and Joint Disorders, 3rd ed. Philadelphia, W.B. Saunders, 1995.

2. CRYSTALLINE ARTHROPATHIES

Steven J. Wees, M.D.

1. What are the major clinical crystalline arthropathies?
- Monosodium urate arthropathy
- Calcium pyrophosphate deposition (CPPD) disease

2. Is there more than one clinical manifestation of gouty arthropathy?
Yes. Gouty arthropathy may manifest clinically as acute inflammatory arthritis or chronic, erosive tophaceous arthritis.

3. What are the clinical features of calcium pyrophosphate dihydrate deposition (CPPD) disease?
- Acute pseudogout
- Several subsets of chronic arthritis (see table).

Subsets of Chronic CPPD

Pseudorheumatoid arthritis
Pseudoosteoarthritis
Pseudoneuropathic arthropathy

4. Describe the common clinical features of acute gouty arthritis and acute pseudogout.
The onset is usually abrupt. Involved joints rapidly become painful, swollen, warm, and tender. Patients are frequently awakened from sleep with gouty attacks. The joint may become so inflamed that the patient will not allow even a sheet to touch it. At times the overlying skin may resemble a bacterial cellulitis. Systemic signs of fever, leukocytosis, and elevated sedimentation rate often are present. Mild attacks may resolve spontaneously without treatment over several hours or 1–2 days. More severe untreated attacks may not subside for 7–10 days or, in the case of pseudogout, for as long as 2–4 weeks. Attacks may be provoked by surgery, trauma, and current illness.

5. What are the most commonly involved joints in acute gout?
In the majority of patients the first attack is monarticular. The first metatarsophalangeal joint is the most common site of involvement. Other frequent sites of initial involvement are the ankles, knees, wrists, fingers, and elbows. Distal and lower extremity joints tend to be involved most often.

6. What are the most commonly involved joints in acute pseudogout?

Larger joints are preferentially affected. Nearly 50% of attacks involve the knees. Other areas commonly involved are elbows, wrists, ankles, and, in contrast to gout, shoulders and hips.

7. What is the significance of hyperuricemia?

Large numbers of the general population have hyperuricemia, yet 19 out of 20 hyperuricemic patients remain asymptomatic throughout life. Hyperuricemia is often associated with other general medical conditions, such as hypertension, obesity, heavy alcohol use, atherosclerosis, ischemic heart disease, and impaired glucose tolerance.

8. List the major considerations in the differential diagnosis of acute gouty arthritis, chronic tophaceous gout, and acute pseudogout.

Acute gouty arthritis
Infectious arthritis, rheumatoid arthritis, acute pseudogout, and acute seronegative inflammatory arthritis (i.e., psoriatic arthritis)
Chronic tophaceous gout
Nodular rheumatoid arthritis and osteoarthritis
Acute pseudogout
Acute gouty arthritis and infectious arthritis

9. Explain the roles of laboratory and radiographic studies in the differential diagnosis of crystalline arthropathies.

Beyond joint aspiration and synovial analysis, all other laboratory studies are superfluous. The most critical diagnostic studies of synovial fluid are (1) cell count and differential; (2) crystal analysis under polarized microscopy; and (3) Gram stain and routine culture and sensitivity. In many patients who present with acute crystalline-induced arthritis, routine radiographs are normal. A helpful clue for the diagnosis of acute pseudogout is the finding of chondrocalcinosis on plain films.

10. What are the definitive diagnostic procedure and the definitive laboratory test for acute gout or acute pseudogout?

The definitive diagnostic procedure is joint aspiration; the definitive laboratory test is analysis of synovial fluid under polarized microscopy for the appropriate crystal (monosodium urate in acute gouty arthritis and calcium pyrophosphate in acute pseudogout).

11. Does the synovial fluid cell count distinguish acute gouty arthritis from acute bacterial arthritis?

No. Although synovial fluid white cell counts > 50,000 cells/mm suggest bacterial infection, they occasionally are seen in crystal-induced arthritis and rheumatoid arthritis. Examination of fluid under polarized light and routine culture are most essential.

12. What is the treatment of choice in acute crystalline-induced arthritis?

The initial treatment is 75–100 mg orally of indomethacin, followed by 50 mg every 6 hours. As the attack subsides, the drug may be gradually tapered off. An equally effective alternative is to aspirate dry the involved joint and to inject a corticosteroid, such as triamcinolone.

CONTROVERSIES

13. What is the relationship of fever to crystal-induced arthritis?

Fever is frequent in acute gout and acute pseudogout, a fact that is frequently unrecognized. Temperatures may be ≥ 39° C. Leukocytosis also is common. Usually joint infection is suspected in the febrile patient, and crystal-induced arthritis is often forgotten as a diagnostic possibility. The fact that approximately 40% of patients with acute polyarticular gout are normouricemic during an attack compounds the problem. In patients hospitalized for serious medical problems, crystal-induced arthritis is often overlooked as a cause of fever, and antibiotics are prescribed for presumed infection. Defervescence occurs when antiinflammatory agents are introduced.

14. Describe the intravenous and oral role of colchicine.

Currently the use of colchicine has few indications. When given orally, colchicine typically induces significant gastrointestinal intolerance before joint symptoms subside. Intravenous colchicine may be strikingly effective but carries the risk of significant hematologic toxicity, particularly in elderly patients with underlying renal or hepatic disease and limited bone marrow reserve.

15. What is the appropriate management of hyperuricemia?

The physician often is faced with the question of whether or not to treat asymptomatic hyperuricemia. Because many years of silent deposition of urate are necessary before the first attack of gouty arthritis, it seems reasonable not to treat hyperuricemia solely to prevent its development.

Controversy also exists about when to begin antihyperuricemic therapy in the patient with gout arthritis. The first issue to resolve is whether the patient is in fact having attacks of acute gout. Hence the patient must be seen during an acute episode and have his or her synovial fluid carefully examined for the presence of intracellular, strongly negatively birefringent crystals (sodium urate). The absence of urate crystals in an attack of acute synovitis makes gout an unlikely cause of acute arthritis. An elevated serum urate level in a patient with acute inflammatory arthritis is not diagnostic of gout; examination of synovial fluid is mandatory.

After the clinician is sure that the patient has suffered acute gout but is now asymptomatic, the decision to begin antihyperuricemic treatment may be made. The large number of patients who have only infrequent gouty attacks even in the absence of therapy probably do not require antihyperuricemic treatment. Patients suffering recurrent acute attacks of gout may find that small daily doses of colchicine (0.5 mg 2 times/day) provide adequate prophylaxis against further attacks. Other patients have found that using indomethacin (25–50 mg 3–4 times/day) at the first sign of an acute attack will abort a full-blown incident. Nevertheless, some patients suffer recurrent gouty attacks despite adequate prophylaxis with colchicine or indomethacin. Such patients are good candidates for long-term treatment with allopurinol. Patients with tophaceous deposits also require long-term treatment with allopurinol. It is important not to administer allopurinol during the acute phase of gouty arthritis, because it typically prolongs the acute attack; wait at least 2 weeks before initiating such treatment.

BIBLIOGRAPHY

1. Kelley WN, Harris ED Jr, Ruddy S, Sledge CB (eds): Textbook of Rheumatology, 6th ed. Philadelphia, W.B. Saunders, 2001.
2. Krey PR, Lazaro DM (eds): Analysis of Synovial Fluid. Summit, NJ, Ciba-Geigy Corporation, 1992.
3. Maddison PJ, Isenberg DA (eds): Oxford Textbook of Rheumatology, 2nd ed. New York, Oxford University Press, 1998.
4. McCarty DJ, Koopman WJ (eds): Arthritis and Allied Conditions, 14th ed. Philadelphia, Lea & Febiger, 2000.
5. Pinals RS: Polyarthritis and fever. N Engl J Med 330:769–774, 1994.

3. INFLAMMATORY ARTHROPATHIES

William R. Palmer, M.D.

1. What are the seronegative spondyloarthropathies?

The seronegative spondyloarthropathies are a group of rheumatic diseases that share common clinical, genetic, and radiologic features. Examples include ankylosing spondylitis, psoriatic arthritis (Reiter's syndrome), juvenile ankylosing spondylitis, and arthropathies that complicate inflammatory bowel diseases (regional enteritis and ulcerative colitis).

2. Name the common features of the seronegative spondyloarthropathies.

1. Predilection for inflammatory lesions of axial skeleton in many (sacroiliitis and spondylitis)
2. Oligoarticular peripheral joint arthritis
3. Enthesitis—inflammation at bony insertion of tendons, ligaments, and articular capsules
4. Frequent extraarticular inflammation of eye (uveitis), heart (aortitis), skin, and mucous membranes
5. Tendency to afflict young adults (mostly men)
6. Strong association with HLA-B27
7. Negative rheumatoid factor

3. What are characteristic features of low-back pain in patients with ankylosing spondylitis (AS)?

Onset before age 40   Prolonged morning stiffness
Insidious onset   Improvement of symptoms with exercise
Daily symptoms for more than 3 months

4. What steps should be taken to diagnose ankylosing spondylitis?

- Compatible history
- Compatible physical exam
- Radiologic demonstration of sacroiliitis— absolutely essential

5. How is sacroiliitis best demonstrated radiographically?

An anteroposterior radiograph of the pelvis usually suffices to demonstrate the bilateral sacroiliitis of AS. Occasionally a computed tomographic (CT) scan of the pelvis and sacroiliac (SI) joints is necessary in early adult disease or juvenile AS.

6. What is the most common extraskeletal manifestation of AS?

Acute uveitis (anterior iridocyclitis), usually unilateral, occurs in 30% of patients.

7. What treatment modalities are commonly used in the management of AS?

- Nonsteroidal antiinflammatory drugs (NSAIDs); indomethacin widely used
- Patient education
- Physical therapy—as important as medical therapy (range-of-motion exercises, back extension, done at home)

8. What is osteitis condensans ilii (OCI)?

OCI is a disorder primarily of young multiparous women, who often are asymptomatic. It is usually discovered radiographically and frequently confused with sacroiliitis. OCI is characterized by a triangular area of dense sclerotic bone limited to iliac bones of the pelvis adjacent to the lower half of normal SI joints.

9. Is disability common in AS?

Fewer than 20% of patients have significant work disability. Those who do frequently have deterioration of the hips and spinal fusion (bamboo spine).

10. Name the clinical features of psoriatic arthritis.

- Psoriasis
- Asymmetric peripheral arthritis with frequent involvement of distal interphalangeal (DIP) joints
- Negative rheumatoid factor
- Sausage digits (dactylitis)
- Spondylitis and sacroiliitis (in a minority of patients)

11. List the five clinical patterns of psoriatic arthritis.

15% Classic psoriatic arthritis confined to DIP joints of hands and feet
5% Arthritis mutilans
15% Symmetric polyarthritis similar to rheumatoid arthritis
60% Asymmetric, oligoarticular involvement of small joints, dactylitis
5% Spondylitis/sacroiliitis with or without arthritis

12. Are nail changes common in psoriatic arthritis?

Yes. Changes include pitting, onycholysis, and transverse ridging. In patients with few psoriatic skin lesions the nail changes may be the most prominent clue to the presence of psoriasis.

13. How many patients with psoriasis develop psoriatic arthritis?

Approximately 5%.

14. Is it advisable to treat psoriasis as part of the comprehensive therapy for psoriatic arthritis?

Yes. The consensus is that the more active and severe the psoriasis, the more severe the psoriatic arthritis.

15. What systemic pharmacologic agents are used in the treatment of psoriatic arthritis?

- Nonsteroidal drugs
- Disease modifiers—hydroxychloroquine, gold, methotrexate, sulfasalazine
- Corticosteroids—low-dose systemic prednisone; intraarticular corticosteroids (e.g., triamcinolone hexacetonide)

16. What are the unique radiographic findings of psoriatic arthritis?

- Lack of paraarticular osteopenia
- "Pencil-in-cup" deformity of DIP or proximal interphalangeal (PIP) joints (pathognomonic)

17. Is the prognosis of psoriatic arthritis similar to that of rheumatoid arthritis?

The prognosis of psoriatic arthritis is actually much better. Five percent or fewer of patients have significant disability; mortality is minimal.

18. What is the most common extraintestinal manifestations of inflammatory bowel disease (Crohn's disease, ulcerative colitis)?

Up to 20% of patients have arthritis in one of two patterns:

1. Peripheral arthritis—oligoarticular involvement of the lower limbs; remitting (parallels activity of bowel disease) and nondeforming

2. Sacroiliitis/spondylitis—identical to that of AS

19. Define reactive arthritis.

Reactive arthritis is joint inflammation initiated by an infection in which the causative agent cannot be isolated from the joint. Reactive arthritis is included in the family of spondyloarthropathies because of a similar pattern of involvement, occurrence of enthesopathy and sacroiliitis, and high association with HLA-B27.

20. Where do the infections that precipitate reactive arthritis usually occur?
   Gastrointestinal (GI) tract
   Urogenital tract (especially in young men)

21. Describe the symptom complex of classic reactive arthritis (Reiter's syndrome).
   • Infection (GI or genital)—may be barely symptomatic
   • Urethritis or cervicitis
   • Conjunctivitis   } Develop 1–4 weeks
   • Mucocutaneous lesions   } after infection
   • Arthritis/spondylitis/enthesitis

22. What is incomplete Reiter's syndrome?
Incomplete Reiter's syndrome is defined as typical reactive arthritis of the musculoskeletal system without other manifestations (e.g., skin, eyes); it occurs in 40% of all patients with reactive arthritis.

23. List the musculoskeletal manifestations of reactive arthritis.
   • Asymmetric oligoarthritis of lower extremities
   • Sausage digits (dactylitis)
   • Enthesitis—Achilles' heel ("lover's heel")
   • Spondylitis/sacroiliitis in 20% (asymmetric)

24. What are the common mucocutaneous features of reactive arthritis?
   • Keratoderma blenorrhagicum—palms, soles, penis
   • Circinate balanitis—penis
   • Oral ulcerations—tongue, palate
   • Nail changes—no pits; onycholysis and yellow color

25. What is Löfgren's syndrome?
Löfgren's syndrome is a benign, self-limited, acute arthropathy that occurs in patients with sarcoidosis. Classic manifestations include (1) hilar lymphadenopathy, (2) erythema nodosum, and (3) symmetric migratory, additive polyarthritis with a predilection for the ankles (erythema), knees, wrists, hands. The syndrome usually resolves within 2–3 months and requires supportive (NSAID) therapy.

26. Name the common viral disorders that may be accompanied by arthritis.

Hepatitis B	Mumps
Parvovirus B19 (fifth disease)	Chickenpox
Rubella	Human immunodeficiency virus (HIV)

27. Define Lyme disease.
Lyme disease is a tick-borne inflammatory disorder caused by the spirochete *Borrelia burgdorferi*. Disease onset frequently is heralded by a characteristic skin lesion (erythema chronicum migrans) at the site of the tick bite. Most untreated patients subsequently develop disseminated infection that results in a variable and occasionally chronic inflammatory process affecting joints, nervous system, heart, or skin.

CONTROVERSIES

28. Are the seronegative spondyloarthropathies related to rheumatoid arthritis?
   No. Although once classified as part of the spectrum of rheumatoid arthritis ("rheumatoid variants"), the seronegative spondyloarthropathies now stand apart on the basis of clinical, ge-

netic, and epidemiologic investigations. This distinction is necessary because of differing articular and nonarticular complications, responses to therapy, and prognosis.

Major Differences between Rheumatoid Arthritis and the Spondyloarthropathies

	RHEUMATOID ARTHRITIS	SPONDYLOARTHROPATHIES
Peripheral arthritis	Symmetric	Asymmetric
	Polyarticular	Pauciarticular
Sacroiliitis	No	Yes
Spondylitis	No	Yes
Enthesopathy	No	Yes
Rheumatoid factor	Present (85%)	Absent
Subcutaneous nodules	Yes	Absent
Associated with HLA-B27	No	Yes

Comparison of Ankylosing Spondylitis and Related Disorders

CHARACTERISTIC	ANKYLOSING SPONDYLITIS	REACTIVE ARTHRITIS (REITER'S SYNDROME)	PSORIATIC ARTHROPATHY	ENTEROPATHIC ARTHROPATHY
Usual age at middle-onset	Young adult age < 40 yr	Young to middle-aged adult	Young to middle-aged adult	Young to aged adult
Sex ratio	Three times more common in males	Predominantly males	Equally distributed	Equally distributed
Sacroiliitis or spondylitis	Virtually 100%	< 50%	~ 20%	< 20%
Symmetry of sacroiliitis	Symmetric	Asymmetric	Asymmetric	Symmetric
Peripheral joint	~ 25%	~ 90%	~ 95%	15–20%
HLA-B27 (in Caucasians)	~ 90%	~ 75%	< 50%	~ 50%
Eye involvement	25–30% (iritis)	~ 50% (conjunctivitis)	~ 20% (conjunctivitis)	≤ 15% (iritis)
Skin or nail involvement	None	< 40%	Virtually 100%	Uncommon

29. Is HLA-B27 a useful test in the diagnosis of AS and other spondyloarthropathies?
Even though HLA-B27 is found in a large percentage of patients with AS and other spondyloarthropathies (see table below), this relatively expensive test is rarely necessary to make an accurate diagnosis. A careful history and physical exam, frequently supplemented by appropriate radiographs (sacroiliitis), are the best and most accurate tools for diagnosis. The HLA-B27 test should be ordered primarily in the following situations:
- Classic history and physical exam for AS but radiographic findings do not permit the diagnosis;
- Suspected juvenile AS; and
- Suspected atypical reactive arthritis.

Frequency of HLA-B27

Normal	2–13%
Ankylosing spondylitis	90%
Reactive (Reiter's) arthritis	75%
Psoriatic arthritis	
Sacroiliitis	50%
Without sacroiliitis	Normal
Enteropathic arthritis	
Peripheral arthritis	Normal
Sacroiliitis	50%

30. Can psoriatic arthritis precede the clinical appearance of psoriasis?

Yes. Psoriatic arthritis precedes the clinical appearance of psoriasis in 10–15% of adult patients. In 15–20% of patients, psoriasis and arthritis occur simultaneously. In the remainder, psoriasis precedes the arthritis.

31. Is there a difference in the outcome of joint replacement surgery in the seronegative spondyloarthropathies?

Many physicians may still believe that the outcome of total joint replacement in patients with AS or psoriatic arthritis is poor. Anecdotal reports have raised the possibility of reankylosis and mechanical failure of total hip replacements. A more optimistic report concluded that 75% of total hip replacements were graded as excellent or good. In another retrospective study, 86% of 87 patients who underwent 150 total hip replacement procedures considered the outcome to be good or very good. Such statistics compare favorably with total hip replacement for other conditions.

Patients with psoriatic arthritis undergoing joint surgery have been thought to be at risk of wound infections from the heavy bacterial contamination of psoriatic plaques. Because the peripheral joints in psoriatic arthritis tend to ankylose, reankylosis and mechanical failure of a replaced joint have been speculated but rarely reported. The problem of infection may be controlled by careful antiseptic skin preparation and perioperative antibiotic therapy against the common psoriasis contaminants (staphylococci and streptococci). On rare occasions psoriasis may occur in the incision site, but is not a major problem.

The indications for joint replacement surgery are the same for psoriatic arthritis, AS, and other spondyloarthropathies. Steps to prevent early postoperative loss of motion and appropriate perioperative antibiotic therapy are appropriate.

32. Can reactive arthritis (Reiter's syndrome) be chronic and disabling?

In years past medical students were taught that reactive arthritis was a self-limited disorder that usually resolved without sequelae. We now know that the course and progression of reactive arthritis are more varied and unpredictable. The majority of patients have an initial episode of arthritis lasting 3–12 months. Many then experience recurrent attacks, frequently after disease-free intervals. Between 20 and 50% of patients have a chronic course of persistent disease activity with the potential for a destructive arthropathy and/or progressive spondylitic change. Several studies have shown that < 15% of patients experience severe disability, which usually is due to severe arthropathy of lower extremities or aggressive spondylitis. The overall prognosis is better than for most other arthropathies. Death is rare.

BIBLIOGRAPHY

1. Arnett FC: Seronegative spondyloarthropathies. Bull Rheum Dis 37(1):1987.
2. Beyer CA, Hanssen AD, et al: Primary total knee arthroplasty in patients with psoriasis. J Bone Joint Surg 73B:258–259, 1991.
3. Calin A, Elswood J: The outcome of 138 total hip replacements and 12 revisions as AS: High success rate after a mean followup of 7.5 years. J Rheumatol 16:955–958, 1989.
4. Calin A, Kaye B, et al: The prevalence and nature of back pain in an industrial complex. Spine 5:201–205, 1980.
5. Kelley WN, Harris ED Jr, Ruddy S, Sledge CB (eds): Textbook of Rheumatology, 6th ed. Philadelphia, W.B. Saunders, 2001.
6. Klippel JH, Dieppe PA (eds): Rheumatology, 2nd ed. St. Louis, Mosby, 1998.
7. McCarty DJ, Koopman WJ (eds): Arthritis and Allied Conditions, 14th ed. Philadelphia, Lea & Febiger, 2000.
8. Maddison PJ, Isenberg DA, Woo P, Glass D (eds): Oxford Textbook of Rheumatology, 2nd ed. New York, Oxford University Press, 1998.
9. Stern SH, Insall TM, et al: Total knee arthroplasty in patients with psoriasis. Clin Orthop 248:108–111, 1989.

4. RHEUMATOID ARTHRITIS

Steven J. Wees, M.D.

1. Give a brief clinical definition of rheumatoid arthritis (RA).

Rheumatoid arthritis is a symmetric inflammatory arthritis, involving small and large joints, of at least 6 weeks' duration.

2. List the seven diagnostic criteria for RA.

1. Morning stiffness
2. Arthritis of at least 3 areas lasting > 6 weeks
3. Arthritis of hand joints lasting > 6 weeks
4. Symmetric arthritis lasting > 6 weeks
5. Rheumatoid arthritis
6. Serum rheumatoid factor
7. Radiographic changes

Establishing a diagnosis of RA requires adherence to the 1987 revised criteria from the American College of Rheumatology. At least four criteria must be fulfilled to diagnose RA.

3. What is the most common pattern of onset?

Most patients have an insidious, slow onset over weeks to months, often accompanied by complaints of fatigue, malaise, anorexia and weight loss, arthralgias, myalgias, and morning stiffness. A smaller number of people have an acute or subacute onset.

4. Name the main sites of joint involvement.

Wrists	Ankles and metatarsophalangeal	Shoulders
Metacarpophalangeal and proximal	joints	Hips
interphalangeal finger joints	Knees	Elbows

5. What are the most common extraarticular manifestations of RA?

Nodules, dry eyes, dry mouth, and carpal tunnel syndrome.

6. What are the four major pharmacologic treatment groups used in the management of RA?

Narcotic analgesics	Corticosteroids
Nonsteroidal antiinflammatory drugs (NSAIDs)	Disease-modifying agents

7. Describe the role of corticosteroids in the management of RA.

Most patients with RA demonstrate significant improvement with conservative use of corticosteroids. Men are given up to 7.5 mg of prednisone and women up to 5 mg each morning. This regimen can be tolerated on a long-term basis with minimal adverse effect. Selective intraarticular installation of corticosteroids is also highly effective. Triamcinolone hexacetonide has the longest-lasting effect.

8. Name the most commonly used disease-modifying drugs.

Plaquenil, methotrexate, and parenteral gold.

9. What is the indication for initiation of disease-modifying treatment?

Patients with uncontrolled synovitis, despite optimal use of low-dose corticosteroids and NSAIDs, need additional medical treatment. The detection of bony erosions on plain films of the hands and feet in a patient with active rheumatoid synovitis also is an important indication for beginning such treatment.

CONTROVERSIES

10. Does a positive rheumatoid factor (RF) test result definitively diagnose RA?

Contrary to widespread belief among physicians, RF is not specific for RA. RF is found in a small percentage of seemingly normal people, and with increasing age a greater percentage of normal people test positive for RF. Positive tests are found in a large number of acute and chronic inflammatory diseases (see table below). In most nonrheumatic diseases and with increasing age, titers of RF are lower than in RA ($< 1:320$). Furthermore, approximately 20% of patients with bona fide RA have negative RF tests and are categorized as having seronegative RA.

Occurrence of Rheumatoid Factor in Selected Conditions

Rheumatic diseases	Acute viral infections	Miscellaneous
Adult rheumatoid arthritis	Infectious mononucleosis	Elderly but otherwise
Sjögren's syndrome	Infectious hepatitis	healthy individuals
Systemic lupus erythematosus	Influenza	Sarcoidosis
Scleroderma	Rubella	Chronic active hepatitis
Mixed connective tissue disease	**Chronic inflammatory diseases**	Chronic persistent hepatitis
Polymyositis	Tuberculosis	Hyperglobulinemic purpura
Juvenile rheumatoid arthritis	Infective endocarditis	After transfusions
	Neoplasms	After renal transplantation

11. Can RA be diagnosed without objective physical evidence of joint inflammation?

No. One may suspect the diagnosis, but a patient with joint pain but no objectively demonstrable synovitis cannot be said to have RA, regardless of the positivity of the serum RF test. Many patients are erroneously diagnosed with RA solely on the basis of joint pain and a positive serum RF test, often as low titer. In essence, RA is diagnosed at the bedside. Laboratory and radiologic tests are ancillary.

12. Does a positive serum antinuclear antibody test result exclude a diagnosis of RA?

No. A large number of antinuclear antibodies are present in patients with RA.

13. Discuss the current role of synovectomy.

Over the past two decades the use of synovectomy has diminished substantially. Although the procedure is still effective in relieving pain, no retardation of radiologic progression is achieved. More intensive pharmacologic management, including earlier institution of disease-modifying agents, is the preferred approach. The major indication for synovectomy at present is extensor tenosynovectomy for prophylaxis of extensor tendon rupture.

BIBLIOGRAPHY

1. Kelley WN, Harris ED Jr, Ruddy S, Sledge CB (eds): Textbook of Rheumatology, 6th ed. Philadelphia, W.B. Saunders, 2001.
2. Maddison PJ, Isenberg DA (eds): Oxford Textbook of Rheumatology, 2nd ed. New York, Oxford University Press, 1998.
3. McCarty DJ, Koopman WJ (eds): Arthritis and Allied Conditions, 14th ed. Philadelphia, Lea & Febiger, 2000.
4. Wees SJ: Practical Points in Rheumatology. New York, Medical Examination Publishing, 1983.

5. SEPTIC ARTHRITIS

Randall D. Neumann, M.D., and Joshua A. Urban, M.D.

1. What is septic arthritis?

Septic arthritis is a bacterial infection of the synovium and joint space that causes an intense inflammatory reaction with migration of polymorphonuclear leukocytes and subsequent release of proteolytic enzymes. Bacterial infection remains one of the most rapidly destructive and potentially lethal forms of arthritis; one-third of affected patients suffer residual loss of function in the involved joint.

2. Describe the process of articular damage in septic arthritis.

Hematogenous infection results from bacterial seeding of the synovium. When the bacteria in the synovium begin to multiply, products from the bacteria stimulate the migration of polymorphonuclear leukocytes into the joint. The leukocytes release proteolytic enzymes, which cause acute damage to the articular cartilage.

3. List the major predisposing conditions for septic arthritis.

Underlying chronic joint disease	Immunosuppressive drug treatment
Trauma	Malignancy
Joint involvement in rheumatoid arthritis	Parenteral drug abuse
Diabetes mellitus	Recent joint infection
Steroid administration	Injection or aspiration
Renal failure	Vascular insufficiency

4. What are the common sites affected with septic arthritis?

In reviews of bacterial arthritis, 443 joints were identified; 85% of cases were monarticular.

Knee	53%	Shoulder	11%	Wrist	9%
Hip	20%	Elbow	17%	Ankle	8%

5. What are the most common sites of bacterial septic arthritis in pediatric patients?

The knee is affected 39% of the time and the hip 32% of the time, with a broad mixture in all other joints.

6. Describe the clinical classification of septic arthritis.

It is helpful to classify cases of septic arthritis based on chronicity and number of joints involved. Acute monoarticular septic arthritis, chronic monoarticular septic arthritis, and polyarticular septic arthritis are the three common types of clinical presentation. Each of these entities has a unique spectrum of potential causative agents and treatment regimens.

7. What percentage of patients with septic arthritis have monarticular disease? What percentage have polyarticular disease?

Ninety percent of patients have monarticular septic arthritis; 10% have polyarticular septic arthritis.

8. Describe the clinical presentation of acute monoarticular septic arthritis?

The presentation of septic arthritis varies with the age and immunocompetency of the patient. In older children and adults, the typical clinical presentation is the acute onset over hours to days of pain, swelling, and limitation of motion of the involved joint. Fever has been reported to be present in 50–78% of cases. In neonates, the immune system is not yet fully mature, and as a result, the inflammatory response that typically accompanies these infections in older patients is absent. Neonates may present with only mild swelling, tenderness, irritability, discomfort with joint motion, and pseudoparalysis of the affected limb. In toddlers, the immune system is fully functional and the typical signs and symptoms of septic arthritis seen in adults are present.

9. Describe the microbiology of acute monoarticular septic arthritis in neonates, children, young adults, and elderly adults.

The organisms that are most likely to be encountered depend on the age of the patient. For a given age group, certain bacteria are more likely to be encountered. When all age groups are considered together, *Staphylococcus aureus* is the most common organism isolated in septic arthritis. Also, when each age group is considered individually, *S. aureus* is the most common, or second most common, infecting organism.

In the neonate, most cases of joint sepsis are caused by *S. aureus* with group B streptococci being the next most common. Gram-negative organisms such as *Neisseria gonorrhoeae* account for 10–15% of infections.

In young children aged 2 months to 2 years, *Haemophilus influenzae* was the most frequently encountered organism before the widespread use of the *H. influenzae* b conjugated vaccine. With the use of this vaccine, the incidence of *H. influenzae* infections has significantly decreased. Currently, the most common organisms in this age group in decreasing order are *S. aureus,* streptococci, and H. influenzae.

In young adults, *S. aureus* and *N. gonorrhoeae* are the most common organisms causing joint sepsis. Although previous reports have shown that *N. gonorrhoeae* is the most frequently isolated organism in this age group, more recent studies have suggested that *S. aureus* may actually be more common. However, this may due to the potential for underrepresentation that can be encountered with *N. gonorrhoeae*—as few as 25% of purulent joint effusions caused by *N. gonorrhoeae may grow positive cultures.*

In the elderly, S. aureus is the predominant causative organism as it is responsible for 43-64% of septic arthritis cases in this population. Gram-negative bacilli are seen in 14-35% of elderly patients.

10. Describe the clinical presentation and microbiology of chronic monoarticular septic arthritis.

Patients with chronic monoarticular septic arthritis typically have indolent signs and symptoms. Early in the course of the disease process, a low-grade synovitis may be present causing only mild-to-moderate manifestations of the typical harbingers of infective arthritis—pain, swelling, warmth, and erythema. Chronic septic arthritis commonly occurs in patients with impaired immune systems. Patients with rheumatoid arthritis, systemic lupus erythematous, renal transplantation, chronic dialysis, and chronic immunosuppressive therapy remain at risk for this clinical entity.

The organism typically responsible for chronic infective arthritis are mycobacteria, fungi, and saprophytic bacteria (*Brucella* species and Lyme disease). These organsism typically seed the joint from remote areas of infection via lymphatic spread, hematogenous spread, and spread along planes of tissue destruction. They may also be introduced into the joint by penetrating trauma, surgery, or athrocentesis. The granulomatous reaction associated with these infections leads to tissue destruction characterized by a mononuclear cell and giant cell infiltrate. Only late in the course of these chronic infections do the signs and symptoms of extensive tissue destruction occur. Because of the likelihood of chronicity prior to diagnosis, radiographic changes are usually evident at the time of initial presentation.

11. Describe patients who present with polyarticular septic arthritis.

Polyarticular infection occures in 5–8% of pediatric cases, and 10–19% of nongonococcal adult cases. In gonococcal arthritis, the majority of patients (70%) present with polyarthralgias, but only 25–50% of these joints yield a positive culture on aspiration. Patients with gonococcal polyarthritis typically are young, healthy, sexually active adults.

Patients with nongonococcal polyarticular disease are usually elderly and chronically ill. They present with multiple sites of infection and have multiple predisposing conditions, including rheumatoid arthritis, prosthetic joints, diabetes, corticosteroid usage, immunosuppressive drug usage, renal failure, and parenteral drug abuse. The mortality rate is approximately 25–50%. The most common organism isolated in these infections is *S. aureus*. Other microbes that have a predilection for polyarticular involvement include *Neisseria* sp., *Streptococcus* sp., *Pneumococcus* sp., and *H. influenzae*.

12. What is the clinical presentation of gonoccal arthritis?

Disseminated gonococcal infection (DGI) is the term used to describe the clinical manifestations of *N. gonorrhoeae* bacteremia (gonococcemia). Only 0.5–3% of individuals with gonorrhea develop the symptoms of DGI. It is reported that 17–33% of patients with DGI develop septic arthrits. The initial symptoms of DGI are usually migratory or additive polyarthralgias (70%), tenosynovitis (67%), dermatitis (67%), fever (63%), and arthritis (42%). The tenosynovitis usually involves multiple joints and is especially common over the wrists, fingers, ankles, and toes. The dermatitis usually consists of multiple (usually painless) skin lesions, usually found on the extremities or on the trunk. Lesions usually are hemorrhagic macules or papules, but pustules, vessicles, and bullae have also been described. Genitourinary symptoms are unusual.

There are two distinct clinical presentations of arthritis in DGI. The first is a monoarthritis characterized by a swollen, tender joint with decreased range of motion. Aspiration usually reveals *N. gonorrhoeae* with leukocyte counts greater than 50,000 cells/mm^3. In up to 75% of cases, joint aspirates are sterile, but the leukocyte count usually remains high. The second clinical presentation of arthritis in DGI is that of a migratory polyarthralgia, which eventually settles into one or more joints and is associated with a pustular dermatitis and tenosynovitis that may also be suppurative.

13. What organisms should be suspected in septic arthritis associated with nail punctures through shoeware?

The MTP joint is most commonly affected in this scenario. Although *S. aureus* is present in a majority of these cases, *Pseudomonas aeruginosa* has been isolated in many of these infections.

14. Describe septic arthritis from an animal bite.

Animal bites are most frequently inflicted by dogs, cats, and rodents. *Pasturella multocida* is commonly associated with cat bites. *S. aureus* and *Streptococcus* sp. also are quite common. Treatment for *P. multocida* infection should include penicillin G and appropriate coverage for other microorganisms. Drainage is commonly necessary.

15. Which bacteria are commonly found in septic arthritis in patients with parenteral drug abuse?

- *S. aureus*
- *P. aeruginosa*
- *Serratia marcescens*

16. What unusual locations of septic arthritis are found in parenteral drug abusers?

- Sacroiliac joint
- Sternal articulations
- Pubic symphysis

17. What common diseases are considered in the differential diagnosis of septic arthritis?

Trauma	Rheumatoid arthritis
Osteoarthritis	Crystalline arthropathies

18. What diagnostic studies should be ordered in the evaluation of septic arthritis?

Complete blood count with differential	Blood cultures
Erythrocyte sedimentation rate	Plain radiographs
C-reactive protein	Joint aspiration

19. What is the most accurate diagnostic study for septic arthritis?
The most accurate diagnostic tool is joint aspiration with joint fluid analysis.

20. Which diagnostic tests should be included in the analysis of the synovial fluid in patients with septic arthritis?

Gram stain	Glucose level
Culture and sensitivity	Crystals
White blood cell count and differential	

21. Describe the analysis of synovial fluid in an aspirate from a patient with septic arthritis.
The white blood cell count is generally over 50,000 cells per mm^3, with 80% being polymorphonuclear leukocytes. The glucose level is low. A positive Gram stain is found in approximately 60% of patients; of these, 60% involve gram-positive cocci. Tests for crystals of uric acid and calcium pyrophosphate are negative.

Caution must be exercised in using 50,000 cells per mm^3 as the threshhold for infection because 55% of joint aspirates from children with bacteriologically proven septic arthritis have counts below this number. This scenario commonly occurs in neonates, infants, and patients taking immunosuppressive medications who have difficulty mounting an effective immune response.

22. Describe the abnormalities seen in the diagnostic tests of the serum.
The erythrocyte sedimentation rate (ESR), C-reactive protein (C-RP), and leukocyte count are often elevated but are nonspecific and may be abnormal in other inflammatory conditions. Approximately 60% of patinets with septic arthritis have normal leukocyte counts. The ESR is elevated above 20 mm/hour in approximately 95% of cases. Comparisons of the ESR and C-RP have shown the C-RP to be more sensitive and to respond more rapidly to infections than the ESR. The C-RP is elevated in nearly every case (if the immune system is not compromised). Blood cultures are positive in approximately 50% of cases.

23. Describe the use of serum inflammatory markers in the diagnosis of septic arthritis in the neonate?
Because if the lack of a mature immune system, laboratory studies that reflect immune response (leukocyte count, ESR, C-RP) are of little value in the neonate. Blood cultures reveal the pathogen in only 50% of cases. Joint aspiration in this population is critical.

24. What additional diagnostic test should be considered in children under 4 who have not been immunized for *H. influenzae*?
Spinal fluid analysis should be considered in this patient population because of the increased risk of developing meningitis. Patients should also be examined for signs and symptoms of meningitis.

25. Describe the findings seen on plain radiographs, both early and late.
Although plain radiographs are usually normal initially, they should be obtained to limit the differential diagnosis and to serve as a baseline for subsequent radiographs. They may show soft-tissue swelling, effusions, and obliteration of normal fat planes but do not demonstrate bone destruction until about 7–14 days into the disease process. Joint space widening, subluxation, and dislocation are also late findings.

26. What other radiographic tests may be helpful in the evaluation of septic arthritis?
Ultrasound, radionucleotide imaging, computed tomography, and magnetic resonance imaging.

27. What is the treatment for septic arthritis?
Septic arthritis constitutes an orthopedic emergency, and prompt surgical drainage is necessary. Empirical intravenous antibiotic therapy is begun after the joint aspirate is obtained. The an-

tibiotic regimen is adjusted once culture and sensitivity results are known. An infectious disease specialist should be consulted to aid in determing the optimal antibiotic regimen. The joint should be temporarily immobilized to avoid the discomfort associated with motion. In 2–3 days, the pain has typically subsided enough to begin to allow passive and active range of motion. A formal physical therapy regimen is encouraged to prevent loss of motion.

28. Discuss the methods that can be used to drain the septic joint.

Needle aspiration. The indications for needle aspiration as the definitive procedure for septic joint drainage and lavage are (1) an acute infection of less than 3 days duration; (2) multiple infected joints; (3) the involvement of joints easily aspirated joints (not the hip); and (4) a systemically ill patient who cannot withstand surgery. This technique should include the use of a large bore needle (14–18 gauge) to evacuate the joint fluid entirely. Once the joint has been drained, multiple syringes of saline should be injected into the joint and reaspirated. In cases in which the effusion recurs, aspiration is repeated at daily or twice daily intervals. If symptoms do not resolve in 1–3 days, a formal arthrotomy is indicated. The major complication of this technique is incomplete drainage of the joint. This complication often results from the formation of loculations within the joint that cannot be drained with a single needlestick or intraarticular debris that impedes flow through the needle. If the aspirate does not flow through the needle freely, it should be assumed that aspiration has not completely drained the joint and the patient should undergo open arthrotomy or arthroscopic drainage and lavage. The sequelae of an inadequately drained joint includes progression of an acute process to a subacute or chronic infection with its associated compromise of articular carilage and destruction of periarticular bone. Because of this potential for failure, repeated aspiration should be used only when all of the above criteria are present.

Arthroscopic drainage and lavage. This technique is appropriate for the treatment of septic arthritis of every joint in the body. The possible exception is the pediatric hip, for which treatment failure is more costly. The use of this technique also affords the opportunity for an examination for intra-articular pathology particularly softening of the articular cartilage and collections of adherent fibrin debris. In many cases, only one arthroscopic procedure is necessary. If the septic process proves refractory to the first drainage, repeat arthroscopic drainage and lavage can be done with minimal additional morbidity.

Open arthrotomy. This technique is the simplest method to ensure the debridement and lavage of the entire joint. The surgical approach is influenced by the joint involved and surgeon's preference, but it must allow adequate visualization of the involved joint. If fibrinous material is found adherent to the articular surface, this material is debrided. Synovectomy is indicated in infections considered subacute, chronic, or caused by anaerobes, gram-negative organsims, mycobacteria, and fungi. In addition to the removal of the synovium, removal of any cartilage overgrowth should be performed. This overgrowth is similar to the pannus seen in rheumatoid arthritis and starts at the margins of the articular cartilage. This overgrowth can be gently curetted from the articular surface. If the infection is chronic, there may be necrotic material and intraosseous cysts, which must also be debrided. After the procedure, the joint is closed in multiple layers over large bore suction drains.

Before arthroscopy, open arthrotomy was the treatment of choice in the treatment of septic joints because of the access it afforded to the entire joint. Since the introduction of arthroscopy, this less invasive procedure has demonstrated similar success to open arthrotomy in the treatment of septic arthritis and is probably the current gold standard in cases involving joints readily accessible to arthroscopy. Most authors still endorse open arthrotomy as the necessary procedure in the treatment of the septic hip in children because of the serious sequelae of incomplete treatment.

29. What is the duration of treatment with intravenous antibiotics?

Duration of treatment remains controversial, but most authors believe that a 2- to 4-week course of parenteral antibiotics is necessary for eradication of bacteria in the joint space. Some authors believe that children may be treated for 7–10 days intravenously followed with high oral dosages.

30. Is physical therapy appropriate in the treatment of septic arthritis?
During the acute phase of bacterial joint infection, motion of the infected joint is exquisitely painful. Therefore, decompression of the joint and external splinting should provide early relief. The optimal time for initiating exercises with passive range of motion is usually within the first week of treatment, followed by active motion as soon as the patient feels comfortable.

31. What is the prognosis in bacterial septic arthritis?
Patients who are not diagnosed and remain untreated for more than 5–7 days appear to do poorly. Other factors associated with a poor outcome are infections with gram-negative rods, positive blood culture results, polyarticular infection, existence of other serious illness, prior arthritis, and old age. After treatment has begun, the persistence of high levels of synovial fluid, high WBC count, or positive synovial fluid cultures points to a poor outcome.

32. Describe the three types of arthritis that have been encountered in patients with sickle cell disease.
The most common form of arthritis in patients with sickle cell disease is an aseptic arthritis that is most likely due to the sickle cell disease process itself. It may be seen during crisis but is more often a transient synovitis that usually involves the knee and resolves within 5 days. The second type of arthritis is also aseptic and is associated with a *remote* infection (often *Salmonella*). The mechanism of this type of arthritis is unclear. The third type is septic arthritis, in which the most likely organism is *S. aureus*. Salmonella is actually a rare organism in septic arthritis, and when it is encountered, it is most often in patients without sickle cell disease. When *Salmonella* septic arthritis does occur in sickle cell patients, it is most likely from a contiguous spread of an adjacent osteomyelitis process.

33. What are the clinical characteristics of patients with septic bursitis?
Septic bursitis causes painful swelling in the bursa overlying the olecranon process or the patella. Joint effusion is normally absent, and the range of motion is normal. Pain may be caused with full flexion of the joint but is due to stretching of the overlying soft tissues. Fever is found only in 30–40% of patients. Local skin abrasions, lacerations, or draining sinuses are frequently noted. Cellulitis surrounds the bursa. In adults, infection of olecranon bursa is 4 times more common than septic prepatellar bursitis. In children, however, the ratio of septic prepatellar bursitis to olecranon bursitis is close to 8:1.

34. Which bursa are most commonly affected by septic bursitis?
The prepatellar bursa and the olecranon bursa are the most common sites.

35. What is the pathogenesis of septic bursitis?
Septic bursitis usually results from transcutaneous inoculation of pathogens, whereas septic arthritis typically results from hematogenous spread. The most common organism in septic prepatellar bursitis is *S. aureus*. The second most common organism is *Streptococcus* sp.

36. Describe the treatment for septic bursitis.
Both parenteral and oral routes of antibiotic administration have been used successfully for the treatment of septic bursitis. Antibiotic levels can be maintained in bursal fluid by both routes, sometimes at levels higher than simultaneous serum levels. Patients with overwhelming bursal infection, which is manifested by extensive local skin infection, marked peribursal cellulitis, or signs of systemic illness, should be hospitalized and given parenteral antibiotic therapy. Proper drainage of the infected bursa is essential for successful therapy. Most cases respond to percutaneous needle aspiration, a procedure that may be performed daily or every other day, depending on the severity of the infection. Open surgical drainage should be done when the infection does not respond to standard treatment. The duration of antibiotic treatment for septic bursitis should

be adjusted for each individual; the average duration of antibiotic therapy, however, is approximately 10 days, which is the length of time necessary to sterilize bursal fluid.

BIBLIOGRAPHY

1. Abrams RA, Botte MJ: Hand infections: Treatment recommendations for specific types. J Am Acad Orthop Surg 4:219–230, 1996.
2. Lane JG, Falahe MH, Wojtys EM: Pyarthrosis of the knee: Treatment considerations. Clin Orthop 252:198–204, 1990.
3. Leslie BM, Harris JM III, Driscoll D: Septic arthritis of the shoulder in adults. J Bone Joint Surg 71A:1515–1522, 1989.
4. Morrissy RT: Bone and joint sepsis. In Morrissy RT, Weinstein SL (eds): Pediatric Orthopaedics. Philadelphia, Lippincott Williams & Wilkins, pp 459–504, 2001.
5. Osmon DR: Diagnosis and management of musculoskeletal infection. In Fitzgerald RH, Kaufer H, Malkani AL (eds): Mosby, St. Louis, 2002, pp 695–707.
6. Ruthberg AD, Ho G: Nongonococcal bacterial arthritis. In D'Ambrosia R, Marier R (eds): Orthopedic Infections. Thorofare, NJ, Slack, 1989, pp—.
7. Schoifet SD, Morrey BF: Treatment of infection after total knee arthroplasty by debridement with retention of components. J Bone Joint Surg 72A:1383–1390, 1990.
8. Shaw BA, Kasser JR: Acute septic arthritis in infancy and childhood. Clin Orthop 257:212–225, 1990.

6. OSTEOMYELITIS

Randall D. Neumann, M.D., and Joshua A. Urban, M.D.

1. What is osteomyelitis?
Osteomyelitis is an infection of bone.

2. What are the three types of osteomyelitis based on pathogenesis?
Hematogenous osteomyelitis. Infection by this route occurs during a bacteremic event and results in seeding of the bone. This type of osteomyelitis is responsible for 20% of cases.

Contiguous osteomyelitis. The bone is seeded from adjacent infections of the surrounding soft-tissues. These infections can result from penetrating trauma or an operative wound and are responsible for 50% of osteomyelitis cases.

Diabetic neuropathic osteomyelitis. The small bones of the feet are almost exclusively involved as a consequence of a local diabetic neuropathic ulcer. Painless tissue breakdown occurs over a prominent bone until seeding of the underlying bone occurs. This type of osteomyelitis is responsible for 30% of cases.

3. In what two age groups are the majority of hematogenous osteomyelitis cases seen?
Children under the age of 15 and adults older than 50. In both groups, the long bones (i.e., tibia, femur, humerus) are the most frequently involved.

4. What are the three clinical classifications for hematogenous osteomyelitis?
Acute hematogenous osteomyelitis is characterized by systemic illness, absence of bony radiologic changes at presentation, duration of less than 10 days, an in most cases, no history of a previous episode.

Subacute hematogenous osteomyelitis is characterized by a lack of systemic illness, established bony radiographic changes at presentation, duration of more than 10 days, and no history of a previous episode.

Chronic osteomyelitis is characterized by the presence or absence of systemic illness, bony radiologic changes, and a history of previous episodes of infection.

5. Describe the pathogenesis and natural history of acute hematogenous osteomyelitis in children.

The infection initially presents in the metaphyseal region of long bones. In the metaphysis, the capillary branches from the nutrient artery progress longitudinally toward the epiphysis. Just before reaching the physis, the capillaries turn 180° and empty into much larger venous sinusoids. These venous sinusoids are an area of slow and turbulent blood flow, which allows bacteria to adhere to exposed matrices adjacent to endothelial gaps in the maturing metaphyseal vessels. Since the capillary loops do not anastomose and, therefore, serve as "end vessels," thrombosis of these vessels can result in avascular necrosis of bone. Another factor that has been postulated to add to the vulnerability of the metaphysis to infection is decreased oxygen tension, which diminishes the phagocyte activity of macrophages and hampers the local host defenses.

Once microinfarcted metaphyseal bone becomes colonized by a bacteremic process, the organisms can proliferate in isolation from host defenses. The infection can spread via pathways of least resistance, including the haversian systems, Volkman's canals, and along thrombosed nutrient vessels. In individuals older than 1–2 years of age, the infection spreads in two general directions. Firstly, the infection can spread to erode the cortex and form a subperiosteal abscess. As the periosteum is elevated from the underlying bone by this abscess, the periosteal blood supply is jeopardized. The other type of infectious spread occurs in the direction of the diaphysis, where the endosteal blood supply to the bone can be jeopardized by thrombosis of the nutrient arteries and from the increases in intramedullary pressure as a result of the involvement of the haversian systems and Volkman's canals.

When both the endosteal and periosteal blood supply are compromised, extensive sequestrum formation results. In this situation, the stripped periosteum, which is provided with its own blood supply from its muscular attachments, lays down new bone (involucrum) around the infected cortex (sequestrum). Acute hematogenous osteomyelitis becomes chronic in about 10% of patients despite early and appropriate treatment. Delayed therapy can increase the incidence of subsequent chronic osteomyelitis.

6. Describe the perimetaphyseal blood supply in the infant and how it relates to the sequela of acute hematogenous osteomyelitis.

In children younger than 1 or 2 years old, transphyseal vessels from the metaphysis to the epiphysis have been demonstrated. This finding explains the increased incidence of epiphyseal involvement and coinciding septic arthritis in this population.

7. Describe the pathogenesis and natural history of acute hematogenous osteomyelitis in adults.

Hematogenous osteomyelitis in adults begins as an acute infection usually within the medullary canal. Edema and breakdown of products increase local vascular compromise and result in the necrosis of fat, hematopoietic tissue, and trabecular bone. Increased osteoclastic activity, induced by hyperemia, enlarges cortical haversian and Volkman's canals. Macrophages, white blood cells, and fibroblasts gain access to the site. The pathogens and/or inflammatory byproducts pass through these channels into the soft tissues to produce induration and periosteal abscesses. The timing and adequacy of treatment, virulence of the organism, condition of the host, and status of the local milieu determine whether the infection is eradicated or chronic osteomyelitis ensues.

8. Describe the pathogenesis and typical clinical picture of chronic osteomyelitis.

The original cortex is replaced by a thickened, reactive involucrum. Necrotic areas of bone become entrapped with the involucrum and form sequestra within the bone. Unless the sequestrum is removed and the organisms eradicated by debridement and antibiotics, a chronic infection ensues. Since bone has a limited resorptive capacity for necrotic mineralized tissue and since antibiotics cannot penetrate this avascular area, the bacteria contained within the sequestrum may persist indefinitely. Commonly the host has long periods of symptomless quiescence separated by sporatic periods of disease exacerbation characterized by an increase in discomfort and occasionally spontaneous drainage from the medullary canal into the soft tissues and from the skin via sinus tracts.

9. What are the clinical findings in acute osteomyelitis?

Patients nearly always describe severe, localized bone pain and can readily identify the affected area. Dramatic local tenderness is present, along with soft-tissue inflammation. Approximately 75–80% of patients have fever. Loss of function around the adjacent joint typically occurs within 12–48 hours after the onset of infection. Painful and tense joint effusion may indicate either septic arthritis or an aseptic sympathetic effusion.

10. What nonradiographic tests should be obtained in the evaluation of osteomyelitis? Describe their likely results.

Complete blood count with differential. Leukocytosis is present in approximately one-third of patients.

Erythrocyte sedimentation rate (ESR) and C-reactive protein (C-RP). An elevated ESR or C-RP is present in more than 90% of cases. Both of these tests are nonspecific inflammatory markers that may also be elevated in rheumatoid arthritis, neoplasms, other infections, recent surgery, and other inflammatory conditions.

Blood cultures may help isolate a causative organism prior to bone aspiration and are positive in 36–76% of cases. In cases of vertebral osteomyelitis, if blood cultures yield a pathogenic organism and there is definitive radiographic evidence of a bone infection, biopsy is not needed.

Aspiration. Aspiration of associated soft-tissue or subperiosteal abscesses or biopsy of the involved bone is diagnostic. Aspiration of an adjacent joint effusion should also be performed if present. Care should be taken to avoid any areas of cellulitis so as not to inoculate what may actually be a sterile joint.

11. What radiographic tests may be helpful in the workup of osteomyelitis?

Plain radiographs should be obtained in every case. These serve to stage the disease with respect to its duration and also serve as a baseline for subsequent films. Plain radiographs are negative in the early part of the infection. The earliest specific changes, minimal periosteal elevation and thickening, can be seen as early as 10 days after the onset of infection. These changes are somewhat subtle and can be easily overlooked. Lytic lesions can be seen 2 to 6 weeks after the onset of infection. Thirty to 50% of the bone must be destroyed before lysis is evident on plain xrays. Sclerotic changes and periosteal new bone formation are late findings and suggest chronicity of infection. Demineralization of the surrounding bone may be present. Soft-tissue edema is present in 35–50% of the cases.

Radionuclide scanning is more sensitive than plain radiographs. Its usefulness is limited by an overall lack of specificity and marginal sensitivity early in the course of osteomyelitis. Magnetic resonance imaging (MRI) has replaced radionuclide scanning as the procedure of choice early in the course of acute osteomyelitis before changes on the plain xrays are evident. However, radionuclide scanning may be more helpful than MRI in cases with possible multiple sites of involvement and when retained hardware will result in substantial artifact on MRI imaging.

Magnetic resonance imaging has replaced radionuclide scanning as the procedure of choice not only in determing the presence of osteolmyelitis but also in evaluating the extent of the infectious process. It is also valuable early in the course of disease (the first 24–72 hours) when the accuracy of bone scans can be unreliable. MRI provides the best anatomic detail and is more accurate in distinguishing soft-tissue infection from osteomyelitis and allows for localization of the infectious process for aspiration or biopsy.

Computed tomography (CT) scans can distinguish between soft-tissue and bone infections and can aid in the determination of optimal sites for biopsy or aspiration. Intraosseous gas, decreased density of infected bone in association with soft-tissue masses, and destructive lesions of bone can be seen on CT. CT scans are not as useful as MRI.

12. If plain radiographs reveal abnormalities of bone, what is the clinical stage of infection?
Abnormalities of bone on plain x-rays signify that the infection is either subacute or chronic. If only a lytic lesion is present, a subacute process is most likely present. If a sequestrum and an involucrum are present, this represents a chronic disease process.

13. What is a sequestrum?
A sequestrum is a necrotic segment of bone without blood supply that acts as the nidus for infection in chronic osteomyelitis.

14. What is an involucrum?
The involucrum is the new cortical bone laid down by the periosteum around the shell of the old cortex (sequestrum).

15. What radionuclide studies can be used to diagnose osteomyelitis?
Several types of radionuclide scans are available for the diagnosis of osteomyelitis including technetium-99m, gallium-67, and indium-111-labeled leukocytes. The uptake of technetium phosphorate is related primarily to osteoblastic activity. Because technetium is rapidly cleared from the blood and absorbed into the bone, maximal uptake occurs within 1 hour of injection. The usual procedure in evaluating areas of suspected osteomyelitis is to perform a three-phase bone scan. The first phase includes a flow study at the time of injection. The second stage is the equilibrium (or intermediate) stage in which increased uptake of tracer aids in the differentiation of superficial nonosseous and joint infections from osteomyelitis. A delayed phase, generally performed 2–4 hours after injection of the radioisotope, shows active osteoblastic activity and is positive in various disease states, including osteomyelitis, tumors, degenerative joint disease, trauma, and postsurgical changes. A focus of osteomyelitis presents as an area of increased tracer uptake on the delayed image. On occasion, a "cold" area may result from decreased delivery of tracer due to edematous occlusion of flow and intramedullary vessels. Indium-labeled leukocytes have been suggested for differentiating between osteomyelitis and reactive involucrum without the necessity for delayed imaging. The test requires drawing approximately 50 cc of venous blood. The leukocytes are separated from the other blood elements and labeled with indium-111. The indium-labeled leukocytes are then reinjected into the patient, and scans are performed 18–24 hours later. The scan is interpreted as positive if a focal accumulation of activity exceeds adjacent normal bone activity.

16. What preexisting conditions may negatively affect the host's response to infection?

Malnutrition	Immune deficiency	Extremes of age
Renal failure	Chronic hypoxia	Steroid therapy
Liver failure	Malignancy	Tobacco use
Alcohol abuse	Diabetes mellitus	

17. Describe the treatment principles of acute osteomyelitis.
Antibiotics represent the primary treatment for acute osteomyelitis. Initially, empiric intravenous antibiotics are started as soon as culture specimens have been obtained. This initial antibiotic should cover the organisms most likely to be encountered based on the patient's age and risk factors. Once the infecting organism is identified, appropriate adjustments in the antibiotic regimen should be made. If no pathogen is identified, the empirically-chosen antibiotic therapy is continued as long as the patient shows signs of improvement. If no improvement occurs after 24–36 hours of empiric treatment, consideration should be given to further investigation, alterations in the antibiotic regimen, or surgical intervention.

18. What is the appropriate duration of antibiotic treatment for acute osteomyelitis?

The duration of antibiotic treatment is controversial. Historically, 4–6 weeks of intravenous antibiotics have been recommended as treatment failures as high as 19% can occur when the duration of therapy is reduced to 3 weeks or less.

Currently, however, the trend has been to shorten the intravenous antibiotic course and start oral antibiotics sooner than previously thought acceptable. Often, intravenous antibiotics are substituted for oral agents after 5–7 days of treatment if the following conditions exist: (1) an oral form of an appropriate antibiotic is available; (2) the infection is resolving; (3) the medication is tolerable at the necessary dose; and (4) adequate serum levels have been demonstrated after compliant administration of the oral antibiotic.

The duration of antibiotic treatment is also dependent upon the infecting organism. In general, the infections caused by group B streptococci or *Haemophilus influenzae* type B can be treated for a minimum of 10–14 days. On the other end of the spectrum, infections caused by S. aureus or by gram negative bacilli should be treated for a minimum of 3 weeks.

In all circumstances, once the patient is on an antibiotic regimen, clinical signs of continuous imporvement should occur (decreasing pain, swelling, erythema, and fever). Sequential laboratory studies should also be obtained and should demonstrate a normalizing pattern (ESR, C-RP). Normalization of these studies (especially the C-RP) should be present before antibiotic treatment is discontinued.

19. What are the common organisms and recommended antibiotics associated with osteomyelitis in neonates? Infants? Older Children?

Neonates. The three most common organisms that cause osteomyelitis in decreasing order are *Staphylococcus aureus* group B streptococci, and gram-negative bacilli. Neonates lack a mature immune system and, therefore, cannot exhibit the usual inflammatory response that characterizes the presence of osteomyelitis. As a result, the clinical signs and symptoms, as well as the usual laboratory markers, that can herald osteomyelitis are often not present. Neonates may present with only mild swelling, pseudoparalysis of the affected limb, and tenderness. Plain radiographs are rarely diagnostic, especially early in the disease process. Given the paucity of clinical, radiographic, and laboratory findings, aspiration is both mandatory and critical in this population. The treating physician should also be vigilant for other sights of infection as this phenomena may occur in up to 40% in this age group. In addition, adjacent septic arthritis often occurs simultaneously due to the transphyseal vessels that are present at this age. Empirical treatment usually involves an antistaphylococcal penicillin (e.g., oxacillin) and gentamicin, or a broad-spectrum third-generation cephalosporin such as cefotaxime.

Infants and children under 2–3 years of age. The most common organisms encountered in this age group (in decreasing order) are *S. aureus,* streptococci, and *H. influenzae* type B. In patients who have received the influenza vaccine, the initial treatment should consist of an antistaphylococcal penicillin (oxacillin, naficillin, methicillin) or a first- or third-generation cephalosporin. For patients who have not been immunized against *H. influenzae* or who have an unknown vaccination history, a second-generation cephalosporin such as cefuroxime should be administered. Signs of coexisting meningitis should be sought for and spinal fluid examination and culture should be performed if indicated.

Older children. As with the other age groups, *S. aureus* is responsible for the majority of osteomyelitis. Initial treatment should consist of an anti-staphylococcal penicillin. Clindamycin is an appropriate choice for patients with allergies to penicillin and cephalosporins. Vancomycin should be reserved only for situations involving methicillin-resistant staphylococcal infections.

20. When is surgical intervention indicated in the treatment of osteomyelitis?

Surgical treatment of osteomyelitis is indicated when joint involvement occurs or when an abscess exists either in the bone or subperiosteally. The goals of treatment are to remove the purulent material by drainage of the subperiosteal abscess, irrigation and debridement of septic joints and abscesses within bone, and removal of avascular and necrotic bone. Culture and histo-logic examination should be obtained in each of these cases as malignant tumors may infrequently be mistaken for infection. An additional indication for surgery includes the lack of improvement after 24–36 hours of intravenous antibiotic therapy. Therefore, in acute osteomyelitis, surgery may not be needed if response to the antibiotic regimen is adequate. By definition, subacute and chronic osteomyelitis are themselves indications for surgery since they do have chronic changes of bone.

21. What are the principal isolates in hematogenous osteomyelitis in patients with sickle-cell disease?

The predominant organisms are *Salmonella* species. Other common organisms include *S. aureus, Streptococcus pneumoniae,* and *H. influenzae.*

22. What are the principal isolates in patients with drug addiction?

S. aureus, Pseudomonas aeruginosa, gram-negative bacilli.

23. What are the common isolates in patients on hemodialysis?

S. aureus and *epidermidis,* and *Mycobacterium tuberculosis.*

24. What classification system is commonly used for chronic osteomyelitis? Describe it.

Cierny and Mader developed the most commonly used classification system for chronic os-teomyelitis in 1981. This system breaks down each case by evaluating the anatomic personality of the osteomyelitis and the medical fitness of the host. It was developed to not only guide treat-ment, but to also serve as a prognostic indicator.

25. What are the four anatomic types of osteomyelitis in the Cierny-Mader classification system?

Type 1. In this type of chronic osteomyelitis, the nidus of infection is medullary; therefore, this is primarily an endosteal disease. Most of the patients in this stage have a hematogenous eti-ology, but type 1 disease can also present as a sequelae of medullary fixation (i.e., an infected fracture union). The extent of disease can be determined by a bone scan or MRI. Soft-tissue ab-scesses and induration may develop as an expansion from involved haversian systems.

Type 2. Also known as superficial osteomyelitis, this type is characterized by an exposed and usually dissecated bone surface as a result of an overlying soft-tissue deficit. As granulation buds penetrate the surface eschar from the deep cortex of the bone, they succumb to the local surface environment of the soft-tissue defect- repeated trauma, exposure, bacteria, etc. The buds die back cyclically. Eventually, the haversian systems are sealed off with a proteinaceous debris and the surface becomes sequestered until it is sloughed by the host.

Type 3. Also known as localized osteomyelitis, it is characterized by a cavitary and well-marginated process that contains a cortical sequestrum. Features of types 1 and 2 may be present. This disease process, by definition, can be completely excised without compromising stability of the bone.

Type 4. Also known as diffuse osteomyelitis, it is characterized by a permeative through and through process with the characteristics of types 1, 2, and 3 with the added feature of instability.

26. What are the three host classifications in the Cierny-Mader system?

A **class A** host is a normal responder to infection and surgery. A **class B** host has either a lo-cal (L), systemic (S), or a combined local and systemic (L/S) condition that compromises the abil-ity to fight infection. Examples of local compromise include chronic lymphedema, venous stasis, major vessel disease, arteritis, extensive scarring, and radiation fibrosis. Examples of systemic compromise include malnutrition, immunodeficiency, chronic hypoxia, malignancy, diabetes mellitus, old age, and renal or liver failure. The **class C** host is not a treatment candidate either because disability is minimal or the morbidity of treatment is in excess of the disease status or metabolic capabilities. The class C host, therefore, receives no treatment or a palliative course or is simply supported to promote a spontaneous arrest.

27. Describe the dual vascular supply to bone. Why is this an important concept in the surgical treatment of chronic osteomyelitis?

The blood supply of the bone is derived from two sources: (1) an intramedullary endosteal network of vessels that supply the inner two-thirds of the cortex and (2) a periosteal network that supplies the outer one-third of the cortex. Any manipulation of bone, especially for the treatment of infection, must keep this dual nature of vascular supply in mind. All exposure of bone should be extraperiosteal in order to preserve the periosteal supply. Exposing the bone subperiosteally strips the bone of the periosteal blood supply. Any surgical plan that involves both intramedullary reaming and plating of the cortex potentially sacrifices both the endosteal and periosteal supply, and therefore, these procedures should be staged and separated by a 6- to 8-week interval to allow for the reconstitution of the damaged blood supply before the second procedure is done.

28. Discuss the surgical principles of the treatment of chronic osteomyelitis with respect to staging of surgery, surgical debridement, accessory sinus tracts, the involucrum and sequestrum, metaphyseal disease, and the use of antibiotic cement.

Most authors agree that the surgical treatment of chronic osteomyelitis should be staged. The first stage should consist of an adequate debridement and placement, if possible, of antibiotic-laden cement depots usually in the form of hand-made beads or dowels. The second stage should consist of cement depot removal, repeat debridement, placement of bone graft and fixation of the bone as needed.

The quality of surgical debridement is the most critical factor in the successful management of chronic osteomyelitis. Debridement must include release of accumulated pus, which is often under pressure and serves to decrease the bacterial load sufficiently to allow host defenses and antibiotics to effectively fight the infection. All dense, adherent overlying scar that cannot contribute to wound healing should be excised.

Accessory sinus tracts distant from the intended course of the incision do not need to be routinely excised, because once the source of drainage is eliminated, they usually close spontaneously.

Efforts should be made to retain as much of the reactive new bone (involucrum) as possible while removing all the necrotic colonized bone (sequestrum).

Intramedullary reaming is an appropriate debridement method for diaphyseal involvement. However, when metaphyseal disease is present, reaming of the intramedullary canal alone is not sufficient. Debridement through a longitudinal trough created in the metaphyseal region is necessary in these cases. Care must be taken to minimize the damage to the periosteal blood supply when exposing the metaphyseal region for the trough. Extraperiosteal dissection and minimizing the area that is dissected will help preserve some blood supply to this region.

The combined use of 3.0 grams and 3.6 grams of vancomycin and tobramycin powder, respectively, covers the majority of organisms typically responsible for chronic osteomyelitis. This amount of antibiotics should not be added to cement intended for structural use (fixation of total joint components). Removal of these antibiotic-laden cement depots (fahsioned into beads or dowels) should be done only after the soft-tissues recover completely (usually 3–4 weeks). If within the medullary canal, it is recommended that they be removed in 10–14 days as the formation of granulation tissue after that period makes subsequent removal difficult.

29. What is dead space? Why is its management critical in the surgical treatment of chronic osteomyelitis?

Dead space is the void that is left after debridement of infected tissue. This void can be in the bone, soft-tissue, or both. The obliteration of dead space is critical in treating chronic osteomyelitis because it minimizes the ability of bacteria to congregate substantially in one location. For example, obliteration of dead space prevents the formation of a hematoma, which is an ideal culture media that can be seeded by bacteria. Dead space can be provisionally obliterated by antibiotic-laden cement during the first stage of surgical treatment. Definitive obliteration usually consists of bone graft, muscle flaps, or both.

30. Describe the role of local muscular flaps in the treatment of chronic osteomyelitis.
Chronic osteomyelitis can be considered as much of an ischemic disease of bone as it is an infectious disease of bone. Blood flow to areas of chronic osteomyelitis is decreased both during the presence of disease and after successful treatment. An ischemic environment may be responsible for the chronicity of these infections as the organisms responsible are known to survive in avascular and marginally vascularized tissues. The addition of a muscle flap to the surgical therapy serves to not only obliterate dead space, but it also enhances the local bone-blood flow which serves to improve the local host defenses and the delivery of antibiotics.

31. Describe the common flaps used for orthopedic infections.
Conventional rotation flaps have very limited place for skin coverage in the extremity.

Rotation muscle flaps. The gastrocnemius flap is by far the most useful and has the least morbidity at the donor site. The muscle with available skin is taken, along with the blood supply branching from the popliteal artery. This flap is most useful for defects of the tibial plateau or in the knee.

Free tissue transfer. The most versatile technique of skin coverage is the free tissue transfer, which includes the scapular, radial arm, groin, and dorsal pedis flaps. Skin and muscle pedicles are transferred with a branch of local artery, and microscopic anastomosis of the transferred vessel to a local vessel results in free blood flow to the musculocutaneous flap.

Osteocutaneous flaps. The most commonly used is the free fibular graft; vascularity is based on the peroneal blood supply. The graft may be taken with or without skin.

Free muscle flaps. The most popular free muscle flaps are the latissimus, gracilis, and rectus abdominis. Vascularity is based on local blood supply and allows coverage of large areas. Skin is then grafted over the muscle.

32. What is the reported success rate for the treatment of chronic osteomyelitis using this surgical philosophy?
The overall success rate is approximately 90%. The likelihood of treatment success in a particular case can be predicted by the Cierny-Mader classification and depends both on the anatomic type of osteomyelitis and on the quality of the host. Success in these studies has been defined as the lack of recurrence at least 2 years after treatment.

33. Describe the surgical treatment and success rate for type 1 (medullary) chronic osteomyelitis.
Treatment of medullary osteomyelitis involves simple dead space management and closure techniques. Debridement of medullary osteomyelitis can be either via intramedullary reaming or local cortical unroofing, but not both in order to preserve as much blood supply as possible. In most cases, cortical unroofing with drainage and curettage of the lesion is performed during the first stage. Antibiotic-laden cement depots are placed in the dead space created by the bone debridement. Intravenous antibiotics are also given for 6 weeks. Removal of the cement, redebridement, and placement of cancellous grafting as needed to fill the dead space is done at the second stage. Using these techniques, success rates for type 1 chronic osteomyelitis have been as high as 100% in class A hosts and 89% in class B hosts.

34. Describe the surgical treatment and success rate for type 2 (superficial) osteomyelitis.
Treatment of superficial osteomyelitis usually does not require dead space management but may involve complex closures. After drainage and curettage of the exposed bone surface, complex closures are generally required. Success rates with class A hosts can be as high as 100%; however, with class B hosts, only 79% success rates have been achieved.

35. Describe the treatment and success rate for type 3 (localized) osteomyelitis.

Treatment of localized osteomyelitis typically involves simple stabilization procedures with complex dead space and closure management. These cases often involve infected unions and refractory pin tract infections. Treatment includes combining the techniques used for types 1 and 2 with simple methods of stabilization. The bone is usually debrided through a local cortical window and all the necrotic bone is removed. An interval stage consisting of antibiotic-laden cement depots is used followed by reconstruction of the defect at a second stage. Treatment of localized chronic osteomyelitis has resulted in a 98% and 92% success rate in class A and class B hosts, respectively.

36. Describe the treatment and success rate for type 4 (diffuse) osteomyelitis.

Treatment for this type of chronic osteomyelitis typically involves complex stabilization, dead space, and closure management. Diffuse osteomyelitis cases often occur in the setting of infected nonunions that require not only the removal of the infected bone but also reconstruction and complex stabilization of the bone. The initial treatment consists of the debridement of all the infected bone (if possible) followed by the standard interval of intravenous antibiotics and antibiotic-laden cement depots. Definitive stabilization can be performed during either the first or second stage but care must be taken not to perform procedures that compromise both the endosteal and periosteal blood supply at the same surgical setting. Treatment of this type of chronic osteomyelitis has resulted in 98% and 80% success rates in class A and B hosts, respectively.

BIBLIOGRAPHY

1. Bateman JL, Pevzner MM: Spinal osteomyelitis: A review of 10 years' experience. Orthopedics 18:561–565, 1995.
2. Cierny G III, Mader JT: Adult chronic osteomyelitis: An overview. In D'Ambrosia RD, Marier RL (eds): Orthopedic Infections. Thorofare, NJ, Slack, 1991, pp 33–47.
3. Cierny G III, Mader JT: Approach to adult osteomyelitis. Orthop Rev 26:259–295, 1987.
4. Carragee EJ, Kim D: The clinical use of erythrocyte sedimentation rate in pyogenic vertebral osteomyelitis. Spine 22:2089–2093, 1997.
5. Fitzgerald Jr. RH, Whalen JL, Petersen SA: Pathophysiology of osteomyelitis and pharmacokinetics of antimicrobial agents in normal and osteomyelitic bone. In Esterhai Jr. JL, Gristina AG, Poss R (eds): Musculoskeletal Infection. Park Ridge, IL, American Academy of Orthopaedic Surgeons, 1992, pp 396–399.
6. Green NE, Edwards K: Bone and joint infections in children. Orthop Clin North Am 18:555, 1987.
7. Gustilo RB (ed): Orthopedic Infections: Diagnosis and Treatment. Philadelphia, W.B. Saunders, 1989.
8. Mader JT, Pennick J: The chemical staging of adult osteomyelitis. Contemp Orthop 10:17–37, 1985.
9. Reilly KE, Linz JC, Stem PJ: Osteomyelitis of the tubular bones of the hand. J Hand Surg 22A:644–649, 1997.
10. Schurman DJ, Fitzgerald RH, Nelson CL, Patzakis MJ: Symposium: Antibiotics in bone and joint infections. Contemp Orthop 15:47, 1987.
11. Spangehl MJ, Younger A, Masri BA, Duncan CP: Diagnosis of infection following total hip arthroplasty. AAOS Instructional Course Lecture 47:285–295, 1998.
12. Tetsworth K, Cierny G III: Osteomyelitis debridement techniques. Clin Orthop 360: 87–96, 1999.
13. Warner WC: Osteomyelitis. In Canale ST (ed): Campbell's Operative Orthopedics, 9th ed. St. Louis, Mosby, 1998, pp 578–800.

7. OPEN FRACTURES

Matthew A. Mormino, M.D., and David A. Peterson, M.D.

1. How are open fractures classified?

Type I   < 1-cm wound, low-energy fracture

Type II   1–10-cm wound, higher energy fracture

Type III   > 10-cm wound, high-energy fracture

Type IIIA   Moderate periosteal stripping, wound closure not requiring soft tissue flap

Type IIIB   Marked periosteal stripping, wound closure requires soft tissue flap

Type IIIC   Any open fracture with a vascular injury that requires repair

This classification system is the source of endless arguments among orthopaedists; do not feel bad if you cannot accurately classify a fracture. Chances are, neither can the attending physician.

2. What is the initial treatment for patients with open fractures?

Many open fractures are associated with motor vehicle accidents, gunshot wounds, falls, and other major trauma. Consequently, all patients with an open fracture should be evaluated by advanced trauma life support protocols. An examination that includes neurologic status, head, spine, abdomen, and pelvis is completed before starting treatment of the open fracture. The wound is coverd by a dry sterile dressing and the extremity is splinted. Tetanus is updated or tetanus immunoglobin is given if imunization status is uncertain. Antibiotics are started.

3. What is the initial objective in the treatment of open fractures?

The initial objective is to remove all contamination from the wound and fracture site. The aphorism "Dilution is the solution to the pollution," describes the role of irrigation in open fractures. Liters (9–12) of normal saline are used to clean fractures of long bones. All foreign material must be removed, including the wadding from gunshot wounds and pieces of clothing driven inward by the force of injury. Necrotic muscle and devitalized bone are excised from the wound.

4. Which tissues are removed during debridement of an open fracture?

The four major principles of debridement are described in a poem by James Learmonth:

On the edges of the skin take a piece very thin (1);

The tenser the fascia, the more you should slash'er (2);

Of muscles much more, 'til you see fresh gore (3);

And the bundles contract at least the impact;

Hardly any of bone, only bits quite alone (4).

Nonviable tissues (i.e., dead muscle, fascia, and small pieces of bone not attached to soft tissue) that provide a focus for infection are removed. Skin should be preserved; only the contaminated edge is removed.

5. In the open fracture, how can you differentiate viable from nonviable muscle tissue?

The four Cs—color, contractility, consistency, and capacity to bleed—help the surgeon to decide which muscles to debride. Pale muscle that does not (1) bleed when cut or (2) contract when touched should be excised.

6. What is the difference in treatment of open fractures between low-velocity and high-velocity gunshot wounds?

High-velocity gunshot wounds (e.g., military rifle) or close-range shotgun wounds result in more disruption and destruction of soft tissue due to the high energy involved. Multiple debridements may be required to ensure that no nonviable tissue is left behind as a focus of infection. Low-velocity wounds may require only local irrigation, debridement of the entry and exit wounds, and supportive oral antibiotic treatment.

7. Which antibiotics are given prophylactically when an open fracture is present?

A first-generation cephalosporin (cefazolin) should be given for all open fractures. Add an aminoglycoside (gentamicin) for type III injuries, and add penicillin for barnyard or heavily contaminated wounds. Tetanus status should be assessed and updated or treated appropriately.

8. What is the best time to close the wounds of type III open fractures?

The ideal time frame is 5–7 days. Closure may be accomplished if no necrotic tissue or contamination is present. Local muscle flaps or vascularized free-tissue transfers may be required for larger soft-tissue defects. The flaps may provide the additional benefit of improved circulation to the area, which assists healing of the fracture site and protects against infection with increased oxygen tension.

9. What type of fixation is used to stabilize open fractures?

This issue is complex and controversial. The surgeon needs to stabilize the fracture site to protect viable soft tissue, but the metal provides a potential source of infection, because bacteria are isolated from the immune system and circulation. In general, external fixation is used when multiple irrigation and debridements are required (e.g., type III) and subsequent soft-tissue transfers may be necessary. Internal fixation with plates and screws may be used in type I open fractures and articular fractures that require anatomic reduction. Primary and delayed intramedullary fixation have been used in types I , II, and III open fractures of the long bones.

10. In a type IIIC fracture, which is completed first—arterial repair or fracture fixation?

Fracture stability, usually with external fixation, is achieved before arterial repair. Occasionally a temporary arterial shunt may be used before skeletal repair, but attempts at achieving fracture fixation after arterial repair may disrupt the vascular reconstruction with the repetitive motion of reduction and correction of alignment.

CONTROVERSIES

11. Which is the better treatment for type IIIC open fractures of the tibia: amputation or salvage?

Amputation may be the better treatment, although it still has disadvantages. The obvious disadvantage is loss of limb and dependence on a prosthesis. Participation in strenuous sports or employment in a job requiring heavy labor or fine foot movements may be impossible. Advantages include shorter hospitalization, fewer operations, and a quick return to work.

Salvage of the leg may require many procedures and more operating time for vascular repair, fracture fixation, soft-tissue transfers, removal of infected bone, nerve repair and reconstruction, and removal of fixation. Amputation may still be required if infection, nonunion, or a painful limb results from attempted salvage. The four Ds—divorce, destitution, depression, and disability— may be the final result of attempted salvage.

12. What factors assist the surgeon in deciding whether to amputate or salvage a type IIIC open fracture of the tibia?

Warm ischemia time over 6 hours and disruption of the posterior tibial nerve are considered to be absolute indications for amputation by Lange. In addition, the Mangled Extremity Severity Score (MESS) may help determine whether amputation or salvage should be performed. A score of at least 7 points indicates that amputation should be strongly considered over salvage.

The Mangled Extremity Severity Score

TYPE	CHARACTERISTICS	INJURIES	POINTS	SCORE
Skeletal and soft-tissue group				
1	Low energy	Stab wounds, simple closed fractures, small-caliber gunshot wounds	1	_____
2	Medium energy	Open or multiple-level fractures, dislocations, moderate crush injuries	2	_____
3	High energy	Shotgun blast (close range), high-velocity gunshot wound	3	_____
4	Massive crush	Logging, railroad, oil-rig accidents	4	_____
			Subtotal	_____
Shock group				
1	Normotensive	Blood pressure stable in field and OR	0	_____
2	Transient hypotension	Blood pressure unstable in field, but responsive to intravenous fluids	1	_____
3	Prolonged hypotension	Systolic blood pressure < 90 mmHg in field hypotension responsive to intravenous fluids only in OR	2	_____
4	Advanced	Pulseless, cool, paralyzed, and numb	3	_____
			Subtotal	_____
Ischemia group (points double if ischemia > 6 hr)				
1	None	Pulsatile leg without signs of ischemia	0	_____
2	Mild	Diminished pulses only	1	_____
3	Moderate	No pulse by Doppler, sluggish capillary refill, paresthesias, diminished motor activity	2	_____
4	Advanced	Pulseless, cool, paralyzed, numb	3	_____
			Subtotal	_____
Age group				
1	< 30 yr		0	_____
2	30–50 yr		1	_____
3	> 50 yr		2	_____
			Subtotal	_____
Total mangled extremity severity score			Total	_____

From Helfet DL, Howey T, Sanders R, Johansen K: Limb salvage versus amputation: Preliminary results of the mangled extremity severity score. Clin Orthop 256:80–86, 1990, with permission.

BIBLIOGRAPHY

1. Bartlett C, Weiner L, Young E: Treatment of type II and type III open tibia fractures in children. J Orthop Trauma 2:357–362, 1997.
2. Bartlett CS, Helfet DL, Hausman MR, et al: Ballistics and gunshot wounds: Effects on musculoskeletal tissues. J Am Acad Orthop Surg 8(1):21–36, 2000.
3. Chapman MW: Open fractures. In Rockwood CA, Green DP, Bucholz RW (eds): Rockwood and Green's Fractures in Adults, 4th ed. Philadelphia, J.B. Lippincott, 1996.
4. Christian CA: General principles of fracture treatment. In Canale ST (ed): Campbell's Operative Orthopaedics, 9th ed. St. Louis, Mosby, 1998, pp 1993–2041.
5. Connolly JF: Management of open fractures. In Connolly JF (ed): DePalma's The Management of Fractures and Dislocations, vol. 1, 3rd ed. Philadelphia, W.B. Saunders, 1981, pp 125–135.
6. Gustilo RB, Anderson JT: Prevention of infection in the treatment of one thousand and twenty-five open fractures of long bones: Retrospective and prospective analyses. J Bone Joint Surg 58A:453–458, 1976.
7. Gustilo RB, Mendoza RM, Williams DN: Problems in the management of type III (severe) open fractures: A new classification of type III open fractures. J Trauma 24:742–746, 1984.

8. Hansen ST Jr: Editorial. The type-IIIC tibial fracture: Salvage or amputation. J Bone Joint Surg 69A:799–800, 1987.
9. Hansen ST Jr: Overview of the severely traumatized lower limb: Reconstruction versus amputation. Clin Orthop 243:17–19, 1989.
10. Helfet DL, Howey T, Sanders R, Johansen K: Limb salvage versus amputation: Preliminary results of the mangled extremity severity score. Clin Orthop 256:80–86, 1990.
11. Henley M, Chapman J, Agel J, et al: Treatment of type II, IIIA, and IIIB open fractures of the tibial shaft: A prospective comparison of unreamed interlocking intramedullary nails and half-pin external fixators. J Orthop Trauma 12:1–7, 1998.
12. Lange RH: Limb reconstruction versus amputation decision making in massive lower extremity trauma. Clin Orthop 243:92–99, 1989.
13. Ordog GJ,etal : Civilian gunshot wounds- Outpatient management. J Trauma 36:106–111.1994.
14. Sanders R, Swiontkowski M, Nunley J, Spiegel P: The management of fractures with soft tissue disruptions. J Bone Joint Surg 75A:778–789, 1993.

8. DEEP VENOUS THROMBOSIS

Scott P. Wattenhofer, M.D., FACS

1. Describe the classic triad for the pathogenesis of venous thrombosis as described by Virchow.

1. **Venous stasis:** prevents clearance of activated coagulation factors, retards inflow of clotting inhibitors, promotes endothelial cell hypoxia and injury, and increases blood viscosity.

Vascular damage: intact endothelial cells inhibit platelet adherence and initiation of blood clotting; injury to the endothelial layer of the vessel wall exposes the underlying tissue that initiates platelet adherence and initiation of the clotting cascade.

3. **Hypercoagulability:** alteration of the normal clotting mechanism that predisposes to thrombus formation (e.g., congenital or acquired hypercoagulable states, hypercoagulability associated with malignancies, and hypercoagulability associated with oral contraceptives).

2. What risk factors are associated with an increased risk of development of deep venous thrombosis (DVT)?
- Previous episode of DVT or pulmonary embolism (most important risk factor)
- Pregnancy (fivefold increase)
- Age > 40 years
- Surgery in the pelvis or lower extremities
- Prolonged immobility
- Congestive heart failure
- Obesity
- Malignancy
- Oral contraceptives (reduce antithrombin III levels)
- Venous valvular reflux and varicose veins
- Hypercoagulable states

3. Where do most DVTs originate?
The calf veins.

4. What is the natural history of calf vein thromboses?
Seventy-eight percent spontaneously lyse with little or no sequelae; 22% propagate into the popliteal and femoral veins, where they have a greater potential for embolization and chronic venous stasis.

5. What is the frequency of DVT after surgery?
- Major abdominal surgery: 30–40%
- Prostatectomy: 38%
- Elective orthopedic operation: 52%
- Emergency orthopedic operation: 70%
- Peripheral vascular procedure: 7%
- Cardiothoracic operation: 3%
- Medical intensive care (nonsurgical): 70%

6. What is the incidence of DVT after total hip arthroplasty and total knee arthroplasty in patients unprotected by anticoagulation therapy?

The incidence of DVT after total hip replacement is 40–70%. Thromboembolic disease is the most common serious complication after total hip arthroplasty. It is the most common cause of death within 3 months after surgery and accounts for > 50% of the postoperative mortality after total hip arthroplasty.

The incidence of DVT after total knee arthroplasty was originally thought to be 1–10% on the basis of clinical diagnosis. Studies using radioactive fibrinogen, however, have reported DVT at rates of 50–70%, indicating that DVT is more common than clinical diagnosis suggests and that prophylactic treatment is warranted.

7. When do most postoperative DVTs occur?

Fifty percent occur within the first 24 hours; 85% occur within the first 4 days.

8. What are the signs and symptoms of DVT?

The clinical findings of DVT can vary from obvious to elusive. The classic signs and symptoms are unilateral pain and swelling (pain is due to venous engorgement and inflammation associated with the thrombus; swelling is caused by venous outflow obstruction). Other signs and symptoms may include warmth, erythema, engorged superficial veins, and low-grade fever.

9. What is Homan's sign?

Homan's sign is a clinical test for evaluation of DVT. With a positive Homan's sign, calf pain is produced with dorsiflexion of the ankle. The absence of Homan's sign does **not** rule out DVT, and a positive sign is not diagnostic of DVT.

10. Describe the clinical picture of phlegmasia alba dolens (milk leg).

Phlegmasia alba dolens is characterized by a swollen, white painful leg secondary to extensive acute DVT of the iliac and femoral veins. Initially it was described in the 18th century in postpartum patients. Physicians attributed the condition to suppression of lactation and accumulation of milk in the blood vessels of the leg, hence the term *milk leg*.

11. Describe the more serious condition phlegmasia cerulea dolens.

This condition presents with a swollen, blue painful leg secondary to extensive acute DVT of the iliac and femoral veins. The popliteal, tibial, and superficial veins may be thrombosed as well. This serious condition has a high risk of limb loss and death. Extensive venous outflow obstruction interferes with arterial inflow and results in leg ischemia.

12. How is DVT diagnosed?

Diagnosis of DVT begins with a high **clinical suspicion**. The greater the number of risk factors, the higher the suspicion for DVT. Because the diagnosis of DVT cannot reliably be made on physical examination, diagnostic study is required.

Radioactive-labeled fibrinogen, Doppler ultrasound, and impedance plethysmography are not currently routinely available for diagnosis of DVT, but they may be used in select circumstances. The two studies currently used to diagnose DVT are contrast venography and venous duplex scan.

Contrast venography remains the gold standard for diagnosis of DVT; however, it has largely been replaced by the venous duplex scan. The venogram is useful when duplex scanning capability is not available or when the duplex scan is not diagnostic or is equivocal. Venography is invasive, uncomfortable for the patient, expensive, potentially may induce adverse reaction to contrast material, and has a small risk of initiating venous thrombosis.

Venous duplex scans have replaced contrast venography because they are noninvasive, cause little or no patient discomfort, and are low-risk and less expensive than venography. The reliability of the duplex scan is dependent on a number of factors, including the quality of the equipment used, the experience, skill, and training of the technologist performing the study, as well as the skill of the physician interpreting the study. When properly performed, the duplex scan can accurately diagnose DVT in the femoral, popliteal, and tibial veins. Due to technical difficulties, accurate diagnosis of iliac vein thrombosis is limited.

13. What is the most serious complication of DVT?

Pulmonary embolism is the most serious complication. The annual incidence of fatal and nonfatal pulmonary embolism is >500,000. Approximately 95% of pulmonary emboli arise from the lower extremity. The risk of embolism is higher with thrombi located above the knee versus below the knee.

14. What are the long-term complications of DVT?

The most common long-term complication of DVT is chronic venous insufficiency. Patients with chronic lower extremity edema eventually develop stasis pigmentation, stasis dermatitis, and stasis ulceration after 10–20 years.

15. What prophylactic measures are recommended to prevent DVT?

- Early ambulation
- Extremity elevation
- Range-of-motion exercises (calf muscles act as a pump to empty he calf veins)
- Graduated elastic stockings (only decrease DVT by 5–10%)
- Intermittent pneumatic compression stockings (highly effective after knee surgery but less effective after hip surgery)
- Anticoagulation

16. Outline the medical treatment for DVT.

1. Obtain baseline coagulation studies
2. Bed rest and lower extremity elevation to reduce swelling and discomfort
3. Begin heparinization:
- Average-sized adult: bolus of 5,000–10,000 U followed by IV infusion at 1,000 U/hr **or** loading dose of 100–150 U/kg IV with a maintenance dose of 10–15 U/kg/hr.
- Check activated partial thromboplastin time (aPTT) every 6 hours initially and adjust heparin infusion to maintain aPTT at 1.5–2.5 times normal.
- Administer until therapeutic level of warfarin achieved.
4. Administer warfarin (Coumadin):
- Daily prothrombin time (PT) and daily maintenance dose of 2.5–10 mg to achieve PT 1.5–2.0 times normal or internationally normalized ratio (INR) of 2–3.
- Continue Coumadin for 3–6 months.
5. Monitor for bleeding complications

17. Which patients require DVT prophylaxis?

The greater the number of risk factors that a patient has, the more they benefit from DVT prophylaxis. Patients < 40 years of age undergoing uncomplicated abdominal or thoracic operations do *not* require DVT prophylaxis.

18. What methods are available for DVT prophylaxis?

Mechanical

- Graduated compression stockings worn before and after surgery. Knee-high stockings are as effective as the thigh-high variety; each decreases the risk of DVT by only 5–10%.
- Intermittent pneumatic compression devices are as effective as low-dose heparin; they are highly effective after knee surgery but less effective after hip surgery.

Anticoagulants

- Low-dose heparin (2 hr SQ before surgery and 8–12 hr after surgery) decreases the risk of DVT by 15–20% with no increased risk of major bleeding episodes, but the risk of wound hematomas increases. Anticoagulants work well for general surgery patients but lower the risk of DVT by only 15% in orthopedic patients.
- Low–molecular-weight heparin has a different mechanism of action than regular heparin, equivalent antithrombotic effect, and less bleeding potential. It is superior to low-dose heparin for orthopedic patients.
- Warfarin (low fixed dose 2 mg/day or adjust PT to achieve mildly prolonged PT) reduces the risk of DVT after elective hip procedures, but has a slow onset and a slow reversal.

BIBLIOGRAPHY

1. Canale ST (ed): Campbell's Operative Orthopedics, 9th ed. St. Louis, Mosby, 1998.
2. Ferree BA, Stern PJ, Jolson RS, et al: Deep venous thrombosis after spinal surgery. Spine 18:515–319, 1993.
3. Greenfield LJ: Venous and lymphatic disease. In Schwartz SI (ed): Principles of Surgery, 6th ed. New York, McGraw-Hill, 1994, pp 989–1003.
4. Kassir JP (ed): Current Therapy in Internal Medicine, 3rd ed. Philadelphia, B.C. Decker, 1991.
6. McNally MA, Kernohan WG, Croal SA, Mollan RAB: Deep venous thrombosis in orthopedic patients. Clin Orthop 295:275–280, 1993.
7. Raju S: Pathophysiology of venous thrombosis. In Ernst CB, Stanley JC (eds): Current Therapy in Vascular Surgery, 3rd ed. St. Louis, Mosby, 1995, pp 874–879.
8. Kumar V, Cotran RS, Robbins SL (eds): Basic Pathology, 6th ed. Philadelphia, W.B. Saunders, 1997.
8. Sumner DS: Diagnosis of deep venous thrombosis. In Rutherford RB (ed): Vascular Surgery, 4th ed. Philadelphia, W.B. Saunders, 1995, pp 1698–1743.
9. Swayze OS, Nasser S, Roberson JR: Deep venous thrombosis in total hip arthroplasty. Orthop Clin North Am 23:359–364, 1992.
10. Vitti MJ, Barnes RW: Nonoperative treatment of acute thrombophlebitis and femoral venous thrombosis. In Ernst CB, Stanley JC (eds): Current Therapy in Vascular Surgery, 3rd ed. St. Louis, Mosby, 1995, pp 888–893.
11. Wilde AH, Colwell CW, Paiement G, et al: Symposium: Advances in the prevention of venous thromboembolic disease in orthopedics: The introduction of LWMH. Contemp Orthop 27:551–577, 1993.

9. PULMONARY PROBLEMS

Matthew T. McLeay, M.D.

1. What are the most common pulmonary problems in orthopedic medicine?

- Atelectasis
- Postoperative pneumonia
- Pulmonary thromboembolism
- Acute respiratory distress syndrome (ARDS)
- Fat emboli

2. What are the postoperative risk factors for atelectasis?
- Upper abdominal surgery
- Thoracotomy
- Smoking
- Chronic obstructive pulmonary disease (COPD)
- Restrictive pulmonary disease
- Obesity
- Age greater than 70-years
- Post operative immobility

Atelectasis is the most common postoperative pulmonary complication and generally resolves spontaneously within 24–48 hours.

3. What methods may be used to improve postoperative pulmonary function?

Deep breathing, incentive spirometer, intermittent positive pressure breathing and continuous positive airway pressure (CPAP). Currently nebulizers with an attached positive expiratory pressure valve are used and are significantly more convenient than nasal or face mask technique for CPAP. Microatelectasis is currently felt to be a likely explanation for postoperative hypoxemia. For all causes of atelectasis, bronchoscopy is rarely required.

4. What perioperative management strategies can be used to reduce the likelihood of pulmonary complications?

Smoking cessation for at least 8 weeks before surgery, management of chronic obstructive pulmonary disease or asthma (with corticosteroids, bronchodilators and antibiotics) and optimizing other comorbidities (e.g., cardiac disease).

5. What is the mortality rate of postoperative pneumonia?

The mortality rate approaches 50% and is caused by either gross or microscopic aspiration of gastric contents. Manual pressure of the cricoid cartilage during intubation, avoidance of oral intake 8–12 hours before the operation, and use of H_2 blockers (which increase gastric pH and decrease volume) may reduce the risk.

6. What are the most common organisms seen in postoperative pneumonia?

Gram-negative rods, specifically *Pseudomonas,* and *Klebsiella* spp. and *Escherichia coli.* The most prevalent gram-positive organism is *Staphylococcus aureus.* A prolonged preoperative stay probably increases risk for Gram negative bacilli.

7. What risk factors increase the risk of deep venous thrombosis (DVT) and pulmonary emboli (PE)?
- Venous stasis (i.e. immobility, bed rest, obesity, cerebrovascular accident)
- Hyperviscosity (polycythemia, low cardiac output states, pregnancy)
- Injury to the vessel wall (orthopedic surgery, trauma)
- Hypercoaguabilty (medications, such as oral contraceptives), disease (malignancy or inherited)

8. What is the risk of DVT and pulmonary thromboembolism in patient undergoing hip surgery?

The incidence of proximal DVT is 15–35%; of pulmonary thromboembolism, 4.5%–25%; and of fatal thromboembolism, 3.5–15% in *untreated* patients undergoing hip fracture surgery. Surgical deaths from pulmonary thromboembolism have shown that 50% of patients had not received any form of preventative therapy.

9. What are the signs and symptoms of pulmonary thromboembolism?

The clinical presentation may be variable, but most often patients have dyspnea, pleuritic chest pain, hypoxemia, and tachypnea.

10. How are DVT and pulmonary thromboembolism diagnosed?

Because 70% of patients with pulmonary thromboembolism have DVT, duplex ultrasonography is often performed to detect proximal DVT. Contrast venography or magnetic resonance imaging (MRI) can also be utilized.

Currently spiral computed tomography (CT) angiography is a common method used for diagnosis of pulmonary thromboembolism. It has a reported sensitivity of approximately 60% and specificity of 81–97%. CT scan of the chest has the advantage of making other pulmonary diagnoses and, therefore, is preferable to VQ scan. MRI of the chest may be used for diagnosis of pulmonary thromboembolism, although it is used less commonly than CT scan.

Plasma levels of D-dimer are frequently ordered to determine the likelihood of pulmonary embolism. The absence of D-dimer is valuable and provides strong evidence against venous thromboembolism. However, D-dimer is elevated in most hospitalized patients, especially those with malignancy or following surgery.

11. What is the treatment for pulmonary thromboembolism?

Anticoagulation with heparin retards additional thrombus formation, allowing endogenous fibrinolytic mechanisms to act on the existing clot. Heparin followed by warfarin results in a greater than 90% reduction in the risk of both recurrent venous thrombosis and death from pulmonary embolism.

Low-molecular-weight heparins are currently under evaluation for treatment of both DVT and PE. They have a predictable and longer plasma half-life and possibly a lower risk of hemorrhage and thrombocytopenia. No monitoring is required because the dosing is based on body weight.

Thrombolytic therapy, such as tissue plasminogen activator, may be used for patients who are hemodynamically unstable despite Heparin therapy. Insertion of vena cava filters may be indicated with patients who a have contraindication to anticoagulation or who have had recurrent embolism despite anticoagulation.

12. Define ARDS.

The American Thoracic Society defines ARDS as a clinical syndrome in a patient with acute respiratory failure with bilateral infiltrates on chest radiograph, a PaO_2/FiO_2 ratio below 300, and no evidence of volume overload for left-sided heart failure. A pulmonary wedge pressure less than 18 is generally used. The recently introduced brain-type naturetic protein (BNP) lab test may be considered to assess volume status in lieu of a pulmonary artery catheter. A normal value suggests the absence of left ventricular failure or volume overload.

13. What is the mortality rate of ARDS?

Mortality rates with ARDS currently range from 35% to 40% but may be as high as 90% when accompanied by sepsis. A significant reduction in ARDS has resulted from changes in mechanical ventilation, with the use of low tidal volumes that are believed to reduce lung injury significantly. No pharmacologic agent has been found to markedly reduce mortality rates. Corticosteroids probably have a benefit later in the treatment of ARDS.

14. What are fat emboli?

Fat emboli characterize a syndrome due to entry of neutral fat into the vascular system. This syndrome usually develops 24–48 hours after the inciting event, which generally is traumatic fracture of the long bones, and is associated with the number of fractures present. Orthopedic procedures as well as trauma to fat tissue, such as a fatty liver, also produce this syndrome.

15. What are the most common signs and symptoms of fat emboli?

Mental status changes along with high fever, marked dyspnea, and petechial rash over the thorax and upper extremities. The lungs have fine crackles and x-ray shows a diffuse alveolar filling pattern throughout both lung fields. Anemia, thrombocytopenia, hypoxemia and hypocapnia are often present.

Current therapy is supportive. Prophylactic corticosteroids have been found to reduce the incidence of fat emboli syndrome, although their role remains controversial.

BIBLIOGRAPHY

1. Claget GP, et al: Prevention of venous thromboembolism. Chest 114 (Suppl):531S, 1998.
2. Coosling H, Pelligrini V: Fat embolism syndrome. Clin Orthop 165:68–92, 1982.
3. Dalen JE, Alpert JS, Hirsch J: Thrombolytic therapy for pulmonary embolism. Arch Intern Med 157:2550, 1997.
4. George RB, Light RW, Matthay MA, Matthay RA: Chest Medicine, 3rd ed. Baltimore, Williams & Wilkins, 1995.
5. Ginsberg JS, et al Sensitivity and specifity of rapid whole blood assay for D-dimer and the diagnosis of pulmonary embolism. Ann Intern Med 129:1006, 1998.
6. Kallenbach J, et al: Trauma 27:1173–1176, 1987.
7. Marini JJ, Pierson DJ, Hudson LD: Am Rev Respir Dis 119:971–978, 1979.
8. Martin, LF, et al: Arch Surg 119:379–383, 1984.
9. Ricksten SE, Bengtsson A, Soderberg C, et al: Chest 89:774–781, 1986.
10. Tierney L: Current Medical Diagnosis and Treatment, 40th ed. New York, Flang Medical Book/McGraw Hill, 2001.
11. Valenti WM, et al: N Engl J Med 298:1108–1111, 1978.

10. SURGICAL NUTRITION

Scott G. Rose, M.D.

1. How is a patient evaluated for nutritional intervention?

Evaluation for nutritional intervention depends on a combination of factors derived from the physical examination, prehospital nutritional deficiencies, expected clinical course, anthropometric measurements, and biochemical tests. The subjective global assessment (SGA) is made at the bedside without the input of sophisticated metabolic, biochemical, or anthropometric measurements. It is based on clinical appearance, history of weight loss preceding the illness, extent of metabolic demands during the illness, and the patient's ability to maintain an adequate oral intake during the hospitalization. Some authors suggest that the SGA alone can adequately identify 60–80% of patients in need of nutritional intervention. The SGA should be undertaken during the admission of any patient to the hospital, and plans for further nutritional testing or nutritional intervention should be entertained early in the hospitalization. Other studies show that if the physician waits until a severe complication develops to begin nutritional support, morbidity and mortality are markedly increased. Early intervention in appropriate patients has been shown to decrease morbidity and mortality. The restoration of normal metabolic activities, the development of an anabolic state, and the return to a normal immune functioning system have been found to be beneficial in patients with nutritional deficiencies.

2. What are the components of a nutritional assessment?

Components of an adequate nutritional assessment generally include a detailed history of a patient's weight changes before hospitalization. The clinical course and expected surgical intervention also are noted. The patient's current weight is evaluated and compared with expected ideal body weight. Although no specific weight loss in an adult is considered critical, the amount of weight lost over a certain period is an important factor in deciding on early intervention. Anthropometric measurements, based on standards recommended by the World Health Organization, include measurement of triceps skinfold and mid-arm circumference. Additional laboratory tests often included are albumin, prealbumin, transferrin, and retinol-binding protein. A decreased lymphocyte count has been found to be an early marker of a catabolic state.

Immune skin testing has been recommended for evaluation of reactivity to delayed cutaneous antigens, but in a study of over 3,000 patients at Methodist Hospital, Omaha, Nebraska, it was not found to be a critical determinant. The tests are so sensitive that >90% of the studied population showed evidence of anergy or relative anergy. Because negative results were so common in the identified population, the test is no longer recommended routinely.

Determination of urine urea nitrogen (UUN) to measure excretion of nitrogen in urine is also recommended. Although the test does not reflect all nitrogen degradation that is excreted, it tends to reflect accurately total urinary nitrogen. Increased losses of UUN are seen in a hypermetabolic state and in patients with closed head injuries and spinal injuries. Sometimes the dramatic increase in UUN in this setting is the normal result of denervation of muscle mass and should not be used as a target for delivery of protein. In most circumstances, however, nitrogen delivery to the patient should be equal to or in excess of nitrogen lost through the urine. Each day the average adult patient loses an additional 4 gm of nitrogen that is not measured in the UUN. This additional loss should be calculated in nitrogen balance studies. In patients on aggressive nutritional support, this author recommends weekly determinations of UUN to adjust nutritional support.

3. What is indirect calorimetry?

Indirect calorimetry is a measurement of caloric demands over time. It is done through the hospital's pulmonary laboratory. The patient's oxygen consumption and production of carbon dioxide (CO_2) are measured over a period through a closed system. When these data are fed into a computer, caloric demand over a 24-hour period can be accurately estimated. Substrate utilization also can be detailed from the same data. A respiratory quotient (RQ) is useful in adjusting total calories during nutritional support. An RQ >1.0 indicates overfeeding of the patient, which not only has metabolic consequences but also is expensive. The author recommends an RQ between 0.7 and 0.9 to keep the patient in a positive caloric balance. The RQ is evaluated each week, along with the UUN, for better adjustment of nutritional balance support products. The RQ is a ration of CO_2 production divided by oxygen consumption and does not take into account activity during the day. Most hospitalized patients, however, are physically inactive and do not require increased nutritional requirements. It was originally thought that caloric demand would exceed 3,500 cal/day in a severely traumatized patient. Experience with RQs, however, has shown that the demand rarely exceeds 1,500–2,000 cal/day. As a standard guideline, the delivery of 2,000–2,500 cal/day parenterally, enterally, or orally is usually sufficient for the hospitalized patient, even in the setting of trauma. This author currently uses a peripheral parenteral solution delivering 1,520 kcal/day for the majority of surgical/trauma patients.

4. Which fuels are used as preferred fuel sources during increased metabolic demands?

The three fuels commonly available for utilization under any circumstances include glucose, fat, and protein. During periods of starvation glucose and glycogen stores are initially the preferred fuel. Because both are generally exhausted in the first day or two, ketosis becomes a prominent fuel source. Ketones are broken down into free fatty acids and glycerol, which are then metabolized as the preferred fuel source in the absence of glucose. Ketosis is followed by a slow but chronic breakdown of visceral and somatic protein stores. Nutritional intervention should help to reduce the amount of ketosis, to eliminate protein degradation, and to supply adequate glucose and fat calories for daily metabolic activity.

5. What routes are available for administration of calories?

In evaluation of a patient, all routes of administration of calories should be considered, including oral delivery and consumption of adequate calories. Sometimes the addition of between-meal snacks and nutritional supplements is sufficient to meet caloric requirements. If oral feedings are not adequate, enteral feedings can be administered through a nasogastric tube, nasoduodenal tube, percutaneous endoscopic gastrostomy tube, laparoscopically placed gastrostomy tube, or surgically placed jejunostomy tube. In general, routes of administration that deliver nutrients directly into the stomach can deliver larger quantities in a bolus fashion. Nutrients delivered directly into the small intestine need to be administered by continuous infusion, because no reservoir function is present. If the GI tract must be bypassed, intravenous options include peripheral total parenteral nutrition and central total parenteral nutrition. Both can deliver adequate parenteral products.

6. When should nutritional support be considered in a patient who is not allowed or not able to eat?

In a healthy adult under maximal stress, parenteral or enteral support can be safely initiated 3–5 days after admission without causing undue risk. Patients with multiple trauma often have a hyperglycemic/hypermetabolic response immediately after injury. Early intervention during a period of rapid volume resuscitation is not indicated. In general, once fluid requirements have stabilized, parenteral or enteral support may be initiated. Some evidence, however, suggests that early enteral nutritional support in burn patients not only decreases morbidity and mortality during hospitalization but also attenuates the acute metabolic response to the burn. The patient should be evaluated for the need for invasive enteral or parenteral nutrition on a daily basis during rounds.

7. What is the most common metabolic abnormality associated with central total parenteral nutrition?

Hyperglycemia remains the main metabolic problem associated with total parenteral nutrition. Most formulas deliver a solution with a 25% concentration of dextrose (comparable to a blood sugar of 25,000 mg/dl). Thus glucose intolerance may develop in some individuals. Close monitoring of serum glucose during the initiation of parenteral nutrition is essential for a successful outcome. Glucosuria and hyperglycemia should be treated by decreasing the glucose concentration of the delivered fluid or by adding insulin to combat the exogenous hyperglycemia. Insulin may be delivered subcutaneously or intravenously by a pump or mixed directly with the parenteral nutritional solution. Blood sugar should generally be < 200 mg/dl. If severe glucose intolerance develops and the glucose content is reduced, the lipid protein portion of nonnitrogen calories may be increased. In a patient who develops hyperglycemia but otherwise has been stable on glucose infusion, evaluation for subclinical sepsis should be considered. Often sepsis is first recognized by newly developed glucose intolerance. If hyperglycemia is not treated, hyperosmolarity may result, leading to dehydration, coma, and death.

8. Describe the appropriate enteral formula.

Although enteral products are currently under intensive investigation, presently they are evaluated in two major categories:

Elemental diets include basic nutrients-amino acids, carbohydrates, and fats-delivered in forms that require little sophisticated change during digestion. Elemental diets are generally recommended for patients who have a short amount of GI tract available for absorption, who have poorly functioning GI mucosa, or who are intolerant of other formulas. These are the most expensive diets.

Non-elemental diets include combinations of proteins, polypeptides, and dipeptides, along with more complex fats and carbohydrates. Most use complete formulas that include the micronutrients, vitamins, minerals, and free water required for normal metabolic activities.

Selection of an enteral formula may be a hit-or-miss proposition. Some patients may tolerate one formula but not another for no identifiable reason. Intolerance of all enteral formulas may be due to poor gastric emptying, which often results from injury, ileus, or drugs. Malabsorption may be secondary to atrophic jejunal villi with inability to digest nutrients appropriately. Intolerance due to diarrhea may be secondary to bacterial overgrowth from use of broad-spectrum antibiotics or histamine blockers that alkalinize the gastric contents. Such problems may require adjustment in the enteral formula.

9. **What is the appropriate ratio of nonnitrogen calories for each gram of nitrogen delivered in parenteral and enteral formulas?**

Most parenteral formulas have a ratio of 150–300 nonnitrogen cal/gm of nitrogen, usually in the form of carbohydrates and lipids. Under normal metabolic activities, this ratio supplies enough nonnitrogen so that nitrogen products can be used for metabolic activities. Because the early posttraumatic period is associated with glucose intolerance, formulas with a ratio of <100 nonnitrogen cal/gm of nitrogen may be appropriate. A similar ratio for enteral formulas has been recommended. If the caloric density of enteral formulas is increased, the solution often becomes hyperosmotic and intolerance develops. In general, enteral formulas with > 1 cal/ml carry a higher risk of intolerance. Most parenteral formulas at full strength deliver 1 cal/ml.

10. **What causes metabolic bone disease associated with total parenteral nutrition? How is it treated?**

Metabolic bone disease is a poorly understood complication of long-term home parenteral nutrition. It is clinically manifested by development of compression fractures, usually of the thoracic and lumbar spine, at some point after the first year of home parenteral therapy. Many theories have been suggested to explain this process, but none has proved consistently true. At one point, aluminum toxicity was implicated because of aluminum salts. After elimination of such salts, however, the incidence does not appear to change. Perhaps a micro- or macronutrient excess or deficiency develops as a result of long-term parenteral nutrition. Levels of trace elements, including copper, zinc, chromium, magnesium, manganese, calcium, and selenium, should be monitored in all patients on long-term home parenteral nutrition. Correcting metabolic serum deficiencies is the only known treatment other than supportive care. Over time metabolic bone disease seems to become less active, and patients complain less of new fractures as the years pass.

11. **What specialty was instrumental in the development of parenteral nutrition?**

Laboratory experiments and the clinical use of parenteral nutrition were begun in the late 1960s by a group of general surgeons at the University of Pennsylvania. Their initial experiments were in beagle puppies. They found that puppies from the same litter could grow and develop at a normal rate whether they received parenteral nutrition or standard puppy formula. The first human patient to be maintained successfully on the new parenteral nutrition formula was a newborn infant.

12. **What are the potential pulmonary complications of hypermetabolic state?**

The end-products of metabolism of carbohydrates are CO_2 and water. The patient who receives excessive glucose may develop an excess of CO_2 that needs to be eliminated through the pulmonary system. Patients with severe pulmonary problems may not be able to excrete the CO_2 and thus may become hyperbaric due to its retention. Because of this potential problem, it is best to decrease the glucose concentration for patients with severe respiratory compromise.

BIBLIOGRAPHY

1. August D, Teitelbaum D, Albina J, et al: J Parent Ent Nutr 26(Suppl), 2002.
2. Fischer JE (ed): Nutrition and Metabolism in the Surgical Patient, 2nd. ed. Philadelphia, Lippincott-Raven, 1996.
3. Silk DBA: Nutritional Support in Hospital Practice. Oxford, Blackwell, 1983.
4. Wright R, Heymsfield S (eds): Nutritional Assessment. Boston, Blackwell, 1984.

11. DIAGNOSTIC RADIOLOGY

Richard A. Kutilek, M.D.

1. What are the usual radiographic views for evaluating shoulder problems?

The anteroposterior view is the most common; it may be taken in a neutral position or in internal and external rotation. A transthoracic lateral view or axillary view assesses positioning of the humeral head in the glenoid.

2. Which is more common—anterior or posterior dislocations of the shoulder?

Anterior dislocations are much more common, occurring in approximately 95% of cases, whereas posterior dislocations occur in 5%. Posterior dislocations can look normal on anteroposterior radiographs. The only clue is that the humerus is usually locked in internal rotation.

3. What radiographic examination best differentiates anterior and posterior dislocations?

Anterior and posterior dislocations are best differentiated by an axillary view of the shoulder (see figure). The x-ray beam is directed from an inferior position through the axilla to a superior plate.

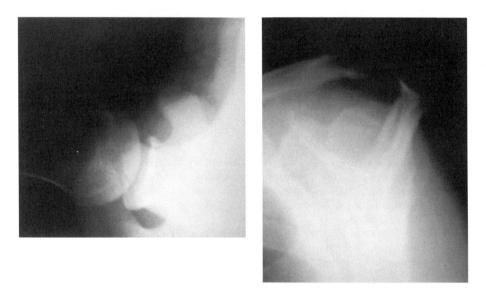

Axillary view of the shoulder. *Left,* This view demonstrates any anteroposterior dislocation. In this radiograph, the humeral head is normally seeded in the glenoid. A small avulsion fracture of the glenohumeral ligament is identified at the superior aspect of the glenoid. *Right,* Supraspinatus outlet view demonstrates the morphology of the acromion.

4. What is a Hill-Sachs lesion?

A Hill-Sachs lesion is a defect of the posterolateral aspect of the humeral head. It occurs with anterior dislocation of the shoulder when the posterior superior surface of the humeral head impinges on the anteroinferior portion of the glenoid. The Hill-Sachs deformity is easily visualized by anteroposterior view of the shoulder with the arm in full internal rotation.

5. What is a Bankart lesion?

A Bankart lesion is an avulsion of the anterior capsular structures with a fragment of bone. This lesion is the hallmark of radiographic findings for recurrent dislocations of the shoulder. It is best seen on an axillary view of the shoulder.

6. What is the radiographic appearance of an acromioclavicular dislocation?

An acromioclavicular dislocation is a disruption of the coracoclavicular and acromioclavicular ligaments. The space between the clavicle and the coracoid is widened. Dissociation of the acromioclavicular joint is complete, and the clavicle is displaced superiorly in comparison with the acromion. The best view to visualize an acromioclavicular dislocation is attained with the patient holding 10–15 pounds of weight in each arm. Anteroposterior radiographs are then taken simultaneously of the affected and nonaffected acromioclavicular joint.

7. What radiographic view is used to evaluate impingement syndrome?

The supraspinatus outlet view is used to evaluate impingement syndrome. In this view the patient is positioned for the scapular lateral radiograph, and the tube is angled inferiorly at approximately 10°. This view shows the morphology of the acromion for the treatment of impingement syndrome.

8. What are the most common views for evaluating elbow symptoms?

Anteroposterior and lateral radiographs are most commonly used. Fractures are common around the radial head with trauma. Loose bodies may be identified in the olecranon fossa or anteriorly in the anterior joint. Osteochondritis dissecans may be seen as irregularities along the capitellum.

9. Is it normal to visualize the anterior fat pad on lateral radiographs of the flexed elbow?

The normal anterior fat pad appears as a lucid stripe paralleling the anterior margin of the supracondylar region. If the anterior fat pad has assumed a "sail-shaped" configuration, the elbow capsule is distended. This finding signifies recent trauma, most likely a hemarthrosis.

10. Is it normal to visualize a posterior fat pad on lateral radiographs of a flexed elbow?

The posterior fat pad is not visible on routine lateral views of the flexed elbow. Visualization of the posterior fat pad indicates capsular distension, most likely due to hemarthrosis and often caused by a nondisplaced radial head fracture.

11. What radiographic examination is invaluable for evaluating patients with rheumatologic diseases?

An anteroposterior radiograph of the hand shows many joints of the wrist and phalanges. Rheumatoid arthritis has a predilection for an entire wrist and metacarpophalangeal joint. Osteoarthritis generally affects the interphalangeal joints and the first carpometacarpal joint. Erosive osteoarthritis is characterized by interphalangeal joint destruction with subluxation and severe erosions. Radiographs of patients with calcium pyrophosphate dihydrate deposition disease (CPDD) may show small subchondral cysts and interarticular soft-tissue calcification, most notably over the radial styloid and triangular fibrocartilage. Erosions in gout may show a characteristic overhanging margin.

12. What radiographic studies should be taken for evaluation of hip disease?

An anteroposterior view of the pelvis, not just the affected hip, should be taken. This view gives clues to the diagnosis of other disease processes by visualizing the pelvic bones, lower portion of the spine, sacroiliac joint, and pubic symphysis. Joint changes may give clues to diagnoses such as ankylosing spondylitis and rheumatoid arthritis. Bone destruction commonly occurs in the pelvis of patients with metastatic disease or multiple myeloma. Fractures generally occur in the ring of the pelvis and can be seen in the contralateral iliac crest and pubic and ischial rami.

13. What are the standard radiographs for evaluation of knee pathology?

The standard radiographs are anteroposterior and lateral views of the knee, which show the metaphyseal bone of the femur and fibula joint surfaces and the surrounding soft tissue. A **tunnel view** shows the intercondylar notch and may visualize loose bodies not seen on the anteroposterior radiographs (see figure). It is also the best view to see osteochondritis dissecans of the medial or lateral femoral condyles. A sunrise Hughston view shows subluxation or dislocations of the patella from the trochlear groove.

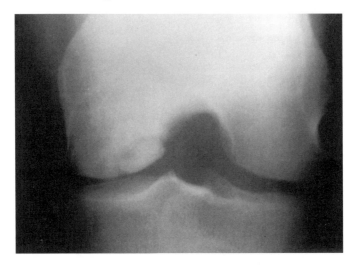

Tunnel view. The tunnel view radially shows osteochondritis dissecans on the medial femoral condyle.

14. What is a Segond fracture?

A Segond fracture is an avulsion fracture of the capsular ligament on the lateral side of the tibia, best seen on the anteroposterior view of the knee (see figure). It is highly suggestive of an anterior cruciate ligament tear because the two are commonly associated.

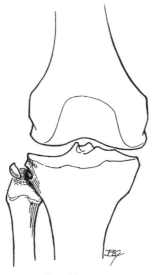

Segond fracture.

15. Which radiographs are used in evaluation of the ankle injuries?

Anteroposterior and lateral radiographs are used in conjunction with a mortise view, an oblique view with approximately 20–30° of internal rotation that attempts to show the ankle mortise. The medial and lateral malleolus are on the same plane in the mortise view, which can be used to evaluate the congruity of the talus as it sits adjacent to the medial and lateral malleolus and the tibial plafond.

16. What talar abnormalities are seen on ankle radiographs?

Fractures of the talar neck or talar dome may be seen on ankle radiographs (see figure). Dome fractures are usually related to inversion or eversion injuries and occur on the superolateral or superomedial portion of the talar dome. The radiographic appearance suggests a small, separated fracture. Dome fractures are sometimes best visualized on an anteroposterior film in full plantar flexion.

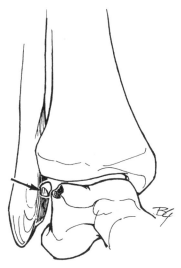

Talar dome fracture (arrow)

17. Describe the radiographic features of an *inversion* injury of the ankle.

With inversion injuries of the foot and ankle, avulsive forces affect the lateral structures and compressive forces affect the medial structures (see figure). Lateral injuries may consist of a sprain or avulsion of the lateral ligamentous complex, neither of which is apparent on radiographs. If, however, a fracture is involved, it is usually a transverse fracture in which the ligaments have been avulsed with bone. Fractures appear on the anteroposterior and oblique views. Medial injuries with inversion sprains may show an oblique fracture of the medial malleolus. In general, oblique fractures are usually due to compressive forces and transverse fractures to avulsion forces.

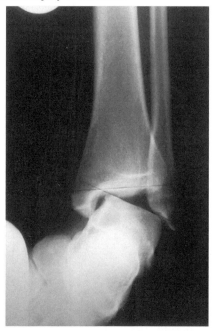

Stress view of the ankle. Stress views of the ankle show the opening on the lateral side of the joint from an inversion stress injury.

18. Describe the radiographic appearance of an *eversion* injury of the ankle.

With eversion injuries of the foot, avulsive forces act on the medial structures and compressive forces on the lateral. Depending on the rotation involved, a sprain or avulsion of the medial deltoid ligament may occur; neither is apparent on radiographs. However, if a fracture is involved, it is usually a transverse fracture of the medial malleolus below the ankle mortise. Lateral injuries consist of an oblique or spiral fracture of the lateral malleolus with rupture of the syndesmosis. The tibiofibular ligament may rupture with or without a fracture of the fibula.

19. What is a Jones fracture?

A Jones fracture is a transverse fracture of the proximal fifth metatarsal shaft (see figure). The fracture is located approximately 1.5–2 cm distal to the tip of the metatarsal and usually is a stress fracture. It is differentiated from a styloid fracture, which occurs in the metaphysis, on an oblique view of the foot (see figures). The normal apophysis may not be entirely fused in children and may give the appearance of a fracture.

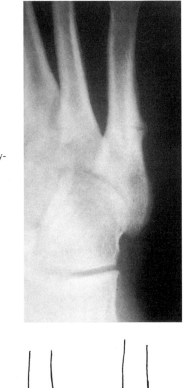

Jones fracture. This typical stress fracture occurs in the diaphyseal portion of the fifth metatarsal.

Fifth metatarsal fractures.

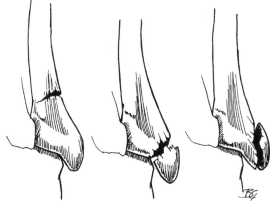

Jones fracture   Styloid fracture   Normal apophysis

20. What types of stress fractures are seen?
Stress fractures generally can be divided into two categories: fatigue fractures and insufficiency fractures. Fatigue fractures are due to repetitive prolonged stress on normal bone. Insufficiency fractures result from normal stresses on abnormal bone, such as that in osteomalacia or osteoporosis.

21. Name the common sites for fatigue fractures.

Tibial shaft	Metatarsals	Patella
Midfibula	Calcaneus	Pars interarticularis
Pubic ramus		

22. Name the major predisposing conditions for insufficiency fractures.

Osteomalacia	Radiation	Osteoporosis
Paget's disease	Fibrous dysplasia	Hyperparathyroidism

23. What is the radiographic appearance of a stress fracture?
Stress fractures generally are seen as transverse fractures in the shaft of the bone. Stress fractures of the metatarsals (see figure) may be seen as a slight, thin, radiolucent line, whereas in larger bones, such as the tibia or the femur, they are better visualized. Some fractures show no lines, but only signs of healing, such as new bone formation. Often callus formation is abundant in metatarsal fractures but minimal in fractures of the tibia and femur.

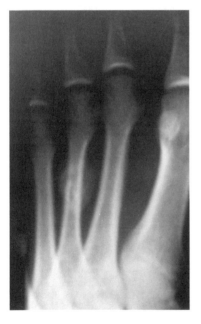

Stress fracture of the third metatarsal. This anteroposterior radiograph of the foot shows the third metatarsal stress fracture. Note the transverse radiolucent line with the formation of new cortical bone.

24. What is avascular necrosis?
Avascular necrosis, also known as osteonecrosis, is bone death caused by vascular insult. The vessels may be damaged directly by trauma or occluded by emboli or elevated marrow pressure. The most common sites include the hips, shoulders, medial femoral condyle, and talus (see figure).

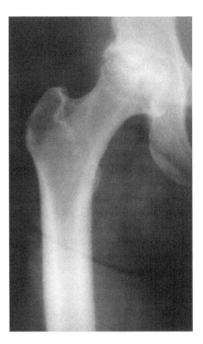

Avascular necrosis of the right hip. This anteroposterior radiograph shows loss of joint space and collapse and sclerosis of the superior segment of the femoral heal.

25. What are the common causes of avascular necrosis?

Steroids	Sickle-cell disease	Emboli
Alcohol abuse	Lupus erythematosus	Caisson disease
Congenital problems such as Gaucher's disease	Radiation therapy	Pancreatitis

26. Which radiographic features suggest a slow-growing or benign process?

See figure:

- Preservation of cortical margin
- Well-demarcated boundary of the lesion
- Sclerotic margin
- Solid, uninterrupted periosteal reaction
- Little or no soft-tissue mass, except in acute osteomyelitis

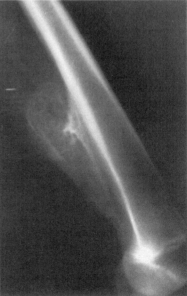

Osteochondroma of femur. Osteochondroma is a slow-growing, benign process. A good cortical margin is present. The boundary of the lesion is well defined. No host reaction is present.

27. What are the radiographic findings in patients with osteonecrosis?

In the early stages radiographs may be nondiagnostic; bone scans may be the only positive test. In the later stages, radiographic changes include (1) bone cysts with sclerotic changes in the bone; (2) subchondral collapse, with or without flattening of the articular surface; (3) narrowing of joint spaces; and (4) other degenerative signs. Degenerative changes may be minimal but generally progress to include joint space narrowing, osteophytes, subchondral cysts, and subchondral sclerosis.

28. List the common radiographic features of a malignant bone lesion.

- Cortical erosion and destruction
- Irregular periosteal reaction, including sunburst, onion peeling, and Codman's triangle
- Indistinct boundaries of the lesion, which seems to permeate into the adjacent soft tissue and bone
- Absence of sclerotic margin
- Associated soft-tissue mass

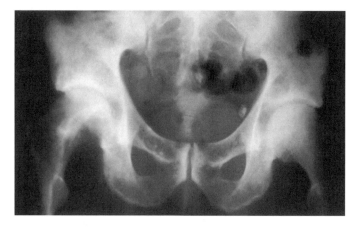

Renal cell carcinoma metastasis to the hip. Complete destruction of the inferior portion of the femoral head is seen on the hip. A stress fracture is noted in the superior cortex of the femoral neck. Note the indistinct margins, along with the moth-eaten appearance and significant destruction of bone.

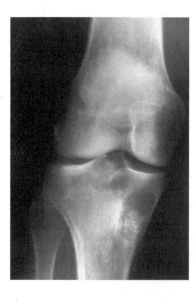

Giant cell tumor of bone. Malignant giant cell tumor of bone is characterized by bone destruction with breach of the medial cortex of the tibia and a soft-tissue mass.

29. What is Codman's triangle?

Codman's triangle is a radiographic pattern, usually in patients with infection or tumor. When infection or tumor elevates the periosteum of the bone, a gap occurs between the periosteum and bone (see figure). Where the gap is elevated, bone is formed, creating a triangular shape on radiographs. Codman's triangle, which denotes soft-tissue extension of the tumor or infectious process, was first described in 1914 by Rubbert. Although long considered to be a manifestation of malignancy, Codman's triangle may result from any disorder that lifts the periosteum, whether benign or malignant.

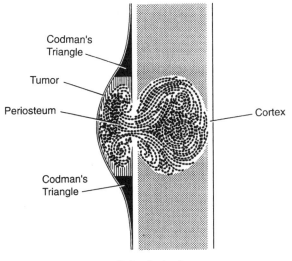

Codman's triangle.

30. What is a pathologic fracture?

A pathologic fracture occurs when the bone has been weakened by infection, neoplasm, or metabolic bone disease (see figure). Common causes include benign tumors, osteomyelitis, and tuberculosis.

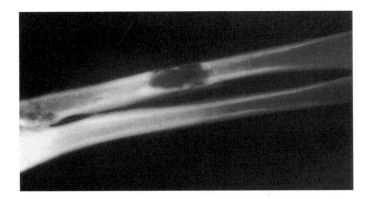

Pathologic fracture of bone. This pathologic fracture is due to multiple myeloma of the radius.

31. What are radiologic features of acute osteomyelitis?
The earliest sign may be blurring or obliteration of soft-tissue fat planes. Soft-tissue changes are followed by intramedullary destruction, usually in a permeative pattern. Subsequent findings are cortical destruction, endosteal scalloping, and periosteal reaction. Radiographic changes lag behind onset of infection by 10–14 days.

32. What is the study of choice in diagnosis of suspected acute osteomyelitis?
Initial radiographic findings may be nonspecific. A three-phase bone scan is useful in diagnosing early acute osteomyelitis. Increased activity on perfusion, blood pool, and delayed images in the areas of bony involvement are compatible with a diagnosis of osteomyelitis. MRI can also be helpful in diagnosing early osteomyelitis. MRI can show marrow edema and early cortical destruction as well as evaluate the soft tissues for abscess.

33. What is a Charcot joint?
Charcot joint, also called neuropathic joint, occurs in patients who have neurologic neuropathy secondary to diabetes mellitus, paraplegia, syphilis, leprosy, and various other peripheral neuropathies. Patients generally have lost sensations of pain and proprioception, but motion is maintained. Subtle fractures occur, along with significant degenerative changes. Radiographic features include joint destruction, significant amounts of bony debris from fractures and loose bodies, and disorganization of the joint with subluxation and dislocation.

34. What is the initial film to obtain in evaluating a patient for cervical spine trauma?
The first film to obtain is a cross-table lateral view. All seven cervical vertebrae and the upper thoracic vertebrae need to be visualized. The cervicothoracic junction is a common site of traumatic injury and potential instability.

35. If the cross-table lateral view is normal, is further imaging needed?
Yes. A standard cervical spine series includes a lateral, anteroposterior and odontoid views. A complete series also includes oblique views. Flexion and extension views can provide useful information regarding ligament injury.

36. Describe the Salter-Harris classification for epiphyseal plate injuries.

Type I   Epiphyseal plate separation—the fracture line is in the cartilage and is not visible radiographically.

Type II   A fragment from the metaphysis is associated with the epiphyseal plate fracture; this is the most common injury.

Type III The fracture runs through the epiphysis and growth plate.

Type IV   A vertically oriented fracture extends through the epiphysis and growth plate into the metaphysis; growth arrest and joint deformities are possible complications.

Type V   Crushing injury to the epiphyseal plate; a frequent complication is shortening or angulation of the bone due to premature closure of the epiphyseal plate.

37. What lines and angle are useful in the evaluation of the pediatric hip for developmental dysplasia?
- Hilgenreiner—line connecting the triradiate cartilages (see figure, *arrow 1*)
- Perkins—perpendicular to Hilgenreiner's line through the lateral acetabular rim (*arrow 2*)
- Shenton—Arc formed by the inferior surface of the superior pubic ramus and the medial surface of the femoral metaphysis (*arrow 3*)
- Acetabular angle—angle between the line drawn from the superolateral ossified acetabular edge to the triradiate cartilage and Hilgenreiner's line; >30 degrees suggests dysplasia (*arrow 4*)

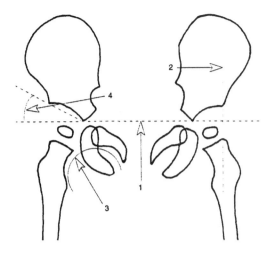

BIBLIOGRAPHY

1. Harris HH, Harris HH, Novelline RA: Radiology of Emergency Medicine, 3rd ed. Baltimore, Williams & Wilkens, 1993.
2. Keats TE: Emergency Radiology. Chicago, Year Book, 1989.
3. Mettler FA, Guiberteau MJ: Essentials of Nuclear Medicine Imaging. Philadelphia, W.B. Saunders, 1991.
4. Resnick D, Niwayama G: Diagnosis of Bone and Joint Disorders, 4th ed. Philadelphia, W.B. Saunders, 2002.
5. Rockwood CA, Green DP, Bucholz RW (eds): Rockwood and Green's Fractures in Adults, 3rd ed. Philadelphia, J.B. Lippincott, 1991.
6. Rockwood CA, Wilkins KE, King RE (eds): Fractures in Children, 3rd ed. Philadelphia, J.B. Lippincott, 1991.
7. Rogers LF: Radiology of Skeletal Trauma, 3rd ed. New York, Churchill Livingstone, 2002.

12. NUCLEAR MEDICINE

Richard A. Kutilek, M.D.

1. What is nuclear medicine?

Nuclear medicine imaging studies demonstrate organ physiology through administration of radiolabeled drugs. Selection of radiolabeled drugs extracted by specific organs allows observation of how the organs function through recorded images of activity distribution.

2. How does nuclear medicine differ from other imaging modalities (plain film, MRI, and CT)?

Nuclear medicine studies provide functional information, while CT, MRI, and plain films provide anatomic or structural information.

3. What is a bone scan?

A bone scan uses a physiologic marker to detect abnormalities of bone metabolism. The imaging agents used are radiolabeled phosphorus-based compounds. Depending on the clinical indication, imaging may include the whole body or be limited to a specific region.

4. What is a SPECT scan?

SPECT is an acronym for single photon emission computed tomography. Conventional nuclear medicine studies use planar images (anterior, posterior, oblique, and lateral views). SPECT studies use a computer to generate tomographic images in the axial, sagittal, and coronal planes. This is much more sensitive to detect subtle or small osseous abnormalities.

5. What is a three-phase bone scan?

A three-phase bone scan consists of the following:

- A radionuclide angiogram centered over the area of interest and performed during injection;
- Blood pool images of the area of interest obtained after injection; and
- Delayed images obtained 2–3 hours after injection.

6. What are the scintigraphic features of osteomyelitis?

A three-phase bone scan is needed for evaluation of possible osteomyelitis (see figure). If osteomyelitis is present, the radionuclide angiogram reveals focally increased blood flow. Blood pool and delay images also show increased activity, which is more focal on the delayed scans.

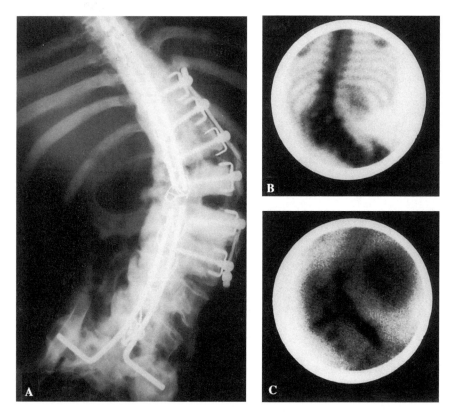

A, Patient with instrumentation of the thoracolumbar spine for scoliosis. Patient complains of fever and back pain. *B*, Bone scan delay images demonstrate multiple sites of abnormal increased activity. *C*, Gallium scan demonstrates abnormal increased activity corresponding to the left psoas muscle. Increased activity is noted in an upper lumbar vertebral body. Findings are consistent with osteomyelitis and left psoas abscess.

7. What scintigraphic features distinguish osteomyelitis from cellulitis?

On a three-phase bone scan, cellulitis presents as increased activity on the perfusion (radionuclide angiogram) and blood pool images. Normal activity is demonstrated on delayed images. Osteomyelitis has abnormal activity in all three phases.

8. What additional nuclear medicine examinations may be performed if bone scan findings for osteomyelitis are equivocal?

Gallium-67 citrate and leukocytes labeled with indium 111 or technetium 99m are useful in the diagnosis of inflammatory and infectious disease of soft tissue and bone (see figure). Labeled white blood cells have a lower sensitivity than gallium in detecting chronic osteomyelitis.

9. Name three bones that are studied more effectively with nuclear medicine than with plain film in cases of trauma.

Nuclear medicine is more effective than plain film for studies of the three S's—sternum, scapula, and sacrum.

10. What does the H-shaped pattern of increased activity in the sacrum indicate?

Bilateral linear areas of increased activity in the sacral alae with transverse increased activity in the mid sacrum are characteristic of sacral insufficiency fractures (see figure). Osteoporosis is the most common underlying etiology. MRI is also very sensitive for detecting stress fractures.

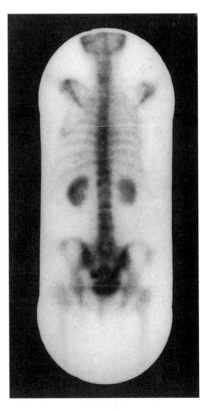

Abnormal increased activity superior to the bladder corresponding to the sacrum. Findings are consistent with a sacral fracture, which may be an insufficiency type.

11. Which is the more sensitive in the detection of stress fractures—plain film or bone scan?

Bone scan is more sensitive in the detection of stress fractures. If the stress injury is acute, angiogram and blood pool images show increased uptake. In both acute and subacute stress fractures, delayed images show increased uptake. The activity is focal and corresponds to the area of pain (see figure next page).

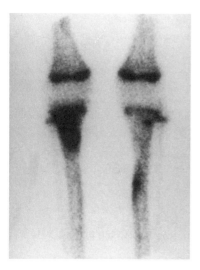

Areas of abnormal increased activity in the right proximal tibia and left tibial shaft consistent with stress fractures in a runner.

12. Shin splints occur in the same location as tibial stress fractures—the distal third of the tibia in the posteromedial cortex. What are the scintigraphic features of shin splints?

The angiogram and blood pool images are normal. Delayed images show longitudinal linear uptake on the posteromedial tibial cortex. Involvement covers approximately one-third of the length of the bone.

13. What is Legg-Calvé-Perthes disease?

Legg-Calvé-Perthes disease refers to primary avascular necrosis of the capital femoral epiphysis. It occurs most frequently between the ages of 5–7 years and is more common in boys. In early disease, radionuclide scanning is used to evaluate the vascular supply to the femoral head. Scintigraphic studies show a cold area in the proximal femoral epiphysis with early disease.

14. Name the other common sites of avascular necrosis.

Other common sites of avascular necrosis include the femoral head (see figure), lunate, scaphoid, body of the talus, and knee.

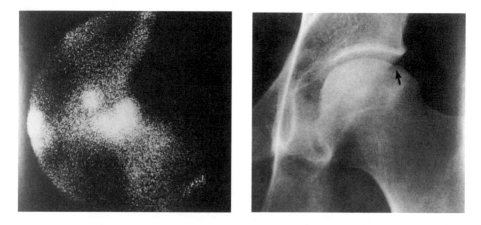

Left, Abnormal increased activity in left femoral head in 30-year-old male on steroids for lupus. Findings are consistent with avascular necrosis. *Right,* Plain film of left hip demonstrates early collapse of the articular surface.

15. Are the scintigraphic features always the same with osteonecrosis?

No. Scintigraphic findings vary with the stage of disease. In early disease, decreased uptake is seen. With reparative process and degenerative changes, increased activity is noted.

16. What is reflex sympathetic dystrophy syndrome (RSDS)?

Reflex sympathetic dystrophy is a syndrome characterized by pain, vasomotor instability, swelling, and dystrophic skin changes. Patients frequently report a history of trauma or injury. RSDS may follow a self-limited course or become chronic and irreversible. RSDS usually involves the upper extremity.

17. What are the scintigraphic features of RSDS?

Three-phase bone scan shows increased blood flow to the affected limb with increased activity on blood pool images (see figure). On delayed images, increased juxtaarticular activity is noted around all of the joints.

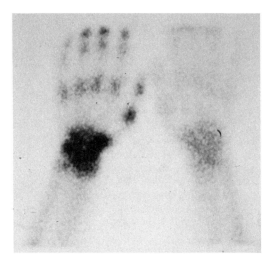

Reflex sympathetic dystrophy. Notice the increased activity in wrist and joints of the right hand.

18. What are the most frequent complications of hip replacement?

The most frequent complications of hip replacement are loosening of the prosthesis and infection. Other complications include dislocation, hematoma, and heterotopic bone formation. Loosening is the most common cause of pain.

19. What are the scintigraphic findings in loosening of a prosthesis?

On a bone scan, loosening of a prosthesis appears as an area of increased activity, usually at the distal aspect of the femoral component or around the shaft of the femur or acetabulum. The bone scan should be correlated with plain films. The bone scan is not reliable in the first 9–12 months after surgery.

20. Name the primary cancers that most frequently metastasize to bone.

A mnemonic for "lead kettle"—PB KTL—can be useful for remembering the common nonosseous tumors that metastasize to bone. The cancers are prostate, breast, bladder, kidney, thyroid, lung, and lymphoma. Bone scans are more sensitive than plain films in identification of metastatic disease because it takes a 30–50% loss in bone density for the lesion to be detected radiographically. Whole bone images show multiple areas of abnormal increased activity (see figure next page). Remember that the most common primary bone tumor, multiple myeloma, commonly has a negative bone scan and should be evaluated by plain films (metastatic bone survey).

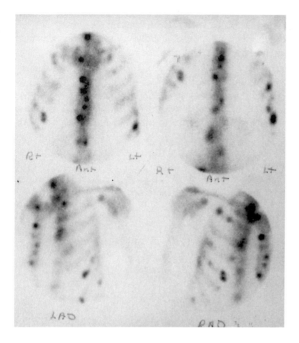

Multiple areas of abnormal increased activity are demonstrated in a random distribution consistent with diffuse bony metastatic disease.

21. What is a superscan?
Diffuse increased uptake of activity is noted throughout the skeleton, along with a lack of renal activity and nearly complete absence of soft-tissue activity.

22. What are the causes of superscans?
Metastatic disease is the most common cause, usually from the prostate or breast. Additional etiologies include hyperparathyroidism, osteomalacia, Paget's disease, and fibrous dysplasia.

BIBLIOGRAPHY

1. Datz FL, Patch GG, Arias JM, Morton KA: Nuclear Medicine: A Teaching File. St. Louis, Mosby, 1992.
2. Freeman LM (ed): Nuclear Medicine Annual 1997. Philadelphia, Lippincott-Raven, 1997.
3. Mettler FA, Guiberteau MJ: Essentials of Nuclear Medicine Imaging, 4th ed. Philadelphia, W.B. Saunders, 1998.
4. Murray IPC, Ell PJ: Nuclear Medicine in Clinical Diagnosis and Treatment, 2nd ed. Edinburgh, Churchill Livingstone, 1998.

13. COMPUTED TOMOGRAPHY

Kevin L. Nelson, M.D.

1. When a complex pelvic fracture is identified on radiographs, what is the best imaging study for further evaluation and surgical planning?
Computed tomography (CT) of the pelvis provides a cross-sectional image to evaluate the degree of displacement of bone fragments as well as soft-tissue injuries, including hematomas.

2. A complex fracture of the hip is best visualized with what imaging modality?

CT provides the orthopedic surgeon with the greatest amount of information about the extent of fractures, displacement, and fracture fragments within the joint space. Three-dimensional CT images may also enhance the anatomic depiction of the fractures.

3. A suspected acute fracture of the sacrum that cannot be defined on plain films is probably best imaged with what modality?

CT is the preferred modality. Acute fractures may not be identified on nuclear medicine bone scans for several days.

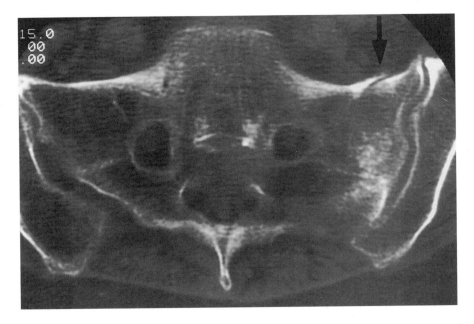

Sacral stress fracture. Axial CT image reveals an acute fracture of the sacrum that could not be demonstrated on radiographs.

4. A fracture dislocation of the sternoclavicular joint is best defined with what imaging modality?

CT is more rapid and accurate in identifying fractures of the sternoclavicular joint than plain radiographs. Subtle fractures or dislocations are easily ascertained, and underlying mediastinal trauma also may be evaluated with CT.

5. Complex fractures of the foot such as the Lisfranc fractures are best evaluated by what imaging methods?

The preferred protocol is plain radiographs followed by CT reformatted in the coronal plane.

6. After radiographs, what additional studies are useful for evaluation of tarsal coalition?

CT is the most appropriate imaging study, particularly to define the bony coalition and to identify facets. CT indirectly images fibrous coalitions by demonstrating irregular or roughened cortical surfaces. Magnetic resonance imaging (MRI) is becoming increasingly useful in tarsal coalition because of its direct multiplanar imaging capabilities.

7. A suspected fracture of the triquetrum not identified on plain radiographs is best defined on what imaging study?

CT is generally more useful in displaying fracture morphology and cortical detail than MRI.

8. What is the best imaging study to obtain in a case of a suspected cartilaginous intraarticular loose body in a joint?

CT arthrography or MRI is the preferred study. MR arthrography is also useful; however, the Food and Drug Administration (FDA) has approved no MR contrast agent for intraarticular use.

9. What is the most sensitive imaging modality for evaluation of glenoid labral tears?

CT arthrography or MR arthrography are probably more sensitive in detecting glenoid labrum tears than routine MRI alone. Sensitivity for detection of glenoid labral tears by CT or MR arthrography is believed to be greater than 95%.

10. What is the imaging procedure of choice for identifying a suspected lumbar disc herniation?

This issue is controversial. There is little disagreement, however, that MRI is more sensitive in identifying early changes in degenerative disc disease and offers the added advantage of direct sagittal imaging. CT, however, is a highly sensitive test for identifying a suspected lumbar disc herniation (see figure, top of next page) and is generally less expensive than MRI. CT offers the added advantage of superior cortical bone detail (see figure, middle of next page). In some instances, the examinations are complementary, and both may be needed.

11. What is the appropriate imaging modality for evaluating the patient with recurrent low back pain after lumbar discectomy?

Contrast-enhanced MRI is more accurate than CT in differentiating recurrent nonenhancing lumbar disc herniation from enhancing postoperative epidural scar. Other etiologies of recurrent low back pain may include spinal stenosis, which is effectively evaluated with MRI, and arachnoiditis, which also is evaluated more effectively with MRI than with CT.

12. What is the most sensitive imaging examination for identifying a cervical disc herniation?

Although MRI is an excellent screening examination, postmyelogram thin-section CT is considered by many to be the most sensitive imaging study to identify subtle cervical disc herniations (see figure, bottom of next page).

13. What imaging modality is appropriate in the clinical setting of cervical spine trauma when plain radiographs are equivocal but suspicious for fracture?

Thin-section CT of the suspected area is the modality of choice.

14. If a spinal cord contusion is suspected after cervical spine trauma, what is the appropriate imaging study?

MRI is the study of choice. Although CT provides high-resolution bone detail of the osseous elements, the intradural structures, including the cervical spinal cord, are best imaged with MRI.

15. What is the best imaging modality for identifying a pseudarthrosis in the patient who has undergone a bone fusion of the lumbar spine?

CT is the modality of choice. Plain radiographs in flexion and extension are also useful to define the degree of instability.

16. What are the two types of spondylolisthesis?

The two types are lytic and degenerative spondylolisthesis. **Lytic spondylolisthesis** is due to bilateral fractures or congenital defects in the pars intraarticularis (classically described as the "collar on the neck of the Scottie dog" on oblique plain radiographs of the lumbar spine). Lytic

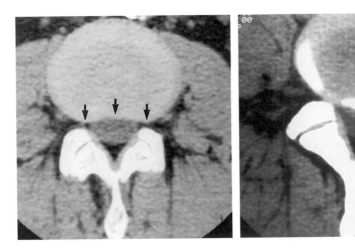

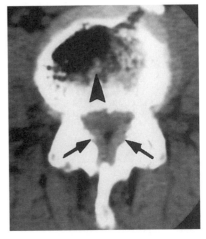

Normal lumbar discs *(top, left).* Axial CT scan at the level of the lumbar intervertebral discs shows the posterior margin of the intermediate density disc *(arrows)* is confined to the posterior margin of the vertebral body with no abnormal protrusion of the disc.

Lumbar disc herniation *(top, right).* Axial CT scan at the level of the lumbar intervertebral disc reveals an abnormal protrusion of the disc *(arrow).*

Central lumbar spinal canal stenosis *(right).* Axial CT scan at the level of the lumbar intervertebral disc shows narrowing of the central spinal canal. There is hypertrophy of the ligamentum flavum *(arrows)* and low-density vacuum *(arrowhead)* in the nucleus pulposus of the degenerated disc. CT is very useful in evaluating suspected lumbar spinal stenosis due to eloquent definition of bony encroachment of the spinal canal.

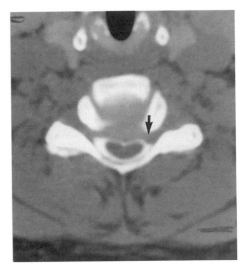

Cervical disc herniation. Axial CT image at the level of the cervical intervertebral disc following myelography reveals a cervical disc herniation *(arrow)* compressing the high-density myelogram contrast agent that has been placed in the intradural space.

spondylolisthesis results in posterior displacement of the superior vertebral body with respect to the inferior vertebral body. **Degenerative spondylolisthesis** is due to degenerative erosion of the superior facet of the inferior vertebral body. Such erosion allows forward movement of the inferior facet of the superior vertebral body and results in spondylolisthesis. CT scanning can document the degree of displacement and the pars intraarticularis defects.

17. A suspected soft-tissue mass in the extremity is best evaluated first with what imaging modality?
With direct multiplanar imaging capabilities and excellent soft-tissue discrimination, MRI is the initial imaging modality of choice in evaluating soft-tissue masses in an extremity. CT usually is reserved for cases that require a clearer depiction of bony detail.

BIBLIOGRAPHY

1. Greenfield GB (ed): Radiology of Bone Diseases, 5th ed. Philadelphia, Lippincott-Raven, 1990.
2. Lee JKT, Sagel SS, Stanley RJ, Heiken JP (eds): Computed Body Tomography with MRI Correlation, 3rd ed. Philadelphia, Lippincott-Raven, 1997.
3. Magid D, Fishman EK, Gregerman MB (eds): Computed Tomography with Multiplanar Reconstructions: An Atlas of the Normal and Abnormal Hip. New York, Field & Wood, 1989.
4. Resnick D (ed): Diagnosis of Bone and Joint Disorders, 3rd ed. Philadelphia, W.B. Saunders, 1995.
5. Stiles RG, Otto MT: Imaging of the shoulder. Radiology 188:603–613, 1993.

14. MAGNETIC RESONANCE IMAGING

Kevin L. Nelson, M.D.

1. What pulse sequences are most commonly used in magnetic resonance imaging (MRI) of the musculoskeletal system?
Conventional spin-echo T1-weighted, proton density, and T2-weighted images are used most often. Gradient-echo and inversion recovery (STIR) images are also common.

2. What are the absolute contraindications to MRI?
Patients with an internal cardiac pacemaker, brain aneurysm clip, metallic foreign body in the eye, cochlear implant, and surgically implanted drug infusion pumps, neurostimulators, or bone growth stimulators cannot undergo MRI.

3. May a patient who has a metallic hip or knee prosthesis undergo an MRI examination?
Yes. Metallic distortion artifact may cause signal void on MR images of anatomic structures in the immediate region of the metal implant. If the patient has a hip or knee prosthesis in place, the contralateral hip or knee can be readily imaged with MRI. Orthopedic screws or wire usually do not cause significant distortion of the MR signal. For example, an anterior cruciate ligament reconstruction stabilized with metallic screws usually can be well visualized with MRI.

4. What is the accuracy rate of MRI in detecting meniscal tears of the knee?
The accuracy rate of MRI in detecting meniscal tears is greater than 90% in most series. With three-dimensional imaging the rate of concurrence between MRI and arthroscopy is 95%.

5. What is the normal MRI appearance of a meniscus?
The intact meniscus demonstrates homogeneous low signal intensity on all pulse sequences.

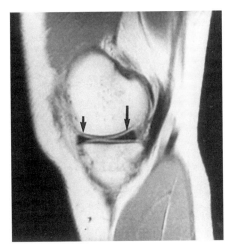

Normal medial meniscus. The normal meniscus demonstrates homogeneous low signal intensity on this sagittal proton-density–weighted image. The anterior *(short arrow)* and posterior *(long arrow)* horns are triangular in configuration and sharply marginated.

6. How many grades of abnormal signal intensity are used to classify an abnormal meniscus on MRI?

There are three grades of abnormal signal intensity. Grade 1, which correlates with globular foci of early mucinous degeneration, may be observed in normal volunteers and has no clinical significance. Grade 2 is a linear horizontal area of increased signal intensity that does not extend to an articular surface but may contact a capsular margin. Grade 1 and 2 menisci are arthroscopically normal. An abnormal signal intensity that extends to an articular surface is considered grade 3, which represents a torn meniscus and is visible at arthroscopy.

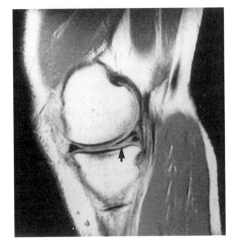

Torn posterior horn medial meniscus. The sagittal proton-density–weighted image reveals abnormal grade III high signal intensity *(arrow)* in the posterior horn of the medial meniscus, which extends in an oblique fashion to the inferior or tibial articular surface of the meniscus. This tear was confirmed at arthroscopy.

7. What is a discoid meniscus of the knee? What are the complications of a discoid meniscus?

A discoid meniscus is a dysplastic meniscus that has a broad, disclike configuration. Lateral discoid menisci are more common than medial discoid menisci. Complications include tears and cysts.

8. What is the appearance of an anterior cruciate ligament (ACL) tear on MRI?

A complete tear results in nonvisualization of the normal low-signal–intensity ACL. If the tear is acute, the MRI usually shows an effusion in the joint space and an edematous pseudomass

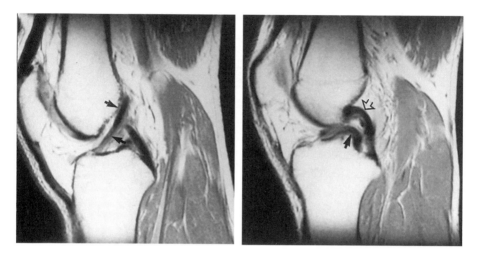

Normal anterior cruciate ligament *(left).* The normal anterior cruciate ligament is identified as a low-signal band *(arrows)* on this sagittal proton-density–weighted image.

Torn anterior cruciate ligament *(right).* As compared with the normal anterior cruciate ligament seen at left, the torn anterior cruciate ligament *(arrow)* is identified lying inferiorly in the knee joint space on the sagittal proton-density–weighted image. The normal posterior cruciate ligament *(open arrow)* is also visualized.

where the ACL is normally visualized. Most tears occur in the mid to proximal portion of the ACL. If the tear is chronic, the ACL is not visualized in its normal oblique course, and the distal portion of the remaining intact ACL may be seen lying inferiorly within the joint.

9. Certain bone contusions of the knee are commonly associated with a complete tear of the ACL. Where are these contusions located?

Bone contusions of the knee commonly associated with a complete tear of the ACL are located on the posterolateral tibial plateau and lateral femoral condyle, presumably because of impaction of the lateral femoral condyle into the posterior tibia during injury.

10. Chondromalacia patella is usually best defined on which MR pulse sequence and plane?

Axial T2-weighted or gradient-echo T2 images usually offer the best depiction of the changes of chondromalacia patella.

11. Which pathologic findings of a lateral patellar dislocation may be demonstrated with MRI?
- Torn medial retinaculum
- Osteochondral fracture of the patella
- Impaction bone bruise of the lateral femoral condyle
- Lateral subluxation of the patella
- Joint effusion and dysplastic patella without a medial facet
- Shallow or hypoplastic femoral groove

12. Where is osteochondritis dissecans of the knee classically located?

Osteochondritis dissecans of the knee is classically located in the non–weight-bearing lateral aspect of the medial femoral condyle. It is usually seen in men, and up to 50% of patients may have a history of trauma. Early osteochondritis dissecans is best visualized with MRI.

13. A complete rupture of the medial collateral ligament is often associated with what other injuries of the knee that can be visualized on MRI?

Complete tears of the medial collateral ligament may be associated with tears of the anterior cruciate ligament, medial meniscus, or medial and posterior capsule of the knee as well as impaction injuries of the lateral femoral condyle and lateral tibial plateau.

14. What is the best imaging modality for evaluation of a suspected popliteal fossa mass?

MRI accurately differentiates most popliteal fossa masses, including cysts, aneurysms, and soft-tissue masses.

15. What is the imaging procedure of choice for early detection of avascular necrosis (AVN) of the femoral head?

MRI is reported to be the most sensitive imaging modality for differentiating AVN from non-AVN of the femoral head with a specificity of 98% and a sensitivity of 97% (see figures, below). In addition to MRI, nuclear scintigraphy with technetium-99m–labeled phosphate compounds is the second most sensitive imaging modality. Radiographs become positive in later stages of AVN (see figure below). Early diagnosis is critical because all treatment procedures are more successful in the initial stages of AVN.

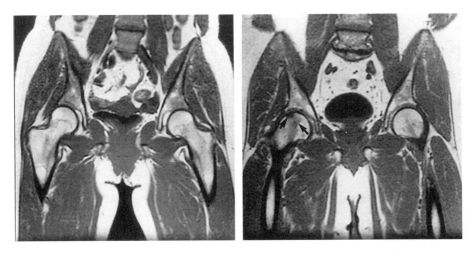

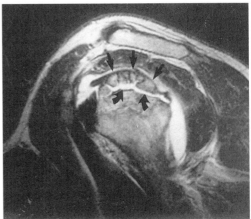

Normal hips *(top, left).* On this coronal T1-weighted image, the normal femoral heads demonstrate high signal intensity fat in the bone marrow space.

Early avascular necrosis femoral head *(top, right).* Compared with the figure at left, this patient shows early changes of avascular necrosis of the femoral head. Abnormal low signal intensity *(arrowheads)* observed in the femoral head is indicative of early avascular necrosis.

Late changes of avascular necrosis humeral head *(right).* More advanced changes of avascular necrosis are demonstrated in the humeral head of this patient. Multiple loose fragments *(arrows),* which are surrounded by a rim of high-signal–intensity fluid *(curved arrows),* are seen on the sagittal T2-weighted image.

16. What imaging study is appropriate when a nondisplaced femoral neck fracture is suspected clinically but radiographs are negative?

MRI is useful in identifying nondisplaced femoral neck fractures that cannot be detected on routine radiographs. Although bone scintigraphy is also useful, it is not as specific. MRI is able to depict the morphology of the nondisplaced fracture more accurately than bone scintigraphy.

17. What nerve is entrapped or compressed in the tarsal tunnel syndrome?

In the tarsal tunnel syndrome the posterior tibial nerve is entrapped or compressed. Etiologies of this compression neuropathy that can be effectively imaged with MRI include neuromas, ganglion cysts, lipomas, varicose veins, and tenosynovitis.

18. What is the most likely tendon to be torn in the patient presenting with a unilateral flat-foot deformity?

The tibialis posterior tendon is the most likely candidate. MRI is the best imaging modality to confirm a partial or complete tear of the tendon.

19. What is the most common site of rupture of the Achilles tendon?

The Achilles tendon is most susceptible to rupture 2–6 cm above the os calcis. Because rupture may be missed on clinical examination in up to 25% of patients, MRI is invaluable in confirming the diagnosis.

20. The rotator cuff comprises which muscles?

The SIT muscles (supraspinatus, infraspinatus, teres minor) and the subscapularis muscle.

21. Which tendon of the rotator cuff is most likely to tear first?

The tear usually begins along the anterolateral leading edge of the supraspinatus tendon at its insertion into the greater tuberosity of the humerus.

22. Describe the difference between a partial-thickness and full-thickness tear of the rotator cuff.

A full-thickness tear extends through the entire width of the tendon and appears as an area of high signal intensity, approximating fluid, on T2-weighted MR images (see figure, top of next page). A partial-thickness tear does not extend through the width of the tendon. It may involve either the inferior or articular surface or the superior or bursal surface of the tendon. Partial-thickness tears can—and probably often do—progress to full-thickness tears.

23. How are abnormal tendons of the rotator cuff classified on MRI?

There are three grades of abnormal rotator cuff tendons. Grade 1 tendinitis demonstrates normal morphology of the tendon with high signal intensity on T1-weighted images and normal low signal intensity on T2-weighted images. Grade 2 lesions are partial-thickness tears on either the articular or bursal surface of the tendon and are seen as high-signal–intensity lesions on T2-weighted images. Grade 3 lesions are full-thickness tears that show a high-signal–intensity gap in the tendon on T2-weighted images.

24. What important abnormal anatomic etiologies of impingement syndrome of the shoulder can be effectively imaged with MRI?

Shape and slope of the acromion process
- Subacromial osteophytes
- Morphology of the acromioclavicular joint

25. Which pathologic bone and soft-tissue lesions of recurrent anterior dislocations of the shoulder can be demonstrated on MRI?

The bone lesions are a Hill-Sachs deformity of the humeral head and a fracture of the inferior glenoid. The soft-tissue lesions are tears of the anterior glenoid labrum and anterior capsule.

26. What is the site of insertion of the biceps tendon in the elbow? What is the appropriate imaging modality when a torn biceps tendon is suspected?

The biceps tendon inserts at the tuberosity of the radius. Partial- or full-thickness tears of the tendon are best imaged with MRI.

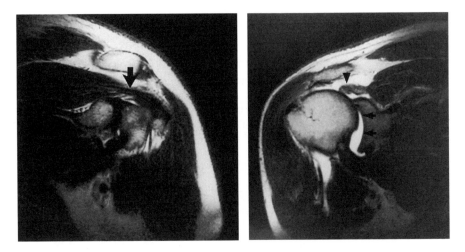

Normal supraspinatus muscle and supraspinatus tendon *(left)*. A normal supraspinatus muscle and low-signal–intensity supraspinatus tendon *(arrow)* are seen on this coronal T2-weighted image.

Full-thickness tear supraspinatus tendon *(right)*. A coronal T2-weighted image demonstrates a large full-thickness tear of the supraspinatus tendon. The torn supraspinatus tendon *(arrowhead)* is retracted from its normal insertion on the humeral head and is surrounded by high-signal–intensity fluid. The humeral head is also noted to be superiorly subluxed in the glenoid fossa *(arrows)*.

27. What is the most common appearance of avascular necrosis of the scaphoid on MRI?

The most common appearance of AVN of the scaphoid is low signal intensity on both T1- and T2-weighted images. Occasionally an increased signal on T2-weighted images may be noted because of marrow edema and local fluid accumulation.

28. What carpal bone is affected by Kienböck's disease?

Kienböck's disease is avascular necrosis of the lunate. MRI is the imaging modality of choice in diagnosing Kienböck's disease.

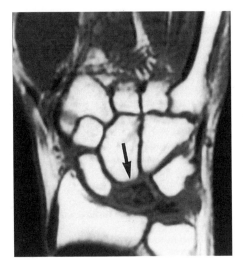

Kienböck's disease. Compared with the other normal high-signal–intensity carpal bones of the wrist on this coronal T1-weighted image, the lunate demonstrates low signal intensity *(arrow)* as a result of avascular necrosis.

29. What is the imaging procedure of choice to identify a suspected lesion of the brachial plexus?

The procedure of choice is MRI.

30. What is the first imaging modality to order in screening for pathology of the cervical or thoracic spine?

MRI provides the most information in a single imaging examination for pathology of the cervical and thoracic spine. Both the extradural structures, including the vertebra and intervertebral discs, and the intradural anatomy, including the spinal cord, are clearly depicted on MRI.

31. For evaluating congenital abnormalities of the pediatric spine, what is the first imaging study to order?

Plain radiographs always should be obtained first to evaluate bony anatomy for such abnormalities as spina bifida, butterfly vertebra, or other congenital bony abnormalities. MRI is commonly used next for evaluating the neural elements of the spine for abnormalities such as myelomeningocele, tethered cord, syrinx, diastematomyelia, and other congenital abnormalities of the neural elements.

32. What is the first imaging modality to order in evaluating spinal infections?

The first imaging modality to order for discitis, vertebral osteomyelitis, and epidural abscess is MRI.

33. What is the best imaging modality for evaluating bone marrow?

MRI directly images bone marrow and is highly sensitive in detecting early disease such as metastases, lymphoma, and myeloma. Nuclear bone scintigraphy is the best modality in screening for metastatic disease in the asymptomatic patient with a known malignancy.

34. Is MRI able to differentiate confidently between benign and malignant lesions of soft tissue and bone?

No. No specific characteristic of MR signal intensity determines whether the lesion is benign or malignant. If the mass is extensive and has poorly circumscribed margins involving soft tissue, bone, and the neurovascular bundle, it is more likely to be malignant.

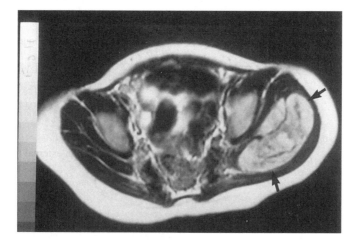

Rhabdomyosarcoma. A large heterogeneous signal intensity mass *(arrows)* is demonstrated in the gluteal muscles.

BIBLIOGRAPHY

1. Berquist TH (ed): MRI of the Musculoskeletal System, 3rd ed. Philadelphia, Lippincott-Raven, 1996.
2. Deutsch AL, Mink JH, Kerr R (eds): MRI of the Foot and Ankle. New York, Raven Press, 1992.
3. Mink JH, Reicher MA, Crues JV III, Deutsch AL (eds): MRI of the Knee. New York, Raven Press, 1993.
4. Reicher MA, Kellerhouse LE (eds): MRI of the Wrist and Hand. New York, Raven Press, 1990.
5. Stoller DW (ed): Magnetic Resonance Imaging in Orthopaedics and Sports Medicine, 2nd ed. Philadelphia, Lippincott-Raven, 1997.
6. Uri DS: MR imaging of shoulder impingement and rotator cuff disease. Radiol Clin North Am 35:77, 1997.
7. Virolainen H, Visuri T, Kuusela T: Acute dislocation of the patella: MR findings. Radiology 189:243–246, 1993.
8. Zlatkin MB (ed): MRI of the Shoulder. New York, Raven Press, 1991.

15. MULTIPLE TRAUMA

Matthew A. Mormino, M.D.

1. How should a patient with multiple injuries be evaluated?

All trauma patients should be evaluated using standard advanced trauma life support protocols, which include the ABCDE of initial evaluation: **a**irway, **b**reathing, **c**irculation, **d**isability (neurologic evaluation), and **e**xposure (undress the patient). The primary survey is followed by a secondary survey to identify non-life-threatening injuries.

2. Which radiographs are required in the initial assessment of a trauma patient?

Initial films include an anteroposterior (AP) view of the chest, an AP of the pelvis, and a lateral view of the cervical spine.

3. What is the "golden hour" of trauma management?

Death from trauma has a trimodal distribution. The first peak is within the first seconds to minutes after injury. Very few such patients can be saved due to the severity of their injuries. The second peak is within the next few hours. The first hour of care following injury is characterized by the rapid assessment and repair of life-threatening injuries. Within this "golden hour" an organized trauma system can have the greatest impact on patient outcome. The third death peak occurs within several days or weeks of injury and is most often due to sepsis and multiorgan failure.

4. How should an unstable pelvic fracture be managed acutely in a patient with hemodynamic instability?

The unstable pelvis is most easily stabilized in the emergency room by binding the pelvis with a sheet. This method may temporarily reduce pelvic volume and promote tamponade until more definitive measures can be taken. The emergent application of an external fixator and angiographic arterial embolization are more definitive ways to address hemodynamic instability in a patient with a pelvic fracture.

5. What does MAST stand for?

Military antishock trousers (MAST) were developed to stabilize shock victims during transport. The idea was to put compression on the lower extremities to shunt blood to more vital organs. The use of MAST is controversial because of associated complications (e.g., compartment syndrome, skin slough).

6. What is the best way to control external hemorrhage?

External bleeding is best controlled by direct pressure. The use of tourniquets and clamping should be avoided.

7. What noninvasive methods are available to evaluate the vascular status of an extremity?

The vascular status of an injured extremity can be evaluated by palpation of pulses, Doppler examination of pulses, and the ankle brachial index (ABI). The ABI is the ratio of the arterial occlusive pressure of the arm versus the ankle. If the ABI is $\leq$ 90%, further vascular work-up should be considered.

8. What should be done with a pulseless and deformed extremity?

The extremity should be gently realigned, the pulses should be re-evaluated, and the extremity should be splinted. If pulses do not return, consider angiography.

9. When should long bone fractures be stabilized?

Several studies have shown that long bone fractures should be stabilized within the first 24 hours. Such studies also demonstrate decreased rates of sepsis, acute respiratory distress syndrome (ARDS), pneumonia, and mortality in patients who had early skeletal stabilization.

10. Describe fat embolism syndrome.

The systemic release of intramedullary fat droplets and the cellular responses to them cause this syndrome. Patients with long bone fractures may develop a syndrome manifested by mental status changes, petechiae, and decreased O_2 saturation. Treatment is respiratory support. The syndrome is prevented by early skeletal stabilization.

11. What is the incidence of deep venous thrombosis (DVT) in patients with multiple trauma and lower extremity or pelvic fractures?

Depending on the screening method, the incidence of DVT in such patients is between 40% and 80%. Early patient mobilization and prophylactic measures, such as sequential compression stockings and subcutaneous low-molecular-weight heparin, have reduced its incidence. The use of vena cava filters to reduce the incidence of fatal pulmonary embolism in selected high-risk patients has gained popularity.

12. How is a patient's cervical spine best immobilized for transport?

In patients with a suspected cervical spine injury, the neck should be immobilized in a Philadelphia-type collar and further supported by sandbags and taping the head to a spine board. A Philadelphia-type collar limits approximately 40% of rotary motion and 60% of flexion/extension motion.

13. List the clinical signs suggestive of a cervical spinal cord injury in an unconscious patient.

In an unconscious patient in whom the mechanism of injury was a fall or a motor vehicle accident, incidence of cervical spine injury is 5–10%. Clinical signs include:
- Flaccid areflexia, especially with flaccid rectal tone
- Diaphragmatic breathing
- Ability to flex but not extend the elbow
- Aresponse to painful stimulus above but not below the clavicle
- Hypotension with bradycardia
- Priapism

14. How is spinal shock characterized?

Shortly after spinal cord injury the cord may appear completely functionless, even though some areas are not completely destroyed. This produces flaccidity and areflexia instead of spasticity and hyperreflexia. Days to weeks later, spinal shock resolves; in areas of permanent loss, spasticity replaces the flaccidity. The return of the bulbocavernosus reflex (anal sphincter contraction with a gentle tug on the Foley catheter) frequently signifies the end of spinal shock.

15. Describe neurogenic shock.

Injury to the descending sympathetic pathways in the spinal cord results in loss of vasomotor tone and sympathetic innervation to the heart, which in turn results in vasodilitation and pooling of the blood in the extremities and viscera. The patient fails to become tachycardic or may become bradycardic as a result of loss of sympathetic innervation to the heart. The hallmark of neurogenic shock is bradycardia in the presence of hypertension.

BIBLIOGRAPHY

1. Alexander RH, Proctor HJ: ATLS Student Manual, 3rd ed. Chicago, American College of Surgeons, 1993.
2. Bone LB, Johnson KD, Weigelt J: Early versus delayed stabilization of femoral fractures: A prospective randomized study. J Bone Joint Surg 71A:336, 1989.
3. Bosse MJ, et al: Adult respiratory distress syndrome, pneumonia, and mortality following thoracic injury and a femoral fracture treated either with intramedullary nailing with reaming or with a plate. A comparative study. J Bone Joint Surg 79A:799, 1997.
4. Hansen Jr ST, Swiontkowski MF: Orthopaedic Trauma Protocols. New York, Raven, 1993.
5. Routt Jr ML, et al: Circumferential pelvic antishock sheeting: A temporary resuscitation aid. J Orthop Trauma 16:45–48, 2001.

16. BONE GRAFTING

Jonathan E. Fuller, M.D.

1. Name five clinical applications for bone grafting.

Spinal fusion, arthrodesis, enhancement of fracture healing and repair of pseudarthroses, reconstructive surgery, and oral and maxillofacial surgery.

2. What are the three customary sites from which autologous bone graft can be harvested?

The anterior ilium, posterior ilium, and fibula. Other sites, less commonly used, include the distal radius and the tibial metaphysis or even a rib.

3. What is the most common complication of iliac crest graft harvest?

Donor site pain (25% of patients).

4. Name five other common complications of iliac crest harvest.

- Injury to the cluneal or lateral femoral cutaneous nerves
- Sacroiliac joint pain or instability
- Injury to the superior gluteal artery
- Hernia
- Hematoma

5 From what area is harvest of iliac crest bone graft safest?

From Ebraheim's zone 1, the region extending anteriorly from the posterior superior iliac spine, perpendicular to the plane of the operating table.

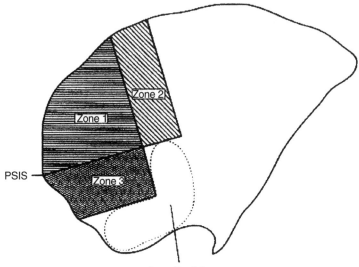

Schematic representation of the zones dividing the posterior iliac region. (From Xu R, Ebraheim NA, Yeasting RA, Jackson WT: Anatomic considerations for posterior iliac bone harvesting. Spine 21(9):1017–1020, 1996; with permission.)

6. Describe two techniques for the harvest of iliac crest bone graft.
    Corticocancellous bone graft can be harvested from the posterior iliac crest by stripping the glutei from the outer table of the ilium and using a gouge to remove strips of bone from the outer table. This technique can also be used on the anterior iliac crest but is used to greatest advantage to harvest graft from the inner table. Another technique used on the posterior ilium is to open a "trap door" from the crest of the ilium and remove cancellous graft from between the inner and outer tables with a curette. This technique is thought by some to entail less morbidity than the technique of stripping the glutei from the ilium. It is also possible to harvest tricortical grafts, most commonly from the anterior ilium to obtain structural autografts, which typically are used in cervical spine reconstructions.

7. Does bone grow back in donor sites?
    No. Costectomies done in the course of a thoracotomy often exhibit rib regeneration in pediatric patients, but bone does not grow back to replace that harvested from the ilium.

8. What is osteoid?
    Osteoid is the nonmineralized precursor of bone. It is formed by osteoblasts induced from precursor cells by fracture hematoma. Osteoid consists of type I collagen (90%) and numerous miscellaneous materials, including glycoproteins and other proteins. As osteoid matures, calcium hydroxyapatite crystals are deposited, imparting strength to the new bone.

9. What is BMP?
    Bone morphogenetic proteins (BMPs) are glycoproteins belonging to the family of transforming growth factor-β (TGF-β). They mediate differentiation and proliferation of a number of cell types and function synergistically in a manner not precisely understood to stimulate endochondral bone formation. TGF-β is released from platelets at the site of hematoma and has a role in recruitment of mesenchymal precursor cells; BMPs are found within bone. The presence of both growth factors at a fracture site stimulates the formation of fracture callus.

10. Who was the first to describe bone morphogenetic protein (BMP)?

Urist and coworkers identified proteins derived from bovine bone that were capable of inducing bone formation in the soft tissue of experimental animals.

11. Name and explain the three processes by which bone grafting lead to bone formation:

The property of **osteogenesis** is found only in fresh autograft in which the cellular elements remain viable. Osteogenesis describes the formation of new bone from viable osteoprogenitor cells or stem cells that retain the capacity to differentiate into bone-forming cells. The vigor of the graft's osteogenetic properties depends on preservation of the viability of the cellular elements; for this reason, the osteogenetic properties of vascularized autografts are superior to those of devitalized autograft.

Osteoinduction describes the ability of the graft to induce stem cells to differentiate into mature osteoblasts and osteocytes. This property depends on the presence of growth factors, such as BMP and TGF-β, that mediate such biologic processes. Osteoinduction must be present for osteogenesis to occur; with use of autograft, the osteoinductive properties are provided by BMP and other growth factors naturally present within autograft.

Osteoconduction describes the ability of a graft to serve as a framework on which the host cells can form living bone. Certain inorganic materials possess the property of osteoconduction, and it has been observed that certain physical properties of the osteoconductive substance (e.g., pore size) play an important role in allowing osteoconduction. Allograft is a classic example of a primarily osteoconductive but minimally osteoinductive substance.

12. What are the three stages of bone healing? Explain each.

The **inflammatory stage** occurs first and lasts 1–3 days. Inflammatory cells and fibroblasts are recruited to the fracture hematoma. Cellular proliferation and vascular ingrowth occur.

In the **repair or induction stage,** the pluripotential stem cells recruited to the area differentiate into bone-forming cells and osteoid is laid down. This process begins at the periphery of the fracture callus and progresses inward within the fracture callus. At the conclusion of this stage a rubbery, minimally calcified woven bone has been laid down, ushering in the third stage of healing.

In the **remodeling stage** the woven bone laid down in the repair stage undergoes refinement. Cutting cones remove woven bone, and osteoblasts lay down trabecular or lamellar bone in response to the loads experienced by the bone in a process that occurs over months to years and concludes with a robust osseous tissue able to withstand the loads to which it is subjected.

13. Which pharmacologic agents can interfere with the biology of bone healing?

Nonsteroidal anti-inflammatory drugs may interfere with the biochemical events of the inflammatory stage, which are mediated by prostaglandins. Likewise, steroids may suppress bone healing by suppression of inflammation. Tobacco has also been shown in several studies to suppress spine fusions, probably because of nicotine's inhibition of vascular neogenesis.

14. What techniques are used in the preparation of allograft?

Fresh-frozen allografts incorporate more quickly but offer greater risks of disease transmission.

Freeze-dried allografts are extremely safe with respect to disease transmission but incorporate less readily. In addition, the strength of lyophilized allograft is inferior in torsion and bending, although similar in compression, compared with fresh-frozen grafts.

Irradiation leads to significant weakening of allograft in all axes.

15. Name and define the three types of bone graft.

Autograft describes bone harvested from one location and placed in another. Autograft has the greatest osteogenic potential, especially in the case of vascularized autograft.

Allograft is bone taken from one member of a common species and transplanted into another. Allograft has much weaker osteoinductive properties but is osteoconductive. No donor site morbidity is associated with allograft, but there is some small, theoretical risk of disease transmission, which can be mitigated by careful tissue banking practices and graft preparation.

Xenograft is bone taken from one species and transplanted into another. Xenograft is not widely used in clinical practice because the ability of xenograft to stimulate bone formation is limited by immunogenicity.

16. When was the first bone-grafting procedure performed?

At the creation. According to Genesis 2:21–22, "So the Lord God caused a deep sleep to fall upon the man, and while he slept took one of his ribs and closed up its place with flesh; and the rib which the Lord God had taken from the man he made into a woman and brought her to the man."

17. Name two major categories of bone graft substitutes.

Bone-derived substitutes. Important examples of demineralized bone matrix (DBM), include Grafton (Osteotech, Inc.) and Osteofil (Regeneration Technologies, Inc.) Demineralized bone matrix consists of bone from which the calcium hydroxyapatite salts have been extracted. It is considered to provide a source of osteoinductive proteins, such as BMP, and therefore to possess osteoinductive properties, although they are weak.

Synthetic (ceramic). These bone graft substitutes consist of mineral salts such as hydroxyapatite, calcium phosphate, calcium sulfate or coralline-derived hydroxyapatite. They can be formed in pastes, blocks or tablets, are readily absorbed, and possess osteoconductive properties.

18. What is the proportion of osteogenic precursor cells to total cells in a sample of autograft?

In young people there is approximately one osteogenic precursor cell to 50,000 total cells. This proportion sinks to one to 200,000 cells in elderly people, explaining the greater reliability of fusions in younger patients.

19. What is the risk of virus transmission with massive allografts? With cancellous chip grafts?

Massive allografts containing blood, processed according to current standards (including serological testing of the donor), entail a 1:1,000,000 risk of virus transmission. In the case of chip grafts this risk becomes negligible.

20. Has use of allograft bone ever resulted in transmission of HIV infection? Of hepatitis C infection?

No HIV infection has ever been transmitted since 1985. No hepatitis C infection has ever been transmitted since 1990.

21. How is human allograft obtained?

Allograft bone is obtained from volunteer donors. Charges reflect costs associated with screening, processing, packaging, warehousing, and distributing the bone. Currently a $13 \times 18 \times 15$ mm tricortical ilium bone graft costs approximately $750.

22. Name important applications for allograft bone.

Massive osteochondral grafts allow the possibility of limb-sparing tumor surgery. These grafts must be fresh to preserve the viability of the articular cartilage. They do not incorporate completely but, depending on the type of graft, unite with a high degree of success.

23. Describe the major types of osteochondral allografts and indications for their use.

- Osteochondral plug grafts, used chiefly for repair of damaged articular surfaces such as osteochondritis dissecans lesions.

- Unicondylar allograft, used chiefly from reconstruction of defects created after the resection of benign tumors about the knee, such as giant cell tumors and chondroblastoma. These grafts are not useful for malignant tumors because tumor margins would be inadequate. Results are excellent with a high union rate.
- Hemijoint allograft, typically used after resection of high grade osteosarcomas. One of the biggest technical problems is the restoration of ligamentous stability after implantation.
- Whole joint allografts. Because results are unreliable, this technique should be considered investigational.

24. How can BMP be delivered to the fusion site?
In the only clinically approved application of rh-BMP-2 at present, the BMP is combined with a collagen sponge in a titanium tapered lumber interbody cage to achieve a lumbar anterior interbody fusion. The proper carrier is critical to the success of fusion stimulation of BMP. An attempt to achieve posterolateral spinal fusion in rhesus monkeys with BMP on a collagen sponge has not met with success, presumably because in the posterolateral fusion model the BMP is squeezed out of the sponge and does not remain in place long enough to achieve a fusion. Use of a hydroxyapatite-tricalcium phosphate carrier, however, gave a 100% fusion rate in rhesus monkeys.

25. What properties determine the osteoconductivity of ceramic bone graft substitutes such as hydroxyapatite or tricalcium phosphate?
Both substances are closely related chemically to the mineral salts of bone itself, rendering them biocompatible. Osteoconductivity also depends on the pore size of the material and the ability to support osteogenic cell populations in culture. Both substances can bind growth factors such as BMP. The capacity to be adsorbed and replaced with bone is important to allow the newly formed bone to experience the mechanical stresses that stimulate remodeling.

26. What is meant by cell-based graft augmentation?
This term describes the concept of augmenting a fusion with populations of mesenchymal stem cells that have the potential to differentiate into osteoblasts. Approaches include implantation of autologous bone marrow cell, implantation of enriched populations of mesenchymal stem cells grown ex vivo in tissue cultures, and implantation of mesenchymal stem cells predifferentiated into osteoblasts in tissue culture.

BIBLIOGRAPHY

1. Boden SD, Martin GJ, Marone MA, et al: Posterolateral lumbar intertransverse process spine arthrodesis with recombinant human bone morphogenetic protein 2/hydroxyapatite-tricalcium phosphate after laminectomy in the nonhuman primate. Spine 24:1179–1185, 1999.
2. Caplan AI: Mesenchymal stem cells. J Orthop Res 9:641–650, 1991.
3. Dimar JR, Ante WA, Zhang YP, Glassman SD: The effects of nonsteroidal anti-inflammatory drugs on posterior spinal fusions in the rat, Spine 21:1870–1876, 1996.
4. Ebraheim NA, Elgafy H, Xu R: Bone graft harvesting from iliac and fibular donor sites: Techniques and complications. J Am Assoc Orthop Surg 9:210–218, 2001.
5. Frakenburg EP, Goldstein SA, Bauer TW, et al: Biomechanical and histological evaluation of a calcium phosphate cement. J Bone Joint Surg 80A:1112–1124, 1998.
6. Heckman JD, Ehler W, Brooks BP, et al: Bone morphogenetic protein but not transforming growth factor-β enhances bone formation in canine diaphyseal nonunions implanted with a biodegradable composite polymer. J Bone Joint Surg 81A:1717–1729, 1999.
7. Helm GA, Dauoub H, Jane JA: Bone graft substitutes for the promotion of spinal arthrodesis. Neurosurg Focus 10(4):1–5, 2001.
8. Hilibrand AS, Fye MA, Emery SE, et al: Impact of smoking on the outcome of anterior cervical arthrodesis with interbody or strut-grafting. J Bone Joint Surg 83A:668–673, 2001.
9. Silcox DH, Daftari T, Boden SD, et al: The effect of nicotine on spinal fusion. Spine 20:1549–1553, 1995.

10. Sim FH, Frassica FJ: Use of allografts following resection of tumors of the musculoskeletal system. American Academy of Orthopedic Surgeons, Instructional Course Lectures 42:405–413, 1993.
11. Summers BN, Eisenstein SM: Donor site pain from the ilium: A complication of lumbar spine fusion, J Bone Joint Surg 71B:677–680, 1989.
12. Tomford W: Bone graft substitutes. Presented at the Annual Meeting of the American Academy of Orthopedic Surgeons, Dallas, Texas, February 14, 2002.
13. Urist MR: Bone: Formation by autoinduction. Science 150:893–899, 1965.
14. Xu R, Ebraheim NA, Yeasting RA, Jackson WT: Anatomic considerations for posterior iliac bone harvesting. Spine 21:1017–1020, 1996.

17. MUSCULOSKELETAL TUMORS

Brian E. Brigman, M.D.

1. What is the difference between a sarcoma and a carcinoma?

A sarcoma (*Sar* = Greek for "fleshy") is a malignancy arising in mesenchymal tissue (fibrous tissue, muscle, bone, adipose). A carcinoma arises from an epithelial cell origin. Sarcomas typically metastasize hematogenously, whereas carcinomas typically metastasize through the lymphatic system.

2. How common are primary malignant musculoskeletal tumors?

They are rare. About 2000 new primary malignant tumors of bone (excluding multiple myeloma) are diagnosed in the United States yearly. About 6500 new soft-tissue sarcomas are diagnosed in the United States yearly. This contrasts with the estimated 165,000 cases of lung cancer, 185,000 cases of breast cancer and 130,000 cases of colon cancer newly diagnosed in the United States yearly.

3. What factors predispose someone to a sarcoma?

Radiation treatment	p53 mutations	Multiple hereditary exostoses
Chemotherapeutic treatment	Retinoblastoma	Langer-Giedion syndrome
Neurofibromatosis-1	Maffuci syndrome	Defect-11 syndrome
Paget's disease	Ollier's disease	Gardner's syndrome
Li-Fraumeni syndrome	Chronic lymphedema	

4. How are tumors of the musculoskeletal system staged?

Enneking developed a system of staging for musculoskeletal tumors based on biologic aggressiveness, anatomic site, and metastases. Biologic aggressiveness, or Grade (G), is an assessment of histologic grade, radiographic classification, and clinical course. Tumors are stratified into benign (G0), low-grade malignant (G1), and high-grade malignant (G2) categories based on these criteria. Anatomic site (T) places tumors into intracompartmental (T1) and extracompartmental (T2) groups. Intracompartmental tumors are contained within an anatomic compartment that serves as a natural barrier to tumor extension. These natural barriers include cortical bone, articular cartilage, joint capsule, and fascia. Extracompartmental tumors span at least one of these natural barriers. Tumors that have either regional or distant metastases are labeled M1, and those with no metastases are designated M0.

Benign lesions (G0) are staged into one of three groups. Benign stage 1 lesions are latent, static lesions. Benign stage 2 lesions are progressive, and may expand a fascial or cortical margin but do not broach it. Benign stage 3 lesions are aggressive and have breached compartments or have metastasized.

Malignant lesions without metastases are grouped into stage I (G1) or stage II (G2). Malignant lesions of either grade with local or distant metastases are grouped into stage III. Each of these malignant stages is further stratified based on anatomic site. Intracompartmental lesions are labeled "A," and extracompartmental lesions are labeled "B."

STAGE	IA	IB	IIA	IIB	IIIA	IIIB
Grade	G1	G1	G2	G2	G1 or G2	G1 or G2
Site	T1	T2	T1	T2	T1	T2
Metastases	M0	M0	M0	M0	M1	M1

5. Name some benign (G0), low-grade malignant (G1), and high-grade malignant (G2) musculoskeletal lesions.

BENIGN (G0)	LOW-GRADE MALIGNANT (G1)	HIGH-GRADE MALIGNANT (G2)
Nonossifying fibroma	Parosteal osteosarcoma	Classic osteosarcoma
Osteoid osteoma	Periosteal osteosarcoma	Telangiectatic osteosarcoma
Osteoblastoma	Secondary chondrosarcoma	Primary chondrosarcoma
Enchondroma	Clear cell chondrosarcoma	Dedifferentiated chondrosarcoma
Osteochondroma	Adamantinoma	Fibrosarcoma
Chondroblastoma	Hemangioendothelioma	Malignant fibrous histiocytoma
Aneurysmal bone cyst	Chordoma	Ewing's sarcoma
Giant cell tumor	Dermatofibrosarcoma protuberans	Liposarcoma
Lipoma	Well-differentiated liposarcoma	Synovial sarcoma
Hemangioma		Epithelioid sarcoma
Schwannoma		
Myxoma		

6. Discuss the principles for biopsy of musculoskeletal tumors.
Biopsy of musculoskeletal tumors should generally be relegated to the surgeon responsible for the final management of the tumor. An improperly placed biopsy incision may compromise the final outcome of treatment. Needle biopsy has the advantages of less morbidity and lower cost, but may not provide sufficient tissue for a diagnosis and is subject to sampling error. Excisional biopsy may be considered with small, benign appearing lesions. Open incisional biopsy should be planned with the definitive surgical procedure in mind, because the biopsy tract will be considered contaminated and necessarily will be removed en bloc with the tumor at the time of tumor excision. Transverse incisions should be avoided, and the biopsy should traverse the minimum number of compartments. Neurovascular structures should be avoided. The biopsy specimen should be taken from the periphery of the soft-tissue extension of the tumor. If there is no soft-tissue extension, a small round or oval window in the cortex should be fashioned to decrease the risk of pathologic fracture. A tourniquet should be used and meticulous hemostasis must be obtained.

7. Do sarcomas have a capsule?
Sarcomas do not have a true capsule. As they grow radially they compress adjacent tissue into a pseudocapsule. This pseudocapsule contains the zone of compression and a surrounding reactive zone made up of neovascular tissue and an inflammatory infiltrate.

8. Describe orthopaedic oncologic surgical margins.
There are four types of musculoskeletal surgical margins. An **intralesional margin** has a plane of dissection through the tumor; by definition, tumor is left behind. A **marginal margin** has a plane of dissection through the reactive zone of the pseudocapsule and may have left microscopic tumor behind. A **wide margin** is through completely normal tissue outside of the reactive zone and potentially may leave "skip" metastases behind. A **radical margin** is a complete *resection* of the affected compartment.

9. What is an osteoid osteoma? How does it present?

An osteoid osteoma is a benign osteoblastic lesion characterized by a well-demarcated central nidus of ≤ 1.5 cm surrounded by dense reactive bone. It typically occurs in the metaphyseal regions of long bones or in the posterior elements of the spine in patients aged 5–30 years. Patients present with pain that increases over time. It is typically worse at night and is characteristically relieved by salicylates or other NSAIDs. Lesions in the posterior elements of the spine can produce a painful scoliosis.

10. What are the treatment options for osteoid osteoma?

Surgical treatment by en bloc excision of the nidus or intralesional curettage has been the mainstay of treatment. A percutaneous radiofrequency ablative treatment has recently been described but is not a viable option for lesions in the spine. Medical treatment with NSAIDs is also an option.

11. Describe the difference between an osteoid osteoma and an osteoblastoma.

An osteoblastoma is larger than an osteoid osteoma and often does not have a rim of reactive bone around it. Both are common in the posterior element of the spine. Treatment of osteoblastoma is surgical excision.

OSTEOCHONDROMA AND ENCHONDROMA

12. Name the benign cartilage-forming tumors of the musculoskeletal system.

Osteochondroma, enchondroma, chondroblastoma, and chondromyxoid fibroma.

13. What is an osteochondroma? How does it present?

An osteochondroma is a benign, cartilage-capped cortical exostosis in the metaphyseal or epiphyseal region of bone. The most common sites are distal femur, proximal tibia, proximal humerus, distal radius, and distal tibia. Osteochondromas are thought to arise as the result of aberrant growth plate cartilage and grow through enchondral ossification until the growth plate from which they arose stops growing. They exist in sessile and pedunculated forms, and in each case the cortical margins of the osteochondroma are continuous with the cortical margin of the underlying bone. Osteochondromas are painless and are usually symptomless unless they are palpable. Occasionally neurovascular compression by an osteochondroma causes symptoms. A painful osteochondroma may signify a fracture of the lesion or malignant degeneration, typically to a low-grade chondrosarcoma. Malignant degeneration occurs in < 1% of osteochondromas. An autosomal dominant hereditary form (multiple hereditary exostoses) represents about 10% of patients with osteochondroma.

14. What is the treatment of osteochondroma?

Surgical excision is necessary only if the lesions become symptomatic or disfiguring.

15. What is an enchondroma?

An enchondroma is a benign island of mature cartilage within a bone, typically in the metaphyseal area. When located on the surface of the bone, it is termed a *periosteal chondroma*. It is the most common primary tumor of bone in the hand, but any bone can be affected. Enchondromas are usually asymptomatic.

16. What is the treatment for enchondroma?

Observation is the mainstay of treatment. If lesions grow or are painful, then en bloc excision or curettage is indicated.

17. What are Ollier's disease and Mafucci syndrome?

Ollier's disease is an eponym for multiple enchondromatosis. Lesions are often unilateral and may result in a dysplastic appearance to bones. A 30% risk of sarcomatous degeneration to chondrosarcoma in patients with Ollier's disease is quoted in the literature, but is probably an overestimate.

Maffuci syndrome is multiple enchondromas with associated soft-tissue angiomas. A 100% risk of sarcomatous degeneration to chondrosarcoma in patients with Maffuci syndrome is quoted in the literature, but again, is likely an overestimate.

Both Ollier's disease and Mafucci syndrome patients carry an increased risk of visceral malignancy, including gastrointestinal adenocarcinoma and astrocytoma.

CHONDROBLASTOMA AND GIANT CELL TUMOR

18. What is a chondroblastoma?
A chondroblastoma is a benign tumor characteristically located in the epiphysis or in an apophysis. Chondroblastomas typically affect people in their second decade of life. They are often painful and may limit joint motion. Histologically, the stromal cells of chondroblastomas are polyhedral with clear halos around the nuclei resulting in the characteristic "chicken wire" appearance. About 2% of chondroblastomas are metastatic to the lungs.

19. What is the treatment for chondroblastoma?
Intralesional curettage with bone grafting or cementage yields an approximate 10% recurrence rate.

20. What other tumor has a predilection for the end of a long bone?
Giant cell tumor.

21. What is the cell of origin for giant cell tumor, Ewing's sarcoma, and adamantinoma?
The cell of origin for each is unknown.

22. The histologic slide has giant cells on it. Doesn't that mean it is a giant cell tumor?
No. Many tumors, ranging from benign osteoid osteoma to malignant osteosarcoma, may contain giant cells.

23. Who gets giant cell tumors?
Giant cell tumor typically affects patients between 20 and 60 years of age. It is one of the few tumors that occur more commonly in women than in men. About one-half occur around the knee. Patients usually present with pain in the affected area. About 2% of giant cell tumors are metastatic to the lung.

24. What is the treatment for giant cell tumor?
Intralesional curettage with cementing or bone grafting gives local control in about 80% of patients.

CHONDROSARCOMA

25. What is a chondrosarcoma? How does it present?
A chondrosarcoma is a malignant, cartilage-forming tumor. It occurs in patients ≥ 30 years of age. Common sites include the pelvis (30%), proximal and distal femur, ribs, proximal humerus, and proximal tibia. Patients typically present with pain or a mass. Pelvic lesions are often misdiagnosed or diagnosed late.

26. What is the difference between a primary and secondary chondrosarcoma?
A primary chondrosarcoma arises de novo in a previously normal bone. A secondary chondrosarcoma arises from preexisting benign cartilage lesion, such as an enchondroma or osteochondroma. Primary chondrosarcomas may be low- or high-grade tumors. Secondary tumors are almost always low grade.

27. What is the most common stage of chondrosarcoma at presentation?
IA.

28. What is the treatment for chondrosarcoma?
Excision with a wide margin is standard treatment. These lesions are resistant to chemotherapy and radiation.

OSTEOSARCOMA

29. What is an osteosarcoma? How does it present?
An osteosarcoma is a malignant tumor that produces osteoid. Osteosarcomas are typically found in metaphyseal locations. More than one-half occur about the knee. Patients present with pain, a mass, or occasionally a pathologic fracture. It typically affects patients in their second or third decade, although there is a second peak of incidence in patients > 60 years old, usually with secondary osteosarcoma. Approximately 1000 new cases of osteosarcoma are diagnosed in the United States yearly.

30. What is the most common stage of osteosarcoma at presentation?
IIB (75%). About 15% are stage III.

31. What is a secondary osteosarcoma?
A secondary osteosarcoma develops in abnormal bone and is usually associated with irradiated bone, Paget's disease, or fibrous dysplasia. Secondary osteosarcomas are typically high-grade malignancies.

32. What are the radiographic findings of osteosarcoma?
Plain films often reveal permeative lesion with cortical destruction. Codman's triangles of bone appear as tumor extension elevates periosteum from the underlying bone. Cortical soft-tissue extension may produce radiating spicules of bone, resulting in the characteristic "sun ray" appearance.

33. What other imaging studies should be ordered?
At a minimum, an MRI of the region (including the entire length of the affected bone) to assess soft-tissue extension and rule out skip lesions and a CT scan of the chest to rule out metastatic disease to the lungs should be obtained. Techniques to evaluate for extrapulmonary metastases include ^{99}Tc scintigraphy or rapid whole body STIR MRI.

34. What is the treatment for osteosarcoma?
Patients with high-grade tumors are subjected to a high-dose chemotherapeutic induction protocol typically including doxirubicin, cis-platin, high-dose methotrexate and ifosfamide. The patients are restaged after the 10–12 week induction protocol then undergo a wide resection of the tumor with limb salvage if deemed viable by the restaging studies. Limb salvage is feasible in about 90% of patients with osteosarcoma. The post-operative adjuvant chemotherapeutic regimen may be adjusted based on the amount of necrosis present in the resected speciment. Low-grade osteosarcomas do not require chemotherapy, only resection.

35. What are the surgical options for osteosarcoma about the knee?
The initial decision is between amputation and limb salvage surgery. Involvement of the neurovascular bundle makes limb salvage difficult. If limb salvage is a viable option, several reconstruction methods are available following tumor resection. Fusion of the knee joint, reconstruction of the knee with a metal prosthesis, or allograft reconstruction are possible. In very young children, these options are less appealing because of the resulting leg length discrepancy at ma-

turity. In these patients an amputation, expandable prosthesis or Van Nes rotationplasty are options. A Van Nes rotationplasty fuses the shortened femur to the shortened tibia after rotation of the tibia 180° to allow the ankle joint to function as a knee joint in a prosthesis.

36. What is the common metastatic pattern found with osteosarcoma?
Like most sarcomas, osteosarcoma most often metastasizes hematogenously. The lungs, by far, are the most common site of metastases, but metastatic disease can be found in liver, brain, bones, kidneys, and regional lymph nodes.

37. What is the prognosis for osteosarcoma?
The prognosis has improved dramatically since the onset of adjuvant chemotherapeutic treatment. Today, 5-year disease-free survival rates in surgically accessible tumors is about 70% following limb salvage surgery.

38. Are there any factors other than stage and adequacy of resection that affect prognosis?
Yes. Tumor size (patients with smaller tumors fare better) and response to chemotherapy (patients with tumors responding to chemotherapy fare better). In a recent meta-analysis of prognostic factors, tumor necrosis in response to chemotherapy was the only variable that remained significant following multivariate analysis.

39. What are MDR-1 and p-glycoprotein?
The MDR-1, or multidrug resistance -1 gene, codes for a 170 kDa membrane protein called p-glycoprotein. This protein functions as an energy-dependent efflux pump which decreases the intracellular concentration of many cytotoxic agents. This gene and its product play a part in the resistance to chemotherapy expressed by some osteosarcomas and other tumors.

EWING'S SARCOMA

40. What is Ewing's sarcoma? How does it present?
Ewing's sarcoma is a primitive small and round blue cell tumor possibly related to primitive neuroectodermal tumors. Patients are usually in their first two decades of life. They present with pain and a mass at the site of the tumor, and they may have constitutional symptoms including fever, anemia, leukocytosis, and an increased sedimentation rate. The tumor is characteristically diaphyseal in location and affects the femur most commonly, but is seen in other long bones and in pelvis in about 20% of cases.

41. What is the radiographic appearance of Ewing's sarcoma?
Ewing's sarcomas typically present as a permeative lesion with cortical destruction and a soft-tissue mass. A periosteal reaction of layers of bone, the so-called "onion skin" appearance, may be present.

42. What genetic derangement is noted in Ewing's sarcoma?
The translocation of chromosome 11 with chromosome 22 [t(11;22)(q24;q12)] is found consistently in Ewing's sarcoma.

43. What is the treatment for Ewing's sarcoma?
The treatment is in evolution. Until recently, radiation treatment alone was used. Problems with recurrence, eventual leg length discrepancy, secondary sarcomas in irradiated limbs, and advances in chemotherapy and surgical techniques have led to protocols of neoadjuvant chemotherapy followed by wide resection and further chemotherapy. Location of the tumor (patients with distal tumors fare better) and its response to chemotherapy (patients with tumors responding to chemotherapy fare better) correlate with long-term survival.

44. What is the most common site of occurrence of adamantinoma?
The tibia.

MULTIPLE MYELOMA

45. What is multiple myeloma? How does it present?
Multiple myeloma is a tumor made up of malignant monoclonal plasma cells. It usually affects patients > 40 years old. Patients often present with malaise, bone pain, or a pathologic fracture.

46. What are the radiographic findings?
The classic radiographic appearance is multiple lytic "punched out" areas in bone. These lesions often do not show uptake of isotope on bone scan, making a skeletal survey the most important radiographic test.

47. What are the laboratory findings associated with multiple myeloma?
A serum protein electrophoresis usually reveals a monoclonal immunoglobulin spike in the a or g region. Light chain immunoglobulins, or Bence-Jones protein, may be found in the urine. Hypercalcemia may be noted. Bone marrow aspirate reveals sheets of "clock-faced" plasma cells.

48. What is the treatment for multiple myeloma?
Multiagent chemotherapy, radiation, and surgical fixation of impending fracture. The average survival is < 2 years.

METASTATIC CARCINOMA

49. What is the most common malignant lesion in bone?
Metastatic carcinoma is by far the most common malignancy in bone.

50. Where do the majority of metastases to bone originate?
Breast, prostate, lung, kidney, and thyroid.

51. What are the most common sites for bony metastases?
Thoracic and lumbar spine, pelvis, femur, rib, proximal humerus, and skull.

52. How common are metastases to the hand?
Acral metastatic disease is very rare. When it does occur, it is usually from lung carcinoma.

53. How are bony metastases treated?
If the primary tumor is unknown, it should be identified. Treatment of metastatic disease is aimed at controlling pain and maintaining function. Local radiation may provide pain relief. Surgical fixation is indicated for impending fractures.

54. What are criteria for an impending fracture?
More than 50% destruction of diaphyseal cortex, a lesion > 2.5 cm in diameter, or persistent pain following irradiation.

SOFT-TISSUE SARCOMA

55. What is the most common soft tissue mass?
Benign soft-tissue masses are approximately 200 times more common than malignant ones. The most common soft-tissue mass is a lipoma. These are usually non-tender, soft, subcutaneous masses.

56. Who gets soft-tissue sarcomas? How do they present?

Soft-tissue sarcoma is predominately a disease of older persons. They typically present with a painless mass. The thigh and buttock are the most common areas of presentation. Many are misdiagnosed as a "pulled muscle."

57. What are the most common soft-tissue sarcomas?

Malignant fibrous histiocytoma is the most common soft tissue sarcoma. Liposarcoma and synovial sarcoma round out the top three.

58. How should a patient with a suspected soft-tissue sarcoma be worked up?

An MRI to evaluate the extent of local disease, a plain film to evaluate for calcification within the lesion and a CT scan of the chest to rule out metastatic disease. Positron emission tomography (PET) scans are being investigated as a means of evaluating for distant metastatic disease. A biopsy is necessary for tissue diagnosis, but should be done after imaging of the lesion.

59. Which soft-tissue sarcomas show calcifications?

Synovial sarcoma shows focal calcification in 15–20% of cases. Epithelioid sarcoma may occasionaly show calcification as well. Other, less common soft-tissue sarcomas which may show calcifications include extraskeletal chondrosarcoma, clear cell sarcoma and ossifying fibromyxoid tumor of soft parts.

60. What is the treatment for soft-tissue sarcoma?

Despite a wide diversity in histogenesis, treatment of soft-tissue sarcoma is relatively uniform. The mainstay of treatment is a wide resection. Pre or post-operative radiation therapy allows for wide local resection with a smaller local recurrence rate. A common regimen for a large (>5 cm) high-grade lesion deep to the fascia would include 50 Gy of pre-operative external beam radiotherapy followed by wide local resection. If close or positve margins are encountered intraoperatively, then intraoperative external beam radiation, brachytherapy catheter placement in the region of concern, or supplemental post-operative external beam radiotherapy of 15 Gy could be used. If wide margins are obtained then no supplemental radiotherapy is necessary. Many institutions are investigating a role for chemotherapy in the treatment of high-grade soft-tissue sarcoma, however no report has shown an increase in patient survival attributable to chemotherapy.

61. What prognostic factors are present with soft-tissue sarcoma?

Several retrospective studies or meta-analyses of prognostic factors in soft-tissue sarcoma have been published. High-grade tumors, tumors deep to the fascia, large tumors (>5 cm), and positive margins have all been shown to adversely affect survival.

BIBLIOGRAPHY

1. Aurias A, Rimbaud C, Buffe D, et al: Chromosomal translocations in Ewing's sarcoma. N Engl J Med 309:496–497, 1983.
2. Bieling P, Rehan N, Winkler P, et al: Tumor size and prognosis in aggressively treated osteosarcoma. J Clin Oncol 14:848–858, 1996.
3. Bridge JA, Schwartz HS, Neff JR: Bone sarcomas. In Abeloff MD, Armitage JO, Lichter AS, Niderhuber JE (eds): Clinical Oncology, 2nd ed. Orlando, FL, Harcourt Brace, 2000, pp 2160–2272.
4. Conrad EU: Multimodality Management of Maligmant Soft-Tissue Tumors. In Menendez LR (ed): Orthopaedic Knowledge Update: Musculoskeletal Tumors. Rosemont, IL, American Academy of Orthopaedic Surgeons, 2002, pp 255–260.
5. Enneking WE, Spanier SS, Goodman MA: A system for the surgical staging of musculoskeletal sarcoma. Clin Orthop Rel Res 153:106–120, 1980.
6. Davis AM, Bell RS, Goodwin PJ: Prognostic factors in osteosarcoma: A critical review. J Clin Oncol 12:423–431, 1994.
7. Harrington KD: Impending pathologic fractures from metastatic malignancy: Evaluation and management. Instr Course Lect 35:357–381, 1986.

8. Kneisl JS, Simon MA: Medical management compared with operative treatment for osteoid osteoma. J Bone Joint Surg 74A:179–185, 1992.

9. Mankin HJ, Mankin CJ, Simon MA: The hazards of the biopsy, revisited. J Bone Joint Surg 78A: 656–663, 1996.

10. Picci P, Sangiorgi L, Rougraff BT, et al: Relationship of chemotherapy-induced necrosis and surgical margins to local recurrence in osteosarcoma. J Clin Oncol 12:2699–2705, 1994.

11. Pisters PW, Leung DH, Woodruff J: Analysis of prognostic factors in 1,041 patients with localized soft tissue sarcomas of the extremities. J Clin Oncol 14:1679–1989, 1996.

12. Rosenthal DI, Hornicek FJ, Wolfe MW, et al: Percutaneous radiofrequency coagulation of osteoid osteoma compared with operative treatment. J Bone Joint Surg 80A:815–821, 1998.

13. Skrzynksi MC, Biermann JS, Montag A, Simon MA: Diagnostic accuracy and charge-savings of outpatient core needle biopsy compared with open biopsy of musculoskeletal tumors. J Bone Joint Surg 78A:644–649, 1996.

14. Winkelmann WW: Rotationplasty. Orthop Clin North Am 27:503–523, 1996.

15. Wunder JS, Bell RS, Wold L, Andrulis IL: Expression of the multidrug resistance gene in osteosarcoma: A pilot study. J Orthop Res 11:396–403, 1993.

16. Wurtz LD, Peabody TD, Simon MA: Delay in the diagnosis and treatment of primary bone sarcoma of the pelvis. J Bone Joint Surg 81A:317–325, 1999.

II. Congenital and Developmental Disorders

18. CONNECTIVE TISSUE DISORDERS (SKELETAL DYSPLASIA)

Deepak V. Chavda, M.D. and Zubin G. Khubchandani, M.D.

1. Who pioneered the work on skeletal dysplasia?
Sir Thomas Fairbank of Edinburgh, Scotland, pioneered the work on skeletal dysplasia in his 1951 book, *An Atlas of General Affections of the Skeleton.*

2. How are the skeletal dysplasias classified?
Most orthopedists follow the classification developed by Rubin, which is based on anatomic distribution of bone changes. Two of the most common forms are multiple epiphyseal dysplasia and spondyloepiphyseal dysplasia.

3. Define the terms dysplasia, dwarfism, midget, dysostosis, malformation, and deformity.
Dysplasia is now the preferred term for dwarfism and is used when the developmental changes in the skeleton are generalized.

Dwarfism denotes a pathologic diminution in stature (below the tenth percentile). Dwarfism is further divided into the proportionate (**midget**) and disproportionate (short-limb or short-trunk) types. The short-limb variety is further subdivided according to the site of maximal shortening: rhizomelic (in the proximal portion), mesomelic (in the middle), and acromelic (in the distal portion).

Dysostosis denotes the developmental changes affecting a single bone or segment of the skeleton.

Malformation means a primary abnormality of development.

Deformity denotes a change in the structure of a previously normal bone.

4. What is multiple epiphyseal dysplasia (MED)?
MED, one of the more common bone dysplasias, is characterized by irregularity in development of the epiphysis. Late appearance or mottling of the ossification centers, knobby joints, stubby digits, and minor shortening of stature is present, with little or no vertebral involvement. The condition is extremely rare (prevalence: 11 per million index cases) and shows no gender predilection.

5. What is chondrodysplasia?
Chondrodysplasia is a heterogeneous group of rare conditions characterized by stippling of the epiphyses, disordered longitudinal bone growth, mental retardation, and cataracts. It is also referred to as chondrodystrophia fetalis ossificans, chondrodystrophia punctata, calcificans punctata, dysplasia epiphysealis punctata, stippled epiphyses, chondrodystrophia calcificans congenita, and Conradi's disease.

6. What is Stickler's syndrome?
Stickler's syndrome is characterized by epiphyseal changes similar to those of MED. The feature that differentiates Stickler's syndrome from MED is severe progressive myopia with retinal detachment and blindness. Patients may have conductive hearing loss and cleft palate. Spinal deformities include minimal platyspondyly and anterior wedging of the vertebrae, causing

thoracic kyphosis (as in Scheuermann's disease). Stickler's syndrome is inherited as autosomal dominant.

7. What is dysplasia epiphysealis hemimelia (DEH)?

DEH is characterized by asymmetric abnormal cartilage proliferation and subsequent enchondral ossification in an epiphysis of a tarsal, carpal, or flat bone. It is limited to the medial or lateral half of a single limb. Other synonyms include tarsomegaly, tarsoepiphyseal aclasis, and benign epiphyseal osteochondroma. Its etiology is unknown.

8. What is the most common type of dwarfism?

The most common type of dwarfism is achondroplasia, a short-limbed disproportionate disorder that results from defective formation of enchondral bone. Formation of intramembranous bone is unaffected. The clinical syndrome consists of short limbs, a large, bulging cranium (especially the forehead), a low nasal bridge, a narrowed spinal canal in the lumbar region, and distinctive pelvic changes. It is autosomal dominant in inheritance, although 80–90% of cases are due to spontaneous new mutations. The most disabling clinical problems are thoracolumbar kyphosis or lumbar spinal stenosis. The latter affects up to 50% of achondroplasts.

Its presence in antiquity is evident from the depiction of the Egyptian goddess Ptah as an achondroplast and from the discovery of an achondroplastic skeleton from the early Egyptian period. In the Middle Ages, court jesters were often achondroplastic dwarfs. Even today they serve in circuses and theaters, where they are incorrectly called "midgets."

9. What is spondyloepiphyseal dysplasia?

Spondyloepiphyseal dysplasia is a group of disorders causing short-trunk disproportionate dwarfism. They are generally autosomal dominant, although the tarda form is x-linked recessive. Clinical features include precocious arthritis, coxa vara, atlantoaxial instability, retinal detachment, and myopia.

10. What is pseudoachondroplasia?

Pseudoachondroplasia is a short-limbed form of dwarfism that involves both the epiphyses and metaphyses. The prevalence is about 4 cases per million population. Clinically it can be distinguished from achondroplasia by the normal face and skull and the absence of interpedicular narrowing of the lumbar vertebrae. Precocious arthritis is a major problem.

11. Is lengthening or angular correction of the lower limbs in patients with skeletal dysplasias a good option?

Yes and no. By using callus distraction (callotasis) surgical technique, it is possible to gain approximately 7 cm in both the femur and tibia. Functioning of the lengthened limbs improves, but malalignment of the mechanical axis of the bones may be present. The rate of complications following the procedure is much higher in children with underlying bone disorders compared with children with normal bone. Correction of angular limb deformities such as genu varum (bow legs) can be achieved by hemichondrodiatasis, in which distraction is applied through only a portion of the growth plate (physis).

12. What is marble bone disease?

Marble bone disease, also called osteopetrosis, is characterized by failure of bone resorption due to functional deficiency of the osteoclasts with persistence of calcified chondroid and primitive bone. On radiographs it appears as a striking opacity of the bones, lack of cortical endosteal margins, and failure of bone remodeling. The only effective treatment is bone marrow transplantation.

13. What is spotted bone disease?

Spotted bone disease, also called osteopoikilosis, is characterized by dense ovoid or circular spots in cancellous bone, usually found in clusters in the metaphyseal or epiphyseal regions of long bones. These 3- to 5-mm densities do not affect the cortex or the contour of the bone and may be present at birth. The common locations are carpals, tarsals, ends of large tubular bones, or around the acetabulum. Spotted bone disease does not cause symptoms, and no treatment is required.

14. What is Caffey's disease?

Caffey's disease, or infantile cortical hyperostosis, is a rare, self-limiting condition of early infancy characterized by swelling of soft tissues, cortical thickening of the underlying bones, and hyperirritability. Roske first noted this disorder in 1930; however, it was thoroughly described by Caffey and Silverman in 1945.

15. What is osteogenesis imperfecta (OI)?

OI is in fact several genetically and clinically heterogeneous syndromes characterized by skeletal fragility. Other manifestations are dentinogenesis imperfecta, blue sclerae, deafness, and ligamentous hyperlaxity. Clinical features include multiple fractures, knee deformities, and scoliosis. It may be difficult to distinguish the tarda form of OI from child abuse.

16. Which clinical finding is a strong predictor of future walking ability in patients with OI?

The ability to sit by the age of 10 months is a good predictor of future walking ability (75% of patients). No patients with OI who have delayed and dependent sitting can walk independently.

17. What are clinically significant features of Marfan syndrome?

The clinically significant features of Marfan syndrome include disproportionately long, thin limbs and digits, scoliosis, generalized joint laxity, dislocation of the lenses, dissecting aortic aneurysm, prolapsed cardiac valves, and increased prevalence of hernias. Marfan, a French pediatrician, originally described the syndrome in 1896. He termed the condition "dolichostemelia," meaning "long, thin limbs." Photographs of Abraham Lincoln suggest that he was afflicted with Marfan syndrome.

18. What is Ehlers-Danlos syndrome?

Ehlers-Danlos syndrome is a group of syndromes caused by defective collagen metabolism and characterized by skin changes of hyper extensibility, fragility, and easy bruisibility with resultant "cigarette paper" scarring, extreme ligamentous laxity of the joints, and bone fragility with osteopenia. There is no specific treatment for this disorder.

19. Define dyschondroplasia, Ollier's disease, and Maffucci's syndrome.

Dyschondroplasia is a rare, nonhereditary developmental defect characterized by the presence of circumscribed masses of cartilage arranged in a linear fashion in the interior of bones.

Multiple enchondromata are due to harmartomatous proliferation of cartilage cells that originate within the bones and from the cambium layer of the periosteum. When the lesions are predominantly unilateral, the eponym **Ollier's disease** is used. Multiple enchondromata with multiple hemangiomas is termed **Maffucci's syndrome**. Both conditions require long-term monitoring because malignant degeneration may occur in up to 25% of those patients with Ollier's disease and nearly 100% of those with Maffucci's syndrome.

20. Describe fibrodysplasia (myositis) ossificans progressiva (FOP).

FOP is a rare disease transmitted in an autosomal dominant inheritance pattern. Defects in the skeletal patterning are present, particularly affecting the big toes. Progressive endochondral or enchondral ossification of the large striated muscles in a specific order ultimately leads to prolonged and severe disability. Painful swelling of the muscles (myositis) further leads to ossification at a mean age of 4.6 years (range: 0–16 years). The muscles of the neck and upper spine are the first to be involved, followed by muscles around the hips, other major joints, and jaws. The rate and extent of involvement and disability has no relationship with the age of onset.

21. How is pseudomalignant heterotopic ossification (PHO) different from FOP?

PHO is a rare, self-limited connective tissue disorder of unknown origin. It usually occurs in the second or third decade (only occasionally during childhood). It may mimic soft tissue sarcoma (e.g., extraosseous osteosarcoma) or FOP. PHO affects the limbs (80% of patients) but often spares the big toes. It is possible that PHO is forme fruste of FOP.

22. What are the clinical and radiographic findings in early degenerative changes in the hip of diastrophic dysplasia patients?

Clinical: Rapid and progressive development of flexion contracture and restriction of rotational movements of hips

Radiographic: Flattening and inferomedial bulking of the femoral head

Double-hump deformation

Delayed (more than 12 years) appearance of the proximal femoral ossific nuclei

BIBLIOGRAPHY

1. Daly K, Wisbeach A, Sanpera I Jr, Fixsen JA: The prognosis for walking in osteogenesis imperfecta. J Bone Joint Surg 78-B:77–80, 1996.
2. Kaplan FS, Gannon FH, Hahn GV, et al: Pseudomalignant heterotopic ossification differential diagnosis and report of two cases. Clin Orthop 346:134–140, 1998.
3. Givon U, Schindler A, Ganel A: Hemichondrodiatasis for the treatment of genu varum deformity associated with bone dysplasias. J Pediatr Orthop 21:238–241, 2001.
4. Herring JA (ed): Tachdjian's Pediatric Orthopaedics, 3rd ed. Philadelphia, W.B. Saunders, 2002.
5. Morrissy RT, Weinstein SL: Lovell and Winter's Pediatric Orthopaedics, 5th ed. Philadelphia, J.B. Lippincott, 2000.
6. Naudie D, Hamdy RC, Fassier F, Duhaime M: Complications of the limb-lengthening in children who have an underlying bone disorder. J Bone Joint Surg 80A:18–24, 1998.
7. Smith R: Fibrodysplasia (myositis) ossificans progressiva. Clinical lessons from a rare disease. Clin Orthop 346:7–14, 1998.
8. Smith R: Osteogenesis imperfecta—Where next? (editorial) J Bone Joint Surg 79B:177–178, 1997.
9. Vaara P, Peltonen J, Poussa M, et al: Development of the hip in diastrophic dysplasia. J Bone Joint Surg 80-B:315–320, 1998.
10. Yasui N, Kawabata H, Kojimoto H, et al: Lengthening of the lower limbs in patients with achondroplasia and hypochondroplasia. Clin Orthop 344:298–306, 1997.

19. METABOLIC AND ENDOCRINE DISORDERS

Katherine K. Brady, B.A., and David E. Brown, M.D.

1. How many types of cartilage are there?

There are three types:
- Hyaline cartilage (articular surfaces, growth plate/physis)
- Fibrocartilage (menisci)
- Elastic cartilage (ear)

2. What are the zones of the growing epiphysis?

Beginning at the epiphyseal side, the four zones are (1) zone of growth, (2) zone of cartilage transformation, (3) zone of ossification, and (4) metaphysis. Some authors still use an older terminology that consists of five zones: (1) resting, (2) proliferative, (3) maturation, (4) provisional calcification, and (5) primary spongiosa.

OSTEOPOROSIS

3. What is osteoporosis?

The World Health Organization has defined osteoporosis as a bone mineral density 2.5 standard deviations below the mean for young, white, adult women. Bone mineral density represents approximately 70% of bone strength. Bone strength is also affected by bone geometry, turnover, and accumulated trauma.

4. What is osteomalacia?

Osteomalacia is an osteopenic condition primarily characterized by insufficient mineralization of bone matrix. The onset can be at any age, but osteomalacia in children is rickets. The most common etiologies of osteomalacia are chronic renal failure, vitamin D deficiency or abnormalities of the vitamin D pathway, and hypophosphatemic conditions. Generalized bone pain is a common symptom.

5. What are the laboratory findings that distinguish osteoporosis and osteomalacia?

	Osteoporosis	*Osteomalacia*
Serum Ca++	Normal	Low or normal
Urinary Ca++	High or normal	Normal to low
Serum P_1	Normal	Low or normal
Alkaline phosphatase	Normal	Elevated
Bone biopsy (tetracycline labels)	normal	abnormal

6. What are the risk factors for osteoporosis?

- Female gender
- Increased age
- Estrogen deficiency
- White race
- Low wieght
- Low body mass index
- Family history of osteoporosis
- Smoking history
- History of prior fracture

7. How do we evaluate bone density in patients?

While traditional x-rays can be used to detect initial osteopenia, they are not the preferred method because a 30% decrease in bone mass must occur before it can be detected on plain films. The dual energy x-ray abosorptiometry, or DEXA, system is currently the preferred method to assess patient baseline bone density. DEXA scans are performed on the femoral heads or lumbar spine. Quantitative computed tomography records trabecular bone density by generating a cross-sectional image of the T12 to L4 vertebral bodies. Meausurements from the center of the five vertebrae are averaged for a mean bone density. Quantitative ultrasound (QUS) is among the newest methods of bone density measurement. It is an appealing option because patients are not exposed to radiation. QUS is also being used to evaluate bone strength directly.

8. How is osteoporosis treated?

- Calcium supplementation of 1000 mg to 1500 mg per day
- Vitamin D intake of 400 to 1000 IU per day
- Physical activity that includes impact, such as weight training. Low-impact exercise (walking) has *not* been shown to increase bone density.
- Bisphosphonates such as etidronate, alendronate, and risedronate
- Hormone replacement therapy. Traditional estrogen replacement is most common. The newer selective estrogen receptor modulators increase bone density while reducing the deleterious effects on the breast and endometrium.

CALCIUM HOMEOSTASIS

9. What is the daily requirement of calcium?

Adult	400–500 mg
Child	700 mg
Adolescent	1000–1300 mg
Pregnant women	1500 mg
Lactating women	2000 mg
Postmenopausal women	1500 mg
Major fracture	1500 mg

10. How much calcium is contained in 8 ounces of milk?
Eight ounces of milk contains 250 mg of calcium.

11. What are the three primary calcitropic hormones?
- Vitamin D
- Calcitonin
- Parathyroid hormone (PTH)

12. What are the biologic effects of vitamin D?
Vitamin D, a steroid hormone, functions to increase calcium resorption from bone by strongly promoting osteoclastic resorption (see figure). Vitamin D also enhances calcium absorption across the intestine lumen. The net effect is increased serum calcium.

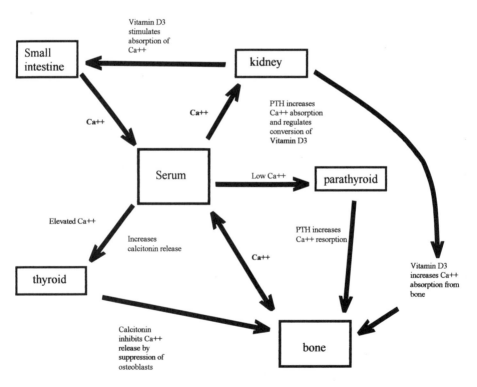

Calcium homeostasis.

13. Describe the biologic effects of calcitonin.

Calcitonin, a peptide hormone produced chiefly by thyroid C-cells, results in lowering of serum calcium, inhibition of osteoclastic bone resorption, shrinking of osteoclasts, and mild stimulation of osteoblasts.

14. What are the effects of parathyroid hormone?

PTH causes the kidney to increase reabsorption of calcium and excretion of phosphate. In bone, osteoclastic resorption is stimulated, releasing calcium and phosphate. The net effect is an increase in serum calcium and a decrease in serum phosphorus.

15. Where is the main storage of calcium and phosphorus in the body?

The skeleton contains 90% of the calcium and 80% of phosphorus in the body.

16. What is a "brown tumor"?

Hyperparathyroidism, primary or secondary, leads to typical changes in bone. Histologic section reveals numerous osteoclasts on the bone surface with characteristic tunneling or dissecting resorption of bony trabeculae (also known as cutting cones). Also evident are resorption of pericellular bone by osteocytes (osteocytic osteolysis), increased woven bone, and marrow replacement by dense fibrous appearing tissue. When the diagnosis of hyperparathyroidism is delayed, such areas become quite large, resulting in a radiolucent lesion in the diaphysis of long bones, jaw, or skull that appears brown because of old and recent hemorrhage. Microscopic examination shows numerous giant cells in the fibrous cellular stroma. These "brown" tumors show dramatic regression both radiologically and histologically when hyperparathyroidism is controlled.

17. What is cretinism?

Congenital or infantile hypothyroidism, which is called cretinism, is recognized by dwarfism and mental retardation. It is more common in girls (male-to-female ratio = 1:3). Other clinical features are dry skin, scanty and coarse hair, enlarged tongue, expressionless face, narrowed palpebral fissures, enlarged abdomen, umbilical hernia, and generalized lethargy. When diagnosed and treated early, prognosis is good for normal bone and mental development. Untreated cretins have increasing mental retardation with age and eventually succumb to infection.

RICKETS

18. What are the four causes of rickets?

Vitamin D deficiency   Chronic renal insufficiency
Renal tubular insufficiency   Hypophosphatasia

19. What is rickets?

Rickets is a disease process characterized by inadequate calcification of bone matrix (osteoid) in the immature skeleton. Osteomalacia is the same process in adults. Because of the growth of the immature skeleton, the disease process is more severe in children.

20. What are the clinical findings of rickets?

Muscular weakness
Lethargy
Protuberant abdomen
Craniotabes (enlargement of the forehead)
Thickening of weight-bearing joints (deformity of metaphyseal-epiphyseal junction)

21. What are the x-ray findings in rickets?

Thickened epiphyseal plate
Brush border of metaphysis

Flaring of metaphysis (trumpeting)
Thickening of osteochondral articulations of ribs (rachitic rosary)
Diminished cortical density
Coarse trabecular pattern, widely spaced and irregular

22. How does renal tubular disease cause rickets?
Renal tubular disease leads to increased renal clearance of phosphate and occasionally to excessive loss of calcium. Serum calcium is normal, whereas phosphate is low (1–3 mg/dl). The result is abnormal mineralization of osteoid. Because large doses of vitamin D (50,000–500,000 IU/day) are required, this group of disorders is called vitamin D–resistant rickets. It is one of the most common metabolic bone diseases of children.

23. What are the late deformities associated with vitamin D–resistant rickets?
Genu varum/valgum   Anterolateral bowing of tibia
Coxa vara   Protrusio acetabuli
Anterior bowing of femur   Kyphoscoliosis

24. How does chronic renal failure cause rickets?
The exact mechanism is unknown, but several factors may play a role, including (1) high levels of PTH, (2) acidosis, and (3) hypocalcemia, factors that alter calcium/phosphorus homeostasis and thus result in abnormal mineralization.

25. How does renal rickets differ from dietary rickets?
In renal rickets the high levels of PTH result in less osteoid and increased osteoclastic resorption of bone. There may be osteosclerosis at the base of the skull. Slipped epiphyses are common in renal rickets. Skeletal maturation is delayed.

26. What are the blood chemistry findings in the four common categories of rickets?

	DIETARY	RESISTANT	RENAL	HYPOPHOSPHATASIA
Phosphate	Low	Low	High	Normal
Calcium	Normal, low	Normal	Normal, low	Normal, high
Creatinine	Normal	Normal	High	Normal, high
Alkaline phosphatase	High	High	High	Very low

27. What is hypophosphatasia?
Hypophosphatasia is a genetically determined error of metabolism with low alkaline phosphatase activity and increased urinary excretion of phosphoryl ethanolamine.

28. How does the radiographic appearance of hypophosphatasia differ from other forms of rickets?
Radiographs show severe osteoporosis and marked widening of the physis. Fractures are common. In milder cases the radiographic findings are difficult to distinguish from dietary rickets.

BIBLIOGRAPHY

1. Boden SD, Kaplan FS: Calcium homeostasis. Orthop Clin North Am 21:31–42, 1990.
2. Buckwalter JA, Einhorn TA, Simon, SR (eds): Orthopaedic Basic Science, 2nd ed. Rosemont, Ill., Am Academy of Orthopaedic Surgeons, 2000.
3. Canale ST (ed): Campbell's Operative Orthopaedics, 9th ed. St. Louis, Mosby, 1998.
4. Doppelt SH: Vitamin D, rickets, and osteomalacia. Orthop Clin North Am 15:671–686, 1984.
5. Eastell R, Riggs BL: Calcium homeostasis and osteoporosis. Endocrinol Metab Clin North Am 16:829–842, 1987.
6. Mankin HJ: Rickets, osteomalacia, and renal osteodystrophy: An update. Orthop Clin North Am 21:81–96, 1990.

20. CEREBRAL PALSY AND NEUROMUSCULAR DISEASE

Marcia E. Bromley, M.D., and Paul W. Esposito, M.D., FAAP, FAAOS

CEREBRAL PALSY

1. Define cerebral palsy.

Cerebral palsy is a nonprogressive insult to the central nervous system during the perinatal period. A broad definition is necessary to address the multiple causes and vast array of clinical presentations.

2. Describe the classification system for cerebral palsy.

- Diplegia—lower extremities involved more than upper extremities, but both are affected.
- Hemiplegic—left-sided or right-sided involvement.
- Paraplegic—lower extremities only affected.
- Quadriplegic—all four extremities involved, plus head, neck, and trunk.
- Tetraplegic—three extremities involved.

3. What are the types of involvement in cerebral palsy?

- Spastic—hyperreflexic stretch reflexes
- Athetoid—involuntary movements, passive resistance to motion, and/or posturing
- Mixed—combination of both motion disorder and spasticity

4. Why is athetoid cerebral palsy less common than in the past?

In the past, most cases of athetoid cerebral palsy were caused by kernicterus (the depositing of bilirubin in the basal ganglia) often due to Rh incompatibility. Screening for Rh incompatibility, medical treatment, and bilirubin-lights have greatly decreased the incidence of athetoid cerebral palsy.

5. What are the common causes for the various types of cerebral palsy?

Diplegia is associated with premature infants, who may develop periventricular hemorrhage. Preventing premature births may avoid this problem. **Hemiplegia** is caused by a variety of unilateral insults to the brain, including trauma, infection, and cerebrovascular hemorrhage. **Quadriplegia,** the most severely involved form, results from an anoxic or severe hypoxic event, or other prenatal problems such as viral infection, which cause global injury. Postnatal causes such as severe diffuse brain trauma or meningitides may also lead to quadriplegia.

6. When do children with cerebral palsy walk?

In children with **hemiplegia,** ambulation frequently occurs at 12–16 months (the time at which the normal child walks). Children with **diplegia** are delayed somewhat, but walking is usually initiated by age 4 years. In those with **quadriplegic** cerebral palsy, onset of ambulation depends on the extent of involvement. If walking is not initiated by age 7 years, it is extremely unlikely that the child will walk.

7. Do all patients show spasticity early in life?

No. In fact, the more severely affected children may be hypotonic or "floppy" early on; only later, when developmental delay is more evident, do they develop signs of spasticity.

8. Does central core disease (CCD) appear clinically the same as cerebral palsy?

No. CCD, like cerebral palsy, is a nonprogressive process—a myopathy that presents at birth with hypotonia and delayed motor milestones. Patients with CCD, however, do not exhibit spasticity. They may exhibit pes cavus, kyphoscoliosis, foot deformities, congenital hip dislocation, and joint contractures, but up to 40% of people with CCD are asymptomatic. The disorder is caused by a defective gene that creates abnormal proteins in the z-band of the muscle fiber, as opposed to cerebral palsy, which is a central nervous system disorder. CCD is an autosomal dominant trait with variable penetrance. The defective gene is also the site for malignant hyperthermia regulation; consequently, such patients often suffer from malignant hyperthermia (in fact, some patients are not diagnosed with CCD until after having had an episode of malignant hyperthermia).

9. How is cerebral palsy diagnosed?

Most patients present to the orthopedist after the diagnosis of cerebral palsy has been made, especially if the patient is a member of a high-risk group, such as premature infants, who are closely monitored for abnormalities. Some children, however, are referred because they are not walking by 18 months of age. Such children retain primitive reflexes and show signs of spasticity. In some cases, computed tomography (CT) and magnetic resonance imaging (MRI) scans of the brain may define the underlying cause. But frequently these congenital myopathies and other neurologic processes that do not cause spasticity may have severe underlying hypotonia associated with developmental delays and, therefore, must be ruled out. Cerebral palsy may be a diagnosis of exclusion when all other possible causes are ruled out.

10. What early problems should the orthopedist look for in a child with cerebral palsy?

In the child with severe spasticity, the hips may dislocate as early as 18 months of age. Therefore, patients should have their hips examined and a pelvic radiograph every 6 months for the first few years, then at variable times depending on many factors such as the degree of spasticity and the development of the hips clinically and radiographically. Early detection of hip subluxation and dislocation, followed by surgical release of the adductor muscles and/or the iliopsoas muscles, frequently prevents the late development of a painful and stiff dislocated hip. After the age of 5 years, the child's course becomes less predictable and the treatment becomes generally more complicated.

11. What are the clinical signs of hip subluxation or dislocation?
- Limited abduction, especially with rapid stretch (grab test)
- Asymmetric knee height with the pelvis level and the knees flexed (Galeazzi sign)
- Windswept posture (one hip adducted and the opposite side abducted)
- Asymmetric leg length
- Severe Hip flexion contractures

12. What is the rationale for treating severely involved patients with dislocating hips?

Even children with severe, total-body involvement have a significant chance for a long life. A dislocated hip can become very painful, make nursing care more difficult, and, as a result, significantly affect the quality of life. A dislocated hip also may contribute to pelvic obliquity and scoliosis, which can make even wheelchair ambulation impossible and potentially cause pressure sores.

13. Should a patient with spastic quadriplegia and a severe scoliosis have surgery for correction of the spinal curvature?

This matter is still debated among orthopedists today. Most agree that pain and loss of function, as measured by decreased ambulation or sitting ability, are indications for surgery. Still some orthopedists believe that the cost, complication rate, and extent of the surgery outweigh the surgical benefits. Benefits of spine stabilization may include improved sitting balance, ease of patient care, decreased pain, increased pulmonary function, and increased level of function. Drawbacks cited are the high cost of the surgery and the high risk of complications such as death, paralysis, wound infection, instrumentation problems, pulmonary complications, and decubitus ulcers. Risks and alternatives must be carefully discussed at length with the patient's family and caregivers. In the appropriately selected patient, spine stabilization surgery may allow the opportunity to sit rather than become bedridden, which also has significant morbidity. The ability to sit greatly enhances the patient's quality of life and comfort.

14. What types of lower extremity deformities are most commonly seen in cerebral palsy?

- Hip adduction and flexion contracture
- Knee flexion contracture
- Equinus of the ankle
- Contractures of the rectus femoris

15. What does tendon lengthening do for spastic contractures?

Muscle contractures frequently do not resolve with stretching or bracing alone especially in patients with significant spasticity. The lengthening procedure attempts to balance muscle forces across the joints and increase the muscle excursion, thereby placing the joints in a more functional position. They do not, however, alter the spasticity of the muscles.

16. What is selective dorsal rhizotomy, and who are the best candidates for the procedure?

Selective dorsal rhizotomy involves a multiple-level lumbar laminectomy, with isolation of the dorsal nerve rootlets and selective sectioning of only those rootlets that cause spastic reflex action when electrically stimulated intraoperatively. This procedure, in effect, reduces spasticity in the patient and allows for better muscle control. The best candidates are approximately 4-year-old, spastic diplegic, ambulatory children with excellent strength whose spasticity interferes with function. This procedure is not done as frequently as in the past because of the potential to result in excessive weakness. Some improvement in fine motor movement has also been noted in the upper extremities after selective dorsal rhizotomy in the lumbar spine. This effect is not predictable though and does not occur in all patients. Risks include sensory abnormalities and persistent back pain in some patients. Rarely, with adequate monitoring and limited number of sacral rootlets release, bowel and bladder dysfunction may also occur.

17. Is there a medical treatment for spasticity in cerebral palsy?

Yes. Treatment of spasticity by intrathecal baclofen has become relatively common. A microinfusion pump placed in the subcutaneous tissues delivers the baclofen via percutaneous catheter to the intrathecal space at a rate determined by the patient's response to the medication. The rate is adjusted until the spasticity improves to an acceptable degree. Intrathecal baclofen pumps do not work for all dystonic patients and higher doses may be necessary in these patients, however, and other surgery may still be necessary. Meningitis is one of the risks of this procedure.

18. Can patients with cerebral palsy benefit from injection of botulinum toxin?

Botulinum toxin type A injection clearly has been shown to be a safe means of at least transiently but significantly improving spasticity and function in selective muscles. Its use is limited by its lack of permanency and its toxicity, which is dose-related. Some patients with functional and not fixed contractures may have permanent improvement when treatment with Botox is coupled with intensive physical therapy, casting, and/or bracing.

19. What is familial spastic paraplegia?

Familial spastic paraplegia is an autosomal dominant disorder that mimics cerebral palsy. Only the lower extremities are involved, however, and in the absence of a family history, the physician is obligated to look for other causes, such as birth trauma to the spinal cord. Complete lack of upper extremity involvement is not typical of cerebral palsy.

20. What factors differentiate the idiopathic and familial toe walkers from the child with mild spastic diplegia?

The child with idiopathic toe walking has a normal birth history, walked at the appropriate time, and has no signs of any other neurologic involvement (spasticity). Frequently a strong family history of toe walking is present. All other causes must be excluded before a diagnosis of mild spastic diplegia is made. Spontaneous onset of toe walking later in development warrants an intensive neurologic evaluation for such diagnoses as brain tumors and muscular dystrophy.

21. Are there any indications for surgery in the upper extremity in children with severe spastic cerebral palsy?

The goals of upper extremity surgery vary based on the severity of contractures, which may cause pain, difficulties in positioning, and hygiene problems, typically in spastic quadriplegics. Tendon releases may relieve these contractures if done prior to the development of severe joint contractures. Botox also has some role in treatment of these patients. Improvement in fine motor control rarely, if ever, occurs after surgical treatment because sensory abnormalities are also present in all of these patients. If arthritis of the wrist has developed, arthrodesis of the wrist may be necessary to alleviate pain.

22. Are there any options to improve upper extremity function in children with spastic hemiplegia?

The arm and hand may be placed in a position for improved function; however, the limiting factors are proprioceptive sensation and the ability of the child to cooperate and operate with a rehabilitation program. Hemiplegic children frequently have a thumb in palm adduction deformity, which may be improved by either injection with botulinum toxin or surgical lengthening of the adductor pollicis. Pronation/flexion deformities of the wrist may be improved with procedures such as transfer of the flexor carpi ulnaris or release of the pronator quadratus. Many other procedures are available, but surgical decision-making is crucial. Improvement in comfort and cosmesis is more common than improvement of function.

MYELODYSPLASIA

23. What are the different types of myelodysplasia?

Meningocele involves only the meninges. Patients usually have normal neurologic function.

Myelomeningocele involves neural elements that are part of an exposed sac and usually are not covered with skin. Arnold-Chiari brainstem involvement and hydrocephalus are also found.

Lipomeningocele is characterized by a lipoma in the thecal sac, with neural elements intertwined. The skin usually is intact, and patients usually are neurologically sound at birth except for foot deformities and/or bowel and bladder dysfunction. Neurologic function deteriorates with growth unless the disorder is treated. Recurrent neurologic problems are common even with appropriate early surgery.

24. What are the common causes of death in children with untreated myelomeningocele?

- Central nervous system infection
- Progressive hydrocephalus

25. What are the common causes of deteriorating function in patients with myelomeningocele?

- Progressive hydrocephalus secondary to shunt malfunction
- Hydromyelia secondary to shunt malfunction
- Spinal cord tethering with growth
- Arnold-Chiari malformation
- Ascending urinary tract infection

26. List the common presenting symptoms in older children with shunt malfunction and increasing hydromyelia.

Irritability	Progressive foot deformity
Decreased motor level	Progressive scoliosis
Worsening bowel or bladder function	Weakness of the upper extremities

27. What is the surgical treatment for patients with significant deterioration of neurologic function?

If the shunt is not functioning and/or hydrocephalus is worsening, the shunt must be repaired or replaced. If hydromyelia is worsening in the presence of a significant Chiari malformation, craniocervical decompression may be necessary.

28. What is the expected cause of an intraoperative anaphylactic reaction in a patient with neuromuscular problems such as myelomeningocele?

Children with cerebral palsy are at an increased risk for developing an anaphylactic reaction to latex. Patients who have undergone multiple surgical procedures or the placement of a ventriculoperitoneal shunt are considered high-risk for latex allergy and should be considered for preoperative latex-sensitivity testing. When obtaining the history of a child with cerebral palsy, all physicians should look carefully for sensitivity (ie. urticaria, facial edema, and bronchospasm) to latex products such as balloons, rubber balls, and rubber gloves. Eighteen to 40% of patients have been reported to be latex-sensitive. Many hospitals insist on latex-free environments for such patients to avoid the consequences of a previously undiagnosed hypersensitivity to latex.

29. What is the role of the orthopedist early in the life of a child with myelomeningocele?

The role of the orthopaedist is twofold: 1) to treat the frequently associated foot deformities, such as clubfeet and congenital vertical talus, and (2) to assist with fitting adaptive devices and bracing to allow weight bearing and ambulation. The height and complexity of the bracing increases with the higher levels of myelomeningocele. Thoracic-level patients, for example, require bracing from the spine to the feet just to stand, whereas a patient with a sacral level lesion may only require advice or shoes that provide adequate support. The spinal cord may need to be detethered (released) with growth. The spinal cord is "tied down" to the meningocele scar; therefore, traction occurs on the spinal cord with growth as the cord because the cord cannot rise up to a higher level in the spinal canal. Detethering may also be necessary if back pain, bladder dysfunction, or lower extremity changes occur.

MUSCULAR DYSTROPHY

30. In classic Duchenne muscular dystrophy, are patients typically male or female?

Duchenne dystrophy is a sex-linked, recessive trait; therefore, patients are typically male. The abnormal dystrophin gene that is the cause of Duchenne muscular dystrophy has been identified and cloned.

31. What are the presenting findings in Duchenne dystrophy?

- Symmetric and progressive proximal muscle weakness
- Deteting gait after delayed ambulation
- Progressive toe walking
- Pseudohypertrophy of the calf
- Hard or rubbery feeling muscle
- Elevation of serum CPK levels

32. What are the goals of treatment in muscular dystrophy?

- To keep the patients ambulatory as long as possible.
- To prevent contractures that interfere with ambulation. Newer pharmacologic treatment primarily with Prednisone is showing some success.

- To begin immediate postoperative ambulation if surgery is necessary.
- To fuse the spine with rigid fixation to maintain a sitting balance. Spine stabilization is considered shortly after the child stops ambulating and when the curve is relatively mild. At this point in the child's life, adequate pulmonary function is maintained to allow safe operative management. Curves that are allowed to progress to 40–50° are usually accompanied by severe pulmonary and, on some occasions, cardiac muscle abnormalities. . (If fusion is delayed until scoliosis is severe, restricted pulmonary function will not allow a safe postoperative course, and the patient may become ventilator-dependent.)

33. What is the cause of death in most patients with Duchenne dystrophy?
Pulmonary failure or cardiomyopathy.

BIBLIOGRAPHY

1. Albright AL, Barry MJ, Painter MH, et. al.: infusion of intrathecal baclofen for generalized dystonia in cerebral palsy. J Neurosurg 88:73–76, 1988.
2. Banta JV, Lonstein JE, Lubicky JP: Resolution: A 15-year-old with spastic quadriplegia and a 60° scoliosis should have a posterior spinal fusion with instrumentation. Dev Med Child Neurol 40:278–283, 1998.
3. Corry IS, Cosgrove AP, Duffy CM, et al: Botulinum toxin A compared with stretching casts in the treatment of spastic equinus: A randomized prospective trial. J Pediatr Orthop 18:304–311, 1998.
4. Delfico AJ, Dormans JP, Craythorne CB, Templeton JJ: Intraoperative anaphylaxis due to allergy to latex in children who have cerebral palsy: A report of six cases. Dev Med Child Neurol 39:194–197, 1996.
5. Evans RA: Orthopedic aspects of neuromuscular disorders in children. Curr Opin Pediatr 5:379–383, 1993.
6. Gamble JG, Rinsky LA, Bleck EE: Established hip dislocations in children with cerebral palsy. Clin Orthop 253:90–99, 1990.
7. Lazareff JA: Limited selective posterior rhizotomy for the treatment of spasticity secondary to infantile cerebral palsy: A preliminary report. Neurosurgery 27:535–538, 1990.
8. Loke J, MacLennan DH: Malignant hyperthermia and central core disease: Disorders of calcium release channels. Am J Med 104:470–486, 1998.
9. McLone, DG: Care of the neonate with myelomeningocele. Neursrg Clin N Am 1:111–120
10. Papariello SG, Skinner SR: Dynamic electromyography analysis of habitual toe-walkers. J Pediatr Orthop 5:171–175, 1985.
11. Scrutton D: The classification of cerebral palsy. Dev Med Child Neurol 35(7):647–648, 1993.
12. Thomas C: Nemaline rod and central core disease: A coexisting z-band myopathy. Muscle Nerve 20:893–896, 1997.
13. Water PM, van Heest A: Spastic hemiplegia of the upper extremity in children. Hand Clin 14(1): 119–134, 1998.
14. Wong V: Use of botulinum toxin injection in 17 children with spastic cerebral palsy. Pediatr Neurol 18:124–131, 1998.

21. MISCELLANEOUS CONGENITAL DISORDERS

Paul W. Esposito, M.D., FAAP, FAAOS and Brian E. Brigman, M.D.

1. What are the orthopedic manifestations of Down syndrome?
Down syndrome affects 1 in 660 live births with a higher incidence with increasing maternal age. Trisomy 21 accounts for 95% of the cases. Common orthopedic sequelae include occipitoatlantal or atlantoaxial instability, hip subluxation-dislocation, patella subluxation-dislocation,

and flexible planovalgus, all possibly related to the ligamentous laxity common in patients with Down syndrome. Other relatively common problems include scoliosis, spondylolisthesis, and slipped capital femoral epiphysis. Patients with Down syndrome have characteristically flat acetabula and flared iliac wings. A polyarticular arthropathy occurs in about 10% of Down syndrome patients, usually affecting the feet. The orthopedist must ensure that the child has been thoroughly evaluated by pediatric cardiologists of the life-threatening cardiac anomalies frequently associated with Down's syndrome before any other treatment.

2. What is arthrogryposis?

Arthrogryposis is a group of nongenetic congenital contracture syndromes of unknown origin. Characteristically the upper extremities, if involved, are adducted and internally rotated at the shoulder. The elbows are extended and the wrists and fingers flexed with the thumb in palm. The lower extremities typically are noted for having flexed, abducted, and externally rotated hips; knees may be in flexion or extension, and clubfeet are common.

3. What is the treatment of choice for congenital muscular torticollis?

Congenital muscular torticollis is a painless contracture of the sternocleidomastoid muscle. Affected infants tilt their head toward and rotate their chin away from the affected sternocleidomastoid muscle. It is usually discovered in the first two months of life. The cause is thought to be ischemia to the muscle. Stretching of the affected muscle (lateral rotation and side bending) is effective about 90% of the time if started before 1 year of age. If stretching is not successful, surgical lengthening or release of the sternocleidomastoid should be considered to prevent facial deformity. Hip dysplasia is associated with this diagnosis and must be looked for diligently.

4. What is Klippel-Feil syndrome?

Klippel-Feil syndrome is a group of deformities that result from failure of segmentation of cervical vertebrae. Classically, patients have a low posterior hairline, short neck, and limited range of motion in the neck, especially with lateral bending. Klippel-Feil syndrome is associated with Sprengel's deformity, scoliosis, urinary tract anomalies, congenital heart disease, and hearing loss.

5. What is Sprengel's deformity?

Sprengel's deformity is characterized by an elevated and medially rotated scapula. It results from an interruption in the normal caudal migration of the scapula. In 30% of patients with Sprengel's deformity the scapula is bound to the cervical spine by fibrous tissue, cartilage, or an omovertebral bone. All patients with Sprengel's deformity have loss of abduction and forward flexion; those with an omovertebral bone generally have less than 90° of abduction. Stretching exercises are not useful. Functional or cosmetic deformities can be treated with surgery.

6. What is von Recklinghausen's disease?

Neurofibromatosis (NF) affects 1 in 3000 newborns. NF is autosomal dominant with 100% penetrance, but about one-half of all cases are spontaneous mutations. Classic NF, or von Recklinghausen's disease (also called peripheral NF or NF1), makes up 85% of cases. Central NF, or NF2, is characterized by bilateral acoustic neuromas.

7. How do I diagnose NF?

The Consensus Development Conference on Neurofibromatosis of the National Institutes of Health concluded that diagnosis of NF1 is dependent on **two or more** of the following criteria:

1. Six or more café au lait macules at least 5 mm in greatest diameter in prepubertal children and at least 15 mm in greatest diameter in adults
2. Two or more neurofibromas of any type or one plexiform neurofibroma
3. Freckling in the axillary or inguinal regions
4. Optic glioma

5. Two or more Lisch nodules, (iris hamartoma)

6. A distinctive osseous lesion, such as sphenoid dysplasia or thinning of long bone cortex without pseudarthrosis

7. A first-degree relative (parent, sibling, or offspring) with von Recklinghausen's disease identified by the above criteria

8. What are the orthopedic manifestations of NF?

Pseudarthrosis of long bones, typically the tibia, but also the ulna, radius, and clavicle, is the most common orthopedic manifestation of NF. Pseudarthrosis of the tibia starts with anterolateral bowing of the tibia in infancy with a fracture when the patient begins walking.

Scoliosis and limb overgrowth are common in NF. Limb overgrowth can range from disproportional overgrowth of a single digit to one or more extremity.

9. Describe the treatment for pseudarthrosis of the tibia.

Spontaneous union is rare. Bracing or casting is not effective in the long term but can be used as palliative treatment. Plating and bone grafting have success rates less than 50%. Successful treatment with free vascularized bone grafts, external fixation and intramedullary rods has been described. Multiple operations are often needed, and shortening, angulation, and stiffness are common. About 5% of patients eventually require amputation, which may be below the knee (above pseudarthrosis), or an ankle disarticulation (Syme's amputation).

10. How do you distinguish benign bowing of the tibia from potential pseudarthrosis of the tibia?

Posteromedial bowing of the tibia is usually benign and does not lead to fracture or pseudarthrosis. A typical long-term sequela is limb length discrepancy. Anterior or anterolateral bowing of the tibia is associated with progressive deformity, fracture, and pseudarthrosis of the tibia.

11. Name another disease process often associated with café-au-lait spots.

Fibrous dysplasia. Café-au-lait spots are tan macules located in the basal layer of the epidermis. They are typically absent during infancy and appear by age 9. Café-au-lait spots associated with neurofibromatosis have smooth margins (so-called "coast of California"), whereas those associated with fibrous dysplasia have jagged edges ("coast of Maine").

12. What defects are associated with VACTERLS?

The nonrandom, but unexplained, association of system defects previously known as VATER is now called VACTERLS. It includes:

- Vertebral anomalies, including failures of segmentation (vertebral bars and blocks), congenital scoliosis, and occult intraspinal pathology
- Anal anomalies, including imperforate anus or anal atresia
- Cardiac abnormalities
- Tracheoesophageal fistula
- Renal anomalies (single kidney)
- Limb anomalies, usually radially based, ranging from hypoplastic thumb to radial clubhand
- Single umbilical artery

13. What are the mucopolysaccharidoses?

The mucopolysaccharidoses are the largest group of lysosomal storage diseases. Lysosomes are enzymes that degrade intracellular molecules into smaller units for cellular metabolism or utilization. Defective activity of any of these enzymes leads to blockage in the breakdown process and intracellular accumulation of semi-degraded compounds. The mucopolysaccharidoses are subdivided into at least 12 types.

Incidence is about 1 in 10,000. Hurler (MPS I) and Morquio (MPS IV) are the most common types. All are autosomal recessive with the exception of the X-linked recessive MPSII or Hunter disease. Orthopedic manifestations include stiff joints, thought to be related to deposition of mucopolysaccharide in the capsule and periarticular structures. Radiographic findings often include oval vertebral bodies with anterior beaking; wide, flat ilia; large acetabula, coxa valga, and an unossified femoral head. The progression of the disease may be halted in Hurler syndrome with bone marrow transplantation but must be considered early in life because the organ damage already done before to transplantation cannot be reversed.

The Mucopolysaccharidoses

TYPE		NAME	ENZYME DEFICIENCY	ACCUMULATED SUBSTANCE
MPS I	Hurler/Scheie	α-L-iduronidase	HS/DS	
MPS II	Hunter	Iduronate-2-sulfatase	HS/DS	
MPS IIIA	Sanfilippo A	Heparan sulfate sulfatase	HS	
MPS IIIB	Sanfilippo B	α-N-acetylglucosaminadase	HS	
MPS IIIC	Sanfilippo C	α-glucosaminide-N-acetyltransferase	HS	
MPSIIID	Sanfilippo D	Glucosamine-6-sulfatase	HS	
MPS IVA	Morquio A	N-acetyl galactosamine-6 sulfate sulfatase	KS/CS	
MPS IVB	Morquio B	β-D-galactosidase	KS	
MPS IVC	Morquio C	Uncertain	KS	
MPS V	Formerly Scheie— no longer used			
MPS VI	Maroteaux-Lamy	Arylsulfatase B, N-acetylgalactosamine-4 sulfatase	DS/CS	
MPS VII	Sly	β-D-glucuronidase	CS/HS/DS	
MPS VIII		Glucoronate-2-sulpitatase	CS/HS	

HS = heparan sulfate; DS = dermatan sulfate; KS = keratin sulfate; CS = chondroitin sulfate.

BIBLIOGRAPHY

1. Aprin H, Zink WB, Hall JE: Management of dislocation of hip in Down syndrome. J Pediatr Orthop. 5:428–431, 1985.
2. Crawford AH, Shorry EK: Neurofibromatosis in children: The role of the orthopaedist. J Am Acad Orthop Surg 7:217–230, 1999.
3. Green WB: Closed treatment of hip dislocation in Down syndrome. J Pediatr Orthop 18:643–647, 1988.
4. Herman, MJ, Pizzutillo PD: Cervical spine disorders in children. Orthop Clin North Am 30:457–66, 1999.

III. The Shoulder

22. SUBACROMIAL SYNDROMES

John P. Furia, M.D., and David E. Brown, M.D.

1. What four muscles make up the rotator cuff? What nerve innervates each muscle? What is the function of each muscle?

MUSCLE	NERVE	FUNCTION
Supraspinatus	Suprascapular	Primary initiator of shoulder elevation
Infraspinatus	Suprascapular	External rotator
Teres minor	Axillary	External rotator
Subscapularis	Upper subscapular Lower subscapular	Internal rotator

2. What is the incidence of rotator cuff tears in humans?

Cadaver dissections reveal high rates of rotator cuff tears. Under age 70, the prevalence of tears is 30%; for ages 71–80, nearly 60%; and over 80 years, nearly 70%.

3. What causes rotator cuff tears?

The exact cause is unknown. A 1989 study revealed that in younger patients with a documented rotator cuff tear, few had had a traumatic event, which suggests that the process was secondary to repetitive microtrauma, degeneration, and/or impingement. Older patients tended to have mild chronic impingement symptoms but then sustained an episode of trauma, after which larger tears of the cuff were found.

4. What are the significant features of the physical examination of subacromial syndromes?

Active and passive range of motion, shoulder strength, and areas of tenderness should be noted. Examination of shoulder stability is important, particularly in younger people. The presence of pain during forward elevation while the examiner stabilizes the scapula is the primary impingement sign. Pain during active abduction of the arm (with the arm in internal rotation) is a secondary impingement sign.

5. How is the strength of the supraspinatus and infraspinatus tested?

The supraspinatus is tested with the shoulder abducted to 90°, flexed 30°, and then maximally internally rotated. Downward pressure exerted by the examiner is resisted primarily by the supraspinatus. The infraspinatus is tested with the shoulder abducted at the side while the elbows are fixed 90°. The examiner resists active external rotation.

6. What are the most common differential diagnoses of exertional shoulder pain?
- Subacromial syndromes (rotator cuff tears, tendinitis, impingement)
- Shoulder instability
- Cervical radiculitis
- Acromioclavicular degenerative disease

- Suprascapular nerve entrapment
- Thoracic outlet syndrome

7. What condition commonly mimics the subacromial syndrome?

"The great mimicker" of shoulder pain is acromioclavicular (AC) arthritis. Patients with AC joint pain usually present with activity related anterior-superior shoulder pain. There is often tenderness directly over the AC joint that is exacerbated with horizontal adduction of the humerus. The pain often radiates to the trapezius, lower cervical region, and anterior acromion. The radiating nature of the pain makes it easy to confuse AC joint pathology with other entities.

8. What are the causes of subacromial syndromes?

- Repetitive overhead use
- Trauma
- Forward sloping acromion or hooked or curved acromion
- Os acromiale
- Shoulder instability
- Technique errors during overhead shoulder sports

9. Describe the treatment of subacromial syndromes.

- Modification of activities, avoiding repetitive overhead use or technique errors
- Ice and nonsteroidal anti-inflammatory drugs (NSAIDs)
- Therapeutic exercises and stretching
- Subacromial injections
- Surgical decompression and repair of rotator cuff tears

10. What are the three types of acromial morphology and their incidence?

Acromial Morphology

TYPE	INCIDENCE IN HEALTHY SUBJECTS	SUBJECTS WITH DOCUMENTED ROTATOR CUFF TEARS
Type I (flat acromion)	17%	3%
Type II (curved acromion)	44%	27%
Type III (hooked acromion)	39%	70%

11. Which radiographic tests are used to evaluate for rotator cuff tears? How useful are they?

Ultrasonography, single- and double-contrast arthrography, and magnetic resonance imaging (MRI) have been used to evaluate rotator cuff tears. Ultrasonography can confirm the presence of a significant rotator cuff tear; however, it is extremely dependent on the individual ultrasonographer. One study found only 30% accuracy compared with surgical confirmation. Arthrography is approximately 85% sensitive and specific in the diagnosis of complete cuff tear but not highly accurate in the diagnosis of partial cuff tear. MRI appears to be 95% sensitive and specific in the diagnosis of complete tears. Intrasubstance degeneration, chronic tendinitis, and partial tearing are imaged by MRI with an accuracy rate of 85%.

12. Describe the technique for rotator cuff repair.

1. Perform acromioplasty (open or closed).
2. Debride end of tendon to fresh tissue.
3. Mobilize tendon laterally. May need to:
   - Release coracohumeral ligament
   - Release capsule (incision above labrum)
4. Use locking suture technique of choice.
5. Secure to greater tuberosity.

13. Describe the steps of arthroscopic rotator cuff repair.

A standard arthroscopic subacromial decompression is performed. Tear size and geometry are assessed. The rotator cuff tendons are mobilized using arthroscopic instrumentation. Releases are performed as needed. When necessary, side-to-side (margin convergence) sutures are placed to decrease the length of the tear. The bone at the intended site of repair is freshened with an arthroscopic burr. Suture anchors are inserted into the prepared bone. The sutures are then passed through the free ends of the rotator cuff tendons. The rotator cuff is then repaired directly to bone using arthroscopic knot tying techniques.

14. What are the results of rotator cuff repair?

Using direct repair or local tendon transposition techniques, surgery has yielded good results in approximately 90% of patients. Pain relief and strength improvements generally follow successful repair. Return of range of motion has been shown to correlate with the timing of surgical repair. Repair within 3 weeks of injury yields the best return of range of motion.

15. Describe the treatment of massive irreparable rotator cuff tears.

Treatment for this entity is controversial. Some authors advocate arthroscopic subacromial decompression and wide debridement of the cuff tear as a means of affording pain relief. In shoulders with normal passive motion and normal deltoid function, humeral prosthetic hemiarthroplasty has relieved pain. Recently, latissimus dorsi transfer has been reported to provide excellent pain relief with marked improvement in flexion and external rotation, yielding approximately 80% of normal shoulder function.

16. What are the causes of failure after rotator cuff repair?

- Persistent impingement
- Acromioclavicular joint pain
- Cervical spondylosis
- Re-rupture of the cuff
- Workers' compensation injury (secondary gain)

17. What is the function of the long head of the biceps tendon?

The tendon has an important contribution as a humeral head depressor. Loss of its function may result in superior migration of the humeral head, which may aggravate or cause rotator cuff impingement.

18. What are the indications for biceps tenodesis?

Indications include significant degeneration or rupture of the tendon found at the time of a shoulder reconstructive procedure. Isolated biceps tenodesis has a high incidence of unsatisfactory long-term results when performed solely for bicipital pain.

19. What is the treatment of proximal biceps rupture?

Most patients do well with conservative management. Gradual return of range of motion and shoulder strength through physiotherapy is expected. Surgical repair by biceps tenodesis affords little improvement in strength. Distal biceps tendon ruptures are generally repaired surgically.

20. Describe the significance of suprascapular nerve entrapment.

Beware the young athlete who presents with vague posterior shoulder pain, loss of rotator cuff strength and muscle atrophy but no history of trauma. Suprascapular nerve entrapment may cause symptoms that mimic the findings associated with rotator cuff tear. Symptoms include the insidious onset of posterior shoulder pain and rotator cuff weakness. The diagnosis is established with electromyographic testing. Treatment consists of decompressing the nerve or excision or decompression of a space-occupying lesion such as a ganglion cyst.

21. Where is the suprascapular nerve usually entrapped?

The suprascapular nerve arises from the upper trunk of the brachial plexus and travels posteriorly through the suprascapular notch just medial to the base of the coracoid. The nerve can be compressed in two locations: in the suprascapular notch and along the neck of the spine of the scapula at the spinoglenoid notch.

22. Describe the treatment of frozen shoulder syndrome.

Most patients show gradual reduction of pain and return of motion for periods up to 18 months. The syndrome itself may be self-limited. Treatment usually consists of physical therapy for range of motion, antiinflammatory medication, and subacromial or intraarticular corticosteroid injections. Patients who fail to improve with such methods may be candidates for manipulation under anesthesia, arthroscopic debridement, or decompression. Diabetics appear to have poor results from surgery.

BIBLIOGRAPHY

1. Arntz CT, Matsen FA, Jackins S: Surgical management of complex irreparable rotator cuff deficiency. J Arthroplasty 6:363, 1991.
2. Bassett RW, Cofield RH: Acute tears of the rotator cuff: The timing of surgical repair. Clin Orthop 175:18, 1983.
3. Burk DL, Karasick D, Kurtz AB, et al: Rotator cuff tears: Prospective comparison of MR imaging with arthrography, sonography, and surgery. Am J Roentgenol 153:87, 1989.
4. Burkhart SS: Arthroscopic treatment of massive rotator cuff tears: Clinical and biomechanical rationale. Clin Orthop 267:45, 1991.
5. Burkhart SS, Danaceau SM, Pearce CE: Arthroscopic rotator cuff repair: Analysis of results by tear size and by repair technique-margin convergence versus direct tendon-to-bone. Arthroscopy 17:905–912, 2001.
6. Cummins CA, Messer TM, Nuber GW: Suprascapular nerve entrapment. J. Bone Joint Surg 82A:415–424, 2000.
7. DiGiovanni J, Marva G, Park JY, et al: Hemiarthroplasty for glenohumeral arthritis with massive rotator cuff tears. Orthop Clin North Am 29:477–489, 1998.
8. Gartsman G: Arthroscopic acromioplasty for lesions of the rotator cuff. J Bone Joint Surg 72A:169, 1990.
9. Gartsman GM, Khan MA, Hammerman SM: Arthroscopic repair of full-thickness tears of the rotator cuff. J Bone Joint Surg 80:832–840, 1998.
10. Gerber C: Latissimus dorsi: Transfer for the treatment of irreparable tears of the rotator Cuff. Clin Orthop 275:152, 1992.
11. Lannotti JP, Zlatkin MB, Esterhai JL, et al: Magnetic resonance imaging of the shoulder: Sensitivity, specificity, and predictive value. J Bone Joint Surg 73:17, 1991.
12. Lehman C, Cuomo F, Kummer FJ, Zuckerman JD: The incidence of full thickness rotator cuff tears in a large cadaveric population. Bull Hosp Jt Dis 54:30–31, 1995.
13. Levine WN, Barron OA, Yamaguchi K: Arthroscopic distal clavicle resection from a bursal approach. Arthroscopy 14:52–56, 1998.
14. Lyons AR, Tomlinson JE: Clinical diagnosis of tears of the rotator cuff. J Bone Joint Surg 74B:414, 1992.
15. Norwood LA, Barrack R, Jacobson KE: Clinical presentation of complete tears of the rotator cuff. J Bone Joint Surg 71:499, 1989.
16. Panni AS, Milano G, Lucania L, et al: Histological analysis of the coracoacromial arch: Correlation between age-related changes and rotator cuff tears. Arthroscopy 12:531–540, 1996.
17. Post M, Silver R, Singh M: Rotator cuff tear: Diagnosis and treatment. Clin Orthop 173:78, 1983.
18. Reed SC, Glossup N, Ogilvie-Harris DJ: Full-thickness rotator cuff tears. A biomechanical comparison of suture versus bone anchor techniques. Am J Sports Med 24:46–48, 1996.
19. Sher JS: Anatomy, Biomechanics, and Pathophysiology of Rotator Cuff Disease. In Iannotti JP, Williams GR (ed): Disorders of the Shoulder: Diagnosis and Management, Philadelphia, Lippincott Williams & Wilkins, 1999, pp 3–31.
20. Sher JS, Uribe J, Posada A, et al: Abnormal findings on magnetic resonance images of asymptomatic shoulders. J Bone Joint Surg 77:10–15, 1995.
21. Snyder SJ, Pachelli AF, Del Pizzo W, et al: Partial thickness rotator cuff tears: Results of arthroscopic treatment. Arthroscopy 7:7, 1991.
22. Tibone JE, Elrod B, Jobe FW, et al: Surgical treatment of tears of the rotator cuff in athletes. J Bone Joint Surg 68:887, 1986.

23. SHOULDER INSTABILITY

Christian Clark, M.D., and David P. Adkison, M.D.

1. What are the primary stabilizers of the shoulder joint?

Stability is achieved through both static and dynamic mechanisms. The stability achieved with the **static** mechanisms is a function of: (1) anatomic elements including articular version, articular conformity and an intact labrum; (2) adhesion-cohesion properties of the synovial fluid; (3) functionally intact and balanced capsular ligaments; and (4) negative intraarticular pressure. **Dynamic** stability is a muscular function that includes: (1) the rotator cuff muscles, which produce the concavity-compression effect; (2) the superficial muscle layer (deltoid, biceps, triceps, pectoralis major, and latissimus dorsi), which balance external torques around the shoulder; and (3) the scapulothoracic muscles, which orient the shoulder on the body for optimal positioning of the glenoid.

2. What are the major capsular ligaments of the shoulder? What directional stability do they impart?

Shoulder ligaments primarily function as restraints at the extremes of motion. The **inferior glenohumeral ligament** (IGHL) complex resists inferior displacement with shoulder abduction; with internal rotation it resists posterior translation; and with external rotation it resists anterior translation. The **middle glenohumeral ligament** resists external rotation in the mid-range of shoulder abduction and anterior translation in the shoulder abducted to 45°. The **superior glenohumeral ligament** resists inferior translation with the arm in neutral position and external rotation at low-range of abduction. The **coracohumeral ligament** resists posterior/inferior humeral head translation.

3. During midrange of motion, which factors provide glenohumeral stability?

During midrange of motion the capsular ligaments are lax and stability is created by the rotator cuff and biceps that maintain a **concavity-compression effect** around the joint. This is a dynamic action in which the rotator cuff compresses the humerus into the congruent glenoid cavity. Lesions that affect this congruency, such as a glenoid rim fracture or labrum detachment, result in a loss of this normal concavity-compression.

4. Is the glenohumeral joint a congruent or incongruent articulation?

The glenohumeral joint articular surfaces are congruent, although the surface area of the humerus is much greater than that of the glenoid. The subchondral bone of the glenoid is less curved than the humerus, but the articular cartilage of the glenoid is thickest at the periphery. The thickness of the cartilage, along with the labrum, deepens the articulating portion of the glenoid and creates a highly conforming joint.

5. What is the difference between laxity and instability?

Laxity is a clinical exam finding and simply refers to the ability to translate the humeral head on the glenoid. A given amount of laxity is required for normal functioning of the shoulder and is affected by age, sex, activities and biologic factors. With certain activities, such as pitching and swimming, a given amount of laxity of the shoulder is beneficial.

Instability is a pathologic condition associated with pain and excessive translation of the joint. Due to the wide spectrum of what is considered normal, it is the inclusion of symptoms with the clinical finding of laxity that implies instability. It is only instability that needs to be treated by physicians.

PATHOANATOMY

6. What is a Bankart lesion? Discuss the pathoanatomy of the IGHL failure and its contribution to joint laxity.

First described by Perthes, the Bankart lesion is the most common lesion in traumatic anterior shoulder dislocations and occurs in about 85% of cases. It is often referred to as the essential lesion of instability after a traumatic dislocation. The Bankart lesion is a detachment of the antero-inferior labrum from the bony glenoid rim and can be associated with a rim fracture. It also represents an avulsion of the glenoid attachment of the inferior glenohumeral ligament. It has been found that before failing at the glenoid insertion, a significant amount of midsubstance strain (plastic deformation) of the IGHL occurs, leading to the concomitant capsular laxity that often accompanies Bankart lesions. Both lesions contribute significantly to shoulder instability.

7. What is a Hill-Sachs lesion? How does it contribute to recurrent shoulder instability?

Caused by impaction of the dislocated humeral head on the glenoid rim, a Hill-Sachs lesion is an osteochondral depression in the posterior humeral head. It may play a causal role in cases of recurrent instability when the lesion is large enough to decrease the humeral head's contribution to passive stability. This is reported to require a depression of about 30% of the articular surface. Larger lesions are associated with dislocations of longer duration, recurrent dislocations, and inferior displacement of the humeral head.

8. Describe the anterior periosteal sleeve avulsion (ALPSA) and the humeral avulsion of the glenhumeral ligament (HAGL) lesions.

The ALPSA lesion was described by Neviaser. It occurs after a traumatic dislocation of the shoulder, with the labrum and the periosteal sleeve of the anterior glenoid being displaced medially. No Bankart lesion is identified, but stability of the joint is compromised. It is a subtle condition that can be difficult to identify on MRI.

The HAGL lesion occurs with a hyperabduction injury to the arm and is also associated with traumatic dislocations. Since this lesion is associated with continued instability, due to the disruption of an important static stabilizer, it is important to recognize and repair anatomically.

9. List the various potential causes of shoulder instability. Discuss why shoulder instability should be thought of as a spectrum of these conditions.

The mnemonics TUBS and AMBRII are helpful:

   Traumatic injury
   Unidirectional instability
   Bankart lesion present
   Surgical treatment

   Atraumatic
   Multidirectional instability
   Bilateral shoulder involvement
   Rehabilitation treatment
   If surgery is needed
   Inferior capsular shift is done

The causes of a patient's instability are often multifactorial and their presentation is better understood as a spectrum. Symptoms may present after an acute traumatic event (unidirectional, less generalized laxity), after multiple episodes of repetitive microtrauma (bidirectional, increased focal laxity), or with no history of trauma (multidirectional, generalized laxity). A careful history and physical exam will help elucidate the etiology, with the understanding that the causes can overlap. Generalized laxity and traumatic capsular avulsion may coexist.

10. What are the most common mechanisms for production of anterior and posterior shoulder dislocations?

Anterior dislocation, which is the direction of 95% of all dislocations, is produced by an external rotation and/or hyperextension force applied to the shoulder that is already in approximately 90° of abduction.

Posterior dislocations can be caused by force applied to the arm when the shoulder is flexed, adducted and internally rotated. The force is usually directed posteriorly along the axis of the arm. This position is often seen when patients fall from a height or grab the dashboard in a motor vechicle accident. Posterior dislocations are often also associated with seizures, electrocutions, and lightning strikes.

11. Describe some of the preferred methods for reducing an anterior dislocation.
- Apply gentle longitudinal traction to the injured arm with countertraction in the axilla. Slow alternation between internal and external rotation is often required to achieve a reduction when performing this manuver. This is considered a safe and reliable method of reduction..
- Place the patient prone with the injured arm lying off the side of the bed. A wrist weight suspended from the unsupported, injured arm is used to apply traction on the arm anteriorly. Rotating the scapula toward the humeral head by application of pressure to the scapular spine is often helpful in achieving a reduction.

12. What is the recurrence rate for patients who sustain an anterior shoulder dislocation?

In a 1987 prospective study by Hovelius, the reported recurrence rates of dislocation over 5 years was noted to vary considerably. Age at the time of initial dislocation was the most important prognostic factor, with recurrence rates of 55% in patients 12–22 years of age, 37% in those 23–29 years, and 12% in those 30–40 years. The recurrence rate after treatment varies depending on the type of treatment and associated injuries.

13. Are any other injuries associated with anterior shoulder dislocations?

Rotator cuff tears are frequently noted in those patiients over the age of 40. Fractures of the greater tuberosity, glenoid, and humeral head are common in the elderly. Major vascular injury to the axillary vessels has been reported in patients with atherosclerotic disease. Brachial plexus injuries, specifically to the axillary nerve, are uncommon but can occur.

14. Which rotator cuff lesions are associated with chronic shoulder instability?

Complete-thickness tears are often seen in older individuals with traumatic shoulder dislocations.

Rotator cuff tendinitis and partial-thickness undersurface tears are very common in patients with chronic shoulder subluxation, whether traumatic or atraumatic. This is thought to be due to abnormal translation of the humeral head increasing the likelihood of rotator cuff impingement and by overworking the cuff in an attempt to keep the head in a reduced positoion. Shoulder subluxation often presents as an "impingement syndrome" and should be suspected in a young, "overhead athlete" (e.g., tennis player, pitcher, swimmer) or a person with a history of traumatic instability who has what appears to be impingement pain.

15. Describe the basis and techniques for the sulcus, apprehension, and relocation tests.

The **sulcus test** demonstrates the degree of inferior laxity and is thought to be a test of the superior glenohumeral and coracohumeral ligaments. It is performed by stabilizing the scapula with the arm in an adducted, neutral positon and the humerus distracted inferiorly. If an asymetric gap beneath the acromion occurs when compared bilaterally or the head is subluxable, the the test is considered positive. The sulcus test measures mid-range stability, i.e., capsular volume.

The **apprehension test** is a provocative exam in which the involved ligament structures are placed in the position of maximal tension, conceptually confirming end-range instability. For the classic apprehension test, the inferior glenohumeral ligament is tested by placing the arm in abduction, external rotation, and extension, also known as the provocative position. In a patient with anterior instability this will cause an abnormal anterior translation of the humeral head, thus producing a sense of impending subluxation.

The **relocation test** is performed by applying a posteriorly directed pressure on the humeral head while performing the apprehension test. If this posterior pressure relieves the subluxation symptoms, it is considered a positive test and is suggestive of anterior instability.

16. Which radiographic views are useful in evaluating shoulder dislocations?

Radiographs taken from perpendicular planes are required: a "true" AP radiograph (which demonstrates the inferior glenoid rim) and either an axillary or transcapular "Y" lateral view. The West Point view may be obtained if an inferior glenoid rim fracture is suspected.

17. Describe a typical rehabilitation plan for a first-time traumatic shoulder anterior dislocation.

In contrast to traditional recommendations for immobilization of up to 6 weeks in young athletes, recent studies indicate that immobilization is required only until adequate pain relief is attained, which typically occurs after 1–3 weeks. Goals of rehabilitation are (1) restoration of a full painless range of motion, (2) avoidance of the "provocative" positions for 6 weeks, and (3) strengthening the cuff and scapulothoracic muscles. Patients start with isometric exercises and gradually progress to isotonic exercises. Scapular stabilizers are strengthened to provide a stable base for humeral rotation and to maintain the glenoid in a position that allows for maximal congruency. Patients >45 years old should have motion restored as quickly as tolerated because their incidence of stiffness is higher, while their risk of recurrent dislocation is lower.

18. List the indications for surgery for traumatic shoulder instability.

- Failed or unstable closed reduction
- Soft tissue interposition by the rotator cuff, capsule, or biceps tendon
- Greater tuberosity fractures that remain displaced >1 cm after reduction
- Large glenoid rim fractures

19. Discuss the effect a glenoid rim fracture has on stability of the glenohumeral joint and how to treat it.

An anteroinferior glenoid rim fracture lessens the stabilizing effect of concavity-compression and may lead to instability. It is also thought to release the negative pressure formed in the glenohumeral joint and makes the labrum an ineffective chock-block anteriorly. If the fracture fragment is > 25%, the fragment should be reduced and repaired in its anatomic position. If the fragment is < 25%, re-establishing the capsular origin at the glenoid rim margin is most important, and the fragment may either be repaired, excised or left displaced.

20. What are the commonly performed shoulder stabilization procedures?

The **Bankart repair** and the various modifications to this surgery involve reattachment of the detached antero-inferior labrum back down to the glenoid, indirectly repairing the inferior glenohumeral ligament complex. When a shoulder develops chronic instability, the capsular ligaments may become incompetent due to interstitial damage. This secondary capsular laxity requires the ligament tension also be addressed with a **capsulorraphy** or **capsular shift,** in addition to the repair of the injured labrum. This can be achieved with a medially, inferiorly, or laterally based shift of the capsule. The lateral-based shifts are currently the most popular due to their effectiveness and reliability. A plethora of other procedures have been described for shoulder instability, that often work by limiting the shoulder's range of motion so that end-range laxity cannot be challenged.

21. What physical findings are typical of an unreduced posterior dislocation?

The arm is usually positioned at the side with an inability to flex or external rotate the shoulder. The anterior shoulder is flattened and the coracoid process may be prominent. The patient may be noted to have a posterior fullness of the shoulder as the head sits trapped behind the glenoid. This type of dislocation is the often missed, usually because of inadequate physical and radiographic exams.

22. What is the current treatment for posterior instability?

The recommended treatment for symptomatic recurrent posterior instability is nonoperative. This includes not only a shoulder strengthening routine, but also avoidance of provocative activities. Various papers have suggested approximately 60% of patients will report success with nonoperative intervention. If after prolonged, dedicated physical therapy the patient continues to have symptoms, surgery should be considered. Surgical intervention can include a capsular shift, a bony block procedure, or a posterior labral repair, if needed. Postoperatively, the patient is splinted in 0 to 10 degrees of external rotation for 4–6 weeks. Recent reports have demonstrated a more satisfactory outcome with surgical treatment.

23. Should patients with voluntary shoulder instability be operated upon?

Many voluntary subluxators or dislocators have underlying psychiatric problems that an orthopaedic surgeon cannot help. Patients who can dislocate voluntarily are considered poor surgical candidates. Any patient with generalized laxity, scapulothoracic instability, or mistracking should be placed in an aggressive rehabilitation program for a minimum of 6 to 12 months before any procedure is considered.

There are other patients who are considered positional dislocators. These are patients who are able to voluntarily dislocate their shoulder when they place their arm in a provocative position, but are generally reluctant to do so. They often will prevent future dislocations by avoiding these positions in their daily activities. These patients are good surgical candidates with historically favorable outcomes.

24. What is the role of arthroscopic repair in the surgeon's armamentarium for shoulder instability?

Long-term follow-up of athroscopic instability procedures have demonstrated failure rates between 5 and 40%, while open capsular repairs have shown success rates of 90–95%. There have been improvements in the results of arthroscopic repairs as experience and fixation methods have improved, but they continue to be considered inferior to the open repair. It is believed that an arthroscopic repair of a Bankart lesion does not directly address the possible concomitant ligamentous laxity often seen with this condition. Even when the laxity is not specifically addressed with a capsular shift during an open Bankart repair, subsequent scarring of the anterior structures at the surgical site is believed to improve the final results with the open repair technique. Evidence shows that the arthroscopic approach works best in a high-demand athlete who has unidirectional instability and no global laxity, generally following a single traumatic episode with associated Bankart lesion. The Bankart capsulorrhaphy is currently *still* the gold standard that all new techniques must be compared to.

BIBLIOGRAPHY

1. American Academy of Orthopaedic Surgeons: Orthopaedic Knowledge Update 6. Rosemont, IL, 1999.
2. American Academy of Orthopaedic Surgeons: OKU Shoulder and Elbow. Rosemont, IL, 1996.
3. Bigliani LU: The Unstable Shoulder. Monograph, American Academy of Orthopaedic Surgeons, Rosemont, IL, 1996.
4. Flatow EL, Warner JJP: Instability of the shoulder: Complex problems and failed repairs. J Bone Joint Surg 80A:122–140, 1998.
5. Iannotti JP, Williams GR: Disorders of the Shoulder, Phildelphia, Lippincott, 1999.
6. Rockwood CA, Matsen FA: The Shoulder, 2nd ed. Philadelphia, W.B. Saunders, 1998.

24. INJURIES OF THE SHOULDER IN THE THROWING ATHLETE

Kirk S. Hutton, M.D.

1. Why is the shoulder so often injured in the throwing athlete?

The glenohumeral joint has more range of motion than any other joint in the human body. Stability of this joint depends on intact muscles and ligaments rather than on bony supporting structures. The forces generated in the throwing shoulder are much greater than the forces generated in the shoulder musculature alone, and, therefore, cause significant stresses around this joint, making it susceptible to acute and chronic inflammatory conditions.

2. List the five phases of pitching.

(1) Wind-up, (2) early cocking, (3) late cocking, (4) acceleration, and (5) follow through.

3. How does throwing form affect the incidence of shoulder injuries in the throwing athlete?

Proper body mechanics require that the thrower use his or her body weight and large leg, trunk, and back muscle groups to generate kinetic energy across the shoulder in the direction of the thrown object. In general, shoulder injuries occur in one of two ways. Improper body mechanics during the wind-up and cocking phases place more dependence on the shoulder muscles to generate the required energy to propel the object, thus leading to fatigue of the shoulder muscles. After the thrown object is released, the retained energy in the throwing arm needs to be dissipated by reversing the initial process, i.e., using the large muscles in the lower limb and back to absorb this energy. An improper follow through results in retention of excessive energy in the soft tissues of the shoulder, subsequently causing tissue damage.

4. What type of injuries may occur in the throwing athlete?

Acute overuse injuries, such as rotator cuff tendinitis and biceps tendinitis, are common. Chronic injuries include impingement syndrome, rotator cuff tears, glenoid labrum tears, and shoulder instability. Inflammation from repetitive stress may injure the acromioclavicular and the sternoclavicular joints. Uncommon causes of shoulder pain in the throwing athlete include quadrilateral space syndrome, suprascapular nerve entrapment, axillary artery occlusion, axillary vein thrombosis, posterior capsular laxity, and glenoid spurs.

5. What are the common presenting symptoms of an athlete with shoulder pain?

The athlete generally reports anterior shoulder pain that becomes worse with increased throwing velocity in his or her throw, stating that he or she cannot obtain maximum velocity in workouts or in a game situation. Occasionally, posterior shoulder pain is present.

6. What are the important positive findings on physical examination of a thrower with shoulder pain?

Most athletes with shoulder pain have positive impingement signs. More important, however, are the signs of subtle instability, such as a positive apprehension sign and a positive relocation test. Posterior capsular tightness manifest by decreased internal rotation of the shoulder also is significant in throwers. Andrews has noted the importance of a total range-of-motion arc of approximately 180° with regard to external and internal rotation. In throwers, a gain in external rotation may come at the loss of internal rotation which would classify as a shoulder "at risk" for injury.

7. Describe the apprehension test.

The apprehension test is used to detect anterior instability of the glenohumeral joint, and involves bringing the involved shoulder into approximately 90° of abduction and externally rotating the shoulder. As external rotation increases, the athlete with anterior instability will feel as if the shoulder is going to "pop out." He or she will guard against further external rotation and become very apprehensive—thus, the apprehension test.

8. Describe the relocation test.

The first part of the relocation test is performed just like the apprehension test. With the patient lying supine, abduct and externally rotate the arm while applying gentle anterior pressure to the posterior aspect of the humeral head. In the athlete with anterior subluxation, this maneuver usually causes pain as opposed to the uncomfortable sensation that the shoulder may dislocate. The second part of the relocation test involves repeating the test, but then applying a posteriorly directed force to the humeral head. This maneuver maintains the head in the anatomic position. A positive test occurs if the athlete experiences relief of pain in maximal abduction and external rotation.

9. Why is it important to distinguish between impingement and instability?

A few years ago, it was believed that most young athletes with anterior shoulder pain had primary impingement. They underwent the standard anterior acromioplasty with repair of the rotator cuff as needed. Tibone et al. reported that the results of this operation in young throwing athletes were very inconsistent. They have now shown that such athletes usually have primary instability with secondary impingement. Thus, an anterior acromioplasty with excision of the coracoacromial ligament in this population may cause more instability of the shoulder and magnify the symptoms.

10. Describe the treatment for primary instability and secondary impingement.

The initial treatment of athletes with this condition involves aggressive rehabilitation. The program should begin with "relative rest," i.e., cessation of the overhead activity that causes the pain. Stretching should be done carefully and only for muscle groups with obvious tightness. Stretching the anterior muscles and capsule in a patient with anterior instability may cause further laxity. Lastly, strengthening exercises concentrating on the rotator cuff and scapular rotators should be performed. The entire program should be continued for 6–12 months with appropriate supervision and documentation before considering any operative procedures.

11. What is the function of the scapular rotators?

Muscles included in the scapular rotator group are the trapezius, serratus anterior, and the rhomboids. Their main function in the throwing athlete is to aid in glenohumeral stability by placing the glenoid in an optimal position for the throwing event.

12. Name the rotator cuff muscles.

Supraspinatus, infraspinatus, teres minor, and subscapularis.

13. What is the function of the rotator cuff muscles?

The subscapularis is a weak internal rotator of the humerus. The infraspinatus and teres minor are external rotators of the humerus. As a whole, the rotator cuff muscles function to center the humeral head in the glenoid, thus adding stability and maximum leverage to shoulder motions.

14. Do ligaments add to the stability of the shoulder?

Yes. The glenohumeral ligaments and the labrum add stability to the shoulder. In the overhead athlete, the inferior glenohumeral ligament is the most important, because it is the prime anterior stabilizer when the arm is abducted >90° and externally rotated. With the arm abducted 45°, the middle glenohumeral ligament is the primary restraint to anterior translation of the humeral head. Other structures important in glenohumeral stability include the labrum (concavity compression), negative intra-articular pressure, and cohesive forces in the glenohumeral joint.

15. How does anterior instability develop in the throwing athlete?

Anterior instability may develop after a high-energy trauma, but in the throwing athlete it more commonly starts as an overuse injury. Chronic overuse can stretch the static stabilizers of the shoulder, thus causing mild instability. Such instability leads to asynchrony in the firing of the scapular rotators and rotator cuff muscles, putting increased stress on the rotator cuff to contain the humerus in the center of the glenoid. As the rotator cuff muscles become weakened from the overload, the head of the humerus subluxes more anteriorly as the arm is abducted and externally rotated. Anterior subluxation then causes secondary impingement of the rotator cuff on the acromion and the coracoacromial ligament.

16. Are imaging studies helpful in the diagnosis of shoulder pain?

Yes. Plain x-rays should be taken to rule out bony pathology such as fractures and osteoarthrosis. Special x-ray views such as the axillary view and West Point may demonstrate signs of instability (spurring or erosion of the anterior glenoid or a Hill-Sachs lesion).

17. Which imaging modality may be the most useful tool in diagnosing the cause of shoulder pain?

Recent studies indicate that MRI is superior to ultrasound and CT arthrography in evaluating shoulder pain due to rotator cuff tears, subacromial impingement, coracoacromial arch stenosis, and osteoarthritis of the glenohumeral or acromioclavicular joint.

18. What other diagnostic tools are helpful?

Selective injections with lidocaine can help pinpoint the painful area in the shoulder. Diagnostic arthroscopy is superior to an open operative procedure because it provides excellent visualization of the glenohumeral joint and subacromial space, causes less soft tissue destruction, and has a shorter rehabilitation period. With newly developed techniques, arthroscopy also may be used to correct or repair many pathologic conditions in the shoulder. Arthroscopy also affords the clinician the opportunity to evaluate for the presence, degree, and direction of shoulder laxity while the athlete is under anesthesia.

19. Is surgery ever necessary?

Yes. If a throwing athlete with instability has faithfully completed 6–12 months of an aggressive supervised rehabilitation program and still cannot participate in throwing secondary to pain, a surgical procedure that addresses the anterior capsule and labrum should be performed. Athletes with documented rotator cuff tears, labrum lesions, or loose bodies should have such lesions repaired or excised.

20. What is a SLAP lesion?

A SLAP lesion is an entity originally described and classified by Snyder in 1990. SLAP (superior labrum anterior and posterior) involves the superior labrum, the biceps anchor, and a portion of the glenohumeral ligament attachment.

21. Describe the mechanism of injury of a SLAP lesion.

Two commonly described mechanisms cause a SLAP injury. In an acute traumatic event, a **superior compression type injury** may represent a fall on an outstretched arm, causing the humeral head to ride superiorly and creating a compression and subsequent avulsion of the superior glenoid labrum. In a thrower, a repetitive microtrauma occurs from rotator cuff disease that results in a chronic or recurrent superior translation of the humeral head on the glenoid rim, thus causing a SLAP lesion.

The second mechanism is **inferior traction**. An acute traumatic event, usually involving carrying a heavy object that causes axial inferior traction on the arm and biceps tendon complex, may cause a SLAP lesion. In the thrower the mechanism is a repetitive torsional overload placed on the labrum and glenohumeral ligaments by the forceful rotation of the humerus during the throwing motion. This force is especially high during the deceleration phase of throwing. Because of the repetitive stress placed on these tissues, a throwing athlete can develop pseudolaxity and posterior shoulder pain secondary to this SLAP lesion.

22. What is a peel-back lesion?

A peel-back lesion is a variant of a type II SLAP lesion that involves the posterior superior portion of the glenoid labrum at its attachment to the glenoid. The laxity in the labrum attachment in this area allows the biceps tendon to change its vector force angle when the arm is brought into an abducted and externally rotated position. This angle change in the biceps tendon transmits a torsional force to the posterior superior labrum which causes the labrum to lift off or peel-back from the posterior superior portion of the glenoid. This causes a pseudoanterior laxity and arthroscopically can be visualized with the arm in abduction and external rotation. Repair of the posterior superior glenoid labrum down to the glenoid rim stabilizes the labrum and corrects the pseudolaxity, thus treating the pain in a thrower's shoulder.

23. What is internal impingement?

Internal impingement was initially described by Walch, and subsequently expanded by Jobe, who described a posterior superior glenohumeral impingement in throwers. Walch and Jobe noted that with the arm in abduction and external rotation, a portion of the rotator cuff contacted the posterior superior glenoid and labrum, which over time, can cause partial tearing and inflammation in the rotator cuff and labrum in this area. Some authors believe that this is a physiologic process, whereas others believe that it is due to hyperexternal rotation and pseudo anterior laxity. The internal impingement could also be exacerbated by the peel-back lesion and treatment of this phenomenon includes glenoid labrum repair if present or possibly a thermal capsular shrinkage of the middle and inferior glenohumeral ligaments in order to reduce the external rotation and obliterate the internal impingement. Humeral head osteotomies to change humeral retroversion may also have a place in the treatment.

24. Describe the four common types of SLAP lesions.

Snyder originally classified slap lesions into four types. A type I SLAP lesion involves degenerative fraying and tearing of the glenoid labrum at its superior attachment usually seen in degenerative or arthritic shoulders. A type II SLAP lesion, which is the most common, involves the biceps anchor. This anchor is unstable anteriorly and posterior from approximately the 10 o'clock to the 2 o'clock position. These lesions are usually treated by repair, whereas type I lesions are treated with debridement. A type III SLAP lesion involves a bucket-handle tear of the glenoid labrum. This is usually seen in a meniscoid type labrum. The biceps anchor is commonly stable and treatment usually is debridement of the bucket-handle fragments. A type IV SLAP lesion involves a bucket-handle tear of the labrum with a longitudinal tear extending into the biceps tendon. Treatment of this lesion is controversial and depends on the stability of the biceps anchor.

BIBLIOGRAPHY

1. Bisson LJ, Andrews JR: Classification in mechanisms ofshoulder injuries in throwers. In Andrews JR, Zarins B, Wilk KE (eds): Injuries in Baseball. Philadelphia, Lippincott-Raven, 1998, pp 47–55.
2. Glousman R, Jobe F, Tibone J, et al: Dynamic electromyographic analysis of the throwing shoulder with glenohumeral instability. J Bone Joint Surg 70A:220–226, 1988.
3. Hurley JA: Shoulder arthroscopy: Its role in evaluating shoulder disorders in the athlete. Am J Sports Med 18:480–483, 1990.
4. Marone PJ (ed): Shoulder Injuries in Sports. Rockville, MD, Aspen Publishers, 1992.
5. Nelson MC, Leather GP, Nirschl RP, et al: Evaluation of the painful shoulder. J Bone Joint Surg 73A:707–715, 1991.

6. Parten PM, Burkhart S: The relationship of superior labral anteroposterior (SLAP) lesions and pseudolaxity to shoulder injuries in the overhead athlete. Op Tech Sports Med 10:10–17, 2002.
7. Rockwood CA, Mattsen FA (eds): The Shoulder, vols. 1 and 2, 2nd ed. Philadelphia, W.B. Saunders, 1998.
8. Snyder SJ, Karzel RP, Del Pizzo W, et al: SLAP lesions of the shoulder. Arthroscopy 6:274–279, 1990.
9. Tibone JA, Jobe FA, Kerlin RF, et al: Shoulder impingement syndrome in athletes treated by anterior acromioplasty. Clin Orthop 188:134–140, 1985.

25. ACROMIOCLAVICULAR AND STERNOCLAVICULAR JOINTS

Jeffrey P. Davick, M.D.

1. What type of joint is the acromioclavicular joint?

The acromioclavicular joint is a diarthroidal (synovial) joint with a fibrocartilaginous disc between the two bones (similar to a meniscus).

2. Name the important ligaments around the acromioclavicular joint.

The acromioclavicular ligament connects the distal end of the clavicle to the acromion, providing horizontal stability. The coracoclavicular ligament connects the coracoid to the clavicle. It is made of two bands that provide vertical stability, the conoid and the trapezoid.

3. Describe the most common mechanism of injury to the acromioclavicular joint.

The acromioclavicular joint is most commonly injured by a direct fall onto the point of the shoulder with the arm adducted.

4. List the types of acromioclavicular sprains.

Type I sprain—a partial injury to the acromioclavicular ligament with no instability or displacement. The coracoclavicular ligament remains intact.

Type II sprain—disruption of the acromioclavicular ligament. The coracoclavicular ligament remains intact, preventing significant superior displacement of the clavicle.

Type III sprain—disruption of both the acromioclavicular and coracoclavicular ligaments, allowing superior displacement of the clavicle.

Type IV sprain—an injury in which the clavicle is displaced not only superiorly but also posteriorly into the trapezius (buttonhole).

Type V sprain—the clavicle is displaced superiorly to the point at which the clavicle is in a subcutaneous position.

Type VI sprain—an extremely rare injury in which both the acromioclavicular and coracoclavicular ligaments are disrupted, with the clavicle displaced inferior to the acromion or coracoid. This is usually the result of a high-energy injury and should arouse suspicion for associated injuries (fractures of the shoulder girdle, brachial plexus injuries, or disruption of the sternoclavicular joint).

5. What type of radiographs are needed to evaluate an injured acromioclavicular joint?

An anteroposterior, axillary, and Zanca view (15° cephalic tilt) are recommended and are usually sufficient to distinguish the type of sprain. Stress radiographs are rarely needed since treatment of a type II sprain and uncomplicated type III sprain is the same.

6. How is an acute incomplete type I or type II acromioclavicular sprain treated?

Ice and immobilization are needed initially. Patients are usually most comfortable in an arm sling. Early range of motion and strengthening exercises are recommended.

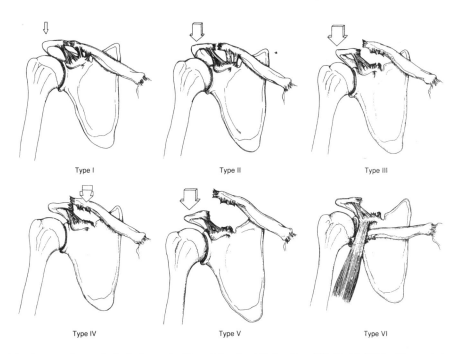

Type I   Type II   Type III

Type IV   Type V   Type VI

The six types of acromioclavicular sprain. (From J Am Acad Orthop Surg 9(1):11–18, 1997; with permission of the American Academy of Orthopaedic Surgeons.)

7. What type of treatment is recommended for an acute complete disruption (type III through type VI)?

Nonoperative treatment (as in types I and II) is used for patients with uncomplicated **type III** injuries and limited functional requirements. Operative treatment for a type III injury is controversial. Functional results (strength and range of motion) are the same with operative and nonoperative treatment. **Type IV** sprains often require operative treatment because the clavicle is buttonholed through the trapezius and remains painful, especially with overhead activities. Operative treatment is recommended for open injuries, **type VI** sprains, and when the clavicle is subcutaneous and in danger of eroding through the skin (**type V**).

Operative treatment consists of repair or reconstruction of the coracoclavicular structures. Pins across the acromioclavicular joint should be avoided; they tend to migrate to undesirable sites such as the mediastinum.

8. What is the recommended treatment for chronically painful acromioclavicular separations?

Excision of the distal clavicle is warranted, followed by reconstruction of the coracoclavicular structures if needed. Coracoclavicular position is maintained by heavy suture or a removable screw. The coracoacromial ligament is detached from the acromion and transferred to the clavicle to act as a new coracoclavicular ligament (the Weaver-Dunn procedure).

9. What type of joint is the sternoclavicular joint?

The sternoclavicular joint, similar to the acromioclavicular joint, is a diarthroidal (synovial) joint with a fibrocartilaginous disc (similar to meniscus) between the clavicle and sternum.

10. Name the important ligaments around the sternoclavicular joint.

The costoclavicular ligaments have anterior fibers that resist upward rotation of the clavicle, and posterior fibers that resist downward rotation of the clavicle. The sternoclavicular ligament is actually a thick portion of the capsule. Its anterior fibers resist upward displacement of the clavicle.

11. What is the usual mechanism of injury to the sternoclavicular joint?
The most common mechanism of injury is a motor vehicle accident. Significant forces are necessary to cause dislocation of the sternoclavicular joint. A direct blow to the clavicle most commonly causes a posterior dislocation of the sternoclavicular joint. An indirect force to the anterolateral aspect of the clavicle can cause an anterior dislocation of the sternoclavicular joint, whereas an indirect force to the posterolateral aspect of the shoulder will cause a posterior dislocation of the sternoclavicular joint.

12. What are the common findings on physical examination of a dislocated sternoclavicular joint?
With **anterior** sternoclavicular dislocation, the medial aspect of the clavicle is prominent and the asymmetry is obvious.
With a **posterior** sternoclavicular dislocation, the findings are subtle. The medial end of the clavicle may be less palpable but more tender when compared with the other side. Patients also may complain of shortness of breath or have difficulty swallowing.

13. Describe the best way to evaluate the sternoclavicular joint radiographically.
AP views of the sternoclavicular joint are often difficult to interpret. Special projections include the serendipity view, which involves a 40° cephalic tilt of the x-ray beam. The medial aspect of both clavicles is seen on this view. Superior displacement of the clavicle represents an anterior dislocation, whereas inferior displacement represent a posterior dislocation. CT scans easily delineate the position of the medial clavicle compared to the sternum. MRI also can be used to provide the same information as the CT scan, but it also shows the soft tissue anatomy and associated mediastinal structures.

14. What are the treatment recommendations for acute sternoclavicular sprains?
With mild sprains that are not dislocated, patients are treated symptomatically with a sling until they are comfortable, followed by early rehabilitation.
Anterior dislocation of the sternoclavicular joint is treated with closed reduction done under either intravenous sedation or general anesthesia. Open reduction has a high complication rate and is generally not necessary.
Acute posterior dislocation is repaired with closed reduction and usually performed under general anesthesia. A towel clip may be required to manually assist reduction of the sternoclavicular joint. An open reduction may be needed for a posterior dislocation, and such injuries should be reduced to avoid late complications from erosion into the underlying mediastinal structures.

15. What is the treatment recommended for chronically dislocated sternoclavicular joints?
For chronic anterior sternoclavicular dislocation, nonoperative treatment is generally preferred. Patients are usually minimally symptomatic and the condition is primarily a cosmetic problem. For chronic posterior dislocation of the sternoclavicular joint, operative treatment may be necessary to prevent potential complications (erosion of the clavicle into the underlying mediastinal structures). Open reduction and stabilization are usually performed with the assistance of a thoracic surgeon.

BIBLIOGRAPHY

1. Bjernfeld H, Hovelius L, Thorling J: Acromioclavicular separations treated conservatively. Acta Orthop Scand 54:747–745, 1983.
2. Clark HD, McCann PD: Acromioclavicular joint injuries. Orthop Clin North Am 31:177–178, 2000.
3. Cox JS: The fate of the acromioclavicular joint in athletic injuries. Am J Sports Med 9:50, 1981.

4. Dias JJ, Steingold RA, Richardson RA, et al: The conservative treatment of acromioclavicular dislocation: Review after five years. J Bone Joint Surg 69B:719–722, 1987.
5. Eskola A: Sternoclavicular dislocation: A plea for open treatment. Acta Orthop Scand 57:227–228, 1986.
6. Galpin RD, Hawkins RJ, Grainger RW: A comparative analysis of operative versus nonoperative treatment of Grade III acromioclavicular separations. Clin Orthop 193:150–155, 1985.
7. Larsen E, Bjerg-Nielsen A, Christensen P: Conservative or surgical treatment of acromioclavicular dislocation: A prospective, controlled, randomized study. J Bone Joint Surg 68A:552–555, 1986.
8. Lee KW, Debski RE, Shen CH, et al: Functional evaluation of the ligaments at the acromioclavicular joint
during anteroposterior and superoinferior translation. Am J Sports Med 25:858–862, 1997.
9. Lemos MJ: The evaluation and treatment of the injured acromioclavicular joint in athletes. Am J Sports
Med 26:137–144, 1998.
10. MacDonald PB, Alexander JM, Frejuk J, Johnson G: Comprehensive functional analysis of shoulders following complete acromioclavicular separation. Am J Sports Med 16:475–480, 1988.
11. Nuber GW, Bowen MK: Acromioclavicular joint injuries and distal clavicle fractures. J Am Acad Orthop Surg 5:11–18, 1997.
12. Phillips AM, Smart C, Groom AF: Acromioclavicular dislocation. Conservative or surgical therapy. Clin
Orthop 353:10–17, 1998.
13. Press J, Zuckerman JD, Gallagher M, Cuomo F: Treatment of grade II acromioclavicular separations. Operative versus nonoperative management. Bull Hosp Dis 56:77–83, 1997.
14. Rawes ML, Dias JJ: Long-term results of conservative treatment for acromioclavicular dislocation. J
Bone Joint Surg Br 78:410–412, 1996.
15. Rockwood CA Jr, Groh GI, Wirth M, Grassi FA: Resection arthroplasty of the sternoclavicular joint. J
Bone Joint Surg Am 79:387–393, 1997.

26. ARTHRITIS, ARTHROPLASTY, AND ARTHRODESIS OF THE SHOULDER

Edward V. Fehringer, M.D.

1. What is glenohumeral arthritis?

Glenohumeral arthritis refers to loss of glenohumeral joint articular cartilage, leading to roughness that frequently manifests itself in shoulder pain and stiffness.

2. What is the differential diagnosis for glenohumeral arthritis?

- Rheumatoid arthritis
- Osteoarthritis
- Posttraumatic arthritis
- Postsurgical arthritis (capsulorraphy arthropathy)
- Cuff tear arthropathy (CTA)
- Avascular necrosis
- Crystalline arthropathy (gout, pseudogout)
- other seronegative arthropathies
- Septic arthritis

3. Describe the typical presentation of a patient with rheumatoid arthritis affecting the shoulder.

Occasionally shoulder pain and stiffness are primary presenting complaints in a patient with rheumatoid arthritis. However, most patients with shoulder pain due to rheumatoid arthritis already carry the diagnosis of rheumatoid arthritis. Shoulder pain due to glenohumeral roughness in such patients is typically insidious in onset and transitory rather than constant and progressive.

4. What is the natural history of rheumatoid arthritis of the shoulder?

During painful inflammatory attacks of the shoulder, patients tyipcally hold the affected arm internally rotated against the chest in a protective position. Inactivity leads to capsular and rotator cuff stiffness and associated weakness. Motion loss has a deleterious effect on the nutrition of the articular surfaces, leading to further arthrosis progression. Progression may also lead to rotator cuff thinning and tears.

5. Does rheumatoid arthritis affect the shoulder in different ways?

The four types of involvement of the shoulder with roughness due to rheumatoid arthritis are dry, wet, resorptive, and bursal. Treatment should be tailored to the patient.

Dry: Marked stiffness and loss of articular surfaces are characteristic. Radiographs typically reveal sclerosis and periarticular cyst formation with small osteophytes. Minimal marginal erosions are generally present.

Wet: Radiographs characteristically reveal evidence of exuberant granulations and marginal erosions with associated narrowing of the proximal humerus. Osteophyte formation is not typically seen. The humeral head may migrate medially due to glenoid erosion.

Resorptive: Typically, increased pain and stiffness are presenting symptoms. Radiographically, dramatic bone destruction and resorption may be seen.

Bursal: Subacromial and subdeltoid bursae may swell with the subacromial bursa filling with rice bodies. Attempts to aspirate fluid generally prove fruitless. The bursal form may spare the glenohumeral joint.

6. Describe the radiographic appearance of glenohumeral arthritis secondary to rheumatologic disease.

When rheumatoid arthritis affects the glenohumeral joint, a central erosion pattern is tyipcal along with periarticular erosions and cystic changes due to the inflmmatory nature of the disease. The large osteophytes seen in osteoarthritis are uncommon in rheumatoid arthritis. Bone loss on either side of the glenohumeral joint may occur which has significant implications when considering shoulder arthroplasty.

7. How do patients with glenohumeral osteoarthritis present?

Patients with glenohumeral osteoarthritis often present with complaints of an insidious onset of aching shoulder pain and stiffness over a period of months to years. Some have a history of heavy labor.

8. Describe the radiographic appearance of glenohumeral osteoarthritis.

In glenohumeral osteoarthritis, humeral head articular surface wear typically begins centrally and is accentuated by peripheral osteophyte formation. This is referred to as the "Friar Tuck" sign. With progression, an inferior humeral head "goat-beard" ostephyte develops as the head flattens. Glenoid articular surface wear typically occurs posteriorly as anterior soft tissue structures tighten, creating obligate posterior translation, glenoid wear and erosion. One may often note posterior glenoid erosion on the essential axillary radiograph.

9. To what does a "biconcave glenoid" refer?

In glenohumeral osteoarthritis, varying amounts of anterior glenoid articular surface remain when posterior erosion is present. Posterior erosion, due to tightness of anterior soft tissues and obligate posterior translation of the humeral head, is manifested by a posterior glenoid concavity where the existing humeral head articulates. This leaves a vertical ridge in the glenoid that separates the posterior concavity from the original glenoid concavity that is made up of remaining anterior glenoid articular surface. Glenoid morphology is noted on an axillary radiograph and is commonly referred to as a biconcave glenoid if two concavities exist. Glenoid concavity and morphology have very important implications in glenohumeral arthroplasty. Bi-concave glenoids are also commonly seen in those with capsulorraphy arthropathy. Glenoid morphology can be difficult to quantify based on an axillary radiograph (because of factors such as projection) and is often underestimated.

10. What is capsulorraphy arthropathy?

Capsulorraphy arthropathy is a glenohumeral arthritic condition that results from previous anterior shoulder capsular surgery. Anterior structures are often tightened in surgery for anterior dislocations. As a result, with external rotation affected shoulders develop obligate posterior tranlsation and subsequent wear. Capsulorraphy arthropathy often leads to some of the most severe cases of posterior erosion.

11. What are the nonoperative treatments for glenohumeral arthritis?

Conservative treatments are directed at diminution of pain and preservation of motion. Patients often present later in the course of glenohumeral disease than they would with a comparable amount of hip or knee arthrosis. However, early radiographic signs of glehomumeral arthritis are frequently overlooked and patient symptoms are attributed to rotator cuff pathology. The distinction between the two is important as their treatments differ. Nonsteroidal anti-inflammatory agents, gentle stretching programs, and occasional intraarticular steroid injections may provide reasonable patient comfort and function.

12. Describe the surgical treatments for glenohumeral arthritis.

Surgical treatment must be tailored to the patient. Options include but are not exclusive to open or arthroscopic synovectomy and/or debridement with or without capsular releases, resection arthroplasty, hemiarthroplasty, total shoulder arthroplasty, and arthrodesis.

13. What is synovectomy of the shoulder?

Synovectomy refers to removal of the diseased synovial lining of the shoulder with an open or arthroscopic technique. It is generally performed in patients with inflammatory arthritidies of the shoulder to alleviate pain and temporarily arrest inflammatory processes. It is typically reserved for early stages of disease in which little articular or osseous destruction has occurred.

14. What is the difference between shoulder hemiarthroplasty and total shoulder arthroplasty?

Shoulder hemiarthroplasty is the surgical resurfacing of the humeral head only with a metallic prosthetic implant. Anatomic resurfacing is the goal. Humeral component fixation may be achieved with a press-fit uncemented humeral prosthesis or with a cemented humeral prosthesis. **Total shoulder arthroplasty** refers to resurfacing the humeral head *and* glenoid surfaces. Glenoid resurfacing is typically performed with a polyethylene prosthesis. After appropriate concentric glenoid reaming, the glenoid component is typically implanted with the aid of methylmethacrylate. Various forms of keeled and pegged polyethelene glenoid components exist. Uncemented metal-backed glenoid components also exist.

15. What are the indications for shoulder arthroplasty?

The main indication for a shoulder arthroplasty is pain and stiffness due to glenohumeral arthritis.

16. How does one decide whether to perform a hemiarthroplasty or a total shoulder arthroplasty in patients with glenohumeral arthritis?

This question is complex and somewhat controversial. In general, hemiarthroplasty may be performed with reliable results in those patients with glenohumeral arthritis and a concentric glenoid; glenohumeral arthritis due to loss the rotator cuff tissues; glehonumeral arthritis with insufficient glenoid bone stock for glenoid resurfacing; glenohumeral arthritis with significant medial erosion and tight soft tissues such that placement of additional hardware increases the risk of joint overstuffing; glenohumeral arthritis due to avascular necrosis in patients without glenoid changes; and in certain three- and four-part proximal humerus fractures. Some patients may not achieve desired pain relief after a hemiarthroplasty and may require conversion to a total shoulder arthroplasty.

Total shoulder arthroplasty should be performed in patients with a bi-concave glenoid. Several recent studies also suggest that total shoulder arthroplasty achieves better pain relief than hemiarthroplasty for cases of glenohumeral arthritis with an intact rotator cuff regardless of glenoid morphology. These studies suggest the glenoid should be resurfaced in cases of glenohumeral arthritis with sufficient bone and an intact rotator cuff. Glenoid resurfacing is technically demanding and should probably be reserved for those surgeons who have had appropriate training in this area.

17. How does one expose the glenoid when resurfacing it?

Glenoid exposure is critical to resurfacing. Subscapularis lengthening by release from the lesser tuberosity (and eventual repair to the humeral neck through bone holes) should be performed in shoulders with internal rotation contractures. A 360°" subscapularis release should be performed, especially releasing the tendon from its coracoid adesions. Finally, an appropriate glenoid-sided 190° capsular release is essential. This is performed from twelve o'clock to seven o'cl,ock in the right shoulder. Posterior capsular releases should be avoided, especially in cases of posterior erosion due to the excess posterior capsular laxity and the risk of creating posterior instability if released. The axiallary nerve should be identified and protected to avoid injury. Appropriate retractors are very helpful.

18. How does one treat a biconcave glenoid?

Affected shoulders require establishment of a concentric glenoid. Often the anterior concavity is preferentially reamed to achieve one concavity for eventual glenoid component placement or for a smooth articulation with the prosthetic humeral component. Posterior bone-grafting has been performed but is somewhat impractical and is used less and less.

19. What are the contraindications to shoulder arthroplasty?

The only absolute contraindication is active infection. Relative contraindications include patients with a neuropathic joint and young heavy laborers who are unwilling or unable to alter their lifestyle. Another relative contraindication is complete incompetence of the rotator cuff and deltoid, which renders the prosthesis highly unstable.

20. What is the youngest age someone may have a shoulder arthroplasty?

This question is difficult to answer. Most surgeons prefer not to resurface the glenoid in patients who are young and active. However, those with a biconcave glenoid must have their glenoid addressed. Glenoid reaming without resurfacing with polyethylene may be an option. In general, patients less than 50 are less satisfied with their shoulder arthroplasty than patients older than 50, regardless of whether a hemiarthroplasty or a total shoulder arthroplasty.

21. What are the different types of shoulder arthroplasty designs?

Constrained design. This original design resulted in an unacceptably high rate of glenoid loosening. The native shoulder is one of the most unconstrained joints in the body and relies on muscular and soft-tissue balancing for stability. Constrained designs are currently unavailable.

Semiconstrained designs. These designs consist of a glenoid component with a superior polyethylene hood to help prevent superior subluxation of the humeral head. They are usually employed with a weak or incompetent rotator cuff or deltoid. Although theoretically appealing, even a small degree of constraint causes increased glenoid keel stresses, which theoretically hasten glenoid loosening. Some designs have been developd for cases of an incompetent cuff but are not yet FDA-approved.

Unconstrained designs. Because they are characterized by a nearly anatomic shape of the humeral head and glenoid surface, reconstruction of the shoulder with unconstrained designs attempts to recreate normal anatomy and biomechanics. Perfectly conforming humeral head and glenoid diameters allow edge loading and subsequent glenoid loosening. Large diameter mismatches lead to central glenoid loading and fragmentation. Currently, most systems recommend a 4- to 6-millimeter diameter mismatch between the head and the glenoid.

22. What surgical approach is used for shoulder arthroplasty?
An extensile anterior approach (deltopectoral) to the shoulder exploits the internervous plane between the deltoid (axillary) nerve and the pectoralis major (medial and lateral pectoral) nerves.

23. What are the complications of shoulder arthroplasty?
- Stiffness. Not frequently recognized in previous studies, shoulder stiffness due to a number of causes is probably th e most frequent complication suffered by patients.
- Component malposition. This can frequently lead to stiffness. Excessive retroversion of the humeral component, excessive humeral head height, "overstuffing," and insufficient glenoid preparation and fixation are common errors.
- Infection. The infection rate of shoulder arthroplasty (0.5–3%) is consistent with that in other joints. Rates are higher in patients with rheumatoid arthritis because of their immunocompromised state.
- Instability. Instability results from soft-tissue imbalance, muscle atrophy, or malposition of components.

24. What results can be expected from shoulder arthroplasty?
Pain relief is the major result. Studies with follow-up for as long as 15 years report relief of pain in 90–95% of patients with osteoarthritis. Hemiarthroplasty yields pain relief in 85–90% of patients, but pain worsens with time due to glenoid arthritis. Pain relief with hemiarthroplasties is much lower in those with biconcave glenoids. Patients with concentric glenoids and intact rotator cuffs obtain the best functional results with hemiarthroplasties. Generally those younger than 50 will have less well-perceived results than those older than 50 regardless of whether they have had a hemiarthroplasty or a total shoulder arthroplasty. Implant longevity is approximately equal to arthroplasties of other joints.

25. Can the shoulder be treated as a "small hip?"
Absolutely not. Hip and shoulder biomechanics are completely different. It should also be understood that shoulder arthroplasty is a soft tissue procedure performed with metal and plastic.

26. What is the role of soft tissue balancing in total shoulder arthroplasty?
Soft tissue balancing is critical to implant stability and motion. To avoid sacrificing stability, it is not uncommon for soft tissues to be either overtightened or insufficiently released.

27. What is "overstuffing" in reference to shoulder arthroplasty?
Overstuffing refers to placing components that are too large for the capsular volume of the shoulder. This is a frequent mistake in shoulder arthroplasty, often made in an attempt to obtain stability. Unfortunately, overstuffing sacrifices motion by tightening soft tissues. This leads to postoperative stiffness, which is often painful, as well as excessive glenoid loads. Thus, anatomic restoration should be the goal with appropriate releases and lengthenings.

28. Can a loose glenoid component be revised?
Glenoid bone stock is limited. At the time of glenoid component resection for symptomatic loosening, rarely does enough bone remain to accept a new glenoid prosthesis. Hemiarthroplasty with resection of the loose glenoid component and cement can reasonably improve pain without re-implantation. Bone grafting of the defect with eventual return to resurface the glenoid again has had variable results.

29. What is the likelihood of treating a patient with an osteoarthritic shoulder that has a full-thickness rotator cuff defect?

The incidence of full-thickness rotator cuff defects in osteoarthritis is ≤ 5%.

30. Are there indications for primary hemiarthroplasty in fractures?

Some 4-part proximal humerus fractures with or without a dislocation as well as head-splitting fractures are indications for primary cemented hemiarthroplasty with fixation of the tuberosities. These fractures can result in disruption of the humeral head blood supply. Primary total shoulder arthroplasty is generally not indicated as the glenoid is usually normal. These arthroplasties generally allow poorer shoulder function than those for arthritis.

31. What is cuff tear arthropathy?

Cuff tear arthropathy refers to arthritic glenohumeral changes due to rotator cuff insufficiency and, therefore, loss of the concavity compression mechanism that the cuff provides. Humeral head elevation with respect to the glenoid and an irregular pebble stone appearance of the articular cartilage are typical. Surgical reconstruction is difficult because of the almost complete loss of the constraining force of the rotator cuff. This condition has been treated with an oversized hemiarthroplasty component as well as with various forms of total shoulder arthroplasty in the past. However, overstuffing often leads to postoperative stiffness and pain; total shoulder arthroplasty has lead to problems with glenoid loosening due to the "rocking horse" phenomenon. As a result, the more recent trend has been to place a smaller, near-anatomic hemiarthroplasty with normal tensioning of the soft tissues. The goal of surgery is pain relief only. Increased function is unreliable except that due to decreased pain.

32. What is shoulder arthrodesis? What are the surgical indications?

Shoulder arthrodesis is surgical resection of the glenohumeral surfaces and fusion with the aid of internal fixation. Relative indications for shoulder arthrodesis include young heavy laborers with osteoarthritis who are unwilling or unable to alter their lifestyle. Arthrodesis is occasionally recommended because of the fear of rapid mechanical loosening of an overused shoulder arthroplasty. Other indications include uncontrolled joint sepsis, complete loss of the rotator cuff and deltoid musculature, brachial plexopathies with functional trapezial and rhomboid musculature, and salvage for failed total shoulder arthroplasty.

33. In what position should the shoulder be fused?

Shoulder arthrodesis should be performed so that the arm rests comfortably at the side without scapular winging and the hand can be brought easily to the mouth and the perineum. Twenty degrees of flexion, 30° of abduction, and 40° of internal rotation has been generally recommended. Because of problems with periscapular muscle fatigue and pain, some authors recommend a position with much less flexion and abduction.

34. What is resection arthroplasty? What are the surgical indications?

Resection arthroplasty is resection of the humeral head. One of the original techniques for treatment of intractable pain due to shoulder arthritis, this procedure is now rarely indicated because it renders a flail shoulder with unpredictable pain relief. Resection arthroplasty is most often used for intractable joint infection, infected nonunion of shoulder arthrodesis, and neoplastic processes of the shoulder.

BIBLIOGRAPHY

1. Arntz CT, Jackins S, Matsen FA: Prosthetic replacement of the shoulder for the treatment of defects in the rotator cuff and the surface of the glenohumeral joint. J Bone Joint Surg 75A:485–590, 1993.
2. Boyd AD Jr, Thomas WH, Scott RD, Thornhill TS: Total shoulder arthroplasty versus hemiarthroplasty: Indications for glenoid resurfacing. J Arthroplasty 5:329–336, 1990.

3. Cofield RD: Instructional course lectures. 34:268–277, 1985.
4. Edwards TB, Boulahia A, Kempf J-F, et al: A comparison of hemiarthroplasty and total shoulder arthroplasty in the treatment of primary glenohumeral osteoarthritis. Proceedings of the 69th Annual Meeting of the American Academy of Orthopaedic Surgeons; Dallas, TX 2002
5. Figgie HE III, Inglis AE, Goldberg VM, et al: An analysis of factors affecting the long-term results of total shoulder arthroplasty in inflammatory arthritis. J Arthroplasty 123:130, 1988.
6. Friedman RJ: Arthroplasty of the Shoulder. New York, Thieme Medical Publishers, 1994.
7. Gartsman GM, Russell JA, Gaenslen E: Modular shoulder arthroplasty. J Shoulder Elbow Surg 6:333–339, 1997.
8. Green A: Current concepts of shoulder arthroplasty. Instr Course Lect 47:123–133, 1998.
9. Matsen FA, Lippitt SB, Sidles JA, Harryman DT: Practical Evaluation and Management of the Shoulder. Philadelphia, W.B. Saunders, 1994.
10. Neer CS II: Shoulder Reconstruction. Philadelphia, W.B. Saunders, 1990.
11. Norris BL, Lachiewicz PF: Modern cement technique and the survivorship of total shoulder arthroplasty. Clin Orthop 328:76–85, 1996.
12. Rockwood CA Jr, Matsen FA III: The Shoulder, vols. 1 and 2, 2nd ed. Philadelphia, W.B. Saunders, 1998.
13. Sledge CB, Ruddy S, Harris ED Jr, Kelley WN (eds): Arthritis Surgery. Philadelphia, W.B. Saunders, 1994.
14. Sperling JW, Cofield RH, Rowland CM: Neer hemiarthroplasty and Neer total shoulder arthroplasty in patients fifty years old or less; Long-term results. J Bone Joint Surg 80A:464–473, 1998.

27. PEDIATRIC SHOULDER

Keith R. Gabriel, M.D.

1. You are called to the nursery to examine a newborn infant who does not spontaneously move one upper extremity. Visually the limb appears normal. What conditions should be included in the initial differential diagnosis?
- Birth palsy (brachial plexus palsy)
- Birth fracture

2. Erb's palsy involves primarily which roots of the brachial plexus?
Erb's palsy involves primarily the upper roots: C4–C6.

3. Which shoulder muscles are usually affected in Erb's palsy?
The shoulder external rotators (supraspinatus, infraspinatus, teres minor) and frequently the deltoid are affected. Occasionally the elbow flexors may be involved.

4. What is the characteristic positioning of the shoulder in Erb's palsy?
The characteristic positioning of the shoulder includes adduction and internal rotation.

5. Are there other types of birth palsy (brachial plexus palsy)?
Yes. The entire plexus may be involved, or only the lower roots, C8 and T1, may be injured (Klumpke's palsy). Erb's palsy is seen four times more frequently than other types.

6. What is the most common birth fracture?
The most common birth fracture involves the clavicle. Such fractures heal readily and are treated simply. Many infants are wrapped in a blanket, which may provide sufficient immobilization. Sometimes the sleeve of the infant's shirt is pinned or loosely sewn to the chest portion of the shirt. Any device (e.g., sling) that encircles the neck should be avoided.

7. During the nursery exam, you palpate what seems to be a clavicle fracture on the right side, but the infant moves the limb normally and does not protest or cry during the exam. A radiograph confirms a small gap in the middle third of the right clavicle. What do you suspect?

The likely diagnosis is pseudarthrosis of the clavicle. A birth fracture of the clavicle should be painful. Pseudarthrosis is a rare congenital condition that almost invariably occurs on the right. The diagnosis is confirmed if no healing reaction is seen on a radiograph at 2 weeks. Orthopedic intervention is usually deferred until age 3–5 years.

8. You are called to the nursery to see a newborn infant who does not spontaneously move the upper extremity. The infant seems to react with pain when you move the shoulder (glenohumeral) joint. Is it dislocated?

Almost certainly not. Shoulder dislocation, either congenital or traumatic, is rare. Birth fracture of the humerus, specifically a fracture through the proximal growth plate, is much more likely. Even when displaced, such fractures usually heal well. Treatment is the same as described for birth fracture of the clavicle.

9. You evaluate an infant with asymmetry at the base of the neck and scapulae. The infant moves the involved upper extremity and shows no sign of pain; yet shoulder abduction, active and passive, is limited compared with the other shoulder. What do you suspect?

The likely diagnosis is Sprengel's deformity (congenital elevation of the scapula). The involved scapula is usually small and displaced upward and forward. Orthopedic intervention depends on functional limitations, which are quite variable. Associated congenital anomalies (scoliosis, cervical fusions, cardiac and renal conditions) should be suspected.

10. A newborn infant has asymmetry of the front of the shoulder. Specifically, one side of the chest seems flat, as though a portion of the pectoralis musculature has not developed. Before talking to the family, what topic should you review?

The likely diagnosis is Poland's syndrome. Examine the infant for cardiac anomalies and syndactyly.

11. A 6-month-old infant seems fussy and has stopped using her shoulder. The child spontaneously moves the elbow, forearm, wrist, and hand. A reliable caretaker observed no trauma. What is your primary and urgent concern?

The urgent concern is infection. Both hematogenous osteomyelitis and septic arthritis may present insidiously. Fever is quite variable. The peripheral white blood cell count may not be elevated initially; the erythrocyte sedimentation rate and C-reactive protein are more sensitive, although nonspecific. Radiographic changes may take a week or more to develop. A high index of suspicion should be maintained.

12. A 13-year-old tennis player or baseball pitcher presents with activity-related pain in the dominant shoulder. The radiograph shows widening and irregularity of the proximal humeral physis. What is the diagnosis?

The disorder sometimes is called little leaguer's shoulder, although other overhead sports may be involved. It is treated symptomatically, and activity restrictions are usually sufficient. Permanent avoidance of the athletic activity is not necessary. The condition is self-limited with no known sequelae.

13. An adolescent swimmer complains of anterior shoulder pain after prolonged workouts. The radiographs are unremarkable. What is a possible diagnosis?

A possible diagnosis is impingement syndrome, sometimes called swimmer's shoulder. The musculotendinous structures of the rotator cuff are pinched repeatedly between the humeral head and the anatomic arch created by the anterior acromion, the acromioclavicular joint, and the coracoacromial ligament. In young athletes, impingement syndrome is usually treated by activity restrictions, physical therapy, and adjustment of the mechanics involved in the sport. In many young athletes, occult instability may be the primary cause of impingement symptoms.

14. What proportion of growth of the humerus is contributed by the proximal humeral physis?
About 80% of growth is contributed by the proximal humeral physis. Proportionately, this is the largest contribution that any growth plate makes to its respective long bone.

15. What bearing does the tremendous growth potential of the proximal humeral physis have on management of fractures of the proximal humerus in juvenile patients?
Moderate angulation or displacement is acceptable because of the tremendous potential for remodeling.

16. A pathologic fracture of the proximal humeral metaphysis in a juvenile patient is often the initial presentation of what benign bone tumor?
A pathologic fracture of the proximal humeral metaphysis is often the initial presentation of a unicameral cyst (simple bone cyst). The proximal humerus is the most common location of this benign tumor.

17. What is the only direct bony connection, or bony strut, between the chest and the shoulder?
The clavicle.

18. What is the most frequently fractured long bone in childhood?
The clavicle.

19. What is the usual treatment for fractures of the shaft of the clavicle?
Fractures of the shaft of the clavicle unite readily and are almost always treated by closed methods. Figure-of-eight bandages, slings, and combinations thereof are usually recommended.

20. What are the indications for open (operative) treatment of a clavicle fracture?
Open fractures must be treated with irrigation and debridement. Exploration may be needed if neurovascular compromise is suspected. A few clavicle fractures are grossly displaced, with the fracture fragments "buttonholed" through the platysma or trapezius; such fractures require open reduction.

21. Fractures and dislocations of the medial clavicle (sternoclavicular joint) are distinctly uncommon in children. When they occur, what is the usual direction of the displacement?
Displacement is usually anterior.

22. What may be the primary concern in a posteriorly displaced fracture-dislocation of the sternoclavicular joint?
The primary concern is compromise of mediastinal structures.

23. Shoulder separations (subluxation and dislocations of the acromioclavicular joint) occur commonly when an adult athlete falls directly onto the point of the shoulder. Would you expect the same injury in a juvenile soccer player?
No. Most distal clavicle or acromioclavicular joint injuries in children are fractures through the distal clavicular physis, with disruption of the periosteal sleeve.

24. A 13-year-old gymnast "pulls" his shoulder while practicing on the rings and now complains that the shoulder blade "pokes backward" when he raises his arm. He has a full passive shoulder range of motion, and radiographs are unremarkable. What is the diagnosis?
Traumatic winging of the scapula. This is an uncommon condition, attributed to injury to the

long thoracic nerve with resultant paralysis of the serratus anterior. The usual treatment is conservative, with spontaneous recovery in 3–6 months.

25. How often do you expect to treat children for traumatic dislocation of the shoulder?
Not often. Traumatic shoulder dislocation is uncommon before adolescence.

26. A child sustains traumatic dislocation of the shoulder, with no neurovascular compromise, and the dislocation is successfully reduced by closed reduction. Why should the prognosis still be guarded?
The recurrence rate is at least 50% when the initial dislocation occurs in childhood or adolescence.

BIBLIOGRAPHY

1. Bak K, Fauno P: Clinical findings in competitive swimmers with shoulder pain. Am J Sports Med 25:254, 1997.
2. Barnett LS: Little league shoulder syndrome: proximal humeral epiphyseolysis in adolescent baseball pitchers. J Bone Joint Surg 67A:495–496, 1985.
3. Busch MT: Sports medicine in children and adolescents. In Morrissy RT, Weinstein SL (eds): Lovell and Winter's Pediatric Orthopaedics, 5th ed. Philadelphia, Lippincott Williams & Wilkins, 2001, pp 1273–1318.
4. Canale ST (ed): Campbell's Operative Orthopaedics, 9th ed. St. Louis, Mosby, 1998.
5. Herring JA: Disorders of the upper extremity. In Herring JA (ed): Tachdjian's Pediatric Orthopedics, 3rd ed. Philadelphia, W.B. Saunders, 2002, pp 379–512.
6. Kay SPJ: Obstetrical brachial palsy. Br J Plast Surg 51:43, 1998.
7. Kwon Y, Sarwark JF: Proximal humerus, scapula, and clavicle. In Beaty JH, Kasser JR (eds): Rockwood and Wilkins Fractures in Children, 5th ed. Philadelphia, Lippincott Williams & Wilkins, 2001, pp 741–806.
8. Mah JY, Otsuka NY: Scapular winging in young athletes. J Pediatr Orthop:12:245–247, 1992.
9. Ogden JA: Chest and shoulder girdle. In Ogden JA: Skeletal Injury in the Child, 3rd ed. New York, Springer, 2000, pp 419–455.
10. Ogden JA (ed): Humerus. In Ogden JA (ed): Skeletal Injury in the Child, 3rd ed. New York, Springer, 2000, pp 456–541.
11. Roberts SW, Hernandez C, Maberry MC, et al: Obstetric clavicular fracture: The enigma of normal birth. Obstet Gynecol 86:978, 1995.
12. Schnall SB, King JD, Marrero G: Congenital pseudarthrosis of the clavicle: A review of the literature and surgical results of six cases. J Pediatr Orthop 8:316, 1988.
13. Wagner KT, Lyne ED: Adolescent traumatic dislocations of the shoulder with open epiphyses. J Pediatr Orthop 3:61, 1993.
14. Waters PM: The upper limb. In Morrissy RT, Weinstein SL (eds): Lovell and Winter's Pediatric Orthopaedics, 5th ed. Philadelphia, Lippincott-Williams & Wilkins, 2001, pp 841–903.

28. SHOULDER ARTHROSCOPY

Kirk S. Hutton, M.D.

1. What areas of the shoulder can be seen during routine shoulder arthroscopy?
Routine shoulder arthroscopy involves evaluation of the glenohumeral joint, including the rotator cuff, biceps tendon, articular surfaces, glenoid labrum, and other recesses where loose bodies may hide. Shoulder arthroscopy also includes evaluation of the subacromial bursa, bursal surface of the rotator cuff, coracoacromial ligament, anatomy of the acromion, and the acromioclavicular joint.

2. What types of procedures can be done arthroscopically in the shoulder?

Shoulder arthroscopy has evolved over recent years to involve many procedures that previously had been done open. It began as a strictly diagnostic procedure and progressed to the point where certain areas of the shoulder could be shaved and debrided. As arthroscopic techniques improved, surgeons performed arthroscopic subacromial decompressions/acromioplasties. Distal clavicle excisions also can be performed arthroscopically with the aid of high-speed burs. Recently, surgeons with advanced arthroscopic skills have performed anterior and posterior stabilizations using various suture and suture anchor techniques and heat-shrinking techniques. Glenoid labrum tears and rotator cuff tears are being completely repaired through the scope with the use of such techniques.

3. What are the indications for shoulder arthroscopy?

Arthroscopy may be used to aid in the diagnosis of any condition in which the preoperative diagnosis is unclear or incomplete. It also is indicated for the treatment of known pathology, such as impingement syndrome, shoulder instability, and rotator cuff pathology.

4. Does shoulder arthroscopy require any special equipment?

Yes. Many special instruments make shoulder arthroscopy easier to perform. In addition to the standard arthroscopic equipment, shoulder arthroscopy requires special guide rods (Wissinger rods and switching sticks) in order to move the portals. A longer arthroscopic probe also is helpful. Operative cannulas with diaphragms to prevent fluid leakage are necessary to reduce significant swelling that may occur during the procedure. Depending on the type of procedure, other specialized instruments may be needed, such as arthroscopic suture anchors and rotator cuff repair systems. An arthroscopic pump, although unnecessary, does help to gauge the pressure settings that aid in hemostasis.

5. What position should a patient be placed in for shoulder arthroscopy?

Two positions are routinely used. The most common position is the lateral decubitus position in which the patient is turned to lie on the nonoperative side and held in place with a bean bag or a type of kidney rest to stabilize his or her position. An axillary roll always is placed beneath the thorax to prevent pressure on the axillary artery. All bony prominences must be padded to prevent skin necrosis during the procedure. Once the body has been placed in this position, the arm may be held in place by a commercial traction unit or one made from pulleys in the operative suite. The position of the arm in the lateral decubitus position depends on the procedure, but in general approximately 20° of abduction and 5–10° of forward flexion is acceptable. The lateral decubitus position allows for easy access to the glenohumeral joint, the subacromial space, and also is an ideal position for performing a mini-open rotator cuff repair.

The lateral decubitus position. The patient lies on the nonoperative side throughout the procedure while the arm is held in place by a traction unit.

The second most commonly used position for shoulder arthroscopy is the beach-chair or semi-Fowler's position, which has the advantage of keeping all structures anatomically oriented. The patient is also in the appropriate position for an open anterior approach, if necessary. An assistant may be needed to place traction on the arm for certain procedures. The beach-chair position also allows for manipulation of the arm during surgery.

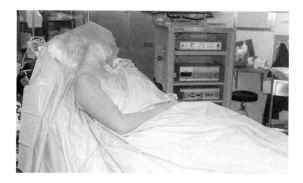

The beach-chair (semi-Fowler's) position. All structures are kept anatomically oriented to allow manipulation of the arm during surgery.

6. How is the examination under anesthesia conducted?

The examination under anesthesia is performed on the shoulder after the patient has received the general anesthetic. The range of motion and stability of the shoulder is tested, including anterior, posterior, and inferior translations. It is important to compare the operative with the non-operative side to document a definitive notation of any type of instability before inserting the arthroscope into the shoulder. This very important part of the arthroscopic and presurgical procedure should be performed on every patient. The examination under anesthesia obviously removes a patient's response to painful motion of the shoulder and also takes away muscle contraction, possibly allowing detection of instability that was not diagnosed preoperatively due to patient guarding or pain.

7. What kind of anesthesia may help with shoulder surgery?

An interscalene block performed by the anesthesiologist may be a helpful regional block given before shoulder surgery. The block involves placing a needle between the anterior and middle scalene muscles and instilling local anesthetic in the area of the brachial plexus. A nerve stimulator helps to ensure the appropriate location of the block, but the paresthesia technique also may be used. It is important to perform the block on an awake patient to avoid potentially disastrous intraneural injections. The interscalene block not only decreases the amount of general anesthetic agent required during surgery, but also gives the patient 12–18 hours of postoperative pain relief.

8. Which portals are commonly used in shoulder arthroscopy?

The **posterior portal** is the most commonly used portal through which the arthroscope is first inserted into the glenohumeral joint. This portal is located 2–3 cm inferior and slightly medial to the posterolateral angle of the acromion and corresponds to the soft spot between the infraspinatus and teres minor muscles posteriorly. The anterior portal is commonly referred to as the working portal for glenohumeral arthroscopy.

The **anterior portal** may be established via an inside-out or an outside-in technique and should remain lateral to the coracoid process, entering the glenohumeral joint above the subscapularis tendon and under the biceps tendon. This area corresponds with the rotator interval in the glenohumeral joint. Numerous other accessory portals can be made anterolaterally and posterolaterally depending on the area of the glenohumeral or subacromial space that needs to be addressed surgically.

9. Which structures should be evaluated during routine shoulder arthroscopy?

Like any other surgical procedure, shoulder arthroscopy needs to be done in a systematic fashion. A technique should allow the surgeon to evaluate every structure within the shoulder and do it the same way every time. Snyder has published a useful 15-point glenohumeral joint evaluation and anatomy review that begins by visualizing from the posterior portal and evaluates the following structures:

1. Biceps tendon
2. Posterior labrum and capsule attachment
3. Inferior axillary recess and inferior capsular insertion to humeral head
4. Inferior labrum and glenoid articular surface
5. Supraspinatus tendon
6. Posterior rotator cuff insertion in the bare area of the humeral head
7. Articular surface of the humeral head
8. Anterior superior labrum, superior and middle glenohumeral ligament, and subscapularis tendon
9. Anterior/inferior labrum
10. Anterior/inferior glenohumeral ligament

The remaining five structures are visualized with the arthroscope in the anterior portal:

11. Posterior glenoid labrum
12. Posterior aspect of rotator cuff, including infraspinatus and supraspinatus
13. Anterior glenoid labrum and inferior glenohumeral ligament attachments to the labrum
14. Subscapularis tendon and recess, as well as middle glenohumeral ligament
15. Anterior surface of the humeral head with subscapularis attachment and biceps tendon passage

10. Is the intraarticular anatomy the same in every shoulder?

No. Many variations are found involving the glenoid labrum and the anterior glenohumeral ligaments that are important for the shoulder arthroscopist to recognize. Less experienced shoulder surgeons may think that some anatomic variants are abnormalities and attempt to repair these normal structures. Two common normal variants include a cordlike middle glenohumeral ligament and the Buford complex, which involves a cordlike glenohumeral ligament with no anterosuperior glenoid labrum.

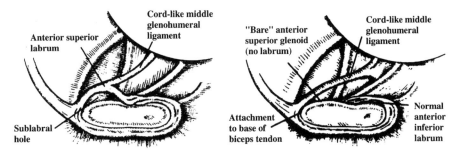

Left, The cordlike middle glenohumeral ligament may attach to the superior labrum, often with an underlying sublabral hole. *Right,* The Buford complex is a rare but important anatomic formation to recognize. It is often mistaken for a pathologic labral detachment. (From Snyder SJ: Shoulder Arthroscopy. New York, McGraw-Hill, 1994, pp 32–33, with permission.)

11. What is the difference between the subacromial bursa and the glenohumeral joint?

The subacromial bursa and glenohumeral joint are anatomically separate areas that are evaluated during routine shoulder arthroscopy. The glenohumeral joint is an area that involves the articular surface of the glenoid, the humeral head, and all other structures mentioned in Snyder's 15-point anatomic checklist for shoulder arthroscopy. The subacromial bursa is a completely separate area in which the arthroscope must be moved superior to the rotator cuff and in a space between the acromion and the superior surface of the rotator cuff. In the subacromial bursa, visualization is generally more difficult and the anatomy is less well defined. The structures involved in this area include the bursal surface of the rotator cuff, the undersurface of the acromion, the coracoacromial ligament, the subdeltoid bursa, and the AC joint. The arthroscopic subacromial decompression is performed in the subacromial bursa. Also, some arthroscopists perform an excision of the distal clavicle while working in the subacromial space.

12. What common abnormalities can be diagnosed during shoulder arthroscopy?

Shoulder arthroscopy is highly useful in the diagnosis and treatment of many shoulder problems. For example, full-thickness or partial-thickness tears of the rotator cuff can be diagnosed. Some surgeons classify rotator cuff tears as partial- versus full-thickness tears, whereas others further classify them as "A" tears, which involve tears on the articular surface; "B" tears, which are seen in the subacromial bursa; or "C" tears, which are complete tears of the rotator cuff. Other abnormalities that can be diagnosed include partial or full biceps tendon tears, glenoid labrum tears, and SLAP (superior labrum, anteroposterior) lesions (SLAP lesions are detailed in chapter 24). A Bankart lesion is another type of glenoid labrum tear that involves an avulsion of the anterior labrum and the glenohumeral ligaments away from the anterior neck of the glenoid. Degenerative changes of the humeral head and glenoid articular surfaces also can be diagnosed, as well as the presence or absence of osteochondral loose bodies, adhesive capsulitis, and other synovial disorders.

13. Describe the glenoid labrum.

The glenoid labrum is a fibrocartilaginous tissue that encircles the glenoid. The biceps tendon attaches to this area, as do the glenohumeral ligaments. The superior labrum often appears loosely attached and may have a meniscoidlike appearance. The glenoid labrum serves as attachment for the glenohumeral ligaments and biceps, and also adds stability to the shoulder by adding depth and concavity to the glenoid socket itself. The glenoid labrum can be damaged in many ways, such as a Bankart lesion from a dislocation or a SLAP lesion from the mechanisms documented in chapter 24, as well as degenerative changes from chronic rotator cuff disease or arthritis.

14. What common complications may occur from incorrect portal placement during shoulder arthroscopy?

Portal placement is highly crucial for proper shoulder arthroscopy. During placement of the posterior portals, the axillary nerve and the descending branch of the suprascapular nerve are at risk. The axillary nerve is approximately 6–7 cm distal to the posterolateral corner of the acromion and spine of the scapula. This distance is some 4–5 cm below the usual posterior portal placement; therefore, the axillary nerve should be safe. The suprascapular nerve is the most commonly injured nerve during shoulder arthroscopy and is located 1.5–2 cm medial to the edge of the glenoid below the area of the spinoglenoid notch. If the posterior portal is too medial, the suprascapular nerve can be injured. It is important to use a blunt trochar and identify the anatomic landmarks before placing this portal to avoid nerve injury.

While making the anterior portals, it is important to always stay lateral to the coracoid process. Structures at risk during anterior portal placement include the cephalic vein, axillary nerve, and musculocutaneous nerve. A common saying in shoulder arthroscopy with regards to the coracoid is that the lateral side is the "safe side," the medial side is the "suicide."

15. What other potential complications may occur during shoulder arthroscopy?
As with any surgical procedure, appropriate positioning and protection of the patient during the procedure is of paramount importance. Appropriate positioning of the head and neck avoids neck or brachial plexus stretch lesions. Padding all bony prominences prevents skin-pressure injuries. In the lateral decubitus position with the arm held in the arthroscopic traction device, stretch or traction injuries may occur to the arm if too much weight is applied over a prolonged period. Shoulder arthroscopy also involves the use of arthroscopic fluid to distend the joint or subacromial bursa; fluid extravasation and compartment syndromes may result if the pressure on the arthroscopic pump and the fluid system is not well managed. Compartment syndrome in the shoulder is very rare but has occurred; prevention is the best form of treatment. Small amounts of swelling and tissue edema should not cause worry, because the body gradually resorbs the arthroscopic fluid within 1–2 hours after the procedure.

16. What is a subacromial decompression? How is it performed?
A subacromial decompression is a procedure initially developed by Neer and performed in an open technique. Recently, shoulder surgeons have advanced to performing this arthroscopically in patients diagnosed with impingement syndrome, rotator cuff tendinitis, or subacromial bursitis. The subacromial decompression is performed in the subacromial bursa. It involves shaving and excising the thickened pathologic subdeltoid bursa, excision of the coracoacromial ligament, and use of a high-speed motorized bur to remove any bone spurs on the anterolateral portion of the acromion. The goal is to create more space in the subacromial subdeltoid bursa and eliminate the impingement process to relieve shoulder pain.

17. How much bone should be removed from the undersurface of the acromion during a subacromial decompression?
The goal of a subacromial decompression is to create a flat (type I) acromion. Bigliani has classified acromion morphology type I as a flat acromion without a slope; a type II acromion has a gentle curve; and type III acromion has a hook along the anterior aspect of the accordion. This anatomy may be seen when viewing from the lateral portal but is more commonly seen on the preoperative outlet x-rays. During the arthroscopic subacromial decompression procedure, a cutting-block type procedure is used in which the bur is placed from the posterior portal along the undersurface of the acromion to verify that no curve or anterior hook remains. Knowing the anatomy of the acromion preoperatively on the x-rays also tells the surgeon how much bone to remove to create a flat acromion.

BIBLIOGRAPHY

1. Beals TC, Harryman DT, Lazarus MD: Useful boundaries of the subacromial bursa. Arthroscopy 14:465–470, 1998.
2. Bigliani LU, Ticker JB, Flatow EL, et al: The relationship of acromial architecture to rotator cuff disease. Clin Sports Med 4:823–838, 1991.
3. Matthews DS, Terry G, Vetter WL: Shoulder anatomy for the arthroscopist. Arthroscopy 1:83, 1985.
4. Morrison DS, Port J: Basics of shoulder arthroscopy. In Hawkins RJ, Misamore GW (eds): Shoulder Injuries in the Athlete. New York, Churchill Livingstone, 1996, pp 87–101.
5. Phillips BB: Arthroscopy of upper extremity. In Canale ST (ed): Campbell's Operative Orthopaedics, 9th ed. St. Louis, Mosby, 1998, pp 1562–1594.
6. Snyder SJ: Diagnostic arthroscopy: Normal anatomy and variations. In Snyder SJ (ed): Shoulder Arthroscopy. New York, McGraw-Hill, 1994, pp 23–39.
7. Snyder SJ, Karzel RP, Del Pizzo W, et al: SLAP lesions of the shoulder. Arthroscopy 6:274–279, 1990.

29. FRACTURES OF THE SHOULDER

Kirk S. Hutton, M.D.

1. What mistake is commonly made when evaluating a patient with a suspected shoulder girdle fracture?

One of the most common mistakes made is not obtaining adequate x-rays. It is mandatory to have two orthogonal views of the glenohumeral joint, such as an AP and an axillary lateral view. When it is difficult to obtain an axillary lateral view, a tangential or scapular Y view will suffice.

2. Name a possible mechanism for a lesser tuberosity fracture.

A posterior glenohumeral dislocation is a known mechanism for causing a lesser tuberosity fracture. The subscapularis attaches to the lesser tuberosity and may cause a bony avulsion of the structure during a posterior dislocation. Posterior dislocations are common after electrocution injuries or with seizures.

3. Describe the major blood supply to the humeral head and proximal humerus.

The major blood supply to the humeral head is from the anterior humeral circumflex artery. The arcuate artery is a continuation of the ascending branch of the anterior humeral circumflex artery, which is the main portion that penetrates the bone and supplies the humeral head. It routinely enters the bone in the area of the intertubercular groove and gives branches to the lesser and greater tuberosities. A small contribution to the humeral head blood supply comes from branches of the posterior circumflex artery and from tendinous osseous and anastomosis from the vascular rotator cuff.

4. Which nerve injuries are commonly associated with fractures about the shoulder?

The most commonly injured nerve is the axillary nerve. The axillary nerve innervates the deltoid muscle as well as the teres minor muscle. It is relatively fixed to the posterior cord of the brachial plexus and to the deltoid; therefore, any abnormal downward pressure on the proximal humerus can result in a traction injury to this nerve. It is also susceptible to injury with any dislocation because it is relatively close to the inferior capsule of the glenohumeral joint. The suprascapular nerve, which innervates the supraspinatus and infraspinatus, also can be injured, but it is much less likely. Injury to the musculocutaneous nerve is very rare.

5. What is the most commonly used classification system for proximal humerus fractures?

In 1970 Charles Neer developed his four-part classification system, which is based on the anatomy and biomechanical forces around the proximal humerus. Four primary fragments involved in proximal humerus fractures are the greater tuberosity, lesser tuberosity, humeral head, and the humeral shaft. Over 80% of humerus fractures are considered nondisplaced, but any fracture with > 1 cm of displacement or any fracture fragment angulated > 45° in the Neer system is considered a displaced fragment. The fracture classification refers to the number of **displaced segments,** not to the number of fragments or lines.

6. How are proximal humerus fractures treated?

Eighty-five percent of proximal humerus fractures are minimally displaced or nondisplaced and may be treated with early functional exercises.

Two-part anatomic neck fractures are difficult to reduce closed. Open reduction and internal fixation are difficult because of inadequate bone purchase for screws. Most authors agree that hemiarthroplasty gives the most predictable results for displaced fractures.

Displaced two-part greater tuberosity fractures may cause impingement under the acromion.

Displacement > 0.5 cm is associated with persistent pain. Open reduction and internal fixation are recommended with displacement > 1 cm.

Two-part surgical neck fractures require 3–4 weeks of sling immobilization if they are minimally displaced. Angulation often occurs after closed reduction without internal fixation. Several forms of internal fixation have been described, including percutaneous pin, intramedullary fixation, tension band wire, and plate fixation.

Three-part fractures in active, young patients are generally best treated with open reduction and internal fixation.

Four-part fractures are associated with avascular necrosis in up to 90% of patients. Immediate hemiarthroplasty has become the accepted method of treatment.

7. Why is the treatment of three- and four-part proximal humerus fractures different from other fractures of the proximal humerus?

Typically, three- and four-part proximal humerus fractures occur in older individuals with osteoporotic bone or in younger individuals who have sustained very high energy trauma. Because of disruption of blood supply, four-part humerus fractures have a very high incidence of avascular necrosis, which has been determined to be between 13 and 34%. These fractures, especially in the elderly, are best treated with a hemiarthroplasty. Three-part fractures in elderly patients with very osteoporotic bone may also require hemiarthroplasty when stable internal fixation is not adequate.

8. What is the treatment of a humeral head impression fracture?

Treatment of impression fractures of the articular surface of the proximal humerus varies according to the percentage of the humeral head involved, as well as the time of diagnosis. If the injury is diagnosed within 2–3 weeks and the humeral head involvement is < 20% of the articular surface, closed reduction may be adequate. If the head defect is > 45% or a dislocation has been missed for six months or more, Hawkins has recommended a hemiarthroplasty of the proximal humerus. Head defects of 20–45% require some type of open reduction and internal fixation or bony transfer, depending on the location of the defect.

9. Why is a head-splitting fracture difficult to treat?

Head-splitting fractures usually occur with a fracture of either tuberosity and involve significant damage of the blood supply to the articular surface. In a young patient with good bone stock, open reduction and internal fixation may be attempted, but this is very difficult and success is low. Most authors recommend treatment of a head split fracture with a hemiarthroplasty.

10. Describe some common complications associated with proximal humerus fractures.

Vascular complications are obviously associated with proximal humerus fractures, and the axillary artery accounts for approximately 6% of all arterial trauma. The most common site of injury to the axillary artery is near the origin of the anterior circumflex artery. Another complication associated with vascular injury, as previously mentioned, is avascular necrosis, especially in three- and four-part humerus fractures. Brachial plexus injuries, primarily the axillary nerve component, have been associated with proximal humerus fractures and may be as high as 6%. The axillary nerve is more commonly injured in dislocations or fracture dislocations. Nonunions and malunions also are a potential complication and must be treated accordingly. Frozen shoulder or adhesive capsulitis is probably a much more common complication and rates are probably higher than noted in the literature.

11. Are there any growth plates or epiphyseal lines around the scapula that may be confused with a scapular fracture?

The os acromiale is probably the best known separate bone in the scapula that results from failure of coalescence of the adjacent ossification centers of the acromion process of the scapula. There are four ossification centers present about the acromion, but the most common site of nonunion is between the meso-acromion and the meta-acromion. An unfused apophysis of the acromion is present in approximately 2.7% of patients and is bilateral in 60% those cases.

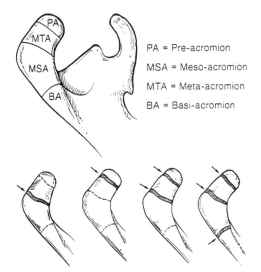

PA = Pre-acromion

MSA = Meso-acromion

MTA = Meta-acromion

BA = Basi-acromion

Ossification centers about the acromion with potential sites of nonunion, creating os acromiale.

12. What is a floating shoulder?

A floating shoulder includes a scapular fracture combined with a proximal humerus fracture or a clavicle fracture. A floating shoulder causes a significantly unstable mid portion in the glenohumeral joint and represents a difficult treatment scenario, which usually requires open reduction and internal fixation of at least one component of the fracture.

13. Describe potential mechanisms of injury for scapular body fractures.

The scapula is well protected, sandwiched between a thick muscle mass posteriorly and the thoracic cavity anteriorly. Because of its anatomic location, scapular fractures are uncommon, constituting only one percent of all fractures. A direct blow is probably the most common cause of injury of the scapular body, but sudden contractures of divergent muscles also may cause fracture. Electrical shock and seizures are included in this mechanism of injury. It should be remembered that of all scapular fractures, scapular body fractures have the highest incidence of associated injuries. Because of their mechanism of injury, up to 95% of scapular fractures are associated with other injuries.

14. Describe the associated injuries that may be found in conjunction with a scapular fracture.

Significant associated injuries can be seen in as many as 98% of individuals with scapular fractures because of the high energy force that is required to fracture the scapula. A pneumothorax may be seen in as many as 38% of individuals with scapular fractures, and the vast majority of these are delayed in onset anywhere from 1–3 days after the injury. Follow-up chest x-rays are mandatory when treating patients with scapular fractures. Other associated injuries include rib fractures, pulmonary contusion, brachial plexus injury, clavicle fractures, arterial injuries, as well as blunt abdominal and spinal cord injuries. It is the associated injuries that may cause the 10–15% mortality rate seen in patients with scapular fractures from blunt trauma.

15. How are scapular fractures evaluated radiographically?

True scapular anteroposterior (AP) and lateral views as well as a glenohumeral axillary projection should be done. The radiographs should be evaluated for fractures of the scapular body and spine, coracoid, glenoid, acromioclavicular joint, glenohumeral joint, and scapulothoracic articulation. Computed tomography (CT) is often necessary to further evaluate the extent of the fracture.

16. What is the classification of scapular fractures?

Scapular fractures are grouped into glenoid, acromion, coracoid, and scapular body fractures. Glenoid fractures may be further divided into glenoid rim, glenoid neck, and fractures through the glenoid cavity. Any fracture line that runs from the posterior scapular spine or acromion to the undersurface of the acromion and the spinoglenoid interval is considered an acromial fracture.

17. What is the most common treatment of scapular fractures?

Greater than 90% of all scapular fractures are treated nonoperatively. Symptomatic treatment includes sling and swathe for comfort. Range-of-motion exercises are initiated early. Return of full function will take several months. The prognosis, in general, is excellent.

Surgical indications for glenoid rim fractures include fractures that will result in persistent subluxation of the humeral head. Such fractures have ≥ 10 mm displacement with involvement of one-fourth of the anterior or one-third of the posterior glenoid rim.

Surgical indications for glenoid neck fractures include translational displacement ≥ 1 cm and/or angulatory displacement ≥ 40° in either the transverse or coronal planes. Significant displacement has been associated with loss of shoulder abduction, weakness, pain, and increased incidence of poor functional outcome.

Isolated fractures of the coracoid and acromion are generally treated nonoperatively as above. Surgical indications include significant displacement resulting in functional compromise.

18. What is the most common clavicle fracture?

Clavicle fractures are common injuries. They account for 5–10% of all instances of adult trauma. Middle third clavicle fractures account for 80% of all clavicle fractures.

19. What is the classification of clavicle fractures?

Allman divided clavicle fractures into three basic groups. Middle third clavicle fractures as classified as Group I and are the most common type. Group II fractures involve the lateral third of the clavicle and are the second most common. Group III fractures are medial third clavicle fractures.

Neer further subdivided the Group II (lateral third) fractures into five subtypes:

Subtype 1: minimally displaced interligamentous fractures
Subtype 2: displaced fractures with the fracture line medial to the coracoclavicular ligament
   insertion
Subtype 3: fractures that enter the acromioclavicular joint
Subtype 4: childhood injuries

These fractures are displaced, but the coracoclavicular ligament remains attached to a periosteal sleeve.

20. What is the treatment of a clavicle fracture?

Most clavicle fractures are treated with figure of eight harness or shoulder sling until pain begins to resolve. Surgical treatment comprises open reduction and internal fixation using Dynamic Compression Plating and screws. Indications for surgical intervention include neurovascular symptoms, skin breakdown due to bony prominence, and nonunion.

BIBLIOGRAPHY

1. Bigliani LU, Flatow EL, Pollock RG: Fractures of the proximal humerus. In Rockwood CA, Matsen FA (eds): The Shoulder, 2nd ed. Philadelphia, W.B. Saunders, 1998, pp 337–389.
2. Boublik M, Hawkins RJ: Clinical examination of the shoulder complex. J Orthop Sports Phys Ther 18:379–385, 1993.

3. Butters KP: The scapula. In Rockwood CA, Matsen FA (eds): The Shoulder, 2nd ed. Philadelphia, W.B. Saunders, 1998, pp 391–427.
4. Craig EV: Fractures of the clavicle. In Rockwood CA, Matsen FA (eds): The Shoulder, 2nd ed. Philadelphia, W.B. Saunders, 1998, pp 428–482.
5. Crenshaw AH: Fractures of the shoulder girdle, arm, and forearm. In Canale ST (ed): Campbell's Operative Orthopaedics, 9th ed. St. Louis, Mosby, 1998, pp 2285–2296.
6. Finkemeier C, Slater R: Fractures and dislocations of the shoulder girdle and humerus. Chapman's Orthopaedic Surgery. Philadelphia, Lippincott, Williams & Wilkins, 2001, pp 431–477.
7. Gerber C, Krushell RJ: Isolated rupture of the tendon of the subscapularis muscle. J Bone Joint Surg 73B:389–394, 1991.
8. Hawkins RJ: Musculoskeletal Examination. St. Louis, Mosby Year-Book, 1995.
9. Hawkins RJ, Hobeika PE: Impingement syndrome in the athletic shoulder. Clin Sports Med 2:391–405, 1983.
10. Hawkins RJ, Mohtadi NG: Clinical Evaluation of shoulder instability. Clin J Sports Med 1:59, 1991.
11. Matsen FA, Arntz CT: Subacromial impingement. In Rockwood CA, Matsen FA (eds): The Shoulder. Philadelphia, W.B. Saunders, 1990, pp 623–646.
12. Matsen FA, Thomas SC, Rockwood CA: Anterior glenohumeral instability. In Rockwood CA, Matsen FA (eds): The Shoulder. Philadelphia, W.B. Saunders, 1990, pp 526–622.

IV. The Elbow and Forearm

30. ELBOW DISLOCATIONS AND INSTABILITY

Edward R. McDevitt, M.D.

1. What is an elbow dislocation?

An elbow dislocation is a disassociation of the joint that connects the humerus with the radius and the ulna.

2. How common are dislocations of the elbow?

Although the elbow is one of the most highly constrained or stabilized joints, dislocations of the elbow are not rare. Only dislocation of the shoulder and the proximal interphalangeal (PIP) joints of the fingers are more common.

3. How do most elbow dislocations occur?

Most occur in sporting events, usually in young people aged 15–25 years. Elbow dislocations also may occur in high-speed motor vehicle or motorcycle accidents.

4. What is the mechanism of injury in most elbow dislocations?

The usual mechanism of injury is a fall on an extended or hyperextended elbow.

5. How are elbow dislocations described?

Like all dislocations, elbow dislocations are described by the position of the distal segment in relation to the proximal segment. Where does the distal segment, the ulna, lie in relation to the proximal segment, the humerus? In > 90% of cases, the dislocation is posterior or posterolateral. The ulna is posterior to the humerus in a posterior elbow dislocation.

6. Describe the other types of elbow dislocations.

Although the most common dislocation is posterior, elbow dislocations also may be anterior, medial, lateral, or divergent. Anterior dislocations are rare and are associated with a high degree of soft-tissue disruption. In a divergent dislocation, which is also rare but very serious, the radius and the ulna dislocate from the humerus in different directions. For a divergent dislocation to occur, the strong musculotendinous complex that binds the ulna and radius together must be completely disrupted.

7. What are the physical findings in an elbow dislocation?

Most patients are in extreme pain. They usually hold the affected forearm with the opposite hand. The elbow is usually held in slight flexion. The forearm appears slightly foreshortened compared with the normal forearm. The olecranon is usually palpable and prominent posteriorly. Swelling of the elbow is usually present and increases with time.

8. How is the presence of a fracture determined?

After documenting the neurovascular status, gently and slowly flex the elbow, carefully feeling for crepitus, which is usually present in a fracture but absent with an elbow dislocation. Obtain radiographs expeditiously.

9. What should be done if a fracture is associated with the elbow dislocation?

Fractures associated with elbow dislocations are not uncommon. Elbow dislocations without associated fractures are called simple dislocations, whereas those associated with associated fractures are called complex dislocations. The fractures most commonly associated with elbow dislocations involve the radial head, the coronoid process of the ulna, and the medial epicondyle. Most complex elbow dislocations are inherently unstable, and most of the associated fractures require surgery. Nevertheless, it is still imperative to reduce the dislocation of the elbow, whether or not an associated fracture is present.

10. What should be done for a patient with a suspected elbow dislocation?

In assessing the patient with an elbow injury, it is critical to check neurovascular function of the forearm and hand *before* an attempt is made to manipulate the joint back into place.

11. How does one check the neurovascular function?

First, check the sensation of pain and light touch distal to the elbow, documenting any paresthesia. Test the median, ulnar, and radial nerves for muscle strength distal to the elbow. Ask the patient to touch the thumb to the fifth finger to assess median nerve function. Ulnar nerve function can be assessed by testing the interosseous muscles, all of which are innervated by the ulnar nerve. Have the patient spread the fingers apart to test for interosseous function. The radial nerve can be assessed by having the patient extend the thumb, fingers, and wrist. Even children can be persuaded to attempt these three muscle tests. The brachial artery should be palpated at the elbow and compared with the unaffected side. The ulnar and radial arteries should be palpated at the wrist. All findings should be documented.

12. What neurovascular injuries are common in elbow dislocations?

In most elbow dislocations the neurovascular examination is unremarkable; the median and ulnar nerves and the brachial artery are most susceptible to injury.

13. What should be done if neurovascular injury is present?

After documentation of the injury, an attempt should be made promptly to reduce the dislocation. Often neurovascular injuries resolve with reduction. Carefully check the neurovascular status after relocation. An arteriogram should be obtained promptly if vascular injury is suspected.

14. Describe the procedure for reducing a dislocation of the elbow.

Elbow dislocations should be reduced as soon as possible. Team physicians covering sports with a high incidence of elbow dislocations are able to quickly and easily reduce the elbow shortly after the injury. If time has elapsed since the injury occurred and soft-tissue swelling is present, reduction is best accomplished under regional or general anesthesia. Intravenous anesthesia, with small doses of diazepam and morphine, is effective and usually allows reduction to be accomplished readily.

Before any reduction maneuver, the neurovascular status *must* be documented. If radiographs have been obtained, they should be examined carefully. Where is the ulna in relation to the humerus? Look for any associated fractures, especially at the coronoid process of the proximal ulna and the radial head. In most cases, the ulna is posterior to the humerus.

Many methods have been described for reduction of elbow dislocations. The easiest and most reliable involves gentle traction applied to the forearm with counteraction applied to the distal aspect of the humerus. The reduction maneuver can be accomplished with the patient either supine or prone. Many prefer the supine position, especially if intravenous anesthesia is used, because it is easier to assess the airway with this position.

If available, an assistant is useful. The assistant stands at the head of the patient, applying steady traction to the upper aspect of the humerus, while the physician applies gentle distal traction to the elbow. As the elbow is gently extended, any medial or lateral displacement of the ulna can be corrected by a counterforce applied to the side of the displacement. Keep one hand on the forearm, applying distal traction, and with the other hand correct the medial/lateral displacement. Then gently flex the elbow to accomplish the reduction. Often a loud "clunk" is palpated and heard. It is often helpful to use one hand to flex the elbow while the other hand pushes the bones back together. In a posterior dislocation, the ulna is posterior to the humerus. While applying a posterior force on the distal humerus with your thumb, wrap your other four fingers around the proximal aspect of the ulna and pull the ulna anteriorly. As you gently flex the elbow with one hand, your opposite hand gently wedges the humerus and the ulna together.

If no assistant is available, a closed reduction of the elbow with the patient in a prone position may be useful. The gravity method of reduction described by Parvin is a gentle method that can be used by the sole practitioner. The patient lies prone on the stretcher while gentle downward traction is applied with one hand to his or her wrist. After a few minutes of traction, the muscle spasm should subside. With your opposite hand apply a gentle upward pressure on the anterior distal humerus, lifting the arm as traction continues to be applied downward. The reduction should occur with an audible "clunk."

After reduction, carefully reassess neurovascular function. Gently flex and extend the elbow to ensure that the reduction is complete. Passive extension within 15–20° of full extension without subluxation implies a stable reduction. Apply a well-padded posterior splint with the elbow held at 90° of flexion. Obtain postreduction radiographs to ensure complete reduction of the dislocation and to rule out any new fractures.

15. What should be done if the elbow dislocation cannot be reduced?

The usual cause of an irreducible dislocation is entrapped fragments within the joint space, most often the fractured medial epicondyle. If the dislocation has not reduced after two gentle attempts under intravenous anesthesia, closed reduction under general anesthesia should be attempted. If the elbow is not reducible even after general anesthesia, open reduction is necessary.

16. Describe the treatment for a patient with an elbow dislocation after reduction.

Recent studies clearly show that prolonged immobilization (>4 weeks) is associated with poor results. Early active motion appears to be the key to successful rehabilitation after dislocation. If the patient demonstrates inherent stability with passive extension to 15–20° without recurrent dislocation, active motion is started within 1 week. Since 1986 at the United States Naval Academy, elbow dislocations without fracture have been treated with an immediate program of active range of motion instead of immobilization. Initial study of the midshipmen shows long-term stability with preservation of range of motion and return to full sports participation.

17. Is there any danger in starting an early active range-of-motion program?

No. Increased instability has not been demonstrated in patients who have been started on an early active range-of-motion program, which actually appears to result in less pain and suffering.

18. What are the late complications of elbow dislocations?

- Recurrent dislocation of the elbow is extremely rare, but when it occurs, it is disabling.
- Almost all patients with dislocations of the elbow have a mild loss of terminal extension. Loss of motion can be minimized through an early range-of-motion program.
- Heterotopic ossification may occur after dislocation of the elbow, but is rarely severe enough to limit motion of the elbow.

19. What is posterolateral instablility of the elbow?

Largely though the research of O'Driscoll, the most common pattern of elbow dislocation has been found to be a posterolateral dislocation. Posterolateral instablility results from a fall on an outstretched hand with the shoulder abducted. An axial compression force is applied to the elbow as the elbow is flexed and the body approaches the ground. A combination of supination and valgus forces leads to posterolateral instability and possibly complete dislocation of the elbow.

20. What is the key ligament injured in posterolateral instablility of the elbow?

The ulnar portion of the lateral collateral ligament is the essential lesion in posterolateral instablility of the elbow.

21. What is the lateral pivot shift test of the elbow for posterolateral instability of the elbow?
The pivot shift test is a clincinal examination maneuver that reproduces the injury pattern of a posterolateral dislocation. A symptomatic elbow demonstrates instability with the maneuver of axial compression, valgus stress, and supination. The test is best performed with the patient in a supine postion with the arm positioned over the head. The examiner stands at the head of the table. One hand holds the wrist with the forearm in full supination. The other hand is positioned on the proximal foream. The arm is held in full extension. To perform the test slowly flex the elbow while simultaneously applying axial compression and a valgus force to the elbow. At approximately 40° of flexion the patient either experiences an audible "clunk" or has such apprehension that he or she aborts the test because the test will reproduce the feeling of instability.

BIBLIOGRAPHY

1. Broberg MA, Morrey BF: Results of treatment of fracture dislocations of the elbow. Clin Orthop 216:109–119, 1987.
2. Cohen MS, Hastings H: Acute elbow dislocation: Evaluation and management. J Am Acad Orthop Surg 6:15–23, 1998.
3. Hotchkiss RN, Green DP: Fractures and dislocations of the elbow. In Rockwood CA, et al (eds): Rockwood and Green's Fractures in Adults. Philadelphia, J.B. Lippincott, 1991, pp 779–793.
4. Josefsson PO, Gentz CF, Johnell O, et al: Surgical versus nonsurgical treatment of ligamentous injuries following dislocation of the elbow joint. Clin Orthop 214:165–169, 1987.
5. Josefsson PO, Gentz CF, Johnell O, et al: Dislocations of the elbow and intraarticular fractures. Clin Orthop 246:126–130, 1989.
6. Jupiter JB, Mehne DK: Trauma to the adult elbow and fractures of the distal humerus. In Browner BE, et al (eds): Skeletal Trauma. Philadelphia, W.B. Saunders, 1992, pp 1141–1145.
7. Kelly BT, Weiland AJ: Posterolateral Rotatory Instability of the Elbow. In Altchek DW and Andrews JR (eds): The Athlete's Elbow. Philadelphia, Lippincott, Williams and Wilkins, 2001, pp 175–190.
8. Mehlhoff TL, Noble PC, Bennett JB, et al: Simple dislocation of the elbow in the adult: Results after closed treatment. J Bone Joint Surg 70A:244–249, 1989.
9. Moehring HD: Traumatic dislocations of the shoulder girdle and elbow. In Chapman MW (ed): Operative Orthopedics, 2nd ed. Philadelphia, J.B. Lippincott, 1993, pp 470–476.
10. O'Driscoll SW: Elbow trauma/fracture/reconstruction. In Orthopaedic Knowledge Update: Shoulder and Elbow. Rosemont, IL, American Academy of Orthopaedic Surgeons, 1997, pp 301–414.
11. Parvin RW: Closed reduction of common shoulder and elbow dislocations without anesthesia. Arch Surg 75:972–975, 1957.
12. Ring D, Jupiter JB: Current concepts review: Fracture-dislocation of the elbow. J Bone Joint Surg 80:566–580, 1998.
13. Ross G, McDevitt ER, et al: Treatment of simple elbow dislocation using a rapid motion protocol. Am J Sport Med May–June 1999.
14. Stanley EA, Mehlhoff TL: Elbow and forearm: Trauma. In Orthopedic Knowledge Update 4. Rosemont, IL, American Academy of Orthopedic Surgeons, 1993, pp 321–322

31. THROWING INJURIES AND OTHER ATHLETIC INJURIES OF THE ELBOW

P. Norman Ove, M.D., and Edward R. McDevitt, M.D.

1. What is the first step in diagnosing an elbow injury?
Examination should begin with a thorough history, including mechanism of injury, location of pain, activities that aggravate or relieve symptoms, and history of prior injuries or treatment. Only then should the examiner proceed with the physical examination.

2. How should one perform the physical examination of the elbow?

Examination should begin with inspection of the elbow and its relationship to the body and comparison of the elbows for swelling or differences in size, shape, or carrying angle. Examination then proceeds with maneuvers that may be more painful. Compare active and passive range of motion, strength, and stability to varus, valgus, and anteroposterior stresses. One may then palpate the anterior, posterior, medial, and lateral aspects of the elbow for tenderness, crepitus, or deformity.

3. How are most athletic injuries similar?

Although acute injuries such as fractures or tendon ruptures occur, most athletic and throwing injuries are secondary to chronic overuse involving repetitive medial tension and lateral compression forces.

4. How does this mechanism of injury affect treatment?

Overuse injuries are most often treated not by surgery but rather by relative rest, anti-inflammatory medications, alteration of mechanics, and careful rehabilitation.

5. List the differential diagnosis for an athlete presenting with anterior elbow pain.

Biceps tendinitis   Anterior capsular strain or tear
Biceps rupture   Median nerve compression syndrome

6. What specific elbow motion should be tested when biceps tendinitis or rupture is suspected?

The biceps is an elbow flexor and forearm supinator. Both conditions can be expected to cause pain and weakness with resisted elbow flexion and supination.

7. Will active elbow flexion and supination be possible after a complete rupture of the biceps tendon?

Yes. The brachialis is the prime flexor of the elbow, and the supinator in the forearm still provides supination. Supination and flexion strength are decreased by 20–50%.

8. What other findings help to diagnose a distal biceps tendon rupture?

Typically the biceps tendon is not palpable, but this finding may be obscured by swelling. Often a deformity in the distal arm is present at the site where the muscle belly has retracted proximally. Ecchymosis in the antecubital area is also suggestive of acute rupture.

9. Should radiographs be obtained?

Yes. They usually are normal, but they may reveal avulsion fragment or degenerative changes at the radial tuberosity. Magnetic resonance imaging (MRI) may be helpful to determine the extent of injury in partial or chronic tears.

10. Which is more common—distal or proximal rupture of the biceps tendon?

Only 3% of ruptures occur at the elbow; 97% occur in the shoulder, often in association with chronic rotator cuff impingement.

11. Do symptoms usually precede acute biceps rupture at the elbow?

Yes. As with Achilles tendon rupture, athletes commonly report preexisting chronic tendinitis. Degenerative changes in the tendon may make it more susceptible to a tear from a traumatic event.

12. Describe the treatment of biceps tendinitis.

As with all overuse syndromes, the first mode of treatment is to decrease the aggravating activity and to rest the inflamed tissue. Ice for acute inflammation or heat for chronic conditions and nonsteroidal anti-inflammatory drugs (NSAIDs) are helpful and usually well tolerated by athletes. Recalcitrant cases may require splinting for 1–2 weeks.

13. Do steroids help biceps tendinitis? Is any risk involved?

Steroid injection around the inflamed tendon may be of benefit in recalcitrant cases but increases the risk of subsequent tendon rupture. Injections should be used sparingly and with caution.

14. What are the predisposing factors for tendon rupture?

History of prior symptoms	Male sex
Steroid injections	Age > 30 years

15. What is the treatment of distal biceps rupture?

The treatment of complete rupture in the athletic population is surgical reattachment of the tendon to the bicipital tuberosity of the radius. After surgery the elbow is immobilized in flexion and supination for 6–8 weeks.

16. How is anterior capsule strain differentiated from biceps injury?

Anterior capsule strain is usually related to hyperextension as opposed to flexion-supination. Ecchymosis and deep tenderness to palpation may be present, but tenderness is usually more diffuse rather than isolated around the biceps tendon.

17. What more significant injury must be ruled out when anterior capsular strain is suspected?

With a hyperextension mechanism the possibility of a spontaneously reduced elbow dislocation should be considered.

18. Should radiographs be obtained in hyperextended elbow injuries?

Yes. Fracture and/or dislocation should be ruled out. With an anterior strain, bony avulsion flecks from the capsular margins may be seen. Later radiographs may reveal heterotopic calcification in the anterior tissues.

19. How long should the injury be splinted or immobilized? Why?

Immobilization should be minimal—perhaps 1 day, if needed for comfort. Prolonged splinting greatly increases the likelihood of developing a flexion contracture at the elbow. Early active range-of-motion exercises are essential to regain full motion.

20. Why should passive range-of-motion (PROM) therapy be avoided or used cautiously?

PROM therapy, especially if painful, leads to further tissue trauma that may result in heterotopic ossification. Gentle, pain-free PROM by a qualified therapist or trainer may be permissible.

21. Give another name for median nerve compression syndrome at the elbow.

Pronator syndrome.

22. How do the symptoms of pronator syndrome differ from those of other causes of anterior elbow pain?

Pain is usually just distal to the elbow in the proximal forearm, may be associated with numbness in the volar forearm or median distribution in the hand, and is often aggravated by resisted pronation activities.

23. What four structures may be responsible for pronator syndrome?

- Ligament of Struthers/supracondylar process
- Lacertus fibrosus
- Pronator teres
- Flexor digitorum superficialis (FDS) arcade

24. What provocative tests may help to identify which structure is responsible?
The following maneuvers should reproduce pain or numbness:
- Supracondylar process—elbow flexion of 120–135°
- Lacertus fibrosus—resisted forearm supination
- Pronator teres—resisted forearm pronation
- FDS arcade—resisted long finger flexion

25. How is pronator syndrome treated?
Most cases respond to modification of activities and physical therapy modalities for stretching and strengthening. Surgical decompression may be required for recalcitrant cases.

26. List the differential diagnosis for an athlete presenting with posterior elbow pain.
- Triceps tendinitis
- Triceps rupture (or olecranon fracture)
- Olecranon impingement syndrome
- Olecranon bursitis

27. What are the common findings in athletes with triceps tendinitis?
- Posterior elbow pain
- Tenderness at the triceps insertion or in the distal part of the tendon
- Resisted elbow extension causes increased pain

28. Should radiographs be obtained?
Yes. Degenerative calcifications or traction spurs may be present. Of greater importance, stress fracture of the olecranon should be excluded.

29. What findings indicate rupture of the triceps mechanism rather than overuse tendinitis?
Tear of the triceps or olecranon fracture is usually associated with an extremely forceful contraction or a fall on the elbow. Other common findings include severe pain and swelling in the posterior elbow and an inability to extend actively. A palpable defect may be present at the site of tendon or bony disruption.

30. Are radiographs useful?
Yes. In addition to excluding an olecranon fracture, radiographs reveal bony avulsion fractures in 80% of triceps tendon avulsions.

31. In what position should a nondisplaced olecranon fracture be immobilized?
Treatment of tendon ruptures and olecranon fractures should be surgical. The pull of the triceps muscle is significant, and even in full extension a well-aligned fracture will become displaced.

32. Define hyperextension overload syndrome of the elbow.
Also called olecranon impingement syndrome, posteromedial impingement syndrome, or boxer's elbow, this condition is an overuse syndrome caused by repetitive valgus extension overload of the elbow. It is common in the throwing motions, which cause the olecranon process to impinge against the medial wall of the olecranon fossa. Athletes commonly complain of pain during the extension phase of throwing and catching or locking in or near extension.

33. What physical findings may suggest the hyperextension overload syndrome?
Typical findings include posterior tenderness or swelling, lack of full extension, pain with forced valgus in full extension, and palpable loose bodies.

34. What is the valgus extension overload test? How is it performed?

The forearm is supinated, and the elbow is forcibly extended as a valgus force is applied. The test is positive if it causes posteromedial pain and crepitus.

35. Are radiographs helpful?

Yes. Anteroposterior, lateral, and axial radiographs may reveal spurring or fracture of the olecranon tip, loose bodies, or hypertrophy of the olecranon.

36. What is the role of arthroscopy in olecranon impingement syndrome?

A loose body or an olecranon osteophyte usually can be removed arthroscopically. Both loose bodies and spurs at times may be quite large, and removal may require a small posterior arthrotomy.

37. What is the leading differential diagnosis for traumatic or chronic olecranon bursitis? How should it be ruled out?

Septic olecranon bursitis is usually much more painful and more impressive on examination but may be confused with the nonseptic conditions in the early stages. It can be ruled out by aspirating the bursa through a sterile field and checking a Gram stain and culture for bacteria.

38. How does treatment of the two types of olecranon bursitis differ?

Chronic bursitis, caused by repetitive trauma or irritation to the bursa, should be treated with NSAIDs and protective padding. Both chronic and acute traumatic bursitis can be decompressed by aspiration, compression, and splinting for a short period. Septic olecranon bursitis should be treated by surgical incision, drainage, and antibiotics.

39. List the differential diagnosis for an athlete presenting with medial elbow pain.
- Medial epicondylitis/flexor-pronator strain
- Ulnar collateral ligament sprain/rupture
- Medial epicondyle fracture
- Cubital tunnel syndrome
- Little leaguer's elbow

40. What is golfer's elbow?

Golfer's elbow is an overuse syndrome of the dominant trailing arm caused by repetitive tension overloading of the flexor-pronator muscle at or near its insertion on the medial epicondyle.

41. What are the likely symptoms and findings in patients with golfer's elbow?

Athletes complain of medial and proximal forearm pain aggravated by golfing, curling, and throwing curve balls. Diagnosis can be confirmed by reproducing the pain with resisted wrist flexion and forearm pronation.

42. What other medial elbow problem is common among pitchers?

Pitchers, quarterbacks, and racquetball and squash players frequently develop chronic sprains of the ulnar collateral ligament (UCL) caused by repetitive valgus stress across the elbow. Long-standing chronic cases may develop UCL laxity with elbow instability.

43. What are the findings in patients with UCL sprains?

The primary finding is tenderness over the anterior oblique portion of the UCL. With the elbow flexed, the UCL is palpable below (more posterior than) the flexor-pronator attachment to the medial epicondyle. Pain is increased by valgus stress of the elbow. More severe cases exhibit valgus laxity.

44. Are radiographs helpful?

In some cases radiographs may reveal calcifications or spurring along the UCL. The gravity stress view can be used to demonstrate UCL laxity. MRI and computed tomography arthrography may be particularly useful in diagnosing UCL injuries. In addition to readily demonstrating complete tears, the "T-sign" is indicative of undersurface partial UCL tears.

45. How is little leaguer's elbow different from the other medial elbow overuse syndromes?

Because children and adolescents still have open growth plates, their joints are subjected to different injuries from those of adults. Repeated tensile stresses on the medial epicondyle can result in inflammation and partial separation of the apophysis. Occasionally an avulsion may occur after a single forceful muscle contraction.

46. What findings may be evident on radiographs?

In early milder cases radiographs are normal. In chronic cases radiographs may show widening or irregularity of the medial apophysis compared with the opposite side. In youngsters presenting with acute severe pain, radiographs may reveal avulsion fracture of the medial epicondyle.

47. What is the management of little leaguer's elbow?

Relatively acute cases should be treated with rest or even splinting for 1–2 weeks. In chronic cases pitching may have to be curtailed for 2–3 months to allow adequate rest. Proper coaching and throwing techniques are imperative to reduce the incidence and to prevent recurrence.

48. When is surgery indicated?

Surgery is *never* indicated for the overuse syndrome. However, in acute injuries with displacement of the epicondyle >2 mm or incarceration of the fragment within the joint, surgical reduction and fixation are required to restore joint congruity and ligament stability.

49. What medial elbow problem may present with vague aching in the forearm and tingling in the fourth and fifth fingers?

Such symptoms suggest cubital tunnel syndrome, an entrapment neuropathy of the ulnar nerve at or about the elbow. It may be the result of a cubitus valgus deformity, but in athletes it is more commonly due to trauma (contusion or subluxation of the ulnar nerve), muscle hypertrophy (especially of the flexor carpi ulnaris from excessive curls), or inflammation from adjacent tissue injury (UCL sprain).

50. List the findings suggestive of cubital tunnel syndrome.

- Positive Tinel's sign at the cubital tunnel
- Decreased sensation in the ulnar forearm and hand
- Increased pain and numbness with forced elbow flexion
- Weakness or atrophy of the first dorsal interosseous muscle (resisted index finger abduction)
- Weakness in grip strength

51. What other conditions must be considered? Name a test for each.

- Cervical radiculopathy — foraminal compression (Spurling's sign)
- Thoracic outlet syndrome (Adson's sign)
- Ulnar nerve compression at the wrist (Tinel's sign at Guyon's canal)

52. What diagnostic test may confirm cubital tunnel syndrome?

Electromyography (EMG) and nerve conduction velocity (NCV) studies may demonstrate slowing of conduction velocity across the elbow.

53. Is surgical decompression necessary?

Surgical decompression may be necessary with a progressive neurologic deficit or with failure of nonsurgical management. Initial treatment should consist of rest, NSAIDs, protective padding, and avoidance of extreme flexion. If symptoms warrant, acute episodes may be treated with splinting at 30–45° of flexion for a few days or at night to relieve compression.

54. List the differential diagnosis for an athlete presenting with lateral elbow pain.
- Lateral epicondylitis
- Radial head fracture
- Radiocapitellar chondromalacia/osteochondritis dissecans
- Posterior interosseous nerve compression syndrome
- Lateral plica
- Posterolateral instability

55. What is tennis elbow? What causes it?
Tennis elbow or lateral epicondylitis is an overuse syndrome due to repetitive tension over-loading of the wrist extensor origins at the lateral epicondyle. Such stresses are increased with pronation or resisted supination of the forearm. The problem is common in racquet sport athletes and is aggravated by vibration (strings too tight, off-center hits), faulty backhand and topspin mechanics, and a grip that is too small. It is also commonly seen in the nondominant leading arm in golfers. Other wrist dorsiflexion and supination activities, such as hammering and using a screwdriver, are also common causes.

56. Besides point tenderness at the lateral epicondyle, what other finding should be present to diagnose tennis elbow?
Increased pain at the lateral epicondyle with resisted wrist dorsiflexion confirms pathology of the origin of the extensor carpi radialis brevis (ECRB).

57. Are steroid injections beneficial in treating tennis elbow?
Yes. Most athletes, however, respond to rest, modification of technique and/or racquet, NSAIDs, and temporary use of a tennis elbow strap or even a wrist cock-up splint.

58. How does a tennis elbow strap work?
The elbow strap results in partial tenodesis of the ECRB at the proximal forearm, which reduces vibratory and tensile stresses at its origin on the epicondyle.

59. A fall on the outstretched arm that results in elbow pain is likely to cause what injury?
Compressive axial loading across the lateral elbow frequently results in a radial head fracture.

60. What is the posterior fat pad sign? What does it suggest?
The posterior fat pad sign is a radiolucency in the posterior elbow joint seen on the lateral radiograph. The posterior fat pad normally rests within the confines of the olecranon fossa and is not visible; however, it can be displaced out of the fossa by blood or other fluid within the joint. Hemarthrosis, which can be confirmed by aspiration, suggests an intraarticular fracture. Oblique views may be necessary to visualize nondisplaced fractures.

61. How are radial head fractures classified? How does classification relate to treatment?
Type I: step-off < 3 mm and angulation of < 30°; treated with brief splinting (1–2 weeks) and early range-of-motion exercises.
Type II: step-off > 3 mm or angulation > 30°; treated surgically with an attempt at open reduction and internal fixation.
Type III: comminuted; usually requires radial head excision.

62. A pitcher being treated for a UCL sprain also complains of lateral elbow pain. What other elbow problem should you suspect? Why?
Tension overloading of the medial structures during throwing and in racquet sports is frequently accompanied by compression overloading of the radiocapitellar joint laterally. Repeated stresses may cause diffuse articular damage (chondromalacia) or more specific lesions, such as osteochondritis dissecans, osteochondral fractures, or loose bodies.

63. What are the expected findings?
Affected athletes frequently cannot achieve extension. Palpation reveals tenderness at the radiocapitellar joint and crepitus with pronation and supination. Radiographs should be evaluated for decreased radiocapitellar joint space, articular spurring, defects or irregularities in the radial head or the capitellum, and loose bodies. Such lesions may require computed tomography, MRI, or arthroscopy for complete evaluation.

64. What other condition coexists in 5% of athletes with tennis elbow and often makes routine treatment unsuccessful?
Posterior interosseous syndrome may coexist with tennis elbow. It is a compression neuropathy of the posterior interosseous branch of the radial nerve at the point where it passes under the edge of (arcade of Frohse) or through the supinator muscle.

65. What structures does the posterior interosseous nerve (PIN) innervate? What findings would you expect on examination?
The posterior motor branch of the radial nerve supplies the extensor carpi ulnaris and the finger and thumb extensors, all of which may show signs of weakness. Radially innervated sensation is normal, because the radial wrist extensors arise proximal to the supinator. Tinel's sign may be positive about 4 fingerbreadths distal to the lateral epicondyle.

66. How does the possibility of concomitant PIN syndrome alter the treatment of tennis elbow?
The initial treatment is unaltered. For both conditions nonsurgical measures are usually successful. Alterations in technique and/or equipment are often helpful, although NSAIDs and a period of rest also may be needed. Occasional steroid injections may be useful. Surgical debridement and release of the inflamed ECRB tendon may be required for recalcitrant cases of tennis elbow. If surgery is contemplated, consideration also should be given to whether exploration and neurolysis of the PIN are warranted.

67. What diagnosis should be considered in an athlete complaining of lateral pain and clicking, snapping, or locking as the arm is extended and the forearm supinated?
Both posterolateral instability and plica syndrome may cause these symptoms. Rotatory stress testing may confirm subtle posterolateral laxity. A palpable snapping band in the lateral gutter may indicate a fibrotic plica band.

BIBLIOGRAPHY

1. Altchek DW, Andrews JR (ed): The Athlete's Elbow. Philadelphia, Lippincott Williams & Wilkins, 2001.
2. Andrews JR: Bony injuries about the elbow in the throwing athlete. In Stauffer ES (ed): Instructional Course Lectures 34. St. Louis, Mosby, 1985.
3. Andrews JR, Holmes SW: Athletic injuries of the elbow. In Norris TR (ed): Orthopaedic Knowledge Update, Shoulder and Elbow, Rosemont, IL, American Academy of Orthopedic Surgeons, 1997.
4. Ciccotti MG. Epicondylitis in the athlete. In Zuckerman JD (ed): Instructional Course Lectures 48. Rosemont, IL, American Academy of Orthopedic Surgeons, 1999.
5. Ciccotti MG, Jobe FW: Medial collateral ligament instability and ulnar neuritis in the athlete's elbow. In Zuckerman JD (ed): Instructional Course Lectures 48. Rosemont, IL, American Academy of Orthopaedic Surgeons, 1999.
6. Gabel GT, Morrey BF: Tennis elbow. In Cannon WT (ed): Instructional Course Lectures 47. St. Louis, Mosby, 1998.
7. Hoppenfield S: Physical Examination of the Spine and Extremities. Norwalk, CT, Appleton-Century-Crofts, 1976.
8. Hotchkiss RN: Fractures of the radial head and related instability and contracture of the forearm. In Cannon WT (ed): Instructional Course Lectures 47. St. Louis, Mosby, 1998.
9. Jobe FW, Nuber G: Throwing injuries of the elbow. Clin Sports Med 5:621, 1986.
10. Morrey BF: The Elbow and Its Disorders. Philadelphia, W.B. Saunders, 1993.

11. Morrey BF. Biceps tendon injury. In Zuckerman JD (ed): Instructional Course Lectures 48. Rosemont, IL, American Academy of Orthopedic Surgeons, 1999.
12. Nirschl RP: Sports and overuse injuries to the elbow: Muscle and tendon trauma. Tennis elbow. In Morrey BF (ed): The Elbow and its Disorders, 2nd ed. Philadelphia, W.B. Saunders, 1993, pp 537–559.
13. Pecina M, Krmpotic-Nemanic J, Markiewitz A: Tunnel Syndromes. Boca Raton, FL, CRC Press, 1991.
14. Posner MA: Compressive neuropathies of the median and radial nerves at the elbow. Clin Sports Med 9:343, 1990.
15. Spinner M: Injuries to the Major Branches of Peripheral Nerves of the Forearm. Philadelphia, W.B. Saunders, 1978.
16. Yocum LA: The diagnosis and nonoperative treatment of elbow problems in the athlete. Clin Sports Med 8:439, 1989.
17. Zarins B, Andrews R, Carson WG Jr: Injuries to the Throwing Arm. Philadelphia, W.B. Saunders, 1985.

32. ARTHROSCOPY OF THE ELBOW

Jason A. Browdy, M.D.

1. How is elbow arthroscopy different from arthroscopy of other joints?

The elbow is highly congruous and tightly constrained, making manipulation difficult. Several portals are therefore required. On average, the normal elbow has about a 30 ± 10 cc capacity. In degenerative and posttraumatic states, it may be as low as 10 cc. In addition, neurovascular structures are in close proximity to portals, making elbow arthroscopy riskier than arthroscopy of other joints.

2. What are the indications for arthroscopy of the elbow?

Loose bodies	Adhesions
Olecranon osteophytes	Osteochondritis dissecans of the capitellum
Synovitis	Chondromalacia of the radial head
Assessment and treatment of instability	Lavage of septic joints
	Miscellaneous

3. What are the contraindications for arthroscopy of the elbow?

The contraindications are bony ankylosis and severe fibrous ankylosis that prevent the introduction of the arthroscope into the elbow joint. A history of transposition of the ulnar nerve or a subluxing ulnar nerve is a contraindication for certain medial portals.

4. What size and angle of an arthroscope are most commonly used for elbow arthroscopy?

A 4-mm, 30°-angled arthroscope is optimal for visualization. A 2.7-mm scope may be used in small or stiff joints or in the direct lateral portal.

5. What are the different patient positions?

Supine, prone, and lateral decubitus.

6. Describe the position of the arm when the patient is supine.

The entire arm is allowed to hang freely over the side of the table with the elbow at 90° and the hand pointed toward the ceiling, directed at a pulley. This elbow position allows the neurovascular structures in the antecubital fossa to be at maximal relaxation. Alternatively, an armboard can be used, while an assistant maitains arm elbow position.

7. What are the advantages and disadvantages of the supine position?

Airway management is simplified for the anesthesiologist. Visualization of the anterior compartment is excellent. If the arthroscopy may need to convert to an open procudure, the supine position is preferred. One of the disadvantages is that the arm is unstable and tends to swing like a pendulum in response to pressure. In addition, access to the posterior aspect of the joint is more difficult. Finally, the use of a pulley may make manipulation of the elbow difficult.

8. Describe the prone position.
The patient is prone on bolsters. With an arm board parallel to the table, the shoulder is abducted to 90° and the elbow is flexed to 90°.

9. What are the advantages and disadvantages of the prone position?
Traction is eliminated, and gravity on the forearm tends to stabilize and assist in distension of the anterior compartment. Access to the posterior joint is good. It is easy to manipulate the elbow from full extension to almost full flexion. With the neurovascular structures displaced anteriorly, it is safer to perform surgery in the anterior compartment. A Kocher lateral approach and a posterior approach can be performed prone, but an anterior approach may require repositioning. A disadvantage is that positioning is more difficult. Airway management may be more difficult for anesthesia. Padding of pressure points and positioning of the head and neck require extra care.

10. Describe the lateral decubitus position.
The patient is placed in the lateral position, the shoulder is flexed forward 90° and internally rotated; the elbow is flexed 90° over a bolster.

11. What are the advantages and disadvantages of the lateral decubitus position?
Many of the advantages are similar to those of the prone position, but patient positioning is easier than the prone position. Airway access is also improved. Conversion to an open procedure may occasionally require repositioning.

12. Name the medial, lateral, and posterior bony landmarks to be outlined before initiation of the procedure.
The medial landmark is the tip of the medial epicondyle; the lateral landmarks are the radial head and the lateral epicondyle; and the posterior landmark is the olecranon.

13. Why is the joint distended prior to portal placement?
Distending the joint with 20–30 cc of saline before portal placement displaces neurovascular structures and makes portal placement safer.

14. Into which area should a needle be inserted to obtain maximal capsular distension?
The location is palpated between the lateral epicondyle, olecranon tip, and radial head. The elbow generally extends and supinates as capsule distends.

15. What are the five most commonly used portals for elbow arthroscopy?
The anteromedial, anterolateral, direct lateral, posterolateral, and straight posterior are the most commonly used portals.

16. What other portals have been described?
The proximal medial and proximal lateral portals.

17. Describe the positions of the various portals.
The anterolateral portal is located 3 cm distal and 2 cm anterior to the lateral epicondyle. The proximal lateral portal is 2 cm proximal and 1 cm anterior to the lateral epicondyle. The anteromedial portal is located 2 cm anterior and 2 cm distal to the medial epicondyle, aiming directly toward the center of the elbow joint. The proximal medial portal is 2 cm proximal to the medial epicondyle and just anteiror to the medial intermuscular septum. The direct lateral portal is the same spot at which the needle was inserted to distend the elbow joint capsule. This portal does

not pose significant risk to neurovascular structures, but the portal may pass within 7 mm of the posterior antebrachial cutaneous nerve. The posterolateral portal is 3 cm proximal to the olecranon tip immediately superior and posterior to the lateral epicondyle and lateral margin of the triceps muscle. This portal is established with the elbow in 20–30° of flexion by aiming toward the olecranon fossa. The straight posterior portal is 3 cm proximal to the olecranon tip and 2 cm medial to the posterolateral portal, directly through the triceps tendon. This portal also should be established with the elbow in 20–30° of flexion.

18. Describe the uses of the various portals.

The **anterolateral portal** is used primarily for instrumentation and viewing of the medial joint. It is a good working portal for the anterior joint while the arthroscope is in the proximal medial portal. One can visualize the coronoid process, trochlea, coronoid fossa, and medial radial head through this portal.

With **the proximal lateral portal**, the anterior joint can be inspected, including the anterior and lateral radial head, capitellum, and lateral gutter. This portal also may be a good initial portal because the thicker soft tissues help minimize soft tissue extravasation. In contrast, the radial capsule has softer, thinner overlying tissue. Some believe that this portal is not only safer than the anterolateral portal, but it also provides a more complete perspective of the anterior joint.

The **antromedial portal** allows visualization of the entire anterior compartment, especially the lateral structures.

With the **proximal medial portal**, one can visualize the entire anterior joint: anterior capsule, trochlea, capitellum, coronoid process, radial head and medial and lateral gutters. Some believe that this is a better portal for viewing the radiocapitellar joint than the standard anteromedial portal. In general, proximal portals are believed to be slightly safer than their distal counterparts. This may be a good starting portal, because of safe access, good visualization and less fluid extravasation than the anterolateral portal.

The **direct lateral portal** provides good visualization of the radial head, the capitellum and the radioulnar articulation. It is the only portal that allows easy access to posterior capitellum and radioulnar joint. This portal can be used along with another posterior portal to work in the posterior joint. One may consider a 2.7-mm scope here. A potential disadvantage of the direct lateral portal is fluid leakage into soft tissues. Again, be aware of the posterior antebrachial cutaneous nerve.

The **posterolateral portal** provides visualization of the posterior joint. One can see the tip of the olecranon, olecranon fossa and both gutters. Also, one can see the posterior aspect of the ulnar collateral ligament with a 4.0-mm 70° scope.

With the **straight posterior portal**, one can see the posterior compartment. It is useful for removing posterior osteophytes and loose bodies. It is needed when a complete synovectomy is performed. This portal affords limited access to the anterior joint. However, n cases of unlnar nerve transposition, the posterior portal can be used for access to the anterior joint. If a foramen between the olecranon and coronoid fossae exists, one can use this to enter the anterior joint from the posterior compartment; otherwise a fenestration must be created. This should be attempted only by practitioners with extensive experience. If the medial elbow is not accessible, then the arthroscope may be placed in the anterolateral portal and instruments may be passed from posterior into the anterior compartment.

19. Describe the risks with each portal.

With the **anterolateral portal**, the radial nerve is at risk. To avoid injuring the radial nerve, one should enter the joint lateral to the joint, and not anterior to it. However, since the anterolateral portal puts the radial nerve at greater risk and have many surgeons use a more proximal entry point; choices include the sulcus between the radial head and capitellum or directly anterior to the lateral epicondyle.

The **proximal lateral portal** puts the posterior branch of the lateral antebrachial cutaneous nerve and the radial nerve at risk. The radial nerve lies further away from this portal than the standard anterolateral portal with the elbow in flexion.

With the **anteromedial portal**, the median nerve and medial antebrachial cutaneous nerve are at risk.

The **proximal medial portal** puts the ulnar nerve, median nerve, brachial artery, and posterior branch of the medial antebrachial cutaneous nerve at risk. To avoid the ulnar nerve, one must

Summary of the Various Portals For Elbow Arthroscopy

PORTAL	LOCATION	USES	RISKS
Anterolateral	3 cm distal and 2 cm anterior to lateral epicondyle	Visualization of coronoid process, trochlea, coronoid fossa, medial radial head and medial capsule Work portal for instrumenting medial joint when camera is medial	Radial nerve Posterior branch of lateral antebrachial cutaneous nerve
Proximal lateral	2 cm proximal and 1cm anterior to lateral epicondyle	Inspection of anterior and lateral radial head, capitellum and the lateral gutter Instrumentation anteriorily Less risk to radial nerve	Posterior branch of the lateral antebrachial cutaneous nerve Radial nerve
Direct lateral	Center of triangle bounded by tip of olecranon, radial head and lateral epicondyle	Initial distention of capsule Visualization of the radial head, capitellum and radioulnar articulation Only portal that allows easy access to posterior capitellum and radioulnar joint Instrumentation Minimal neurovascular risks	Fluid extravasation into soft tissues Posterior branch of lateral antebrachial cutaneous nerve Limited access to anterior joint
Posterolateral	3 cm proximal to olecranon tip and just lateral to lateral edge of triceps tendon	Visualization of tip of olecranon and olecranon fossa posteriorily and both gutters Visualization of ulnar collateral ligament	Ulnar nerve at risk when working in medial gutter Medial brachial cutaneous nerve Posterior antebrachial cutaneous nerve
Anteromedial	2 cm anterior and 2 cm distal to the medial epicondyle	Visualization of entire anterior compartment, especially the lateral structures Inflow portal Instrumentation	Median nerve Medial antebrachial cutaneous nerve.
Proximal medial	2 cm proximal to medial epicondyle and just anterior to medial intermuscular septum	Visualization of anterior capsule, trochlea, capitellum, coronoid process, radial head and medial and lateral gutters Possibly better for viewing the radiocapitellar joint than standard anteromedial portal Instrumentation anteriorily	Ulnar nerve Median nerve Brachial artery Posterior branch of the medial antebrachial cutaneous nerve
Straight posterior	3 cm proximal to olecranon tip and in the midline, through the triceps	Visualization and instrumentation of posterior compartment Option of transhumeral approach	Limited access to the anterior joint Ulnar nerve Posterior antebrachial cutaneous nerve

identify the intermuscular septum and make sure to stay anterior to it. While the trocar is being advanced toward the radial head, one must maintain contact with the anterior surface of the humerus to avoid injury to the median nerve and brachial artery. There are several hazards with the **posterolateral portal.** The ulnar nerve lies superficial to the capsule medially; thus, when working in the medial gutter, one must be aware of this. When the cannula is kept lateral to the posterior midline, the risk to the ulnar nerve is minimal. Other nerves that can be harmed include the medial brachial cutaneous nerve and the posterior antebrachial cutaneous nerves.

With the **straight posterior portal,** one must be aware of the ulnar nerve and posterior antebrachial cutaneous nerve. But it is generally a safe portal.

20. From which portal are the capitellum and radial head best seen?

The anteromedial or proximal medial portal.

21. Through which portals can the coronoid process of the ulna be seen?

The anteromedial and anterolateral portals. The proximal portals can also provide good visualization of these structures.

22. What two types of pathology are most commonly found in the posterior compartment of the elbow?

Loose bodies and olecranon osteophytes.

23. What are the signs and symptoms of loose bodies?

Pain, swelling decreased range of motion (usually extension), catching, clicking, and possibly locking. Not all loose bodies are seen on radiographs.

24. Where are the loose bodies found?

Location may be predictable based on the diagnosis. In osteochondritis dissecans, the fragment is often found near the radiocapitellar joint. Loose bodies from synovial chondromatosis are most often found anteriorily.

25. What are the indications for arthroscopy in the arthritic elbow?

Atraumatic osteoarthritis of the elbow is uncommon and often responds to conservative measures. Patients who fail conservative treatment or those who have significant reduction in range of motion can be considered for arthroscopic debridement and possibly anterior capsular release.

26. What is the normal and functional range of motion of the elbow?

The normal range of motion is defined as $0-146°$. Ninety percent of activities of dailing living may be performed with a $100°$ arc: from $30°$ to $130°$. Certain activities require better than $30°$ of extension; thus, a flexion contracture of $30°$ or greater may be an indication for sugery.

27. How can osteoarthritis be treated arthroscopically?

Arthroscopy can allow excision of osteophytes from the olecranon, coronoid, and olecranon and coronid fossae. Loose bodies are excised; however, this alone is not believed to be effective for treating arthritis. If the arthritis is associated with capsular contracture, some advocate capsular release arthroscopically. This approach is not universally agreed upon, because neurovascular injury is a possible complication. If indicated, the radial head can be excised arthroscopically.

28. What risk is associated with excision of osteophytes?

Damage to articular cartilage and injury to a nerve. The posteromedial osteophyte is close to the ulnar nerve. The ulnar nerve is also close to the prominance of the osteophyte on the trochlea and therefore removal of osteophytes from this region should be done with care.

29. Is capsular release necessary to improve range of motion in osteoarthritis?

Usually not. More typically, oseophytes are the reason for loss of motion. Capsular release may be necessary if osteophytes are not impinging when directly visualized.

30. What risks are associated with arthroscopic capsular release?

Capsular release is perhaps the most dangerous arthroscopic procedure. Injury to the radial and less likely the median nerve is possible with anterior capsular release. The radial nerve lies close to the capsule at the level of the radial neck. Posterior release puts the ulnar nerve at risk.

31. Describe the role of arthroscopic synovectomy.

This procedure is often perfomed in rheumatoids. The elbow is involved in 20–50% of rheumatoids, and about half of these patients have pain and loss of motion. Most patients respond to conservative treatment. Those that do not may respond well to arthroscropic synovectomy. The thin capsule in rheumatoids makes this procudure risky.

32. When and where does osteochondritis dissecans of the elbow occur?

It is a condition seen typically in a throwing athlete or gymnast. The lesion is usually on the capitellum but also may be seen on the radial head.

33. What are the indications for arthroscopic treatment of osteochondritis dissecans?

Failure of conservative treatment, loose bodies, and an elbow that is locked.

34. How is osteochondritis dissecans treated arthroscopically?

Loose, detached cartilage is excised, and a bleeding surface in the crater is created with curettement and drilling.

35. What is the valgus extension overload syndrome?

It is a condition typically seen in baseball pitchers in their mid-20s. It is caused by repetitive valgus stresses associated with pitching. Patients develop an osteophyte on the posteromedial aspect of the tip of the olecranon with impingement in the olecranon fossa. A "kissing lesion", or an osteochondral defect on the trochlea of the humerus, may develop. Soft tissue contractures may also occur. Ultimately, the patient develops a mechanical block to motion demonstrated by a flexion contracture, with loss of full extension.

36. What are the exam and radiographic findings of the valgus extension overload syndrome?

Pain to palpation of the tip of the olecranon, pain with valgus stress and extension, and a flexion contracture. Radiographs show a posterior osteophyte on the tip of the olecranon seen on the lateral view. An axial view may show the posteromedial osteophyte.

37. How is the valgus extension overload syndrome treated?

Rest, NSAIDs and gradual strengthening. If the patient fails this regimen, arthroscopic or open debridement is indicated. The posteromedial osteophyte is resected. It is essential to be cognicent of the ulnar nerve during debridement. Recurrence is not uncommon.

38. Describe the role of arthroscopy in managing trauma.

Persistant pain after minimally displaced radial head fractures may respond to arthroscopic treatment of loose bodies or cartilage irregularities. Some displaced two-part radial head fractures may benefit from arthroscopically aided fixation. Some coronoid and capitellar fractures with large fragments can be fixed arthroscopically. Some unicondylar distal humerus fractures can be fixed with the aid of an arthroscope

39. Describe the role of arthroscopy in managing instability.

Chronic medial or lateral instability may lead to secondary changes such as plica formation, loose body formation, and chondromalacia, all of which may be treated arthroscopically. Complete disruption of the ulnar collateral ligament can be diagnosed arthroscopically. Partial tears involving the important anterior bundle cannot be seen but may be diagnosed with the arthroscopic valgus instability test. This test is done by direct visualization of the medial ulnohumeral articulation while a valgus stress is applied. An opening of 1–2 mm indicates disruption of the anterior bundle. Varus stress may also demonstrate insufficency of the lateral collateral ligament. Subluxation of the radial head can be seen directly in cases of posterolateral rotatory instability.

40. Name two of the miscellaneous conditions treated by arthroscopy.
Lateral epicondylitis and olecranon bursitis.

41. What are the potential complications from elbow arthroscopy?
Neurovascular injury, infection, synovial fistula, and cartilage injury; less commonly, arthrofibrosis, heterotopic bone, and hematoma. The capsule is very close to the skin in certain areas and may predispose to chronic portal drainage and infection. Of note, most neurologic injuries are transient, but some are not.

42. What is the incidence of complications?
A survey done by the Arthroscopy Association of North America found 0.2% complication rate and a review of the literature found a 5% rate of complications. Both of these figures are thought to be underestimations. A preliminary report of the Mayo experience reports a 1% incidence of complications and a 10% rate of minor problems.

43. What nerve is at greatest risk?
The radial nerve is generally regarded as the most vulnerable. Following the radial nerve are the ulnar and median nerves.

44. How can the incidence of complications be reduced?
To avoid the most serious complications, injury to surrounding nerves, landmarks should be defined before distention. The joint should be distended with fluid, and the elbow should be flexed to 90° during insertion of anterior portals. Whenever possible, a needle may be used to located proper portal placement, or an inside-out technique may be used. Sharp incisions are made through the skin only, hemostats are used to spread longitudinally, and a blunt trocar is used to create the portal. Accurate portal placement is essential, because the nerves lie within millimeters of the described portal sites. The more proximal portals are generally safer than the more distal ones. Pronating the arm protects the posterior interosseous nerve. Knowledge of local anatomy helps prevent neurologic injury even after creating the portals. For instance, when using the shaver to excise the radial head in the anterior compartment, the blade should be directed posteriorily, as the posterior interosseous nerve is adjacent to the capsule at that level. In addition, a retractor may be used to lift the capsule away from the instrument during debridement. Suction should not be used when near a nerve, as this can suck the nerve into the field. Some recommend avoiding pressurized inflow. Drains may be used when extensive debridement may lead to hematoma formation. Suturing the posterolateral portal closed may help prevent synovial fistual formation.

45. What rehabilitation instructions are given to the patient for the immediate postoperative period?
The patient should wear a sling for comfort and begin active-assistive range-of-motion exercises on the first postoperative day, progressing to full range of motion as tolerated.

BIBLIOGRAPHY

1. Andrews JR, Craven WM: Lesions of the Posterior Compartment of the Elbow. Clin Sports Med 10: 637–652, 1991.
2. Andrews JR, St. Pierre RK, Carson WG: Arthroscopy of the elbow. Clin Sports Med 5:653–662, 1984.
3. Baker CL, Brooks AA: Arthroscopy of the Elbow. Clin Sports Med 15:261–281,1996.

4. Baker CL, Cummings DC: Arthroscopic Management of Miscellaneous Elbow Disorders. Op Tech Sports Med 6:16–21, 1998.
5. Baumgarten TE, Andrews JR, Satterwhite YE: The arthroscopic classification and treatment of osteo-chondritis dissecans of the capitellum. Am J Sports Med 4:520–523, 1998.
6. Day B: Elbow Arthroscopy in the Athlete. Clin Sports Med 15:785–797, 1996.
7. Esch JC, Baker CL: Atrthroscopic Surgery: The Shoulder and Elbow. Philadelphia, J.B. Lippincott, 1993.
8. Field LD, Savoie FH: The Arthroscopic Evaluation and Management of Elbow Trauma and Instability. Op Tech Sports Med 6:22–27, 1998.
9. Lyons TR, Field LD, Savoie III FH: Basics of Elbow Arthroscopy. Inst Course Lec 49:239–246, 2000.
10. McGinty JP: Operative Arthroscopy. New York, Raven Press, 1991.
11. Morrey BF: Complications of Elbow Arthroscopy. Inst Course Lec 49:255–258, 2000.
12. Morrey BF: The Elbow and Its Disorders. Philadelphia, W.B. Saunders, 1993.
13. Norberg FB, Savoie FH, Field LD: Arthroscopic Treatement of Arthritis of the Elbow. Inst Course Lec 49:247–253, 2000.
14. Phillips BB, Strasburger SE: Arthrofibrosis of the Elbow. Arthroscopy 14:38–44, 1998.
15. Plancher KD, Peterson RK, Brezenoff L: Diagnostic Artrhroscopy of the Elbow: Set-up, Portals and Technique. Op Tech Sports Med 6:2–10, 1998.
16. Woods G: Elbow arthroscopy. Clin Sports Med 6:557–564, 1985.

33. ARTHRITIS OF THE ELBOW

Edward V. Fehringer, M.D.

1. What are the major types of arthritis that involve the elbow?

In order of frequency, the most common types of elbow arthritis are: rheumatoid, posttrau-matic, and osteoarthritis.

2. Describe the epidemiology and typical presenting history of elbow arthritis.

Patients with rheumatoid arthritis generally present to their primary physician or rheumatol-ogist with a painful, stiff elbow and a previous diagnosis of rheumatoid arthritis. Patients that do not have rheumatoid arthritis typically present between the third and eighth decades of life with a history of a previous fracture or dislocation of the elbow, repetitive elbow trauma, or an occu-pation that requires heavy upper extremity physical labor.

3. What are the physical examination findings of a patient with elbow arthritis?

Stiffness is quite common with elbow arthritis, especially loss of extension. Roughness is pal-pable with flexion/extension and pronation/supination. Pain is often elicited with extension and flexion, especially at the extremes of motion.

4. Describe the radiographic appearance of osteoarthrosis of the elbow?

Anteroposterior and lateral radiographs typically reveal osteophytes of the olecranon and coronoid processes as well as osteophytes in the coronoid and olecranon fossae. Loose bodies may be present. Anteroposterior radiographs are difficult to obtain in elbows with flexion contractures. An anteroposterior view of the distal humerus as well as an anteroposterior view of the proximal radius and ulna should be obtained separately to gain a true appreciation of the anatomy of each distinct side of the joint.

5. What are the nonoperative treatments options for elbow arthritis?

Nonoperative treatment of elbow arthritis centers around pain relief and maintenance of mo-tion. Nonsteroidal anti-inflammatory agents, gentle stretching programs, and occasional cort-ciosteroid injections may help provide satisfactory elbow comfort and function for many patients.

6. Name the surgical options for osteoarthritis of the elbow.

Elbow capsular releases, loose body removal, and bony excision: open or arthroscopic. Combinations of these three parts are generally performed. Increased motion and decreased mechanical pain are predictable. Decreased pain at rest is not. Arthroscopic techniques are challenging. Ulnar nerve symptoms should be recognized pre-operatively with a low threshold for transposition, especially when correcting for significant flexion contractures.

Interposition/distraction arthroplasty. This procedure may be considered for osteoarthritis but is generally reserved for young patients with post-traumatic elbow arththritis without other reasonable options.

Total elbow arthroplasty. Total elbow arthroplasty may be performed for elbow arthritis but has led to early failures in osteoarthritis due to high demand and resultant early loosening.

7. What approach should be used for performing an open elbow capsular release and/or bony excision for osteoarthritis?

Various approaches have been described. The lateral approach is probably the most common, allowing release of anterior and posterior capsules as well as excision of bone from the coronoid and olecranon processes and fossae, respectively. The lateral ligamentous complex should be maintained or repaired if taken down. The medial approach is also popular, allowing isolation and protection the ulnar nerve. Either the lateral approach or medial approach alone may make releases on the opposite side of the joint difficult. Therefore, combined medial and lateral approaches may be necessary, especially if an ulnar nerve transposition is needed. Some surgeons prefer to use a straight posterior skin incision, elevating large flaps medially and laterally to allow medial and lateral deep approaches. Wound complications may increase with this approach but the incidence of cutaneous nerve injury decreases.

8. Describe the typical radiographic presentation of rheumatoid arthritis.

There are four distinct stages: stage 1, normal radiograph with the possibility of osteoporosis and active synovitis; stage 2, symmetric joint narrowing and normal architecture; stage 3, distinct alteration of subchondral architecture that may be relatively mild (type A) or extensive (type B); and stage 4, gross destruction of most or all of the articular architecture and characterized clinically by instability and severe pain.

9. What is the natural history of rheumatoid arthritis in the elbow?

1. Synovitis is the first, prominent pathologic process. Biomechanics remain normal. Osteoporosis is present but without gross articular destruction.

2. Joint narrowing generally occurs with progressive osteoporosis.

3. Joint architecture becomes distorted. Osteoporosis worsens, subchondral cysts form, and clinical complaints of instability begin, distinguishing rheumatoid arthritis from osteoarthritis.

4. Finally, gross destruction results in loss of articular surfaces and gross instability.

10. What are the surgical options for treatment of rheumatoid arthritis of the elbow?

Stage, age, and other joint involvement determine one of two choices:
- Synovectomy with or without radial head excision.
- Total elbow arthroplasty.

11. What has been the experience with arthroscopic synovectomy for elbow arthritis?

It is technically demanding and difficult to perform a complete synovectomy without causing neurovascular injury. Early success has been achieved with somewhat diminished 3-year satisfactory results. It is unclear whether it is superior to open synovectomy. Arthroplasty surgeons tend to prefer replacement over synovectomy because of the more predictable long-term results.

12. What are the indications, advantages, and disadvantages of radial head resection?

Resection is recommended for pain relief when the radiocapitellar joint is involved and the ulno-humeral involvement is relatively mild or moderate. This procedure is recommended for pain relief, not for increased motion. Postoperative motion is variable with 50% unchanged, 30% improved, and 20% worse compared with preoperative motion. Radial head resection is not offered as a long-term solution to the patient with rheumatoid arthritis because the disease most likely will progress to involve the ulnohumeral joint.

13. What is the current role of Silastic radial head replacement in elbow surgery?

Although Silastic radial head replacement is advocated by a few authors, the increasing concern about silicone particulate synovitis and lymphadenitis with a subsequent autoimmune response has lessened the enthusiasm. The procedure is currently not recommended by most elbow surgeons.

14. What is interposition/distraction arthroplasty of the elbow? What are its indications?

Interposition arthroplasty refers to resecting the diseased articulating surfaces and filling the joint with interposed materials in hopes of relieving pain. Many materials have been tried with muscle flaps, fascia being the most recent. An external fixator is placed on either side of the elbow to allow joint distraction as healing occurs. The technique is not universally accepted and, because of its technical complexity, is used by relatively few surgeons. It is preferred in a heavy laborer. Its disadvantages include unpredictable pain relief and unpredictable stability. It is used in select patients to avoid elbow arthrodesis or total elbow arthroplasty.

15. What is total elbow arthroplasty?

Total elbow arthroplasty involves replacement of the articulating surfaces of the distal humerus and the proximal ulna. The radial head is not currently included in the reconstruction, but attempts are being made to do so

16. When is total elbow arthroplasty indicated?

Most surgeons agree that the indications for total elbow arthroplasty are narrow. The primary indication is for advanced elbow arthritis in patients with rheumatoid arthritis or other inflmmatory arthritidies that render the elbow functional demands as low. There may also be some select cases of elbow ostoearthritis and posttraumatic arthritis in low-demand patients in whom total elbow arthroplasty may be considered. Acutely, total elbow arthroplasty may also be used in cases of severe supracondylar and intracondylar fractures of the elbow in elderly patients. In addition, it may be indicated for intracondylar and supracondylar nonunions of the distal humerus in elderly patients.

17. What are the contraindications for total elbow arthroplasty?

Active infection in the joint is an absolute contraindication. Relative contraindications are young patients with an active lifestyle or heavy laborers unwilling or unable to alter their lifestyle.

18. What elbow arthroplasty designs are currently used?

There are two types of prosthetic elbow joint designs in current use: unlinked or "unconstrained" and linked or "semiconstrained." Excellent results have been achieved with both at different institutions with similar indications.

19. List the major complications of total elbow arthroplasty.
- Wound problems and infection.
- Component loosening.
- Instability, including dislocations, subluxations, or maltracking (all primarily with the unconstrained).
- Ulnar nerve injury.

20. Identify the main technical considerations in elbow arthroplasty.
- Arthroplasty is usually performed through a posterior approach. The ulnar nerve must be explored and may be transposed anteriorly. The triceps may be "peeled" from the olecra-

non, split, or preserved. Preservation is more technically challenging but may allow for better triceps function, an important detail in patients with rheumatoid arthritis that use their arms to push themselves out of bed and chairs. Meticulous soft tissue handling is paramount.
- Careful attention must be given to soft-tissue balancing and elbow axis restoration and component rotational alignment. Soft tissue reconstruction are especially important with the unconstrained design where ligamentous and capsular reconstructions may be difficult due to the poor tissue often found in patients with rheumatoid arthritis.
- Careful handling, reaming, and preservation of bone is essential.

21. What are the results of total elbow arthroplasty?
Ninety percent of patients are highly satisfied with pain relief. Survivorship analysis predicts a failure rate of approximately 20% at 10 years.

22. Is there an indication for elbow arthrodesis?
Arthrodesis of the elbow is an unsatisfying operation for both patient and surgeon. Most agree that there is almost never an indication for it. It has been performed for intractable elbow sepsis when no other reconstruction is possible. No optimal position of fusion exists as any significantly limits patients in performing activities of daily living.

BIBLIOGRAPHY

1. Azar FM, Wright PE II: Arthroplasty of shoulder and elbow. In Canale ST (ed): Campbell's Operative Orthopaedics, 9th ed. St. Louis, Mosby, 1998, pp 497–513.
2. Figge HE III, Inglis AE, et al: Current concepts review: Total elbow arthroplasty. J Bone Joint Surg 70A: 778–783, 1983.
3. Frymoyer JW (ed): Orthopedic Knowledge Update, No. 4. Chicago, American Academy of Orthopedic Surgeons, 1993.
4. Lee BP, Morrey BF: Arthroscopic synovectomy of the elbow for rheumatoid arthritis: A prospective study. J Bone Joint Surg 79A:770–772, 1997.
5. McKee, MD, Pugh, DMW, Schemitsch, EH, Pederson, ME, Jones, C, Richards, R: Elbow Extension Weakness Following Semi-Constrained Total Elbow Arthroplasty: A Cause for Concern? Proceedings of the 69th Annual Meeting of the American Academy of Orthopaedic Surgeons, Dallas, 2002.
6. Morrey BF: Post-traumatic contracture of the elbow: Operative treatment, including distraction arthroplasty. J Bone Joint Surg 72A:601–618, 1990.
7. Morrey BF: Primary degenerative arthritis of the elbow: Treatment of ulno-humeral arthroplasty. J Bone Joint Surg 74B:409–413, 1992.
8. Morrey BF: Semiconstrained elbow replacement for distal humeral nonunion. J Bone Joint Surg 77B: 67–72, 1995.
9. Morrey BF: The Elbow and Its Disorders, 3rd ed. Philadelphia, W.B. Saunders, 2000.
10. Norris TR (ed): OKU Shoulder and Elbow. Chicago, American Academy of Orthopaedic Surgeons, 1997.
11. O'Driscoll SW: Elbow arthritis: Treatment options. J Am Acad Orthop Surg 1:106–116, 1993.
12. Sledge CB, et al: Arthritis Surgery. Philadelphia, W.B. Saunders, 1994.

34. COMPARTMENT SYNDROMES OF THE UPPER EXTREMITY

David E. Brown, M.D.

1. Define compartment syndrome.
Compartment syndrome is a condition in which elevated pressure in an enclosed space can damage irreversibly the contents of the space.

2. What are the major causes of compartment syndrome?

The causes of compartment syndrome are divided into two categories: those that decrease or constrict the compartment and those that increase the contents of the space. Closure of fascial defects or application of compressive dressings, a tight cast, or military antishock trousers (MAST) may limit the compartment's ability to expand to accommodate an increased volume. Compartment volumes may be increased by hemorrhage after a fracture, surgery, or blunt injury, or by post-ischemic swelling resulting from arterial injury or restoration of blood flow after arterial injury.

3. How does compartment syndrome occur?

Increased compartmental tissue pressures obstruct venous return initially, resulting in vascular congestion and further increase in intracompartmental pressure. Capillary beds become occluded, and blood is shunted away from occluded areas, resulting in muscle and nerve ischemia. Capillary basement membranes become leaky, allowing transudation of fluid into the surrounding tissues and thus compounding the problem. If the condition is uncorrected, arterial flow to the affected compartment becomes so impaired that the muscle and nerve tissues within the compartment die.

4. What are the five Ps of compartment syndrome?

Pain, pallor, paresthesias, paralysis, and pulselessness are the classic signs of compartment syndrome. Paralysis and pulselessness are late findings. If the process has progressed to this point, the limb is less likely to be salvageable.

5. What is the earliest and most sensitive finding in compartment syndrome?

Pain is usually the earliest sign and is often out of proportion to what may be expected from the extent of the injury. Pain with passive stretch of the muscle in the compartment is the most reliable clinical test.

6. Is compartment syndrome possible in a patient without pain?

A patient without pain still may have a compartment syndrome. Pain may be diminished or absent in the late stages as a result of nerve ischemia. A central neurologic deficit or unconsciousness should lower the threshold for prompt treatment.

7. Name the five most common causes of compartment syndrome.

The five most common causes are fracture, soft-tissue injury, arterial injury, prolonged limb compression, and burns.

8. What is Volkmann's contracture?

In 1881 Richard von Volkmann described the contracture and paralysis caused by tissue damage that occurs as a sequela of compartment syndrome. He blamed the ischemia on tight bandaging of the extremity. The term is often used synonymously with compartment syndrome, ischemic muscle damage, and the characteristic position of the hand after forearm compartment syndrome.

9. How is pressure in a compartment measured?

Several methods are available, and anyone dealing with patients at risk should be familiar with at least one. Whitesides popularized an infusion technique that uses supplies available in any hospital. Matsen advocates a similar technique but modifies it for continuous monitoring by using and infusion pump and a blood pressure transducer. Mubarak's wick catheter technique directly measures compartment pressures. In addition, a commercially available device made by the Stryker company is simple and reliable.

10. When should compartment pressures be measured?

Measurements should be obtained in any unresponsive or unreliable patient who has sustained a fracture or other injury to the forearm, especially if the compartment feels tense. In the alert patient, the clinical findings for compartment syndrome often are inconclusive. Pressure readings in such cases help to determine which patients require fasciotomy. As a general rule, if one merely considers compartment pressure measurements, they should be obtained.

11. What is the threshold for intracompartmental pressures?

The threshold for intracompartmental pressures is debatable. Some advocate fasciotomy for all patients who demonstrate a resting pressure > 30 mmHg, whereas others suggest waiting until the pressure is > 45 mmHg. Still others believe that it is more important to relate the intracompartmental pressure to the patient's systolic, diastolic, or mean arterial pressures; i.e., intracompartmental pressure raised to within 20 mmHg of the patient's diastolic pressure indicates the need for fasciotomy. In general, whenever compartment pressures are > 30 mmHg, the patient should be followed closely. Fasciotomy should be performed whenever pressures are > 40 mmHg or fall within 20 mmHg of the diastolic pressure and are associated with clinical findings suggestive of impending compartment syndrome.

12. What is the proper initial management of a responsive patient demonstrating the signs of early impending compartment syndrome?

All constrictive dressings should be removed or split down to the skin. Any circumferential cast should be bivalved, with the underlying cast padding split down to the skin. The limb should not be elevated but placed at the level of the heart to promote arterial inflow.

13. Describe the definitive treatment for acute compartment syndrome.

The definitive treatment is fasciotomy, the open release of the restrictive fascial compartment dividers. In performing this procedure, the skin and fascia are left open; skin is grafted at a later date.

14. How many compartments are in the forearm?

The forearm consists of the volar compartment, dorsal compartment, and a compartment of the mobile wad (brachioradialis, extensor carpioradialis brevis, and extensor radialis longus). The three compartments of the forearm differ from those of the leg in that they are interconnected. Fasciotomy of the volar compartment may decompress the other two. This possibility should not be relied on, however, and any clinically involved compartment should be released.

15. What are the compartments in the hand?

There are 10 compartments in the hand: 1 for each of the 4 dorsal interosseous muscles, 3 for the volar interossei, 1 for the adductor pollicis, and 1 each for the thenar and hypothenar muscles.

16. Can compartment syndrome occur in a finger?

Yes. Although there is no muscle in the finger, nerves and soft tissue can become ischemic because of excessive swelling. The finger has a tight investing fascia that is relatively unyielding.

17. Which muscles are most often involved in compartment syndrome of the forearm?

The muscles closest to the bone are affected first. Therefore, the flexor digitorum profundus and flexor pollicis longus are most often involved, followed by the flexor digitorum superficialis and pronator teres.

18. What is the characteristic position of the hand in Volkmann's contracture?

In a classic Volkmann's contracture, the fingers and thumb are fixed in flexion with the wrist in slight flexion. The position of the hand and degree of flexion contracture depend on the extent of muscle damage.

19. What is the treatment of established Volkmann's contracture of the forearm?

Treatment of established contractures depends on the level of involvement but generally includes tendon release and tendon transfers to restore function.

BIBLIOGRAPHY

1. Eaton RG, Green WT: Epimysiotomy and fasciotomy in the treatment of Volkmann's contracture. Orthop Clin North Am 3:175, 1972.
2. Feliciano DV, Cruss PA, Spjat-Patrinely V, et al: Fasciotomy after trauma to the extremities. Am J Surg 156:533, 1988.
3. Garfin S, Mubarak S, Evans K, et al: Quantification of intracompartmental pressure and volume under plaster casts. J Bone Joint Surg 63A:449, 1981.
4. Green DP (ed): Operative Hand Surgery, 4th ed. New York, Churchill Livingstone, 1998.
5. Hargens AR, Mubarak SJ: Current concepts in the pathophysiology, evaluation and diagnosis of compartment syndrome. Hand Clin 14:371–383, 1998.
6. Lagerstrom CF, Reed RL II, Rowlands BJ, Fischer RP: Early fasciotomy for acute clinically evident post traumatic compartment syndrome. Am J Surg 158:36, 1989.
7. Mabee JR, Bostwick TL: Pathophysiology and mechanisms of compartment syndrome. Orthop Rev 22:175, 1993.
8. Matsen FA III: Compartment syndrome: A unified concept. Clin Orthop 113:8, 1975.
9. Ortiz JA Jr, Berger RA: Compartment syndrome of the hand and wrist. Hand Clin 14:405–418, 1998.
10. Rockwood CA Jr, Green DP, Bucholz RW (eds): Rockwood and Green's Fractures, vols. 1 and 2, 4th ed. Philadelphia, Lippincott-Raven, 1996.
11. Sundararaj GD, Mani K: Pattern of contracture and recovery following ischemia of the upper limb. J Hand Surg 10B:155, 1985.
12. Whitesides TE Jr, Haney TC, Morimoto K, Harada H: Tissue pressure measurements as a determinant for the need of fasciotomy. Clin Orthop 113:43, 1975.

35. NERVE ENTRAPMENTS OF THE ELBOW AND FOREARM

Jeffrey J. Tiedeman, M.D.

1. How are nerve injuries classified?

Seddon classified nerve injuries as neurapraxia, axonotmesis, and neurotmesis. **Neurapraxia** is caused by localized ischemic demyelination often from compression or contusion. **Axonotmesis** results in interruption of the axons and their myelin sheaths but the endoneurial tube remains intact. Stretching or compression is a common cause of axonotmesis. **Neurotmesis** is caused by anatomic disruption of the axons, the myelin sheath, and the endoneurial tube (e.g., from a laceration or severe stretching injury). Spontaneous recovery cannot be expected in neurotmesis; surgical repair or grafting is necessary to maximize function. Complete recovery of nerve function is not expected in adults with neurotmesis.

2. What is pronator syndrome?

Pronator syndrome is essentially a high carpal tunnel syndrome (CTS) because it represents another entrapment neuropathy of the median nerve. Like CTS, it may produce numbness and paresthesias in the median innervated digits, weakness in the thenar muscles, and pain in the wrist and forearm. Unlike CTS, pronator syndrome typically does not cause nocturnal symptoms. Tinel's sign is negative at the wrist, and although nerve conduction studies of the median nerve may be delayed, the delay does not occur at the wrist.

3. What structure can cause entrapment of the median nerve in pronator syndrome?

As the name indicates, the most common source of compression is the pronator teres muscle. Pronator teres compression can be elicited by resisted forearm pronation with the elbow extended. The lacertus fibrosus also has been implicated as a possible cause; compression is elicited by resisted flexion of the elbow with the forearm in supination. Lastly, the arch of the flexor digitorum superficialis also may be responsible for median nerve compression. This muscle is tested by resisted flexion of the proximal interphalangeal (PIP) joint of the middle finger.

4. Describe anterior interosseous syndrome.

Anterior interosseous syndrome is compression of the anterior interosseous nerve, which branches from the median nerve approximately 4–6 cm below the elbow. It functions entirely as a motor nerve and supplies the flexor pollicis longus (FPL), the FDP to the index and middle fingers, and pronator quadratus muscles. Despite its motor function, pain in the forearm is a commonly presenting problem.

5. Where is Gantzer's muscle?

Gantzer's muscle is an accessory head to the FPL muscle and may be responsible for compression of the anterior interosseous nerve.

6. What is the Kiloh-Nevin sign?

The Kiloh-Nevin sign, which is elicited by asking the patient to form an "O" with the tips of the thumb and index finger, is used to test terminal function of the digits against resistance. In a patient with anterior interosseous syndrome, fine-pinch posture is abnormal. The index finger is extended at the distal interphalangeal (DIP) joint as it makes contact with the pulp of the thumb (which is also hyperextended at the IP joint level).

7. What is a Martin-Gruber anastomosis?

A small minority of patients may have crosslinks among the three main nerves of the upper limb. The Martin-Gruber anastomosis is an anomaly in which motor nerve fibers normally carried entirely in the ulnar nerve enter the ulnar nerve from the median nerve via branches in the forearm. In patients with this anomaly, dysfunction or disruption of the ulnar nerve above the level of the anastomosis may not result in motor loss of muscles in the hand typically innervated by the ulnar nerve.

8. What is cubital tunnel syndrome?

Cubital tunnel syndrome refers to entrapment of the ulnar nerve in its passage around the medial aspect of the elbow. The ulnar nerve normally passes through the anatomic cubital tunnel, which is a fibroosseous ring formed by the medial epicondyle and the proximal part of the ulna; it is bridged by a specific fascial sheet known as Osborne's fascia.

9. What causes ulnar nerve entrapment of the elbow?

Ulnar nerve entrapment can result from both pathologic as well as physiologic responses to repetitive trauma. Mechanical factors that have been implicated include compression and traction. The ulnar nerve can be compressed proximal to the cubital tunnel at the level of the arcade of Struthers or by the medial intermuscular septum. Compression at the level of the cubital tunnel may result from osteophytes, loose bodies, synovitis, or a thickening of Osborne's fascia. Compression may also occur distal to the cubital tunnel at the flexor carpi ulnaris aponeurosis or at the deep flexor-pronator aponeurosis. Individual's most at risk include those who perform repetitive elbow flexion activities or overhead throwing athletes.

10. The ulnar nerve supplies which structures?

The ulnar nerve provides motor supply to the flexor carpi ulnaris and one-half of the flexor digitorum profundus (FDP), the palmar and dorsal interosseous muscles, the hypothenar muscles, the ulnar two lumbrical muscles, the adductor pollicis, and the deep head of the flexor pollicis brevis (FPB). The ulnar nerve also supplies sensation to the small finger and the ulnar half of the ring finger. Through its dorsal sensory branch it also supplies sensation to the dorsal ulnar aspect of the hand.

11. What provocative tests are used to substantiate a diagnosis of cubital tunnel syndrome?
Tinel's sign is invariably positive over the ulnar nerve in the cubital tunnel, producing a tingling sensation that radiates to the ulnar two fingers. The elbow flexion test is performed by maximally flexing the elbow. Pain and paresthesias in the ulnar nerve distribution within 60 seconds constitute a positive test and are virtually diagnostic of cubital tunnel syndrome.

12. How is Froment's sign elicited?
The patient is asked to pull on a sheet of paper with the index finger and thumb while the examiner withdraws it strongly. The patient with normal function maintains maximal contact of the digital pulp with the paper by extending the IP joint of the thumb. In ulnar nerve dysfunction, the control of the metacarpophalangeal (MCP) joint is lost through paralysis or weakness of the adductor pollicis and the deep head of the FPB. Consequently, the MCP joint collapses into hyperextension and the IP joint flexes to compensate for the resulting lack of pinch strength.

13. What is radial tunnel syndrome?
Radial tunnel syndrome, or resistant tennis elbow, is entrapment or compression of the posterior interosseous nerve in the lateral aspect of the proximal forearm. Patients may present with motor weakness in the radially innervated muscles of the forearm, pain in the lateral aspect of the elbow region, or both. Because of its close proximity to the lateral epicondyle, this problem is sometimes difficult to differentiate from lateral epicondylitis or tennis elbow.

14. Which structures are typically responsible for posterior interosseous nerve compression?
The mnemonic **FREAS** is useful for remembering the structures that compress the posterior interosseous nerve:
F = Fibrous bands
R = Recurrent radial vessels (the leash of Henry)
E = Extensor carpi radialis brevis
A = Arcade of Frohse
S = Supinator (the distal border)

15. What is Wartenberg's syndrome?
Originally described as cheiralgia paresthetica, Wartenberg's syndrome is an entrapment neuropathy at the point where the sensory branch of the radial nerve emerges from beneath the edge of the brachioradialis tendon, 6–8 cm proximal to the radial styloid. The condition typically arises as a result of previous trauma or from repeated pronation and supination of the forearm.

16. What is Wartenberg's sign?
The inability to adduct the extended small finger to the extended ring finger is referred to as Wartenberg's sign. The patient's ring and small fingers will form a "V" that they are unable to close. It is a sign of ulnar nerve dysfunction with inactivity of the interossei and hypothenar muscles. The small finger remains abducted due to the unopposed activity of the extensor digiti minimi.

17. How does lateral antebrachial cutaneous neuropathy present?
The lateral antebrachial cutaneous nerve is the terminal sensory branch of the musculotaneous nerve. It supplies sensation over the radial half of the forearm from the elbow to the wrist. Compressive neuropathy may occur in persons who perform repeated overhead motions such as throwing (racquet sport athletes and swimmers). It is thought to occur from forced repeated pronation with the elbow extended. Compression occurs at the lateral margin of the biceps aponeurosis. A positive Tinel's sign may be elicited immediately lateral to the biceps tendon. Initial treatment consists of relative rest and/or corticosteroid injection at the site of the Tinel's sign. This should be coupled with elbow splinting in moderate flexion. Surgical release is occasionally necessary.

BIBLIOGRAPHY

1. Blacker GJ, Lister GD, Kleinert HE: The abducted little finger in low ulnar nerve palsy. J Hand Surg 1A:190–196, 1976.
2. Chen FS, Rokito AS, Jobe FW: Medial elbow problems in the overhead-throwing athlete. J Am Acad Orthop Surg 9:99–113, 2001.
3. Dellon AL: Review of treatment results for ulnar nerve entrapment at the elbow. J Hand Surg 14A: 688–700, 1989.
4. Eversmann WW Jr: Entrapment and compressive neuropathies. In Green DP (ed): Operative Hand Surgery, 3rd ed. New York, Churchill Livingstone, 1993, pp 1341–1385.
5. Gelberman RH, Eaton R, Urbaniak JR: Peripheral nerve compression. J Bone Joint Surg 75A:1854–1878, 1993.
6. Idler RS: General principles of patient evaluation and nonoperative management of cubital syndrome. Hand Clin 12:397–403, 1996.
7. Lister GD: Compression. In Lister GD (ed): The Hand: Diagnosis and Indications, 3rd ed. New York, Churchill Livingstone, 1993, pp 283–322.

36. ELBOW AND FOREARM FRACTURES

Brian P. Hasley, M.D., and David E. Brown, M.D.

1. Define and distinguish supracondylar, transcondylar, and intercondylar fractures of the distal humerus.

Supracondylar fractures occur in the distal humeral metaphysis above the joint capsule, and are completely extraarticular. **Transcondylar** fractures, more commonly seen in the elderly osteoporotic population, are a variation of the supracondylar fracture in that the fracture plane occurs within the capsule of the elbow. **Intercondylar** fractures involve a fracture line that splits the medial and lateral condyles, usually associated with a supracondylar fracture.

2. How does treatment differ for the three types of fracture?

Supracondylar fractures occur from an extension injury. Nondisplaced fractures may be treated by splint alone, whereas displaced fractures usually require open reduction and internal fixation.

Transcondylar fractures occur in osteoporotic bone; thus fixation is difficult. Closed reduction with percutaneous pinning is often the best treatment choice. Poor bone quality makes rigid internal fixation difficult to achieve.

Intercondylar fractures, if nondisplaced, can be treated by cast immobilization. The much more common displaced and comminuted fractures require accurate open reduction and rigid internal fixation followed by early range-of-motion therapy. Bone grafting is advisable in comminuted fractures.

3. What is the classification system for intercondylar fractures?

Ryseborough and Radin developed a classification system that involves four types:

Type I: Completely nondisplaced with a transverse supracondylar fracture
Type II: Separation of fractures without rotation
Type III: Significant displacement and malrotation of the condylar fracture fragments
Type IV: Central comminution, regardless of the fracture pattern

4. What is the most common mechanism of radial head fracture?

The most common mechanism is a fall on the outstretched arm. Associated injuries include elbow dislocations and fractures of the distal radius and proximal humerus.

5. What is the classification system of radial head fracture?
Mason's classification system is the most widely used:
Type I: Nondisplaced fracture that can be easily missed without sufficient clinical suspicion
Type II: Marginal radial head fracture with minimal displacement, depression, or angulation
Type III: Comminuted or significantly displaced radial head fracture
Type IV: Radial head fracture associated with an elbow dislocation

6. What is the treatment for a radial head fracture?
Treatment depends on the fracture type. Types I and II generally are treated with short-term splinting and early therapy designed to achieve return of full range of motion. Such fractures are stable. However, type II fractures with > 2 mm of displacement and a mechanical block to extension should be treated with anatomic reduction and internal fixation. Type III fractures should be treated with open reduction and internal fixation. If there is too much comminution to allow adequate fixation, excision of the radial head is performed. The radial head component of type IV fractures are treated by the above guidelines, except that simple excison of the radial head is unacceptable. The excised radial head should be replaced. Metallic implants are now preferred.

7. What is the Essex-Lopresti lesion?
The Essex-Lopresti lesion is a comminuted fracture of the radial head, with disruption of the interosseous membrane and distal radioulnar joint. Thus, excision of the radial head leads to disastrous results, because the entire radius migrates proximally. Treatment involves open reduction and internal fixation or replacement arthroplasty of the radial head followed by accurate reduction and pinning of the distal radioulnar joint. The surgical pin is removed in 6 weeks once the interosseous membrane and distal radioulnar joint ligaments and capsule have healed.

8. Describe the two types of capitellum fractures.
Type I fractures occur in the coronal plane and usually involve the entire capitellum. They are usually displaced and rotated. Open reduction and rigid internal fixation are preferred. Excision of the fracture fragment also has been shown to give satisfactory results, although it is generally reserved for low-demand patients or patients in whom accurate reduction and rigid fixation cannot be achieved.
Type II capitellum fractures involve the articular cartilage and a small shell of subchondral bone. Thus, the chances of satisfactory healing after internal fixation are slight. Excision is advised.

9. What is the mechanism of olecranon fractures?
Olecranon fractures usually result from a fall directly onto the olecranon.

10. Describe the treatment recommendations for olecranon fractures.
Splinting or casting is indicated for nondisplaced olecranon fractures that are stable with elbow motion. The recommended degree of flexion in which to immobilize the elbow ranges from 40° to 90°. However, most olecranon fractures are displaced necessitating open reduction and internal fixation. Two techniques are commonly used: Tension band wiring and plate fixation. Tension band wiring with longitudinal K-wires or screws and figure-of-eight tension banding is advocated for noncomminuted avulsion or transverse fractures. Plate fixation is generally preferred for oblique fractures distal to the midpoint of the trochlear notch or comminuted fractures. Excision of the proximal fragment is reserved for low demand or osteoporotic patients when this fragment involves less than 50% of the articular surface.

11. What are the common mechanisms of injury for diaphyseal fractures of the radius and ulna?
A fall on the outstretched hand or a direct blow.

12. How much angulation can be accepted in an adult diaphyseal radius and ulna fracture?
Cadaveric studies indicate that malangulation of 0–10° results in little loss of rotational motion, whereas 10–15° may result in up to 20° of rotational loss. Malangulation > 20° restricts rotation by ≥ 50%.

13. What is the treatment of radial and ulnar shaft fractures in adults?
The treatment of choice is anatomic reduction and rigid internal fixation using AO principles of interfragmentary compression. A 3.5-mm dynamic compression or limited contact dynamic compression plate is recommended with a minimum of six cortices of purchase on both sides of the fracture.

14. What are the indications for bone grafting of diaphyseal fractures of the radius and ulna?
1. Comminution of more than one-third of the diameter of the shaft
2. Segmental defects
3. Fracture nonunion
The bone graft should not be placed along the interosseous membrane. Grafting of the radius and ulna must be performed through separate incisions to minimize the risk of radioulnar synostosis.

15. When should the plates and screws be removed after internal fixation of forearm fractures?
Timing is controversial because of the risk of refracture of the diaphysis after plate removal. Many surgeons advise leaving the plates in place unless they are causing symptoms. The rate of refracture varies from 10% to 20% in published series. If the plates are to be removed, the fracture must be completely healed, and the arm must be protected from heavy activities for at least 6 weeks.

16. List the risk factors for refracture after plate removal.
- Early plate removal (< 18 months after surgery)
- Use of 4-mm rather than 3-mm compression plates
- Failure to protect the forearm after plate removal
- Marked comminution of the original fracture

17. What is a Monteggia fracture?
Dislocation of the radial head with a diaphyseal fracture of the ulna.

18. What is a Galleazzi fracture?
Dislocation of the distal radioulnar joint (DRUJ) with fracture of the diaphysis of the radius.

19. Give three other names for a Galleazzi fracture.
- Fracture of necessity (it is necessary to perform internal fixation with this fracture pattern)
- Piedmont fracture (Hughston and colleagues in the Piedmont Orthopaedic Society originally described the poor results from nonoperative management)
- Reverse Monteggia fracture

20. What is the treatment of Monteggia fracture?
- Anatomic reduction of the radial head dislocation—usually closed
- Open reduction and rigid internal fixation of the ulnar fracture

21. What is the treatment of Galleazzi fracture?
- Anatomic reduction and rigid internal fixation of the radial fracture
- Management of the distal radioulnar joint (DRUJ) disruption

The radius fracture is to be fixed before addressing the DRUJ. Once completed, closed reduction of the DRUJ is performed. The DRUJ is rarely irreducible by closed measures. However, in such a case, open reduction through a dorsal incision is required. After reduction, the stability of the DRUJ must be assessed. This assessment determines whether simply immobilizing the forearm in supination is sufficient or if further augmentation with K-wires is necessary to achieve adequate stability.

22. What is a night-stick fracture?
A night-stick fracture is an isolated fracture of the ulnar diaphysis, typically in the distal one third of the shaft. These fractures often result from a direct blow to the ulna, so-called because it was originally described in victims of beatings with police night-sticks. Treatment of a nondisplaced night-stick fracture consists of cast immobilization or functional bracing. However, when fracture displacement exceeds 50% or 10° of angulation, open reduction and rigid internal fixation is recommended.

PEDIATRIC FRACTURES

23. Describe types of supracondylar humerus fractures.
Extension-type (Incidence = 96%)
Flexion-type (Incidence = 4%)

24. What is the mechanism of injury for supracondylar humerus fractures?
Extension-type fractures are caused by a fall on a hyperextended elbow. Flexion-type fractures result from a fall on or direct blow to the olecranon with the elbow flexed.

25. What is the classification for extension-type supracondylar humerus fractures?
The Gartland classification is the most widely used system for this fracture.
Type I: Nondisplaced.
Type II: Displaced with an intact posterior cortex.
Type III: Completely displaced. Type III fractures are further divided into posteromedial and posterolateral which describes the relation of the distal fragment to the humeral shaft.

26. What is the Baumann angle?
The Baumann angle is a radiographic assessment to determine the coronal plane deformity of supracondylar humerus fractures. This angle is obtained from an anteroposterior (AP) radiograph of the elbow. It is the angle formed by drawing a line through the long axis of the humerus and the growth plate of the capitellum. The Baumann Angle ranges from 64° to 81° in normal elbows. Because of this variability, most advocate comparison with the uninjured contralateral elbow. A difference of 5° or more is considered significant.

27. What is the most common nerve injury associated with supracondylar humerus fractures?
The anterior interosseus branch of the median nerve is the most commonly injured nerve, followed by the radial nerve.

28. What is the most common iatrogenic nerve injury associated with supracondylar humerus fractures?
Ulnar nerve. Injury to this nerve is commonly associated with medial K-wire placement during percutaneus cross-pinning of this fracture.

29. What are the complications of pediatric supracondylar humerus fractures?
- Fracture malunion/cubitus varus (most common).
- Nerve injury (5–19%).

- Vascular compromise (5–17%).
- Volkmann's ischemic contracture (rare with current treatment techniques).

30. Describe the treatment for supracondylar humerus fractures in children.
Type I fractures can be treated with cast immobilization in 90 degrees of elbow flexion. Type II and III fractures have a higher incidence of complications with casting alone (e.g., cubitus valgus, Volkmann's ischemic contractures). Therefore, closed reduction and percutaneus pin fixation is recommended.

31. What is the recommended mode of pin fixation for supracondylar humerus fractures?
Two pin configurations are commonly advocated for treatment of displaced supracondylar humerus fractures in children: crossed-pin fixation and parallel lateral pin fixation. Cross-pinning has been shown to be the more biomechanically stable of the two pin configuations. However, recent clinical evidence demonstrates equal efficacy in maintaining fracture reduction between the two modes of fixation. In addition, lateral pin fixation avoids the potential iatrogenic ulna nerve injury associated with placement of the medial pin.

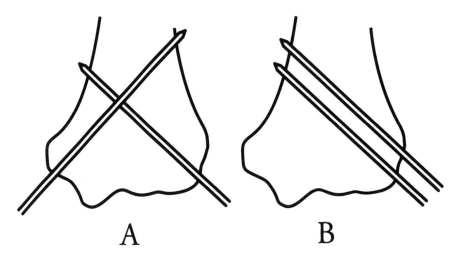

Modes of pin fixation for supracondylar humerus fractures. **A,** Crossed-pin fixation. **B,** Parallel lateral pin fixation.

32. What are the indications for open reduction of supracondylar humerus fractures?
- Open fractures
- Fractures irreducible by closed means
- Fractures with vascular compromise refractory to reduction
- Postreduction nerve palsy

33. Describe the types of Monteggia lesions in children.
Type I: Anterior dislocation of the radial head; ulna fracture with apex anterior angulation
Type II: Lateral dislocation of the radial head with apex radial angulation of the proximal ulna fracture
Type III: Posterior dislocation of the radial head with apex posterior angulation of ulna fracture
Type IV: Anterior dislocation of the radial head with concomitant fracture of the proximal radial shaft. The ulnar fracture has apex anterior angulation.

34. What is the treatment for medial condyle fractures?

Treatment of this uncommon fracture depends on the degree of displacement. Nondisplaced or minimally displaced fractures are treated with splint or cast immobilization for 3–4 weeks. Displacement greater than 2–3 mm requires open reduction and internal fixation.

35. Which is more common, medial or lateral condyle fractures?

Lateral condyle fractures, which account for more than 50% of all distal humeral physeal injuries.

36. Describe the Milch classification for lateral condyle fractures.

Type I: Lateral to the trochlea. The less common of the two, Type I fractures are typically Salter-Harris IV fractures extending through the capitellum and entering the joint lateral to the capitello-trochlear groove. The presence of an intact trochlea acts as a buttress to help maintain the stability of the elbow joint.

Type II: Extension into the trochlea. This Salter-Harris II fracture extends along the capitellar physis and crosses into the trochlear groove. Extension into the trochlea can result in loss of joint stability and, thereby, permit lateral subluxation of the ulna.

Milch classification for lateral condyle fractures.

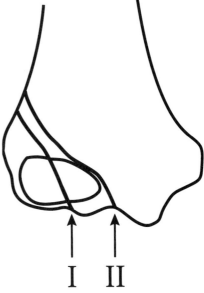

I   II

37. Describe the treatment for lateral condyle fractures.

Casting or splinting with close follow-up is recommended for nondisplaced lateral condyle fractures. When displacement exceeds 2 mm, open reduction through a lateral approach and internal fixation with smooth K-wires is advocated.

38. What are the complications associated with lateral condyle fractures?

Cubitus valgus deformity is one of the most common complications of lateral condyle fractures. This deformity can be caused by malunion, partial growth arrest, or avascular necrosis. In addition to the cosmetic deformity, cubitus valgus has been associated with the development of a tardy ulnar nerve palsy. Other complications include nonunion, avascular necrosis of the trochlea (fishtail deformity), cubitus varus, and lateral spur formation (common).

39. What is the treatment for a tardy ulnar nerve palsy?

Anterior transposition of the ulnar nerve has demonstrated efficacy in improving motor and sensory symptoms. Best results are obtained with early intervention.

40. Describe the treatment of radial neck fractures in children.

These Salter-Harris type II fractures are generally nondisplaced and can be treated with short-term immobilization and early range of motion. Closed reduction should be performed with angulations between 30° and 60° and/or 3 mm to 50% displacement. Beyond that, open reduction and K-wire fixation is recommended. *Note:* Significant displacement or angulation should also prompt concern about a possible spontaneously reduced elbow dislocation.

41. What are the indications for radial head excision in children?

None. Excision of the radial head is commonly associated with cubitus valgus, proximal migration of the radius, and proximal radioulnar synostosis. Markedly comminuted radial head fractures are uncommon in children. The fracture generally occurs at the radial neck, thus leaving sufficient residual bone in the head to allow closed or open reduction or K-wire fixation of the fracture fragments.

42. What is a medial epicondyle fracture?

A medial epicondyle fracture is usually an avulsion fracture of the apophysis of the medial epicondyle. It occurs in adolescents, usually as the result of a forced valgus injury to the elbow. It is also seen in throwing athletes, because the flexor pronator mass is forcefully contracted at ball release. Nondisplaced fractures may be treated with immobilization. Any displacement in the dominant arm of a throwing athlete mandates anatomic reduction and internal fixation.

43. What is the treatment for diaphyseal fractures of the radius and ulna in children?

Treatment includes closed reduction and cast immobilization. Diaphyseal fractures heal more readily in children than in adults; children are more tolerant of short-term immobilization and more accepting of malangulation and translocation.

44. How much angulation or displacement is acceptable for diaphyseal forearm fractures in children?

The acceptable degree of angulation or displacement depends on the age of the child. In children up to 6 years of age, as much as 15° of angulation can be accepted. In older children, only 10° should be accepted. Even complete translocation (bayonet apposition) is tolerated in a child because of the tremendous healing potential of the pediatric periosteum.

45. What are the limits of reduction for physeal fractures of the distal radius?

- 50% apposition
- 25° angulation
- 0° of rotation
- Greater than 1 year of growth remaining

BIBLIOGRAPHY

1. Aronson DD, Prager BI: Supracondylar fractures of the humerus in children: A modified technique for closed pinning. Clin Orthop 219:174–184, 1987.
2. Badelon O, Bensahel H, Mazoa K, et al: Lateral humeral condylar fractures in children: A report of 47 cases. J Pediatr Orthop 8:31–34, 1988.
3. Beaty JH: Fractures and dislocations about the elbow in children. In Eilert RE (ed): American Academy of Orthopedic Surgeons Instructional Course Lectures, 41. Park Ridge, IL, American Academy of Orthopedic Surgeons, 1992, pp 373–384.
4. Case SL, Hennrikus WL: Surgical treatment of displaced medial epicondyle fractures in adolescent athletes. Am J Sports Med 25:682–686, 1997.

5. Chapman MW, Gordon JE, Zissimos AG: Compression plate fixation of acute fractures of the diaphyses of the radius and ulna. J Bone Joint Surg 71A:159–169, 1989.
6. Crenshaw AH Jr: Fractures of shoulder girdle, arm, and forearm. In Canale ST (ed): Campbell's Operative Orthopaedics, 9th ed. St. Louis, Mosby, 1998, pp 2309–2323.
7. Edwards GS Jr, Jupiter JB: Radial head fractures with acute distal radioulnar dislocation: Essex-Lopresti revisited. Clin Orthop 234:61–69, 1988.
8. Esser RD, Davis S, Taavo T: Fractures of the radial head treated by internal fixation: Late results in 26 cases. J Orthop Trauma 9:318–323, 1995.
8. Geel CW, Palmer AK, Ruedi T, et al: Internal fixation of proximal radial head fractures. J Orthop Trauma 4:270–274, 1990.
9. Hak DJ, Golladay GJ: Olecranon fractures: Treatment options. J Am Acad Orthop Surg 8:266–275, 2000.
10. Heim D: Forearm shaft fracture. In Ruedi TP, Murphy WM (ed): AO Principles of Fracture Management. New York, AO Publishing, 2000, pp 341–355.
11. Henley MB, Bone LB, Parker B: Operative management of displaced intraarticular fractures of the distal humerus. J Orthop Trauma 1:24–35, 1987.
12. Huurman WW: Lateral humeral condylar fracture. Nebr Med J Sept: 300–302, 1983.
13. Jupiter JB, Kellam JF: Diaphyseal fractures of the forearm. In Browner BD, Jupiter JB: Skeletal Trauma, 2nd ed. W.B. Saunders, Philadelphia, 1998 pp 1438–1443.
14. Kurer MH, Regan MW: Completely displaced supracondylar fracture of the humerus in children: A review of 1708 comparable cases. Clin Orthop 256:205–214, 1990.
15. Lyons ST, Quinn M, Stanitski CL: Neurovascular injuries in type III humeral supracondylar fractures in children. Clin Orthop 376:62–67, 2000.
16. McGowan AJ: The results of transposition of the ulnar nerve for traumatic ulnar neuritis. J Bone Joint Surg 32-B:293–301, 1950
17. Milch H: Fractures and fracture dislocations of the humeral condyles. J Trauma 4:592–607, 1964.
18. Mirsky EC, Karas EH, Weiner LS: Lateral condyle fractures in children: Evaluation of classification and treatment. J Orthop Trauma 11:117–120, 1997.
19. Otsuka NY, Kasser JR: Supracondylar fractures of the humerus in children. J Am Acad Orthop Surg 5:19–26, 1997.
20. Reitman R, Waters P, Millis M: Open reduction and internal fixation for supracondylar humerus fractures in children. J Pediatr Orthop 21:157–161, 2001.
21. Reynolds RA, Mirzayan R: A technique to determine proper pin placement of crossed pins in supracondylar fractures of the elbow. J Pediatr Orthop 20:485–489, 2000.
22. Ring D, Jupiter JB: Current concepts review. Fracture dislocation of the elbow. J Bone Joint Surg 80:566–580, 1998.
23. Skaggs DL, Hale JM, Bassett J: Operative treatment of supracondylar fractures of the humerus in children: The consequences of pin placement. J Bone Joint Surg 83A:735–740, 2001.
24. Wilkens KE, O'Brien E: Fractures of the distal radius and ulna. In Rockwood CA, Wilkens KE, Beaty JH (ed): Fractures in Children, 4th ed, Lippincott, Philadelphia, 1996, pp 451–515.
25. Williamson DM, Coates CJ, Miller RK et al: Normal characteristics of the Baumann angle: An aid in assessment of supracondylar fractures. J Pediatr Orthop 12:636–639, 1992.
26. Wolfgang G, Burke F, Bush D, et al: Surgical treatment of displaced olecranon fractures by tension band wiring technique. Clin Orthop 224:192–204, 1987.
27. Worlock P: Supracondylar fractures of the humerus: Assessment of cubitus varus by the Baumann Angle. J Bone Joint Surg 68B:755–759, 1986.
28. Zionts LE, McKellop HA, Hathaway R: Torsional strength of pin configurations used to fix supracondylar fractures of the humerus in children. J Bone Joint Surg 76A:253–256, 1994.
29. Zych GA, Latta LL, Zagorski JB: Treatment of isolated ulnar shaft fractures with prefabricated functional fracture braces. Clin Orthop 219:194–200, 1987.

V. Hand and Wrist

37. ANATOMY OF THE HAND

Stephen M. Hansen, M.D., MBA

1. Name the bones of the proximal and distal carpal rows.
The bones of the proximal carpal row, from radial to ulnar, are the scaphoid, lunate, triquetrum, and pisiform. The distal row comprises the trapezium, trapezoid, capitate, and hamate.

2. How much of wrist flexion and extension occurs at the midcarpal joint?
Wrist kinematics are quite complex, and the exact amount of motion that occurs at the radiocarpal and midcarpal joints is debated. In the simplest terms, 50% of wrist motion occurs at the midcarpal level. A greater proportion of flexion occurs at the midcarpal joint, whereas most of wrist extension occurs at the radiocarpal joint.

3. List the contents of the carpal tunnel.
The normal carpal tunnel contains the median nerve and nine flexor tendons: the four sublimis tendons, the four profundus tendons, and the flexor pollicis longus.

4. What is Guyon's canal?
Guyon's canal is the triangular canal immediately ulnar to the carpal tunnel in the wrist. The ulnar nerve and ulnar artery traverse the canal, which may be a site of ulnar nerve entrapment.

5. List the contents of the six dorsal wrist compartments.
The dorsal wrist compartments are numbered from radial to ulnar and contain the extensor tendons. The contents of the compartments are listed in the table below. A helpful mnemonic to remember the number of tendons in each compartment is 2–2–1–2–1–1.

Dorsal Wrist Compartments

COMPARTMENT	CONTENTS
1	Abductor pollicis longus
	Extensor pollicis brevis
2	Extensor carpi radialis longus
	Extensor carpi radialis brevis
3	Extensor pollicis longus
4	Extensor digitorum communis
	Extensor indicis proprius
5	Extensor digiti minimi
6	Extensor carpi ulnaris

6. How much motion occurs at the fifth carpometacarpal joint?
The fifth carpometacarpal joint is a saddle joint and the most mobile of the carpometacarpals. Cadaveric studies demonstrate 15° of motion, but many authors give 20–30° as a functional range of motion for the ulnar side of the hand.

7. How much motion occurs at the third carpometacarpal joint?

No motion occurs at the third carpometacarpal joint. It acts as a central stable post for the hand, and its axis is used as the reference for adduction and abduction of the digits.

8. What muscles are innervated by the median nerve distal to the carpal tunnel?

The mnemonic **LOAF** may be helpful. The median nerve supplies motor branches to the lateral two **l**umbricals, **o**pponens pollicis, **a**bductor pollicis brevis, and the superficial head of the **f**lexor pollicis brevis. Opposition of the thumb is tested easily and reliably by having the patient touch the tips of the small finger and thumb.

9. Why is the recurrent motor branch of the median nerve at risk during carpal tunnel release?

The recurrent motor branch has a variable course across the wrist. It may leave the median nerve proximal (most common) or distal to the transverse carpal ligament, or it may pass through the ligament (up to 30% in some series).

10. What is the action of the interosseous muscles?

The dorsal interossei abduct the digits and assist in metacarpophalangeal (MCP) flexion. The palmar interossei adduct and assist in MCP flexion. While the interossei are the primary flexors of the MCP joints, they also assist lumbricals with extension of the iinterphalangeal (IP) joints through their attachment to the dorsal aponeurosis.

11. What is unique about the lumbrical muscles?

The lumbrical muscles are unique in that they take their origin from a tendon. Arising from the tendons of the flexor digitorum profundus in the palm, these muscles join the dorsal aponeurosis and act primarily as extensors of the IP joints. Because of their tendinous origin, the lumbricals are the only muscles that relax an antagonist (flexor digitorum profundus [FDP]) with contraction. The lumbricals also assist the interossei in MCP flexion. They emerge from the radial side of FDP tendons only.

12. What are the borders of the anatomic "snuff box"?

The snuff box lies just distal to the radial styloid process. The radial border is composed of the abductor pollicis longus and extensor pollicis brevis. The ulnar border is the extensor pollicis longus. The floor of the snuff box is the scaphoid bone.

13. What is Allen's test?

Allen's test evaluates the circulation of the radial and ulnar arteries in the hand. The patient opens and closes the fist several times; then the examiner occludes the radial and ulnar arteries at the wrist with the fist closed. Next the patient opens the fist, and the examiner releases one of the arteries. The hand should flush immediately. The procedure is repeated, with release of the other artery. Failure to flush or slow return of color to the hand suggests occlusion of one of the arteries.

14. Which artery is dominant?

Although the radial artery is more easily palpated, the ulnar artery is usually the dominant source of blood to the hand. Radial artery puncture for blood gases and blood pressure monitoring might not be done so liberally if the radial artery were the dominant source of blood.

15. Where is "no man's land" of the hand?

Bunnel first described no man's land, the area in which *both* flexor tendons of the fingers pass through a tight fibrous tunnel. Designated as zone II, it is the area between the distal palmar crease and the insertion of the flexor superficialis at the midportion of the middle phalanx. Repair of tendon lacerations in this region requires meticulous technique and knowledgeable postoperative management.

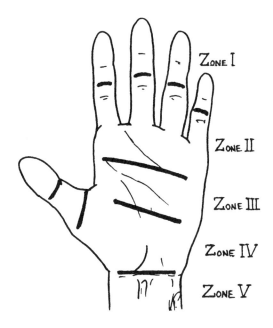

Zones of flexor tendon injury. Zone II: "no man's land."

16. What are the vincula tendinum?

The vincula are thin fibrous slips, covered by synovial membrane, that transmit blood vessels to the flexor tendons. Each tendon has a vinculum brevis and a vinculum longus.

17. What structure is involved in Dupuytren's contracture?

Dupuytren's contracture is a progressive contracture of the fingers into the palm caused by cords of palmar fascia. It commonly begins with the fourth and fifth fingers and may involve the entire palm. Baron Dupuytren is given credit for identifying the cause of the contracture and for the first successful surgical release. The disease is hereditary, and its gene has recently been mapped.

18. What deformity is caused by rupture of the central slip of a finger's long extensor?

Rupture of the central slip, with an attenuated triangular ligament, allows the lateral bands to drop volar to the axis of the proximal interphalangeal (PIP) joint. The lateral bands then become flexors of the PIP as the joint "buttonholes" through the rupture. The distal interphalangeal (DIP) joint then undergoes a compensatory hyperextension. This loss of extension of the PIP and hyperextension of the DIP is called a boutonnière (buttonhole) deformity.

19. What deformity is caused by volar plate laxity at the PIP joint?

A swan neck deformity results from a lax PIP joint volar plate with accompanying hyperextension of the PIP joint. When the PIP joint hyperextends, the dorsal terminal tendon becomes loose, and the DIP joint falls into flexion. Because the PIP joint is hyperextended and the DIP joint is flexed, the deformed finger's profile resembles that of a swan's neck.

20. Where do most wrist ganglia originate?

The most common ganglion is the dorsal wrist ganglion, which originates from the scapholunate ligament and accounts for approximately 60–70% of all hand ganglia. The second most common is the volar ganglion (18–20%). Ganglia of the flexor tendon sheath at the A-1 pulley are the third most common (10–12%).

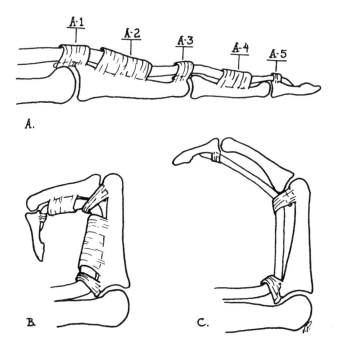

Retinacular pulley system. *A,* Annular pulley, with flexor digitorum superficialis omitted. *B* and *C,* Demonstration of function of annular pulleys and tendon bowstringing with absent A-2 and A-4.

21. Which of the annular pulleys of the flexor tendon are the most important in preventing bowstringing?

Five annular fibrous tissue bands overlie the synovial sheath of the flexor tendons. They are numbered from proximal to distal. Although biomechanical studies have shown the A-1 pulley to be the strongest, the A-2 and A-4 pulleys are the most important for preventing the tendons from bowstringing. Often patients with bowstringing flexor tendons have ruptured multiple pulleys, including A-3

22. What role do the cruciform pulleys play?

The three cruciform pulleys are also numbered from proximal to distal and are found between A-2 and A-3, A-3 and A-4, and A-4 and A-5. They act as accordions, taking up slack in the sheath with flexion of the finger.

BIBLIOGRAPHY

1. American Society for Surgery of the Hand: The Hand: Examination and Diagnosis, 3rd ed. New York, Churchill Livingstone, 1990.
2. Landsmeer JMF: Atlas of Anatomy of the Hand. Edinburgh, Churchill Livingstone, 1976.
3. Lichtman DM, Alexander AH (eds): The Wrist and Its Disorders. Philadelphia, W.B. Saunders, 1997.
4. Matloub HS, Yousef NJ: Peripheral nerve anatomy and innervation patterns. Hand Clin 8:201, 1992.
5. Netter FH: Atlas of Human Anatomy. Summit, NJ, Ciba-Geigy, 1989.
6. Palmer AK, Werner FW, Murphy D, Glisson R: Functional wrist anatomy: A biomechanical study. J Hand Surg 10A:39, 1985.
7. Romanes GJ: Cunningham's Manual of Practical Anatomy, vol 1: Upper and Lower Limbs, 15th ed. Oxford, Oxford University Press, 1986.
8. Seiler, JG III, Fraser, JLL Digital flexor sheath: Repair and reconstruction of the annular pulleys and membranous sheath. J South Orthop Assoc 9(2):8190, 2000.

9. Smith, RJ: Intrinsic muscles of the fingers: Function, dysfunction, and surgical reconstruction. Instructional Course Lectures, vol xxiv. St. Louis, Mosby, 1975.
10. Tubiana R (ed): The Hand, vol v. Philadelphia, W.B. Saunders, 1999.

38. FRACTURES AND DISLOCATIONS OF THE HAND AND WRIST

Stephen M. Hansen, M.D., MBA

1. What is a mallet finger? How is it treated?

Mallet finger describes a flexion deformity of the distal interphalangeal (DIP) joint due to loss of continuity of the extensor tendon with the distal phalanx. It may be due to an avulsion of the tendon or avulsion fracture at the tendon insertion. Splinting of the DIP in extension is the preferred method of treating both types of injury. Many authors advocate surgical treatment if the fracture involves a significant portion of the articular surface and the joint is subluxed or if the patient's occupation prohibits splinting.

2. What structure is frequently injured in crush injuries of the distal phalanx?

The nailbed is frequently involved in crush injuries but often neglected. Care should be taken to repair the nailbed with a fine, absorbable suture. Fractures of the distal phalanx rarely require more than simple splinting for protection.

3. What are the indications for open reduction and internal fixation of proximal and middle phalangeal fractures?

Indications for surgery on proximal and middle phalangeal fractures, which do not differ significantly from indications for other fractures, include unstable fractures that cannot be reduced and maintained by closed means, most intraarticular fractures, multiple fractures in an extremity, and open fractures with associated soft-tissue injury.

4. What methods of fixation are available for fractures of the metacarpals and phalanges?

The most common method of fixation of small bones is by Kirschner wires, either with open or closed reduction. Intraosseous, tension-band, and cerclage-wiring techniques are also useful. Intramedullary fixation has been described but is less popular. Small-plate and screw fixation (as described by the AO group) is technically demanding and recommended only for those very familiar with the technique.

5. What structure is ruptured in dorsal dislocations of the proximal interphalangeal (PIP) joint?

The volar plate is always ruptured in dorsal dislocations (the most common dislocations of the PIP joint). To protect the volar plate injury, some authors recommend splinting the PIP in 20–30° of flexion for 2–3 weeks. Others advocate early mobilization and buddy taping.

6. What is a boxer's fracture?

A boxer's fracture is a fracture of the fifth metacarpal neck. It is one of the most common hand fractures and is usually seen in brawlers or persons who strike a wall or other unyielding object in anger.

7. How is a boxer's fracture treated?

Considerable variation exists in the literature regarding treatment of boxer's fractures. Recommendations range from minimal immobilization with no attempt at reduction to closed reduction and pin fixation; occasionally open reduction also is recommended. Because of the mobility of the carpometacarpal joint of the fifth finger, dorsal angulation of up to 40° appears to be well tolerated. Rotational malalignment, however, is not acceptable. Acute fractures are generally treated by closed manipulation and immobilization in a plaster splint for 3–4 weeks.

8. How can rotational malalignment be evaluated?

Even very small rotational discrepancies at the base of the finger can be magnified at the finger tips, causing overlap or divergence of the digits with flexion. To evaluate rotational alignment, have the patient flex the metacarpophalangeal (MCP) and PIP joints, and look at the alignment of the fingers. They should point toward the scaphoid bone. Subtle differences sometimes can be seen by looking at the semiflexed fingers end-on and comparing the planes of the fingernails with those of the unaffected.

9. What is a "fight bite"? Why is it significant?

Fight bite refers to a laceration over the knuckles caused by a clenched fist striking a tooth. These initially innocuous-appearing wounds lead to serious and rapidly progressive infections from oral flora. All wounds on the dorsum of the fist sustained during a fight should be considered human bites, whether or not the patient admits to striking the teeth. Treatment includes prompt surgical debridement, irrigation, and initiation of appropriate antibiotics.

10. What is the safe position for hand immobilization?

The safe position, also called the intrinsic-plus position and the James position, can be used for many fractures of the metacarpals and phalanges as well as soft-tissue injuries. In this position, the MCPs are in 70° of flexion, the PIPs in 15–20° of flexion, and the DIPs in 5–10° of flexion. Due to the cam shape of the metacarpal head, the MCPs tend to become stiff when immobilized in extension. The interphalangeal (IP) joints are more likely to become stiff in flexion and, therefore, are placed in relative extension. Additionally, the intrinsic plus position minimizes deforming forces of the intrinsics across fracture sites.

11. What is a complex dislocation of the MCP joint?

Dorsal dislocations of the MCP are divided into simple or complex dislocations. Both are caused by hyperextension injuries. Simple dislocations may be treated by closed reduction and splinting or buddy taping. Complex dislocations require open reduction because of the interposition of the volar plate between the metacarpal head and the proximal phalanx. Improper reduction of simple dislocations may convert them to complex dislocations.

12. How can I tell the difference between a simple and a complex dislocation?

Simple dislocations present with the proximal phalanx hyperextended (60–90°) on the dorsum of the metacarpal head. The joint surfaces are still partially in contact on a lateral radiograph. Complex dislocations present with the digit in a less dramatic position. The MCP is slightly hyperextended, and the IPs are slightly flexed. A hollow can be felt proximal to the dorsal base of the proximal phalanx, and the metacarpal head is prominent in the palm. Skin is often puckered in the palm. On radiographs the joint space is widened and the proximal phalanx is usually displaced toward the central digits. A pathognomonic finding is the presence of a sesamoid within the joint space on a radiograph. The sesamoid is in the volar plate, which is interposed between the phalanx and the metacarpal head.

13. What is a Bennett fracture?

A Bennett fracture is actually a fracture-dislocation of the base of the thumb metacarpal joint. Described by Edward Halloran Bennett in 1882, it consists of an intraarticular fracture separating a volar lip fragment from the metacarpal shaft. The shaft is displaced radially and dorsally at the base by the abductor pollicis longus. The pull of the adductor pollicis on the distal shaft increases the displacement of the base in abduction.

14. How is Bennett's fracture treated?
Multiple treatment methods have been reported to produce good results. The most common current recommendation is attempted closed reduction and percutaneous pinning of the metacarpal to the trapezium. If adequate reduction cannot be obtained, then open reduction and pin fixation are advised. A small AO cortical screw also can be used if the fragment is large enough. An external fixator may be required with excessive comminution and instability.

15. Name the other fracture at the base of the thumb.
Rolando described an intraarticular fracture at the base of the first metacarpal in 1910. Rolando's fracture can be viewed as a Bennett's fracture with a second large dorsal fragment in creating a T- or Y-shaped pattern. True Rolando's fractures are less common than more severely comminuted intraarticular fractures. Such fractures are more difficult to treat and have a less favorable outcome.

16. What is gamekeeper's thumb?
The term *gamekeeper's thumb* has come to mean almost any injury of the ulnar collateral ligament of the thumb MCP. It was coined by Campbell in 1955 to describe a chronic stretching of the ulnar collateral ligament, causing instability. Specifically it refers to an occupational deformity of the hands of British gamekeepers due to their methods of killing rabbits. Skier's thumb is a more appropriate name for an acute injury. It is commonly seen in skiers because of forced abduction of the thumb against a planted ski pole. It is also frequently seen in ball-handling athletes.

17. What is a Stener lesion?
Stener reported a series of cases in which the adductor pollicis aponeurosis was interposed between the avulsed ulnar collateral ligament of the thumb MCP joint and its site of insertion. He pointed out that healing of a ligament cannot be expected to occur under these circumstances. Repair of complete tears of the ulnar collateral ligament gives the most predictable results.

18. Which carpal bone is fractured most often?
The scaphoid (carpal navicular) is the most commonly fractured bone in the carpus. After distal radius fractures, it is the most common fracture of the wrist. Its function as a link between the proximal and distal carpal rows makes it vulnerable to injury. Approximately 80% of such fractures occur at the waist of the scaphoid.

19. Fractures at which location in the scaphoid have the lowest rate of healing? Why?
Fractures of the proximal third of the scaphoid have nonunion or avascular necrosis rates in the neighborhood of 30%. Fractures of the tuberosity or distal third have healing rates approaching 100% and waist fractures heal in 80–90% of cases. The major blood supply to the scaphoid is a branch of the radial artery that enters the dorsal ridge distally. The remaining 30% of the distal scaphoid is supplied by a second group entering the tuberosity.

20. What should be done if no fracture is seen on the radiograph but the snuff box area is tender?
It is best to assume that there is a fracture in the presence of significant tenderness. The wrist and thumb should be immobilized if a fracture is suspected. The radiographs should be repeated in 2–3 weeks. Normal resorption along the fracture site may make the fracture line evident at that time.

21. What is scapholunate dissociation? Why is it important?
Tears of the scapholunate interosseous ligament lead to separation of the scaphoid and lunate. A scapholunate interval $\geq$ 3 mm (Terry Thomas sign) is confirmatory. This lesion also presents with persistent snuff box tenderness and should be considered in all cases of suspected scaphoid fractures. It may lead to progressive carpal collapse and disability.

22. What should be done if no fracture is visible at 3 weeks but tenderness remains?

Special radiographic views, including the clenched-fist view, can help to delineate fractures from ligamentous injury. Tomography and bone scans are also useful. More recently, magnetic resonance imaging (MRI) has been shown to be a highly sensitive test for fractures of the scaphoid.

23. How is a scaphoid fracture treated?

Nondisplaced scaphoid fractures are generally treated in a thumb spica cast. Debate persists regarding the merits of immobilizing the elbow. Long arm casts appear to reduce the time to healing compared with short arm casts. A long arm cast for 6 weeks, followed by a short arm cast until radiographic evidence of healing is seen, is an acceptable method. Displaced or unstable fractures require percutaneous pin fixation or compression screw fixation.

24. What should be done if a scaphoid fracture does not heal?

The treatment of choice for nonunion of the scaphoid is bone grafting. Volar grafting, as popularized by Russe, is the most common procedure.

25. What is a chauffeur's fracture?

A fracture of the radial styloid is known as a chauffeur's fracture or back-fire fracture. It was commonly seen in the early 1900s when a car back-fired on starting, causing the crank to strike the distal radius or to wrench the hand back violently. A chauffeur's fracture is generally treated by closed reduction and percutaneous pin fixation.

26. What is a Colles' fracture?

A Colles' fracture is a metaphyseal fracture of the distal radius that is dorsally angulated. It may extend into either the radiocarpal and/or the radioulnar surface.

27. What is a Smith's fracture?

A Smith's fracture is a volar angulated fracture of the distal radius. It is also called a reverse Colles' fracture. A type I Smith's fracture is extraarticular. A type II fracture enters the dorsal rim of the articular surface. A type III fracture enters the middle of the radiocarpal surface.

28. What is a Barton's fracture?

A Barton's fracture is actually a fracture-dislocation of the distal radius. It may be displaced either volarly or dorsally. A type III Smith's fracture is equivalent to a volar Barton's fracture.

29. What is the Frykman classification of distal radius fractures?

The Frykman classification distinguishes between extraarticular and intraarticular fractures involving either the radiocarpal joint or the distal radioulnar joint. It is further modified by the presence of a distal ulnar fracture. (See figure next page.)

30. What is the universal classification of distal radius fractures?

The universal classification system can be used for all distal radius fractures. It is more useful in making treatment decisions than the Frykman classification.

Type I	Extra-articular, nondisplaced
Type II	Extra-articular, displaced
Type III	Intra-articular, undisplaced
Type IVa	Intra-articular, reducible, stable
Type IVb	Intra-articular, reducible, unstable
Type IVc	Intra-articular, irreducible, unstable

31. How is a Colles' fracture treated?

Types I, II and III Colles' fractures are treated by closed reduction and application of a sugar-tong plaster splint, which is later converted to a standard plaster or fiberglass cast. The reduction maneuver usually requires a combination of pronation rotation with a volar and ulnar-directed force. If a satisfactory reduction cannot be achieved or maintained, then surgical methods should be employed.

Primary external fixation (possibly including percutaneous pin fixation) should be considered for type IVa and type IVb fractures.

Other treatment methods include percutaneous pin fixations (radius only, Kapandji intrafocal pinning or transulnar) and open reduction with internal fixation. Combinations of any of the above methods are common.

32. What is an acceptable reduction?

The goal is to restore the distal radius length, radial slope, and palmar tilt. Length should be compared with the contralateral side. Radial slope averages 22° and palmar tilt averages 11°. Poor results are anticipated if length is not restored to at least the level of the ulna, if there is articular step-off of > 2 mm, or if there is dorsal tilt of > 20°.

33. How long should a Colles' fracture be immobilized if cast treatment is used?

The usual course of treatment consists of 1–2 weeks in a sugar-tong splint followed by another 3–5 weeks in a cast. It is imperative that radiographs of the fracture be obtained at 1–2 weeks, or fracture reduction may be lost in plaster. At 1–2 weeks a repeat reduction or conversion to another treatment method is still possible.

34. How should a Smith's fracture be treated?

Types I and II fractures follow the guidelines outlined in questions 30 and 31. Type III Smith's fractures usually require primary open reduction and volar buttress plate fixation.

35. What is Kapandji intrafocal fixation?

Intrafocal fixation involves percutaneous K-wire fixation in which at least one of the wires is inserted into the fracture, and is used to manipulate the displaced fragment as well as prevent later loss of reduction. Studies demonstrate that it is best used alone only in younger individuals with mild comminution.

36. What structure can be injured in fractures or dislocations of the distal radioulnar joint?

The triangular fibrocartilage complex may be damaged in injuries to the distal ulna. The complex consists of a triangular fibrocartilaginous structure and the ulnocarpal ligament. Its base is along the sigmoid notch of the radius, and its apex is attached to the ulnar styloid process.

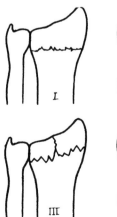
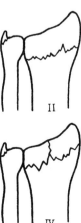
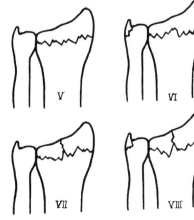

Frykman classification.

37. What value does arthroscopy have in the treatment of distal radius fractures?
Wrist arthroscopy enables surgeons to directly visualize and improve the articular reduction. Arthroscopy also facilitates the diagnosis and treatment of associated ligament and cartilage injuries, including those to the triangular fibrocartilage complex (TFCC).

BIBLIOGRAPHY

1. Ark J, Jupiter JB: The rationale for precise management of distal radius fractures. Orthop Clin North Am 24:205, 1993.
2. Ashkenaze DM, Ruby LK: Metacarpal fractures and dislocations. Orthop Clin North Am 23:19, 1992.
3. Barton N: Conservative treatment of articular fractures in the hand. J Hand Surg 14A:386, 1989.
4. Carter PR, Frederick HA, Laseter GF: Open reduction and internal fixation of unstable distal radius fractures with a low-profile plate: A multicenter study of 73 fractures. J Hand Surg 23A:300–307, 1998.
5. Cooney WP III, Dobyns JH, Linscheid RL: Non-union of the scaphoid: Analysis of the results from bone grafting. J Hand Surg 5:343, 1980.
6. Ford DJ, Ali MS, Steel WM: Fractures of the fifth metacarpal neck: Is reduction or immobilization necessary? J Hand Surg 14B:165, 1989.
7. Green DP (ed): Operative Hand Surgery, 4th ed. New York, Churchill Livingstone, 1999.
8. Hastings H II, Lebovic SJ: Indications and techniques of open reduction and internal fixation of distal radius fractures. Orthop Clin North Am 24:309, 1993.
9. Hubbard LF: Metacarpal phalangeal dislocations. Hand Clin 4:39, 1988.
10. Kaur JM: The distal radioulnar joint: Anatomic and functional considerations. Clin Orthop 275:37, 1992.
11. Knirk JL, Jupiter JB: Intra-articular fractures of the distal end of the radius in young adults. J Bone Joint Surg 68A:657, 1986.
12. Livesley PJ: Conservative management of Bennett's fracture-dislocation: A 26 year follow-up. J Hand Surg 15B:291, 1990.
13. Lubahn JD: Mallet finger fractures: A comparison of open and closed technique. J Hand Surg 14A:394, 1990.
14. Rikli DA, Kupfer K, Bodoky A: Long-term results of the external fixation of distal radius fractures. J Trauma 44:970–976, 1998.
15. Bucholz RW, Heckman JD (eds): Rockwood and Green's Fractures in Adults, vols. 1 and 2, 5th ed. Philadelphia, J.B. Lippincott, 2001.
16. Royle SG: Rotational deformity following metacarpal fracture. J Hand Surg 15B:124, 1990.
17. Russe O: Fractures of the carpal navicular: Diagnosis, non-operative and operative treatment. J Bone Joint Surg 42A:759, 1960.
18. Trumble TE, Wagner W, Hanel DP, et al: Intrafocal (Kapandji) pinning of distal radius fractures with and without external fixation. J Hand Surg 23A:381–394, 1998.
19. Vaccaro AR, Kupcha PC, Salvo JP: Accurate reduction and splint of the common boxer's fracture. Orthop Rev 19:994, 1990.
20. Koval KJ (ed): Orthopedic Knowledge Update Seven. Rosemont, IL, American Academy of Orthopedic Surgeons, 2002.

39. CARPAL INSTABILITY

Jeffrey A. Rodgers, M.D.

1. Name the bones of the proximal and distal carpal rows.
The proximal row consists of the scaphoid, lunate, and triquetrum, whereas the distal row consists of the trapezium, trapezoid, capitate, and hamate. The pisiform is not considered a part of either row. It is of clinical importance to note that the scaphoid spans the midcarpal joint.

2. How many sets of joints compose the wrist joint?
The wrist joint is composed of four distinct joints: the distal radioulnar joint, radiocarpal joint, midcarpal joint, and carpometacarpal joint.

3. Are there any muscles that directly motor the carpal bones?

No muscles or tendons originate or insert on the carpal bones. The proximal and distal carpal rows are intercalated segments with no muscle or tendon attachments. The scaphoid functions as a "slider-crank" control that links motion at the radiocarpal and intercarpal joints.

4. How is relative carpal motion affected in the proximal and distal carpal rows?

With radial deviation, flexion occurs in the proximal carpal row through a mechanism that is not completely understood. However, it is thought that the flexion of the scaphoid is transmitted to the lunate by the scapholunate interosseous ligament. With ulnar deviation, the proximal row extends under the influence of the hamate-triquetral interaction.

5. Compare a normal versus functional range of motion of the wrist.

Normal range of motion of the wrist consists of 70° extension, 80° of flexion, 20° radial deviation and 30° ulnar deviation. Functionally, however, only 10° of flexion and 30° of extension are required for adequate hand function, grip strength and activities of daily living.

6. What is the most common form of carpal instability?

The most common form of carpal instability is dorsiflexion-intercalary segment instability (DISI), which usually is associated with an injury to the scapholunate ligament that results in loss of the normally coordinated motion of the proximal carpal row. The diagnosis of DISI deformity is based on a lateral radiograph. The lunate translates volarly and extends while the scaphoid flexes. The normal scapholunate angle is 30–60°. With DISI, however, this angle exceeds 70°. The capitolunate angle is usually less than 20°.

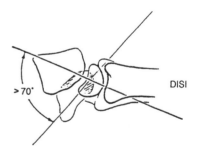

In dorsiflexion–intercalated segment instability (DISI), the lunate extends and the scaphoid flexes, resulting in a scapholunate angle > 70°. (From Cooney WP, Linscheid RL, Dobyns JH: Carpal instability: Treatment of ligament injuries of the wrist. AAOS Instructional Course Lectures 41:33–44, 1992, with permission.)

7. Who was Terry Thomas and what does he have to do with wrist instability?

Terry Thomas was a famous comedian with an all-star spitting gap between his incisors. The Terry Thomas sign is an eponym describing a scapholunate disassociation on the anteroposterior (AP) radiograph of the wrist. By definition, a diastasis > 3 mm is pathognomonic for scapholunate disassociation. Another sign of the DISI deformity on the AP radiograph is the double cortical ring of the scaphoid produced by the overlay of the distal pole on the palmar-flexed scaphoid when viewed end-on.

8. Describe Mayfield's classification of perilunate instability.

Mayfield described a sequential pattern of injury after a fall on the outstretched hand, using a cadaver model in which the wrists were loaded in extension, ulnar deviation, and intercarpal supination. He described progressive perilunate instability in four stages: stage 1, scapholunate diastasis; stage 2, dorsal dislocation of the capitate; stage 3, disruption of the lunotriquetral interosseous ligament; and stage 4, complete dislocation of the lunate. Such injuries represent "lesser arc" injuries. "Greater arc" injuries involve fracture of one or more of the carpal bones; i.e., transscaphoid perilunate dislocation.

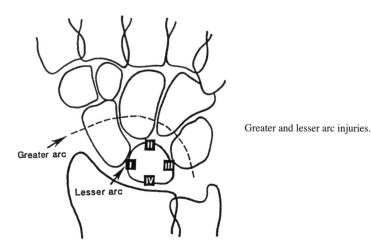

Greater and lesser arc injuries.

9. Describe additional x-ray views of the painful wrist when standard radiographs are normal.

In the setting of an acute wrist injury with normal AP and lateral radiographs, stress radiographs should be obtained, including PA views in ulnar and radial deviation and a clenched fist-supination view to demonstrate dynamic instability of the scaphoid.

10. What is the scaphoid shift test?

The scaphoid shift test as described by Dr. Kirk Watson is a provocative maneuver in which the examiner may reproduce the patient's sensation of instability or even cause subluxation of the proximal pole of the scaphoid by stabilizing the scaphoid palmarly while bringing the wrist from ulnar to radial deviation. A palpable click and pain with this maneuver indicate dynamic rotatory subluxation of the scaphoid.

The exam should be considered abnormal only if different from the uninjured wrist.

11. What other special studies or procedures can be used to evaluate the painful wrist?

A three-phase bone scan is helpful to rule out occult carpal bone fracture or other cause of wrist pain like early avascular necrosis of the lunate. Arthrography, including injection of the radiocarpal, midcarpal joint, and distal radioulnar joints may reveal interosseous ligament tears or injury to the triangular fibrocartilage. The test has a high false-positive rate, and many hand surgeons recommend diagnostic wrist arthroscopy instead. Magnetic resonance imaging does not reliably image the interosseus ligaments and is more valuable in assessment for avascular necrosis or tumor.

12. What pattern of instability is found with injury of the lunotriquetral ligament?

Although much less common than DISI, volar intercalated segment instability (VISI) occurs with injury to the lunotriquetral (LT) ligament in combination with injury to the extrinsic

In volar flexion–intercalated segment instability (VISI), the lunate is flexed and the scaphoid remains in neutral to slight flexion, resulting in a scapholunate angle of 30° or less. (From Cooney WP, Linscheid RL, Dobyns JH: Carpal Instability: Treatment of ligament injuries of the wrist. AAOS Instructional Course Lectures 41:33–44, 1992, with permission.)

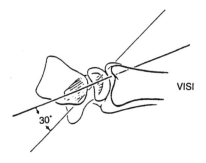

scaphotriquetral and radiotriquetral ligaments. Radiographs show a scapholunate angle $< 30°$, and volar flexion of the lunate results in a capitolunate angle $> 20°$. Diastasis is uncommon between the lunate and the triquetrum. LT ligament injury alone usually does not result in static radiographic instability. Unlike scapholunate ligament injury, this pattern of instability usually occurs following a fall on the outstretched hand in pronation, extension and radial deviation.

13. What is midcarpal instability?
    Midcarpal instability consists of either congenital laxity or ligament attenuation between the scaphoid and capitate and/or the triquetrum and capitate. VISI deformity usually results, with a painful "clunk" during activities that involve ulnar deviation and pronation of the wrist.

14. How is the diagnosis of midcarpal instability confirmed?
    Standard radiographs show a VISI deformity. During cineradiography, as the wrist is taken into ulnar deviation, the proximal carpal row snaps suddenly from a palmarflexed to a dorsiflexed position, reproducing the patient's symptoms.

15. What is the natural history of untreated, chronic scapholunate disassociation?
    Chronic scapholunate disassociation results in osteoarthritis in a predictable pattern termed *scapholunate advanced collapse* (SLAC). Degeneration begins between the radial styloid and the scaphoid and later in the unstable capitolunate joint as the capitate subluxes dorsally in the lunate. The radiolunate articulation is usually preserved until late in the process.

16. What treatment options are available for scapholunate disassociation?
    Injuries are classified as acute (< 4 weeks from time of injury), subacute (> 4 weeks from time of injury), and chronic (> 12 months from time of injury). Treatment options include arthroscopic reduction and percutaneous pinning in the acute phase, open repair techniques in the subacute phase, and open repair or limited intercarpal fusion for chronic instability.

BIBLIOGRAPHY

 1. Cooney WP, Linscheid RL, Dobyns JH: Carpal instability: Treatment of ligament injuries of the wrist. AAOS Instructional Course Lectures 41:33–44, 1992.
 2. Cooney WP, Linscheid RL, Dobyns JH: Fractures and dislocations of the wrist. In Rockwood CA, Greene DP, Bucholz RW (eds): Rockwood and Greene's Fractures in Adults. New York, J.B. Lippincott, 1991, pp 563–678.
 3. Gelberman RH, Cooney WP, Szabo RM: Carpal instability. J Bone Joint Surg 82-A:578–594, 2000.
 4. Kleinman WB: Long term study of chronic scapho-lunate instability treated by scapho-trapezio-trapezoid arthrodesis. J Hand Surg 14A:429–445, 1989.
 5. Lichtman DM, Schneider JR, Swafford AR, et al: Ulnar midcarpal instability: Clinical and laboratory analysis. J Hand Surg 8:515–523, 1981.
 6. Linscheid RL, Dobyns JH, Babout JW, Bryan RS: Traumatic instability of the wrist: Diagnosis classification in pathomechanics. J Bone Joint Surg 54A:1612–1632, 1972.
 7. Reagan DS, Linscheid RL, Dobyns JH: Lunotriquetral sprains. J Hand Surg 9(A):502–514, 1984.
 8. Ritt MJ, Linscheid RL, Cooney WP, Bergen RA, Kai-Nau A: The lunotriquetral joint: Kinematic effects of sequential ligament sectioning, ligament repair and arthrodesis. J Hand Surg 23(A):432–445, 1998.
 9. Shin AY, Battaglia MJ, Bishop AT: Lunotriquetral instability: Diagnosis and treatment. J Am Acad Orthop Surg 8:170–179, 2000.
10. Walsh JJ, Berger RA, Cooney WP: Current status of scapholunate interosseous ligament injuries. J Am Acad Orthop Surg 10:32–42, 2002.
11. Watson HK, Ballet FL: The SLAC wrist: Scapholunate advanced collapsed pattern of degenerative arthritis. J Hand Surg 9A:358–365, 1984.

40. TENDON INJURIES OF THE HAND AND WRIST

John A. Miyano, M.D.

FLEXOR TENDONS

1. How do you test the function of the flexor digitorum profundus (FDP) tendon?

Active flexion of the distal interphalangeal (DIP) joint with the proximal interphalangeal (PIP) joint held in passive extension indicates an intact FDP tendon.

2. Does active flexion at the PIP joint rule out a flexor digitorum superficialis (FDS) laceration?

No. The PIP joint can be flexed using the pull of the FDP tendon. To isolate the FDS, the PIP joint must be actively flexed with the other fingers held in full extension to limit FDP activity.

3. Define the zones of injury of the flexor tendons in the hand and wrist.

Zone I: Insertion of the FDP at the distal phalanx to the middle of the middle phalanx

Zone II: Middle of the middle phalanx to the distal palmar crease

Zone III: Distal palmar crease to the distal edge of the carpal tunnel

Zone IV: Carpal tunnel

Zone V: Proximal edge of the carpal tunnel to the musculotendinous junction

4. Which zone is referred to as "no man's land"? Why?

Historically, it has been most difficult to obtain successful repairs of flexor tendon lacerations in zone II, in which the FDP and FDS tendons run together in a tight, fibroosseous tunnel. Adhesions to the tunnel and between the tendons may develop, compromising tendon gliding.

5. When repairing a flexor tendon in the finger, which pulley(s) of the tendon sheath is/are the most critical to preserve?

The pulleys keep the tendons from bowstringing during active flexion. A2 and A4 are over the shafts of the proximal and middle phalanges, respectively, and must be preserved for normal function.

6. What is the main factor that determines the strength of repair of a flexor tendon at the time of surgery?

The number of strands of suture crossing the repair site is roughly proportional to the strength of repair. Four strands of suture in the core of the tendon are generally needed to be able to withstand the stress of an early active motion therapy program.

7. What is a jersey finger?

A jersey finger is an avulsion of the FDP tendon from its insertion on the distal phalanx. It is commonly a sports injury that occurs when a player tries to make a tackle by grabbing another player's jersey. The resisted, forceful flexion causes the tendon to avulse. Treatment is early surgical repair.

8. What percentage of people do not have a palmaris longus tendon of the wrist?

Roughly 10–15% of people are missing the palmaris longus bilaterally. Approximately the same percentage are missing the tendon unilaterally.

9. What is a Mannerfelt lesion?
A Mannerfelt lesion is an attritional rupture of the FPL over an osteophyte arising from the scaphoid within the carpal tunnel. It is most commonly seen in rheumatoid arthritis.

EXTENSOR TENDONS

10. Describe mallet finger.
A mallet finger is a flexion deformity of the DIP joint caused by rupture or avulsion of the terminal extensor tendon from the distal phalanx.

11. What is the treatment for mallet finger?
Full-time immobilization of the DIP joint only in extension for a minimum of 6 weeks is required, which may be accomplished with a molded plastic splint (Stack splint), aluminum and foam splint, or surgical pinning across the DIP joint.

12. What is the most common extensor tendon problem associated with fractures of the distal radius?
Rupture of the extensor pollicis longus tendon can be seen following fractures of the distal radius. It is probably secondary to compression and attrition of the tendon within the third dorsal compartment. It is more common with minimally displaced fractures in which the third dorsal compartment is still intact.

13. What is the difference between a swan-neck deformity and a boutonnière deformity?
A swan-neck deformity is hyperextension of the PIP joint combined with flexion of the DIP joint (creating the appearance of the head and neck of a swan). A boutonnière deformity is flexion of the PIP joint combined with extension of the DIP joint.

14. What are the deforming forces in a boutonnière deformity?
The initial problem is disruption of the extensor tendon insertion into the middle phalanx, known as the central slip. Over time, the lateral bands migrate volar to the axis of rotation of the PIP joint, thereby becoming PIP flexors instead of extensors.

BIBLIOGRAPHY

1. Doyle JR: Extensor tendons: Acute injuries. In Green DP (ed): Operative Hand Surgery, 4th ed. New York, Churchill Livingstone, 1999, pp 1950–1987.
2. Geyman JP, Fink K, Sullivan SD: Conservative versus surgical treatment of mallet finger: A pooled quantitative literature evaluation. J Am Board Fam Pract 11:382–390, 1998.
3. Strickland JW: Flexor tendons: Acute injuries. In Green DP (ed): Operative Hand Surgery, 4th ed. New York, Churchill Livingstone, 1999, pp 1851–1897.
4. Leddy JP, Packer JW: Avulsion of the profundus tendon insertion in athletes. J Hand Surg 2A:66–69, 1977.
5. Mannerfelt L, Norman O: Attrition ruptures of flexor tendons in rheumatoid arthritis caused by bony spurs in the carpal tunnel. J Bone Joint Surg 51B:270–277, 1969.
6. Siegel D, Gebhardt M, Jupiter JB: Spontaneous rupture of the extensor pollicis longus tendon. J Hand Surg 12A:1106–1109, 1987.
7. Strickland JW: Flexor tendon injuries: Part I and part II. J Am Acad Orthop Surg 3:44–62, 1995.

41. SOFT-TISSUE INJURIES AND DISORDERS OF THE HAND

John A. Miyano, M.D.

FINGERTIP INJURIES

1. Discuss the treatment for a subungual hematoma.

Painful hematomas may be decompressed by perforating the nail with a heated paper clip, a battery-powered cautery, or a large needle (16-gauge) used like a drill. Some advocate nail plate removal and nail bed repair if the hematoma is larger than 25–50% of the nail surface.

2. What is the treatment for nail bed lacerations?

Nail bed lacerations should be repaired primarily with a fine (6–0) absorbable suture, such as plain gut. Part or all of the nail plate may have to be removed to allow adequate visualization and access. After the repair is completed, the nail plate should be reinserted beneath the eponychial fold to prevent scarring of the eponychium to the nail bed.

3. After avulsion of a fingernail, how long does it take for the new nail to regrow completely?

Approximately 3 months

4. In fingertip crush injuries, what additional injury must you look for in pediatric patients?

Growth plate fractures can occur in the distal phalanx of children. Especially when the proximal end of the nail plate has been avulsed, the distal portion of the phalanx may be fractured through the physis and displaced in flexion. When the fracture is reduced, the partially avulsed nailbed may become entrapped in the fracture site.

5. What size fingertip avulsions or amputations will heal without skin grafting or flaps?

Defects up to 1 square cm will heal with dressing changes over a period of 3–6 weeks. Larger defects may require local skin flaps (e.g., V-Y advancement flaps, cross-finger flaps).

6. Describe the treatment for a distal phalangeal tuft fracture.

Commonly the result of fingertip crush injuries, most tuft fractures can be treated symptomatically with a brief period (2–3 weeks) of protection. Aluminum and foam splints may be used to make a "bumper" over the tip of the finger.

7. Describe the difference between a paronychia and a felon.

A paronychia is an infection of the eponychial fold (around the edge of the nail plate). A felon is an infection of the fingertip pulp.

8. Describe the treatment of a paronychia or felon.

Both require incision and drainage. A paronychia can be drained by incising and sometimes elevating the eponychial fold. A felon can be drained through an incision on the side of the fingertip that extends into the pulp, thereby opening the septal compartments.

9. What is the initial treatment for frostbite?

Initial treatment is rapid rewarming in a water bath at approximately 40°C. Blisters should be left intact.

BURNS

10. Define the different degrees of burns.

A first-degree burn is superficial and characterized by pain and erythema; a second-degree burn is a partial-thickness burn characterized by pain and blistering; and a third-degree burn is a full-thickness burn characterized by painless, blanched skin secondary to nerve death and thrombosis.

11. Describe is the treatment for most small and medium-sized second-degree burns.

Most can be treated with local wound care, including topical antibiotics (e.g., silver sulphadiazine) and dressing changes. Tetanus status should be checked for all patients.

12. What is the best way to limit edema in burned extremities?

Elevation and early mobilization are important in the reduction of postburn swelling. Compression dressings are generally contraindicated, especially if the circulation is already compromised.

13. What is the clinical significance of a circumferential burn?

Circumferential burns often cause vascular compromise due to tissue edema and loss of skin elasticity (eschar). Even noncircumferential burns are at risk. Escharatomies and fasciotomies are performed if any compromise is detected.

14. What are the two most common mechanisms of injury in an electrical burn? Which is usually more serious?

Injury is usually caused by either surface burns from the initial flash and fire or deep burns from electrical current conducting through the tissues. Conduction burns occur when an individual is grounded (e.g., standing in a pool of water) and usually cause more severe damage to both superficial and deep tissues.

15. In evaluating patients with conduction electrical burns, what must be examined besides the point of contact?

An exit point also must be sought. Unless the area of exit is broad enough to dissipate the energy, a second burn results.

16. Why must urine output be measured in patients with conduction electrical burns?

Conduction burns are associated with significant muscle necrosis and secondary myoglobin release (rhabdomyolysis). If untreated, this may result in acute renal failure. Hydration to maintain a urine output of at least 75 ml/hr is recommended until the breakdown products have cleared.

17. What is the initial treatment for most chemical burns?

Unless a specific neutralizing agent is known, most chemical burns should be irrigated copiously with water.

18. What acid burn classically continues to damage tissue long after exposure?

Hydrofluoric acid, used in industry for such tasks as etching glass, continues to burn unless the tissues are infiltrated with calcium gluconate or calcium chloride.

DUPUYTREN'S CONTRACTURE

19. What is Dupuytren's contracture?

Dupuytren's contracture is a proliferative fibroplasia of the subcutaneous tissues of the palm and fingers, often leading to progressive flexion contractures.

20. What ethnic group is most commonly affected?

Most people presenting with Dupuytren's disease are of Northern European ancestry, suggesting a strong genetic component to its development.

21. Which fingers are most commonly involved?

The ring and small fingers are most commonly involved. Occasionally, the long finger, thumb, and index finger also may be involved.

22. Who develops Dupuytren's disease more frequently, men or women?

Men develop the disease more frequently than women, at a ratio of 7:1.

23. Which tissues are primarily affected?

Dupuytren's disease is primarily a fibroplasia of palm and finger fascia (e.g., the pretendinous band, natatory ligament, spiral band, lateral digital sheet, Grayson's ligament). Secondary thinning of the subcutaneous fat, as well as thickening and dimpling of the overlying skin, may occur.

24. What other connective tissue disorders are associated with Dupuytren's?
- Plantar fibromatosis (Lederhose's disease)
- Knuckle pads (Garrod's nodes)
- Peyronie's disease

25. Involvement of which portion of the palmar fascia causes contracture of the metacarpophalangeal (MCP) joint?

The pretendinous band.

26. Name the three main cords that develop and cause contracture of the PIP joint.

The central, lateral, and spiral cords. The retrovascular cord is less often the primary lesion, but may be involved in recurrence or incomplete correction.

27. What is the indication for surgical intervention for involvement of the MCP joint?

Consideration for surgery is usually given for contracture > 30°. The MCP joint is tolerant of contracture, and even long-standing deformity > 30° can be reliably corrected. As a general rule, if the patient can place his or her palm flat on a table, operative intervention is not required.

28. What is the main surgical risk of contracture release around the PIP joint? Why?

The neurovascular bundles are at increased risk around the PIP joint. The diseased fascia will often form a "spiral" cord that wraps around the artery and nerve, pulling them more palmar and towards the midline.

29. What is the recurrence rate after surgical intervention?

The recurrence rate may be > 50%, depending on the technique used. However, recurrence may not be rapid or require reoperation. Generally, correction of contracture at the MCP joint is more reliable.

BIBLIOGRAPHY

1. Benson LS, Williams CS, Kahle M: Dupuytren's contracture. J Am Acad Orthop Surg 6:24–35, 1998.
2. Green DP: Operative Hand Surgery, 4th ed. New York, Churchill Livingstone, 1999.
3. Lister G: The Hand: Diagnosis and Indications, 3rd ed. New York, Churchill Livingstone, 1993.

42. ARTHRITIS AND ARTHROPLASTY OF THE HAND AND WRIST

Jeffrey J. Tiedeman, M.D.

1. Which joints are most commonly involved in a patient with osteoarthritis of the hand and wrist?

The joints most prone to osteoarthritis in the hand and wrist include the distal interphalangeal (DIP) joints and the carpometacarpal (CMC) joint of the thumb. The signs and symptoms are usually localized to the involved joints. Pain is common after joint use and is relieved by rest. In contrast to patients with rheumatoid arthritis, patients with osteoarthritis usually have little problem on rising in the morning, but pain increases as the day progresses. Night pain is also common and may interfere with sleep. On physical examination pain with passive motion and crepitus in the joint are prominent findings. Joint enlargement from synovitis and ligamentous laxity are also common features.

2. What are Heberden's nodes?

Heberden's nodes are bone spurs that form on the dorsal aspect of the DIP joints of the fingers. Although typically small, such exostoses around the DIP are readily apparent and give the joint a knobby appearance. Similarly, Bouchard's nodes are osteophytes that develop at the proximal interphalangeal (PIP) joint, which is a much less frequent site of osteoarthritis.

3. Which patients are at risk of developing degenerative arthritis after a fracture of the distal radius?

Patients with intraarticular extension of the fracture either into the radiocarpal joint or the distal radioulnar joint are at greatest risk for developing degenerative arthritis. Specifically, fractures that extend into the radiocarpal joint and subsequently heal with > 2 mm of intraarticular incongruity have been shown to be at increased risk for developing degenerative arthritis. Consequently, the goal of treatment for this particular type of fracture is restoration of normal anatomy with reduction of the intraarticular component, particularly in young active individuals.

4. What is a SLAC wrist?

SLAC wrist refers to scapholunate advanced collapse, which is the most common form of arthritis in the wrist. The degenerative change typically goes through a specific sequence and is caused by articular alignment problems among the scaphoid, the lunate, and the radius. The degenerative arthritis initially involves the radioscaphoid joint. The radiolunate joint is generally spared as the process progresses to the capitolunate joint.

5. Describe the treatment options for CMC arthritis of the thumb.

The CMC joint is the second most frequently involved joint in osteoarthritis of the hand after the DIP joint. The disease process, also known as basal joint arthritis, has a predilection for postmenopausal women and is 10 times more common in women, usually after the fifth decade of life. Conservative treatment includes oral antiinflammatory medication, splints, thenar strengthening exercises, and modification of activity. Pain unresponsive to conservative measures and subsequent loss of function or joint instability are the primary indications for operative intervention. Surgical options include CMC joint arthrodesis or trapezial excision, with either silicone implant arthroplasty or tendinous interpositional graft. An arthrodesis or fusion is a suitable option in a patient with arthritis confined to the CMC joint, particularly in a young person with a demanding occupation. With pantrapezial arthritis good results have been obtained by excising the trapezium and filling the space either with silicone arthroplasty or a tendon graft.

RHEUMATOID ARTHRITIS

6. Who was Küntscher? What innovation did he bring to hand surgery?
Gerhard Küntscher was a German investigator and educator who stood out as a pioneer in orthopedic surgery. His innovations revolutionized fracture management and also have proved to be beneficial for a variety of other applications. He is credited with the development of Küntscher wires or K-wires, as they are more commonly known. K-wires are frequently used in hand surgery for fracture fixation or to stabilize arthritic joints during an arthrodesis procedure.

7. What is caput ulnae syndrome?
Caput ulnae syndrome refers to the destructive process initiated by synovitis of the distal radioulnar joint. Characteristic findings include loss of wrist rotation (pronation/supination) and dorsiflexion, weakness, dorsal prominence and instability of the distal ulna, soft-tissue swelling over the distal ulna secondary to synovitis, loss of normal action of the extensor carpi ulnaris tendon, and occasionally loss of extension of the small, ring, and long fingers as a result of extensor tendon ruptures.

8. Name the indications and contraindications for total wrist arthroplasty.
The **major indication** for total wrist arthroplasty is rheumatoid arthritis with wrist pain secondary to advanced destructive changes in the radiocarpal joint. The operation is best suited for patients who also have involvement of several other joints in the upper extremities with resultant limitation of forearm rotation, elbow flexion, shoulder motion, and motion of the digits. Total wrist arthroplasty is desirable in such patients because the only surgical alternative is wrist arthrodesis, which unfortunately eliminates remaining wrist motion and typically diminishes rather than improves overall upper extremity function. Wrist arthrodesis, however, is the preferred procedure for the vast majority of patients with advanced radiocarpal arthritis not due to rheumatoid arthritis, because it generally provides predictable pain relief with a relatively low complication rate.

The **only true contraindication** for total wrist arthroplasty is active infection. In rare cases of juvenile rheumatoid arthritis the diameter of the medullary canal of the distal radius is too narrow to accommodate the stem of the prosthesis, thereby precluding total wrist arthroplasty.

9. What are the most common complications of total wrist arthroplasty?
The most common complication of total wrist arthroplasty is loosening of the distal component, which has been found in approximately 20% of wrists over a 5-year period postoperatively. A second potential complication is dislocation of the prosthesis. Both complications may cause further problems, such as carpal tunnel syndrome. Failure of total wrist arthroplasty occasionally requires conversion to a wrist fusion.

10. Which flexor tendon most commonly ruptures in rheumatoid arthritis?
The flexor pollicis longus is the tendon that most commonly ruptures in rheumatoid arthritis (Mannerfelt syndrome). The rupture is usually due to attrition as the tendon passes over a bony spur or erosion in the carpal scaphoid. Treatment usually consists of surgical reconstruction with a tendon graft or a tendon transfer using a superficial digital flexor tendon.

11. What is a boutonnière deformity? Why does it occur?
A boutonnière deformity is a progressive condition that occurs frequently in patients with rheumatoid arthritis. The deformity has three components: (1) flexion of the PIPjoint, (2) hyperextension of the DIP joint, and (3) hyperextension of the metaphalangeal (MP)joint. The primary inciting event is synovial proliferation within the PIPjoint, which stretches the extensor mecha-

nism. As a result, the patient is unable to maintain full extension of the PIP joint. The lateral tendinous bands subsequently displace volarward and become fixed in this position. Shortening of the oblique retinacular ligaments then results in hyperextension and limited active flexion of the DIP joint. Patients compensate for the flexion deformity of the PIP joint by hyperextending the MP joint. The deformity tends to progress from a supple and passively correctable condition to a fixed condition that may be functionally disabling.

12. What is swan-neck deformity?

Like the boutonnière deformity, swan-neck deformity is common in but not unique to rheumatoid arthritis. Swan-neck deformity is characterized by hyperextension of the PIP joint, flexion of the DIP joint, and weakening of the periarticular structures of the PIP joint due to synovitis. Tightness of the intrinsic musculature then creates an abnormal force across the joint, resulting in swan-neck deformity.

13. What is a Brewerton view?

A Brewerton view is a variant of an anteroposterior radiograph of the hand. It should be obtained in all patients evaluated for rheumatoid arthritis. The fingers are placed flat on the radiographic plate, and the metacarpals are inclined at a 65°. The radiographic tube is then inclined 15° toward the ulnar side of the hand. The Brewerton view may show bony erosive changes beneath the collateral ligaments of the MCP joints early in the course of rheumatoid arthritis, when standard anteroposterior radiographs of the hand show little change.

14. In advanced rheumatoid arthritis, what MCP joint deformity is typically seen? What are the underlying causes?

The classic deformity seen in rheumatoid arthritis is ulnar drift of the digits and volar dislocation of the proximal phalanges. Various factors are responsible for the pathophysiology, including MCP joint synovitis, articular cartilage erosion and bony destruction, extensor tendon subluxation or dislocation (secondary to selective stretching of the support structures on the radial side), ligamentous and volar plate disruption, intrinsic tightness, and finally the forces of gravity and pinch. The ulnar drift of the fingers is often accompanied by radial deviation of the wrist, creating the characteristic Z-plasty deformity of the hand and wrist often seen in patients with rheumatoid arthritis.

15. What potential complications are associated with silicone MCP joint arthroplasty?

The most common complications are infection, prosthetic breakage, prosthetic dislocation, recurrent deformity, limited motion, and pain. Silicone synovitis, a common problem after carpal bone silicone replacement, is relatively infrequent in MCP joint arthroplasty. Despite these complications, MCP arthroplasty has proved to be an effective, predictable, and long-lasting procedure with high patient satisfaction.

UNUSUAL ARTHRITIS DISORDERS

16. What characteristic manifestations are found in the hands of patients with systemic lupus erythematosus (SLE)?

SLE is a connective tissue disorder that occurs primarily in young adult women. A common clinical feature of SLE is polyarthritis, usually in the small bones of the hands and feet. Ligamentous laxity with subsequent instability of the distal radioulnar joint, intercarpal joints, MCP joints, and all three thumb joints is a distinctive feature of the disease. Raynaud's phenomena may also exist in up to 50% of patients.

17. What is Jaccoud's syndrome?

Jaccoud's syndrome, a classic condition associated with SLE, involves flexion deformities and ulnar deviation of the MCP joints and swan-neck deformities of the digits. As is typical of

SLE, the major problem is soft-tissue attenuation with resultant ligamentous laxity. In this particular syndrome the involved tissue includes the radial portion of the dorsal capsular hood of the MCP joint with ulnar subluxation of the extensor digitorum communis tendons and hyperextension of the PIP joints. The resultant deformity may appear quite similar to that seen in rheumatoid arthritis; radiographs, however, usually reveal preservation of the joint space, which is consistent with the nonerosive synovitis of SLE.

18. What are the typical manifestations of psoriatic arthritis?
Approximately 5% of patients with psoriasis develop arthritis that involves mainly the small bones of the hand and feet. Patients classically present with diffuse swelling throughout an entire digit, which is termed a "sausage digit." Joint involvement is most frequent at the DIP and PIP levels. Erosive articular destruction is common and results in pencil and cup deformities of the joints, which may be seen radiographically. Progressive distal phalangeal osteolysis with tuft resorption is also highly suggestive of psoriatic arthropathy. Spontaneous fusion of the DIP joint and intercarpal joints is also common. The severity of joint destruction often parallels the degree of accompanying fingernail deformities, which include pitting, ridging, thickening, and detachment of the nail.

BIBLIOGRAPHY

1. Azar FM: Arthrodesis of shoulder, elbow, and wrist. In Canale ST (ed): Campbell's Operative Orthopaedics, 9th ed. St. Louis, Mosby, 1998, pp 203–206.
2. Beer TA, Turner RH: Wrist arthrodesis for failed wrist implant arthroplasty. J Hand Surg 22A:685–693, 1997.
3. Gelberman RH:The Wrist:Total Wrist Arthroplasty. New York, Raven Press, 1994, pp 253–278.
4. Green DP: Operative Hand Surgery, 2nd ed. New York, Churchill Livingstone, 1993.
5. Knirk JL, Jupiter JB:Intra-articular fractures of the distal end of the radius in young adults. J Bone Joint Surg 68A:647–658, 1986.
6. Lins RE, Gelberman RH, McKeown L, et al: Basal joint arthritis: Trapeziectomy with ligament reconstruction and tendon interposition arthroplasty. J Hand Surgery 21A:202–209, 1996.
7. Swanson AB, deGroot Swanson G: Flexible implant resection arthroplasty. In Strickland JW (ed): Master Techniques in Orthopaedic Surgery: The Hand. Philadelphia, Lippincott-Raven, 1998, pp 421–438.

43. ARTHRODESIS OF THE HAND AND WRIST

Ian D. Crabb, M.D.

1. What two main symptoms may lead a clinician to consider wrist arthrodesis?
Severe wrist pain or carpal instability/subluxation are the indications for wrist arthrodesis. Numerous etiologies may lead to such symptoms. The most common is a ligamentous or bony injury to the wrist that leads to subsequent degenerative arthritis. The arthritis often begins in the radioscaphoid articulation and ultimately progresses to carpal arthritis. Other etiologies of a painful, unstable wrist include infection, inflammatory arthritis (such as rheumatoid arthritis), or after tumor resection.

2. When is wrist fusion more appropriate than performing an arthroplasty?
The need for wrist stability and strength often outweighs the need for range of motion in the wrist. Complete wrist fusion is a reliable, durable, and functional solution to end-stage wrist arthritis. In contrast, wrist arthroplasties have many complications and are rarely recommended in a high-demand hand.

3. What is the optimal position for wrist fusion?

The optimal position for wrist fusion is continually debated. Clearly some tasks are better served with extension and some with flexion. Perineal care is aided by slight wrist flexion, whereas grip strength is better in extension. In practice, a neutral flexion extension and slight ulnar deviation is best.

4. Name the two main complications of wrist arthrodesis.

The main complications of wrist arthrodesis are nonunion and delayed union.

5. Can patients return to work after wrist arthrodesis?

Successful wrist arthrodesis yields a stable and pain-free arm. Most patients can return to even heavy work. The impairment rating for a wrist arthrodesis in 0° of flexion and 0° radioulnar deviation is 30% of the upper extremity or 18% of the whole person.

6. Define limited carpal arthrodesis.

The definition of a limited carpal arthrodesis is fusion between one or several carpal bones. Many combinations are used.

7. When should a limited wrist arthrodesis be considered?

Limited wrist arthrodesis is best used for localized carpal arthritis. Limited arthrodeses also may be used to treat instability patterns of the wrist that are not amenable to soft tissue reconstruction. By their nature, limited wrist arthrodeses shift stresses from one articulation to another. Load shifting may lead to accelerated degeneration of the more stressed joint.

8. Discuss the advantages and disadvantages of limited carpal arthrodesis.

The main advantage of a limited carpal arthrodesis is the ability to retain some wrist motion. The average postoperative range is approximately one-half of the normal range of motion. The ability to retain some motion is of significant psychological benefit to patients contemplating this type of surgery. The main disadvantage of limited carpal arthrodesis is that the full force of carpal loading is transmitted over a smaller surface area, which leads to increased pressure and the potential for cartilage wear and failure.

9. Describe the common sequence of radiocarpal degenerative arthritis.

The common sequence of arthritis at the radiocarpal joint begins with an instability pattern, which develops between the scaphoid and the lunate after disruption of the scapholunate ligament. Because of the abnormal rotation of the scaphoid, the radioscaphoid articulation will then develop into degenerative arthritis with wear of the articular cartilage, swelling, and pain. Mechanical instability and collapse may persist for years before painful arthritis ensues.

10. How is the common pattern described in question nine used in planning limited carpal arthrodesis?

The pattern of radiocarpal degeneration tends to exclude the radiolunate articulation until very late in the disease. The articulation can thus be used as a base for a limited carpal fusion. The most commonly used arthrodesis currently is the four-corner arthrodesis, in which the lunate capitellum triquetrum and hamate are fused and the scaphoid is excised.

11. What is a four-corner fusion?

A four-corner fusion involves the lunate, capitate, triquetrum, and hamate.

12. What is a triscaphe fusion?

Triscaphe fusion is the fusion of the scaphoid, trapezius, and trapezoid.

13. When is arthrodesis considered in the fingers?

The primary indication for arthrodesis in the finger joints is pain. As a practical matter, arthrodesis in any one of the finger joints causes significant functional morbidity and is a procedure of last resort.

14. Which finger joints are most amenable to fusion?

Fusion of the distal interphalangeal (DIP) joint causes the least functional disability. Fusion of the proximal interphalangeal (PIP) joints and the metacarpophalangeal (MCP) joints causes significant functional disability. The one exception is the thumb MCP joint, which in most people can be fused with very little residual morbidity.

15. How does one choose between arthroplasty or fusion in the hand?

As a general rule, you would fuse the DIP joints, fuse the index and middle PIP joints if absolutely necessary, and may consider arthroplasty for the small and ring finger PIP joints. Arthroplasty may be considered for the MCP joints, with the exception of the thumb.

16. What are the complications of finger arthrodesis?

- Nonunion
- Delayed union
- Malunion with a rotational or angular deformity

17. Which thumb joint can be fused with little consequence for overall function?

The MCP joint of the thumb can be fused with little affect on grip strength or mobility of the hand.

18. What are the indications for thumb carpometacarpal (CMC) joint fusions?

A thumb CMC joint fusion may be considered in a younger patient or one who is involved in heavy labor. The thumb CMC joint is a critical joint that allows the thumb to move from the plane of the palm to a position of opposition. Many arthritic conditions in the CMC joint are handled by a ligament reconstruction and arthroplasty of the basal joint. Young or very active patients are candidates for fusion. The advantage of fusion is that it is durable and gives reasonably good function. The limitation of the thumb CMC fusion is the inability to fully flatten the hand to reach into small spaces or pockets.

19. Is arthroplasty or fusion a better treatment for basal joint arthritis?

Several recent studies have shown ligament-based arthroplasty and arthrodesis of the thumb CMC joint to yield equivalent functional results. Arthrodesis has a slightly higher complication rate owing principally to the difficulty of obtaining fusion at the carpometacarpal joint.

20. What arthrodesis options are available for painful arthritis of the distal radioulnar joint?

The Sauve-Kapandji procedure fuses the distal radioulnar joint and creates an osteotomy in the distal ulna. The forearm rotates at the site of distal ulnar osteotomy.

21. How does proximal row carpectomy compare with four-corner arthrodesis in the treatment of wrist DJD?

Both procedures preserve rotation without total wrist arthrodesis. The functional results are similar; the four-corner arthrodesis can yield slightly greater strength by virtue of maintaining carpal height. New fixation options may allow for faster postoperative recovery.

22. Why is scaphotrapeziotrapezoid (STT) arthrodesis used for Kienböck's?

In Kienböck's disease the lunate undergoes avascular necrosis and progressive collapse. STT arthrodesis is utilized to protect the lunate from axial loading and to maintain carpal height.

BIBLIOGRAPHY

1. Beer TA, Turner RH: Wrist arthrodesis for failed wrist implant arthroplasty. J Hand Surg (Am) 20: 965–970, 1995.
2. Cohen MS, Kozin SH: Degenerative arthritis of the wrist. Proximal row carpectomy versus scaphoid excision and four-corner arthrodesis. J Hand Surg [Am] 26(1):94–104, 2001.

3. Damen A, Dijkstra T, van der Lei B, et al: Long-term arthrodesis of the carpometacarpal joint of the thumb. Scan J Plast Reconstr Surg Hand Surg 35(4):407–413, 2001.
4. De Smet LA, Van Ransbeeck H: The Sauve-Kapandji procedure for posttraumatic wrist disorders: Further experience. Acta Orthop Belg 66(3):251–254. 2000.
5. Hartigan BJ, Stern PJ, Kiefhaber TR: Thumb carpometacarpal osteoarthritis: Arthrodesis compared with ligament reconstruction and tendon interposition. Bone Joint Surg Am 83-A(10):1470–1478, 2001.
6. Kuschner SH, Lane CS: Surgical treatment for osteoarthritis at the base of the thumb. Am J Orthop 25:91–100, 1996.
7. Larsen CF, Jacoby RA, McCabe SJ: Nonunion rates of limited carpal arthrodesis: A meta-analysis of the literature. J Hand Surg (Am) 22:66–73, 1997.
8. Leibovic SJ: Internal fixation for small joint arthrodesis in the hand. The interphalangeal joints. Hand Clin 13:601–613, 1997.
9. Mih AD: Limited wrist fusion. Hand Clin 13:615–625, 1997.
10. Mureau MA, Rademaker RP, Verhaar JA, et al: Tendon interposition arthroplasty versus arthrodesis for the treatment of trapeziometacarpal arthritis: A retrospective comparative follow-up study. J Hand Surg [Am] 26(5):869–876, 2001.
11. Sauerbier M, Trankle M, Erdmann D, et al: Functional outcome with scaphotrapeziotrapezoid arthrodesis in the treatment of Kienböck's disease stage III. Ann Plast Surg 44(6):618–625, 2000.
12. Weiss AP, Hastings H: Wrist arthrodesis for traumatic conditions: A study of plate and local bone graft application. J Hand Surg (Am) 20:50–56, 1995.
13. Wyrick JD, Stern PJ, Kiefhaber TR: Motion-preserving procedures in the treatment of scapholunate advanced collapse wrist: Proximal row carpectomy versus four-corner arthrodesis. J Hand Surg (Am) 20:965–970, 1995.
14. Zachary SV, Stern PJ: Complications following AO/ASIF wrist arthrodesis. J Hand Surg (Am) 20:339–344, 1995.

44. KIENBÖCK'S DISEASE

David M. Lichtman, M.D.

1. Describe the pathologic changes in Kienböck's disease.

The pathologic changes in the lunate are due to avascular necrosis. Decreased lunate vascularity, fragmentation, and osseous necrosis are consistent histologic findings.

2. What causes Kienböck's disease?

The exact cause is unknown. It is thought to be due to repeated stress or an acute fracture that leads to interruption of blood supply in a susceptible or "at-risk" lunate.

3. What is the role of trauma in the etiology of Kienböck's disease?

Numerous authors, including Kienböck himself, have implicated trauma or acute fracture as a cause of the avascular necrosis (AVN). Some series have reported an incidence of fracture lines in the lunate as high as 82%. It is not clear, however, whether the fractures are the cause or the result of AVN.

White and Omer pointed out that classic AVN of the lunate is rare after fracture/dislocation or dislocation of the carpus. Their series of cases demonstrated transient vascular ischemia of the lunate after such injuries, along with radiographic density of the lunate consistent with Kienböck's disease. The clinical course, however, was resolution rather than progression.

4. Discuss the three basic patterns of extraosseous blood supply to the lunate.

In his cadaver experiments Lee noted three predictable patterns of extraosseous blood supply:

- A single volar or dorsal vessel supplying the entire bone;
- Several vessels, volar and dorsal, without central anastomosis;

• Several vessels, volar and dorsal, with central anastomosis.

Lee theorized that patients with patterns 1 and 2 are at greater risk for developing Kienböck's disease.

5. Discuss the three basic patterns of intraosseous blood supply to the lunate.

Gelberman found three basic patterns of intraosseous blood supply:

      Y pattern in 59%
      I pattern in 31%
      X pattern in 10%.

His study revealed that the least vascular zone was in the proximal subchondral area adjacent to the radial articular surface, where subchondral fractures and early collapse are most commonly noted.

6. What is the incidence and effect of ulnar variance on predisposition for the development of Kienböck's disease?

Hulten reported a 78% incidence of short ulna (ulnar minus variant) in his patients with Kienböck's disease compared with an incidence of 23% in the normal population. Numerous authors subsequently confirmed the increased incidence of ulnar minor variance. In Japan, however, ulnar positive variance is equally common in the normal population. In the Netherlands, D'Hoore showed an insignificant difference in ulnar variance between people with normal wrists and those with Kienböck's disease.

7. How does ulnar variance predispose to Kienböck's disease?

A short ulna causes increased shear forces on the lunate, predisposing it to injury with repetitive stress. Originally a theory, this has been confirmed by laboratory studies.

8. What radiographic view is required to define the true degree of ulnar variance? Describe how the patient is positioned.

The neutral position posteroanterior (PA) view is the standard view used to determine variance. The patient is positioned so that the shoulder is abducted 90°, the elbow is flexed 90°, and the palm of the hand is placed flat on the cassette.

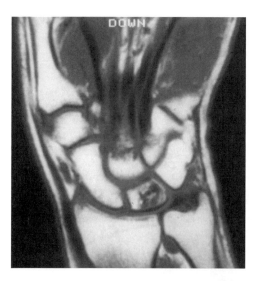

Stage I Kienböck's disease.

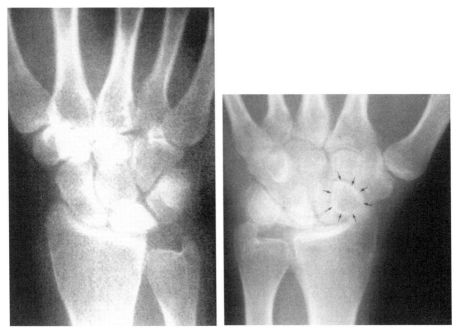

Stage II Kienböck's disease.   Stage III Kienböck's disease.

9. Describe the lunate at risk for Kienböck's disease.
- Lunates with a single extraosseous nutrient vessel
- Lunates with poor intraosseous vascular anastomoses
- Lunates subject to increased shear stress (e.g., negative ulnar variance)

10. What are the criteria for diagnosing Kienböck's disease?
Kienböck's disease is a radiographic diagnosis based on characteristic radiographic density changes in the lunate. Increased density is later followed by fracture lines, fragmentation, and collapse. Kienböck's disease should be included in the differential diagnosis of any chronic wrist pain.

11. Describe the radiographic findings in stage I Kienböck's disease.
Radiographs are normal except for the possibility of a linear or compression fracture of the lunate. Bone scan shows increased uptake around the lunate; magnetic resonance imaging (MRI) shows loss of signal intensity on T1-weighted images.

12. Describe the radiographic findings in stage II Kienböck's disease.
Stage II is characterized by a definite increase in the density of the lunate relative to the other carpal bones (see figure, top of page). Late in stage II there may be some loss of height on the radial side of the lunate.

13. Describe the radiographic findings in stage III Kienböck's disease.
Stage III is a transitional stage in which the disease begins to affect the carpal structure. Radiographs show collapse of the lunate in the frontal plane and elongation in the sagittal plane. The capitate shows proximal migration. Scaphoid foreshortening and scapholunate dissociation may or may not be present. (See figure, top of page.)

14. Describe the radiographic findings in stage IV Kienböck's disease.

All of the radiographic findings of stage III are present along with generalized carpal degenerative arthritis.

15. What is the difference between stages IIIA and IIIB Kienböck's disease?

Stage IIIA is characterized by lunate collapse without fixed scaphoid rotation. In stage IIIB, lunate collapse is accompanied by fixed scaphoid rotation (radioscaphoid angle > 60°) and other secondary carpal derangements.

16. How is the carpal height ratio measured? What is its significance?

The carpal height ratio, as described by Youm, is a measure of the degree of collapse of the wrist related to lunate collapse and proximal migration of the capitate. Carpal height is the distance between the distal articular surface of the third metacarpal and the distal radial articular surface. The carpal height ratio is defined as the carpal height divided by the length of the third metacarpal. The normal value is 0.54 ± 0.03.

17. What is the treatment of stage I Kienböck's disease?

For newly diagnosed cases, immobilization is the treatment of choice. Some authors apply an external fixator to relieve compression across the lunate. If symptoms persist after 2–3 months of immobilization, it is probably best to proceed with treatment as in stage II or IIIA. Some physicians consider lunate edema (increased signal on T2-weighted MRI) a sign of revascularization and will continue conservative treatment for longer periods.

18. Discuss the treatment options for stage II Kienböck's disease.

For stage II with ulnar minus variance, an equalization procedure decreases shear and compressive forces across the lunate and allows possible revascularization. Radial shortening is currently the most popular method, but excellent results also have been reported with ulnar shortening. **For stage II with ulnar positive or neutral variance,** a lunate revascularization procedure is indicated. Popular methods of revascularization include vascular pedicle bone graft and direct implantation of a dorsal metacarpal vessel.

19. Discuss the treatment options for stage IIIA Kienböck's disease.

For **stage IIIA with ulnar minus variance,** an equalization procedure is still acceptable, although some authors recommend limited intercarpal fusion across the midcarpal row. For **stage IIIA with an ulnar positive or neutral variance,** revascularization of the lunate is indicated, although some authors again recommend limited intercarpal arthrodesis.

20. Discuss the treatment options for stage IIIB Kienböck's disease.

For stage IIIB disease, limited intercarpal arthrodesis is indicated to restore carpal stability and to prevent further degeneration. Triscaphe fusion is preferred, although scaphocapitate and scaphocapitolunate fusion accomplishes the same objectives. In addition, if significant synovitis and local fragmentation is present, excision of the lunate is recommended.

21. Discuss the treatment options for stage IV Kienböck's disease.

For stage IV disease salvage operations are indicated. Good results have been reported with both proximal row carpectomy and wrist arthrodesis. The choice of procedure depends on the needs of the patient and the integrity of the articular surfaces of the lunate fossa and the capitate.

22. What is the role of silicone replacement arthroplasty in the treatment of Kienböck's disease?

Once a widely used procedure, silicone lunate replacement arthroplasty has been abandoned; particulate synovitis has been described in many recipients because of stress erosion of the implant.

CONTROVERSIES

23. Should Kienböck's disease be treated conservatively or aggressively?

The precise pathogenesis and natural history of Kienböck's disease are still undetermined. It is possible for progression of the disease to arrest at any stage and for revascularization to occur spontaneously. Some authors, therefore, recommend a nonoperative approach, using cast immobilization to treat symptomatic stages. Most cases, however, continue to progress over time and result in carpal instability and arthritis. We recommend a more aggressive approach, basing our treatment plan on the stage of the disease and ulnar variance.

24. What is the role of venous congestion in the etiology of Kienböck's disease?

In a recent study, the intraosseous venous pressure in Kienböck's disease was significantly higher than in the normal lunate. If venous pressure is higher than the arterial inflow pressure, ischemia will result. Therefore, venous anomalies may represent another form of an at-risk lunate.

25. What is the role of wrist arthroscopy in the management of Kienböck's disease?

The exact role of arthroscopy in Kienböck's disease is still not defined. However, it does provide direct visualization of the lunate surface and surrounding ligaments. A yellowish discoloration as well as detachment of the cartilaginous surface has been identified. Such findings may aid in diagnosis and surgical decision-making.

26. What is the appropriate role of revascularization procedures?

The positive results following most types of revascularization procedures are based on empirical observation rather than laboratory evidence. Clinical studies have not been well controlled. Most reported cases have been done as a supplement to another, more accepted procedure (e.g., radial shortening).

27. What is the appropriate role of external fixation?

Some authors believe that the application of an external fixator decompresses the lunate and enhances revascularization, especially when combined with a revascularization procedure. This concept must be tested by long-term follow-up of a sufficient number of cases before it can be universally recommended.

28. What are the surgical treatment options for Kienböck's disease in a patient with ulnar neutral or positive variance?

In Japan, where many cases of Kienböck's disease have ulnar positive variance, opening- or closing-wedge osteotomies have become popular. Recent evidence has shown that capitate shortening (Almquist procedure) can also effectively decrease shear stress across the lunate.

BIBLIOGRAPHY

1. Almquist EE: Capitate shortening in the treatment of Kienböck's disease. Hand Clin 9:505–512, 1983.
2. Beckenbough RD, Shives TC, Dobyns JH, et al: Kienböck's disease: The natural history of Kienböck's disease and consideration of lunate fractures. Clin Orthop 149:98–106, 1980.
3. D'Hoore K, De smet L, Verellen K, et al: Negative ulnar variance is not a risk for Kienböck's disease. J Hand Surg (Am) 19:229–231, 1994.
4. Gelberman RH, Bauman TD, Menon J, et al: The vascularity of the lunate bone and Kienböck's disease. J Hand Surg 5A:272–278, 1980.
5. Gelberman RH, Szabo RM: Kienböck's disease. Orthop Clin North Am 15:355–367, 1984.
6. Goldfarb CA, Hsu J, Gelberman RH, Boyer MI: The Lichtman Classification for Kienbock's disease: An assessment of reliability. J Hand Surg (Am) 28:74–80, 2003.
7. Lichtman DM, Alexander AH: The Wrist and its Disorders, 2nd ed. Philadelphia, W.B. Saunders, 1997.
8. Lichtman DM, Alexander AH, Mack GR, et al: Kienböck's disease: Update on silicone replacement arthroplasty. J Hand Surg 7A:343–347, 1982.
9. Lichtman DM, Degnan GG: Staging and its use in the determination of treatment modalities for arthroplasty. Hand Clin 9:409–416, 1993.

10. Miura H, Sugioka Y: Radial closing osteotomy for Kienböck's disease. J Hand Surg (Br) 21:1029–1034, 1996.
11. Schiltenwolf M, Martini AK, Mau HC, et al: Further investigation of the intraosseous pressure charac-teristics in necrotic lunates (Kienböck's disease). J Hand Surg (Am) 21:754–758, 1996.
12. Sheetz KK, Bishop AT, Berger RA: The arterial blood supply of the distal radius and ulna and its poten-tial use in vascularized pedicle bone graft. J Hand Surg (Am) 20:902–914, 1995.
13. Sundberg SB, Linscheid RL: Kienböck's disease—Results of treatment with ulnar lengthening. Clin Or-thop 187:43–51, 1984.
14. Trail IA, Linschid RL, Quenzer DE, Scherer PA: Ulnar lengthening and radial recession procedures for Kienböck's disease. Long term clinical and radiographic follow-up. J Hand Surg (Br) 21:169–176, 1996.
15. Viola RW, Kiser PK, Bach AW, et al: Biomechanical analysis of capitate hamate fusion in the treatment of Kienböck's disease. J Hand Surg (Am) 23:395–401, 1998.
16. Watson HK, Ryu J, DiBella A: An approach to Kienböck's disease: Triscaphe arthrodesis. J Hand Surg 10A:179–187, 1985.
17. Weiss AC, Weiland A, Moore JR, et al: Radial shortening for Kienböck's disease. J Bone Joint Surg 73A:384–391, 1991.

45. NERVE ENTRAPMENTS OF HAND AND WRIST

Jeffrey J. Tiedeman, M.D.

1. What is the most commonly encountered compressive neuropathy of the upper ex-tremity? In whom does it occur?

The most common compressive neuropathy of the upper extremity is carpal tunnel syndrome (CTS) or median nerve compression at the wrist. The carpal tunnel is a narrow, fibroosseous canal rigidly bound by the carpal bones and roofed by the transverse carpal ligament, containing the median nerve and the nine extrinsic flexors of the fingers and thumb with their synovial sheath. CTS is most commonly encountered during middle or advanced age; > 80% of patients are more than 40 years of age at the time of diagnosis. It is twice as frequent in women.

2. What are the most common causes of CTS?

Median nerve compression may occur with decreased canal size or increased volume of the contents in the canal. Consequently, a multitude of clinical entities can give rise to the condition. Nonspecific tenosynovial proliferation in otherwise healthy individuals is the most common cause of increased canal contents. The mnemonic **PRAGMATIC** can be used to remember the other common causes of CTS:

P = Pregnancy
R = Rheumatoid arthritis
A = Arthritis (degenerative)
G = Growth hormone abnormalities (acromegaly)
M = Metabolic (hypothyroidism, gout, diabetes mellitus)
A = Alcoholism
T = Tumors
I = Idiopathic
C = Connective tissue disorders (amyloidosis, hemochromatosis)

3. What are the most common symptoms associated with CTS?

The median nerve is responsible for sensory innervation of the thumb and index and long fin-gers as well as the radial border of the ring finger. It also supplies the thenar musculature at the base of the thumb and the two radial lumbrical muscles. The most frequent complaint is numbness, which typically involves the fingers innervated by the median nerve. Patients also may complain of numbness and tingling in the entire hand. Pain also may occur over the same distribution or more proximally in the forearm as the result of median nerve compression in the carpal tunnel. Nocturnal symptoms are common and frequently awaken patients from sleep. Clumsiness or lack of dexterity with the hand is a frequent complaint because of sensory loss or weakness of the thenar musculature.

4. Name the provocative tests used to substantiate the diagnosis of CTS.

A **median nerve percussion** test is performed by percussion with a finger or reflex hammer over the median nerve in the wrist or palm. A positive test produces paresthesias in the median nerve distribution (Tinel's sign). **Phalen's test** is performed with the wrist in full, unforced flexion, which is achieved by putting the dorsum of one hand against the dorsum of the other while the fingers are held dependent. This position increases carpal canal pressures and decreases local median nerve blood flow. A positive test produces paresthesias or sensory disturbances mimicking the patient's symptoms within 60 seconds.

5. What other diagnostic studies should be performed to evaluate a patient for CTS?

Laboratory studies should be obtained to screen for diabetes mellitus, gout, and renal, thyroid, and collagen vascular diseases. Radiographs of the wrist should be obtained to document a fracture, tumor, or arthritis as a possible cause of median nerve compression. Finally, electrodiagnostic studies are the most sensitive and objective tests for the diagnosis of CTS. They always should be obtained before surgical treatment of CTS to corroborate the diagnosis, to rule out other disorders, and to provide baseline nerve function data. Up to 10% of patients with clinically evident CTS, however, produce normal electrodiagnostic studies.

6. Describe the most common complications resulting from carpal tunnel release.

The results from surgical decompression of the median nerve at the carpal tunnel are reliably good. The complication rate is low, ranging from 2% to 15%. Complications include incomplete release of the transverse carpal ligament, injury to the palmar cutaneous branch or recurrent motor branch of the median nerve, reflex sympathetic dystrophy, finger stiffness, decreased strength, and persistent tenderness in the palmar scar.

7. What is an endoscopic carpal tunnel release? What are the reported advantages compared with an open surgical technique?

With endoscopic surgery one or two small incisions are made in the hand, and then an endoscope is used to divide the transverse carpal ligament. Endoscopic carpal tunnel release can reduce patient morbidity and overall recovery time, which allows an early return to activities of daily living and work.

8. Should bilateral carpal tunnel surgery always be done in a staged fashion?

In patients who require bilateral carpal tunnel surgery, the traditional approach has been to do surgeries in a staged fashion because of concerns about ability to perform personal hygiene and activities of daily living in the postoperative period. Recent studies have shown, however, that simultaneous bilateral endoscopic carpal tunnel releases are well tolerated with mild restrictions, high degree of patient satisfaction, and a decrease in overall cost.

9. What is Guyon's canal?

Guyon's canal is a fibroosseous tunnel bound by the hamate and pisiform. The roof is the transverse carpal ligament. The ulnar artery and nerve pass through Guyon's canal. Unlike the carpal tunnel, no tendons pass through Guyon's canal.

10. What causes compressive neuropathies in Guyon's canal?

(1) Trauma, (2) ganglia, (3) lipomas, and (4) fractures of the hamate or pisiform. The most common traumatic mechanism is pressure from bicycling. Sensory neuropathy is usually from a distal canal lesion, whereas motor weakness is from a lesion proximal to or within the canal.

11. What is bowler's thumb?

Bowler's thumb is a traumatic neuropathy of the ulnar digital nerve to the thumb. It is due to repeated friction or compression of the nerve by the edge of the thumb hole at the bowling ball. Early ball adjustment is necessary. The size, fit, spacing, and angulation of the holes should be altered. On rare occasions, transposition or neurolysis is required for relief of severe symptoms.

Digital compression neuropathy also may occur in racquet sports (pressure on the thumb ulnar digital nerve from the grip) or handball (direct compression from the ball strike). Digital nerve compressions will usually occur where the nerve passes near a sesamoid bone.

12. Can posterior interosseous nerve (PIN) compression occur at the wrist?

Yes. Repeated forceful wrist dorsiflexion (as in gymnastics) may irritate PIN. The diagnosis is one of exclusion. Carpal instability, ganglia, and dorsal osteophytes must be excluded. Rest, splinting, and nonsteroidal anti-inflammatory drugs should alleviate the symptoms.

13. How does palmar cutaneous nerve compression occur?

Blunt trauma results in transient neurapraxia. Patients have pain over the thenar eminence and may have a Tinel's sign at the proximal edge of the transverse carpal ligament. Conservative treatment usually suffices.

14. What is double crush syndrome?

Simultaneous compression of a peripheral nerve at more than one location is referred to as double crush syndrome. In fact, a compressive lesion at one point on a peripheral nerve lowers the threshold for development of compression neuropathy at another location (distal or proximal) on the same nerve. For instance, less compression of the median nerve is necessary at the carpal tunnel level to produce symptoms when coexistent cervical nerve root compression is present.

BIBLIOGRAPHY

1. Carr D, Davis P: Distal posterior interosseous nerve syndrome. J Hand Surg 10A:873, 1985.
2. Dobyns JH, O'Brien ET, Linscheid RC, et al: Bowler's thumb: Diagnosis and treatment. A review of seventeen cases. J Bone Joint Surg 54A:751, 1972.
3. Eversman WW: Compression and entrapment neuropathies of the upper extremity. J Hand Surg 8:759, 1983.
4. Glowacki KA, Breen CJ, Sachar K, et al: Electrodiagnostic testing and carpal tunnel release outcome. J Hand Surg 21A:117–122, 1996.
5. Gonzalez del Pino J, Delgado-Martinez AD, Gonzalez Gonzalez I, et al: Value of the carpal compression test in the diagnosis of carpal tunnel syndrome. J Hand Surg 22B:38–41, 1997.
6. Agee JM, McCarroll HR, Tortosa RD, et al: Endoscopic release of the carpal tunnel: A randomized prospective multicenter study. J Hand Surg 17A:987–995, 1992.
7. Szabo RM, Steinberg DR: Nerve entrapment syndromes in the wrist. J Am Acad Orthop Surg 2:115–123, 1994.
8. Watchmaker GP, Weber D, Mackinnon SE: Avoidance of transection of the palmar cutaneous branch of the median nerve in carpal tunnel release. J Hand Surg 21A:644–650, 1996.
7. Fehringer EV, Tiedeman JJ, Dobler K, McCarthy JA: Bilateral endoscopic carpal tunnel releases: Simultaneous versus staged operative intervention. Arthroscopy 18:316–321, 2002.

46. TENOSYNOVITIS OF THE HAND, WRIST, AND FOREARM

David E. Brown, M.D.

1. How many dorsal compartments are found at the wrist? What do they contain?

The six dorsal compartments at the wrist contain the extensor tendons to the wrist and fingers and the abductors to the thumb.

2. Name the tendons in each dorsal compartment.

1st: Abductor pollicis longus
Extensor pollicis brevis

2nd: Extensor carpi radialis longus and brevis

3rd: Extensor pollicis longus

4th: Extensor digitorum
Extensor indicis

5th: Extensor digiti minimi

6th: Extensor carpi ulnaris

One way to remember the number of tendons in each compartment is to remember the sequence 2–2–1–2–1–1.

3. What is de Quervain's disease?

De Quervain's disease is stenosing tenosynovitis of the first dorsal compartment at the wrist. It is most commonly seen in women between 30 and 50 years of age.

4. What are the chief complaints in de Quervain's disease?

Most patients complain of pain and tenderness localized to the radial aspect of the wrist. The pain is worsened with thumb movement because the thumb extensor and abductor travel in this compartment.

5. What is the differential diagnosis for de Quervain's disease?

Arthritis of the first carpometacarpal joint may mimic de Quervain's disease. It can be differentiated by radiographs and physical exam, with a positive grind test. The two lesions, however, commonly coexist. Another possibility is a **scaphoid fracture or arthrosis** involving the radiocarpal or intercarpal joints. Finally, **intersection syndrome** may resemble de Quervain's disease.

6. What causes de Quervain's disease?

The most common cause is an overuse injury of the wrist and hand. The disorder is also seen in patients with inflammatory arthritis.

In some patients the first dorsal compartment is subdivided by a septum, with the extensor pollicis brevis on the ulnar side. This phenomenon has been seen in 20–30% of reported cases. Some patients also have an anomalous tendon in a third tunnel. These septi cause stenosis and are thought to be a cause of de Quervain's disease.

7. Describe the treatment of de Quervain's disease.

Nonoperative therapy consists of rest, thumb and wrist immobilization, local steroid injections, and systemic anti-inflammatories. If this regimen fails, surgical release of the compartment is recommended.

8. Which nerve and artery are at risk during surgical release of the first dorsal compartment?

The superficial sensory branch of the radial nerve has two or three terminal divisions that are located directly over the first dorsal compartment. Transection of these nerves may lead to a painful neuroma. The radial artery is also at risk, because it passes through the anatomic snuff box.

9. What is intersection syndrome?
Tenosynovitis of the second dorsal compartment.

10. What are the symptoms of intersection syndrome?
The most common symptoms are pain and swelling approximately 4 cm above the wrist as the extensor pollicis brevis and abductor pollicis longus cross or intersect the extensor carpi radialis longus and brevis. In severe cases, audible crepitus may be present.

11. What is the cause of intersection syndrome?
Intersection syndrome is frequently associated with repetitive use of the wrist.

12. What is the treatment of intersection syndrome?
Nonoperative therapy consists of rest, work modification, and local steroid injections. The vast majority of cases respond to nonoperative treatment, but occasionally the second dorsal compartment requires surgical release.

13. What are the symptoms of stenosing tenosynovitis of the flexor tendons (trigger finger)?
Patients complain of catching or triggering of the finger with locking in flexion. They often complain of pain at the proximal interphalangeal (PIP) joint, but the lesion occurs at the metacarpophalangeal (MCP) joint. Often there is a palpable nodule on the flexor tendon proximal to the MCP joint. Most commonly the ring and middle fingers are affected, but any digit may be involved.

14. Where is the anatomic lesion that causes trigger finger?
The fingers have four annular (A-1–A-4) and three cruciform (C-1–C-3) pulleys in the fingers that prevent the flexors from bowstringing. The A-1 pulley becomes thickened and narrowed from chronic inflammation and entraps the flexor tendon. A reactive nodular fusiform enlargement of the tendon sheath may compound the entrapment.

15. What other problems caused by stenosing tenosynovitis of the hand are commonly seen with trigger finger?
De Quervain's disease and carpal tunnel syndrome are caused by stenosing tenosynovitis and frequently coexist with trigger finger.

16. In what age group is trigger finger most common?
Two age groups are commonly affected: middle-aged women and neonates. Of congenital trigger fingers, 25% are noted at birth. The condition may present as late as 2 years of age. Unlike the adult type, congenital trigger finger presents with a persistent flexion deformity without triggering. Spontaneous resolution occurs in approximately 30% of cases that present in the first year of life.

17. What is the treatment for trigger finger?
Nonoperative treatment consists of splinting and local injection of steroids into the flexor sheath. Surgical treatment simply involves incising the A-1 pulley. Care must be taken to avoid cutting the A-2 pulley. Studies have shown that the A-2 pulley, attached to the proximal phalanx, and the A-4 pulley, attached to the middle phalanx, are the most important pulleys for prevention of bowstringing.

18. Does the location of a corticosteroid injection for trigger finger really matter?
No. Subcutaneous injection of the corticosteroid has been shown to be as successful as an injection in the tendon sheath.

19. Describe the surgical techniques for trigger finger release.
Open incision. A transverse incision is made on the flexor surface of the metacarpalphalangeal joint. The A-1 pulley is identified and cut longitudinally with a no. 15 blade.

Percutaneous technique. Two methods have been described. The needle technique involves advancing a 19-gauge, 1-inch needle to the proximal margin of the A-1 pulley and "cutting" the pulley with the needle tip. Incomplete release and tendon damage are common. A push-knife technique also has been developed. The knife is a straight blade with a tapered leading flanged edge. Complete release is possible through a 2-mm incision.

20. How does the treatment of stenosing tenosynovitis differ in rheumatoid patients?
In rheumatoid patients the surgeon should preserve the A-1 pulley to prevent bowstringing and ulnar drift. Therefore, the tendon sheath is explored with removal of any nodules within the flexor tendons. A complete tenosynovectomy is performed. Some authors suggest removing one arm of the sublimis tendon to create room for the flexor as they pass through the pulleys. This method is not universally accepted.

BIBLIOGRAPHY

1. Canale ST (ed): Campbell's Operative Orthopaedics, 9th ed. St. Louis, Mosby, 1998.
2. Dunn MJ, Pess GM: Percutaneous trigger finger release: A comparison of a new push knife and a 19-gauge needle in a cadaveric model. J Hand Surg 24-A:860–865, 1999.
3. Green DP (ed): Operative Hand Surgery, 3rd ed. New York, Churchill Livingstone, 1993, pp 2217–2134.
4. Taras JS, Raphael JS, Pan WT, et al: Cortisteroid injections for trigger digits: Is intrasheath injection necessary? J Hand Surg 23A:717–722, 1998.

47. PEDIATRIC HAND AND WRIST

Keith R. Gabriel, M.D.

1. What is the time frame for development of the arm bud?
The arm bud begins to develop at about the fourth week after fertilization and is essentially complete by the eighth fetal week.

2. What group of genes regulates limb development?
Limb development is guided by the "homeobox" or (*HOX*) genes.

3. Define polydactyly, macrodactyly, and syndactyly.
Polydactyly is duplication of one or more digits. **Macrodactyly** is an enlarged digit. **Syndactyly** is fusion of digits.

4. Does postaxial (ulnar-side) polydactyly have a racial predilection?
Yes. Duplication of the small finger is 10 times more common in African-Americans than in Caucasians. Postaxial polydactyly in Caucasians may indicate serious associated abnormalities.

5. Does preaxial (thumb) polydactyly have a similar racial predilection?
The incidence is similar in African-Americans and Caucasians but slightly higher in Asians and Native Americans.

6. Is there a significant association between preaxial polydactyly and other congenital disorders?
Although syndactyly may occur, most duplicated thumbs present as an isolated anomaly and do not demonstrate the same frequency of serious associated abnormalities as postaxial polydactyly in whites.

7. In central polydactyly, which finger is most commonly duplicated?
The ring finger is most commonly duplicated. Duplication of the index finger is rare.

8. How common is macrodactyly?
Macrodactyly is one of the rarest congenital malformations of the upper extremity. It is usually caused by conditions such as neurofibromatosis, Proteus syndrome, lymphangioma, or arteriovenous malformation.

9. An infant presents with absence of one thumb. The index finger is short, and the entire hand deviates toward the radial side of the forearm. The distal end of the ulna is quite prominent. What is the likely diagnosis?
The likely diagnosis is radial dysplasia, commonly called radial club hand. The degree of radial deficiency and the resulting appearance and function are quite variable.

10. How is the stethoscope helpful in evaluating the patient with a radial deficiency?
Radial defects are frequently associated with cardiovascular defects. Gastrointestinal (GI) and genitourinary systems must be carefully evaluated. Aplastic (Fanconi) anemia and platelet defects also should be considered.

11. What interventions are usually recommended for the initial treatment of radial club hand?
Initial treatment usually consists of passive stretching and splinting of the wrist and hand toward a central or even ulnarly deviated position.

12. An infant presents with absence of the small finger, ulnar deviation of the hand and wrists, and a shortened forearm that is bowed toward the ulnar side. What are the major differences between this entity and radial club hand?
Ulnar club hand is less common (reported ratios range form 1:4 to 1:10) than radial club hand. The expression in the limb is even more variable and may include absence of radial rays, limitation of elbow motion, and humeral shortening. Associated anomalies are usually restricted to the musculoskeletal system.

13. Central deficiency of the hand (cleft hand) may be associated with what other cleft deficiencies?
Cleft hand is usually bilateral. Frequent associations are cleft foot, cleft lip, and cleft palate. Noncleft anomalies often are seen in the cardiac and GI systems.

14. Describe symbrachydactyly.
This abnormality includes transverse deficiencies of the central digits and simple syndactyly.

15. How does a trigger digit in the infant differ from a trigger digit in the adult?
In the infant the thumb is more commonly involved, the condition is frequently bilateral, and the presentation is likely to be fixed-flexion posture rather than clicking or "triggering."

16. What is the management of trigger thumb in the infant (> 1 year of age)?
Initial treatment consists of splinting in extension. Perhaps 30% of cases resolve without surgery. After 1 year of age, most thumbs require surgical release.

17. What is the difference between camptodactyly and clinodactyly?
Strictly speaking, both terms mean "bent finger." Both conditions usually occur in the small finger. **Camptodactyly** is angulation in the anteroposterior plane; that is, a flexion contracture. **Clinodactyly** is angulation in a radioulnar direction.

18. In what age groups does camptodactyly usually present?
Camptodactyly usually presents in infancy or adolescence.

19. Mild clinodactyly is common in normal children. Marked clinodactyly is associated with what condition?

Mental retardation.

20. The nursery discharge note says the infant has a simple, incomplete syndactyly between the ring and long fingers. Describe the deformity.

A web of skin joins the fingers (simple), extending from the commissure but not reaching the fingertips (incomplete). In most cases the web extends to the middle of the proximal phalanx.

21. Describe a complex, complete syndactyly.

Complex indicates that the bones of the adjacent fingers are fused together. *Complete* means that the syndactyly extends to the fingertips.

22. What factors influence the timing of surgery to separate syndactyly.

Expected differential growth of the involved digits is a key factor. For instance, the thumb and index must be separated early, whereas syndactyly of the ring and long fingers may be delayed for 2 or 3 years. In practice, most separations are done between 6 months and 1 year of age.

23. When should a surgical procedure to alter prehensile patterns be performed?

Prehensile patterns begin to develop at about 1 year of age and are well established by the age of 3 years. Therefore, a surgical procedure to alter prehensile patterns should be done before the age of 3 years.

24. What is Streeter's dysplasia?

Streeter's dysplasia is a syndrome of congenital constriction bands that may affect any part of the body. In the fingers the constriction may range from simple indentation to congenital amputation. In many cases, surgical release by Z-plasty is necessary to relieve distal circulatory embarrassment.

25. What is Madelung's deformity? Where is the growth disturbance?

The articular surface of the distal radius becomes progressively tilted in an ulnar and palmar direction because of growth disturbances at the ulnar-palmar aspect of the distal radial physis.

26. A young female gymnast presents with bilateral wrist pain. Radiographs show widening and irregularity of the physis of the distal radius. What is the likely diagnosis?

The likely diagnosis is epiphysiolysis of the distal radius. This condition, which is seen almost exclusively in young gymnasts, is analogous to a stress fracture. It is treated symptomatically, with restriction of activity or splinting. In severe cases, premature closure of the physis of the distal radius has been reported.

27. Hyperflexion injury to the distal interphalangeal joint in the adult may cause disruption of the extensor tendon ("mallet finger"). What is the analogous injury in the preadolescent?

The analogous injury in the preadolescent is a displaced Salter-Harris type I or II separation of the physis of the distal phalanx. The nail bed remains firmly affixed to the distal fragment; thus any bleeding around the nail indicates an open injury. This injury is sometimes called the **Seymour fracture.**

28. The term *extra-octave fracture* refers to which injury?

An extra-octave fracture is a Salter-Harris type I or II fracture at the base of the proximal phalanx of the small finger, angulated so that the small finger points toward the ulna, as if the patient had been trying to span a few too many piano keys. This injury is also called a pencil fracture, because physicians place a small pencil or pen between the small and ring fingers to assist with the reduction maneuver.

29. Are fractures of the carpal bones equally common in preadolescents and adults?
No. Such fractures are uncommon in preadolescents. Apparently the thick cartilaginous construction of the growing carpals gives them sufficient resilience to avoid most fractures.

30. Dislocations of the proximal interphalangeal (PIP) joint usually occur in what direction?
Such dislocations usually occur dorsally, in response to a hyperextension force. Specifically, the base of the middle phalanx dislocates dorsal to the tip of the proximal phalanx. Lateral dislocations also occur. In the child, a volar dislocation is rare.

31. How long do you expect to see soreness and swelling after a jammed finger or after reduction of a simple PIP dislocation?
Soreness and swelling persist for 3–6 months. It is imperative that the patient and the parents be properly informed when such injuries are first diagnosed.

32. What is the characteristic hand position in spastic cerebral palsy?
The thumb is clasped into the palm, the fingers flexed at the metacarpophalangeal joints, the wrist flexed, and the forearm pronated.

33. Surgery of the upper extremity (hand) is most often indicated in what general category of patients with cerebral palsy?
Surgery is most often indicated in patients with spastic hemiplegia.

34. What congenital bony connection between the radius and ulna, usually located proximally, prevents forearm rotation?
Radioulnar synostosis.

BIBLIOGRAPHY

1. Albanese SA, Palmer AK, Kerr DR, et al: Wrist pain and distal growth plate closure of the radius in gymnasts. J Pediatr Orthop 9:23–28, 1989.
2. Askins G, Ger E: Congenital constriction band syndrome. J Pediatr Orthop 8:461–466, 1988.
3. Busch MT: Sports medicine in children and adolescents. In Morrissy RT, Weinstein SL (eds): Lovell and Winter's Pediatric Orthopaedics, 5th ed. Philadelphia, Lippincott Williams & Wilkins, 2001, pp 1273–1318.
4. Graham TJ, Waters PM: Fractures and dislocations of the hand and carpus in children. In Beaty JH, Kasser JR (eds): Rockwood and Wilkins' Fractures in Children, 5th ed. Philadelphia, Lippincott Williams & Wilkins, 2001, pp 269–379.
5. Herring JA: Disorders of the upper extremity. In Herring JA: Tachdjian's Pediatric Orthopedics, 3rd ed. Philadelphia, W.B. Saunders, 2002, pp 379–512.
6. Koman LA, Gelberman RH, Toby EB, Poehling GG: Cerebral palsy. Management of the upper extremity. Clin Orthop 253:62–74, 1990.
7. Rao SB, Esposito PW, Crawford AH: Congenital and developmental wrist disorders in children. In Lichtman DM, Alexander AH (eds): The Wrist and its Disorders. Philadelphia, W.B. Saunders, 1997, pp 509–539.
8. Slakey JB, Hennrikus WL: Acquired thumb flexion contracture in children: Congenital trigger thumb. J Bone Joint Surg 78B:481–483, 1996.
9. Waters PM: The upper limb. In Morrissy RT, Weinstein SL (eds): Lovell and Winter's Pediatric Orthopaedics, 5th ed. Philadelphia, Lippincott Williams & Wilkins, 2001, pp 841–903.

VI. The Spine

48. CERVICAL SPINE DISEASE

Stephen R. Pledger, M.D.

1. In what phase of embryo life do the somites develop into cervical vertebrae?

At 5–6 weeks the embryo begins to resegment, and the somites become vertebrae. Resegmentation occurs when the right and left somites at each level fuse across the midline, incorporating the notch cord.

2. In the third week of embryonic life the embryonic spinal cord is developed. What mesenchymal tissues form the notch cord?

In the third life of embryonic life, ectodermal cells sink into the dorsal surface of the caudal end of the embryo and push forward between the ectoderm and endoderm to form mesoderm. In the middle the mesoderm coalesces into an axial segmental rod called the natal cord.

3. How many vertebrae make up the cervical spine?

The cervical spine consists of the first seven vertebrae of the spinal column.

4. Do any of the cervical vertebrae have bifid spinous processes?

The spinous processes at the third, fourth, and fifth cervical vertebrae are bifid.

5. The articulations between the vertebral arches of the cervical spine are maintained by what anatomic structures?

The articulations between the vertebral arches are maintained by (1) the supraspinous ligaments, which in the cervical spine have evolved into the ligamentum nuchae; (2) the interspinous ligaments; (3) the ligamentum flavum at each level; and (4) the synovial facet joints.

6. What artery has an intimate relationship with the cervical spine and serves as the major source of blood to the cervical cord and cervical spine?

The vertebral artery is the major source of blood for the cervical cord and cervical spine. The vertebral arches originate from the subclavian artery on each side and are usually the first and largest branches of the subclavian artery.

7. Which elements of the cervical spine are responsible for its mobility?

The elements primarily responsible for the mobility of the spine are the discs in the apophyseal joints. Each of these elements provides a relative contribution to degree and pattern of motion, such as flexion/extension and rotation.

8. Which vertebrae are responsible primarily for the rotation of the cervical spine?

The atlantoaxial joints (C1 and C2) are responsible for right and left lateral rotation.

9. Which vertebrae are responsible for flexion/extension?

Primary flexion of the cervical spine is determined from C3 to C7 with the primary movement coming from the C2–C3, C3–C4, and C4–C5 vertebral spaces.

10. Is the atlantoaxial joint (C1, C2) a stable or unstable joint?

The atlantoaxial joints are unstable because of their opposed convexity with a small contact area between the joint surfaces. This configuration is necessary for the joint to perform movements in all directions; flexion/extension, lateral flexion, and rotation. Stability between the atlas and axis depends on the transverse ligament.

11. Which type of injuries are responsible for the majority of cervical spine fractures from C2 to C7: flexion, extension, or axial compression?

Extreme cervical compression is the major cause of cervical spine fractures from C2 to C7. Such compression may occur from diving, American football, and trampoline injuries; automobile accidents; and emergency aircraft egress (ejection-seat injuries). Compression forces are responsible for the majority of nonfatal cervical fractures.

12. The teardrop fracture of the cervical spine is caused by what type of injury: hyperflexion, hyperextension, or compression?

The mechanism of injury is hyperflexion. The term teardrop reflects the sadness often associated with a neurologic sequela.

13. The unilateral facet dislocations are caused by what external forces?

The unilateral facet dislocation is assumed to occur from axial rotation movements as well as flexion movements and distraction. Tearing of the interspinous ligaments and variable amounts of ligamentum flavum and capsule in one of the facet joints leads to facet dislocation.

14. Which cervical arthrosis is the most effective in controlling flexion/extension, rotation, and lateral bending?

The halo vest or cast is the most effective in controlling rotation, flexion/extension, and lateral bending. The second most effective device is a rigid cervicothoracic brace, followed by a four-poster brace. The least effective is a soft cervical collar.

15. What is the recommended cervical orthotic device for cervical strain?

Philadelphia collar.

16. What is the most commonly recommended orthotic for most cervical spine fractures?

The halo vest or cast is recognized for most cervical spine fractures. The cervicothoracic brace is used for less unstable fractures.

17. In cervical trauma, which radiograph should be obtained, before anything else is done, to evaluate the stability of the cervical spine?

The initial radiograph is a lateral radiograph of the cervical spine, preferably made with the patient still on the transportation stretcher. All handling should be postponed until the results of the radiographic examination are known. If handling is necessary, the patient should be lifted "as one piece" by at least four persons to avoid cervical cord injury, especially in the unconscious patient.

18. When the fracture is not obvious on a lateral radiograph of the cervical spine, what is initially evaluated to help determine whether fracture has occurred?

Because swelling is noted in the prevertebral soft tissue after cervical spine fractures, the mid-position of C3–C7, where most fractures occur, should be evaluated. At C3, 3.5 mm is standard; at C4, 5.0 mm; and at C5, C6, and C7, approximately 15 mm, with up to 20 mm at the distal portion. If abnormal widening is noted at any area along the anterior cervical spine, fracture should be suspected.

19. What other radiographs are helpful in determining cervical fractures or dislocations?

The oblique views are essential in evaluation of the apophyseal joints, which indicate either unilateral or bilateral facet dislocation. Tomograms are also helpful in determining odontoid fractures.

20. Is there a normal subluxation (spondylolisthesis) or stepped-off formation in the cervical spine of children?
Yes. Normal variants of a type of subluxation that occurs in the posterior borders of vertebral bodies at C2, C3 and C3, C4 often have led to the diagnosis of subluxation in children. Understanding that this phenomenon is a normal variation or pseudosubluxation is important. Evaluation of vertebral swelling helps to determine whether or not an acute injury is involved.

21. What type of spinal instability is commonly found in children with Down syndrome?
The incidence of C1, C2 subluxation is 20%. This lesion is found in all age groups, with no preponderance at any age.

22. Which radiographic imaging study is the most helpful in determining herniated discs of the cervical spine?
The gold standard is the myelogram with subsequent computed tomographic (CT) scan. However, magnetic resonance imaging (MRI) is quickly becoming the gold standard. The CT scan alone, without contrast or myelogram, is contraindicated.

23. Is the CT scan contraindicated for any cervical spine abnormalities?
No. The CT scan is indispensable in determining bony problems of the cervical spine, whether tumors or fractures are involved. CT is the imaging study of choice for all victims of trauma.

24. In evaluating a cervical spine problem, what abnormal findings are expected with a C5, C6 nerve abnormality (e.g., herniated disc, trauma)?
Expected findings include decreased sensation in the thumb and index finger, with weakness of the deltoid and biceps muscles, absence of the biceps reflex, and weakness of the extensor carpi radialis longus.

25. What abnormalities are expected with a C7 abnormality (e.g., herniated disc at C6, C7)?
Expected findings include numbness in the long finger and potentially in the index finger, slight weakness of the triceps, and absence of the brachioradialis reflex.

26. What abnormality is expected with a C8 nerve abnormality (e.g., herniated disc at the C7, T1 area)?
Expected findings include numbness in the ulnar nerve distribution of the little finger and ring finger, a claw-hand deformity, weakness of the triceps muscle, and absence of the triceps reflex.

27. What is os odontoideum?
Os odontoideum is a congenital anomaly of the odontoid. Patients may present clinically with no symptoms, local neck symptoms and transitory episodes of paresthesia after trauma, or frank myelopathy. Clinical manifestations are limited to neck pain and torticollis; depending on the severity, frank brainstem abnormalities may be present.

28. How is os odontoideum treated when patients present with transitory myelopathy?
Nonoperative treatment is sufficient for the patient presenting with a relatively stable os odontoideum and little compromise of the spinal cord. For marked instabilities, however, a cervical fusion of C1 and C2 is the procedure of choice.

29. What are the most common clinical findings in Klippel-Feil syndrome?
The classic clinical findings are a short neck, a low posterior headline, and a limited range of neck motion. However, fewer than 50% of patients have all three elements of the triad.

30. What are the most common radiographic findings of Klippel-Feil syndrome?

The most common findings are congenitally fused vertebrae from C2 to C7. The fusions may be multiple-level or single-level.

31. Do patients with Klippel-Feil syndrome have any auditory abnormalities?

Yes. Deafness was first associated with Klippel-Feil syndrome by Jalladeau in 1936. The incidence in Klippel-Feil syndrome is approximately 30%.

32. What other spine abnormality is most commonly associated with Klippel-Feil syndrome?

Scoliosis is the most commonly associated spinal abnormality in Klippel-Feil syndrome. Approximately 50% of patients report cases of scoliosis, either alone or in combination with kyphosis.

33. What is the most common congenital abnormality found in patients with quadriplegia due to football injury?

Torg reported that the most common congenital abnormallity is stenosis of the cervical spine canal, with the quadriplegia occurring at the stenotic level. Any football player with transient neurologic abnormalities should be evaluated; if cervical stenosis is found, it is recommended that the patient quit playing football.

34. The Jefferson fracture involves what type of injury to the cervical spine?

The Jefferson fracture is a unique fracture of the first cervical vertebra. Axial loading directly downward on the ring of C1 causes multiple fractures of the ring and usually a spreading of the fragments.

35. The hangman's fracture involves what lesion of the cervical spine?

The hangman's fracture is scientifically termed a traumatic spondylolisthesis of the axis or C2. The weakest length of the vertebrae is the pars interarticularis of C2, a narrow isthmus located between the superior and inferior facets. This injury usually occurs during rapid deceleration in a motor vehicle accident, when the victim is thrown forward with the head striking the windshield. The accident usually involves head-on collision with another vehicle or with a fixed object.

36. Give the most common signs and symptoms of hangman's fracture.

The most common symptoms are not highly specific. The patient often feels marked apprehension and fear with a sense of subjective instability. Pain radiating along the course of the greater occipital nerve (C2), so-called occipital neuralgia, is frequent and leads to marked guarding of neck motion. Another common finding is direct trauma to the top of the forehead of the skull.

37. In an unconscious patient with obvious blunt trauma to the forehead, what type of injuries must be ruled out immediately?

With obvious head trauma and unconsciousness, one needs to rule out a cervical spine fracture. This is best done with a scout lateral radiograph of the cervical spine.

38. Where is the most common injury to the cervical spine in children?

Injuries to the cervical spine are rare in children. The most common, however, occur from the occiput to C3. Lesions at the atlantoaxial joint are noted in 70% of children < 15 years of age but in only 16% of adults.

39. Athletic injuries to the cervical spine associated with quadriplegia are the result of what mechanism?

Athletic injuries to the cervical spine associated with quadriplegia most commonly occur as a result of axial loading. Examples include spearing in football (when a player strikes an opponent with the crown of his helmet); a poorly executed dive into a shallow body of water; with the head striking the bottom; or pushing a hockey player into the boards headfirst. The fragile cervical spine is compressed between the rapidly decelerated head and the continued momentum of the body.

40. In C4 quadriplegia, with lesion between C4 and C5 vertebrae, what changes in motor function, sensory function, or reflexes are expected?

In C4 quadriplegia, you expect the patient to breathe spontaneously because C4 innervates the diaphragm. The patient is able to shrug the shoulders independently but lacks functional abdominal muscles. Sensation is present in the upper anterior chest wall but not in the upper extremities. All reflexes are absent.

41. In C5 quadriplegia, what motor, sensation, and reflex changes are expected?

In C5 quadriplegia, the deltoid muscle and a portion of the biceps muscle are functioning. The patient is able to perform shoulder abduction and flexion/extension as well as some elbow flexion. However, all these functions are weak. Sensation is normal over the upper portion of the anterior chest wall and the lateral aspect of the arm from the shoulder to the elbow crease. The biceps reflex may be normal or slightly decreased.

42. In C6 quadriplegia, what motor functions, sensations, and reflexes remain intact?

Both the biceps and rotator cuff muscles continue to function.

Motor: The most distal functional muscle group is the wrist extensor group. The extensor carpi radialis longus and brevis and extensor carpi ulnaris may not be functioning. The patient has almost full function of the shoulder, full flexion of the elbow, full supination and partial pronation of the forearm, and partial extension of the wrist. The strength of wrist extension is normal, because some power for the extension is supplied predominantly by the extensor carpi radialis longus and brevis.

Sensation: The lateral side of the entire upper extremity as well as the thumb, index, and half of the middle finger have normal sensory power.

Reflexes: Both the biceps and the brachioradialis reflexes are normal.

43. In C7 quadriplegia, what motor functions, sensations, and reflexes remain intact?

C7 quadriplegia involves the vertebral level of C7, T1.

Motor: With the C7 nerve root intact, the triceps, wrist flexors, and long-finger extensors are functional. The patient can hold objects, but the grasp is extremely weak. Although still confined to a wheelchair, the patient may be able to attempt parallel bar and brace function for general exercise.

Sensation: C7 has little pure sensory representation in the upper extremity. No precise zone for C7 sensation may be mapped.

Reflexes: The biceps, brachioradialis, and triceps reflexes are normal.

44. What is a central cord injury?

A central cord injury is an incomplete spinal cord lesion that most commonly occurs in the elderly and results from an extension injury. This type of quadriplegia involves the upper extremities more than the lower extremities. Seventy-five percent recover and are ambulatory.

45. What is Brown-Séquard syndrome?

The syndrome results from an incomplete spinal cord injury in which ipsilateral motor loss, contralateral pain, and temperature loss are found. The recovery rate is 90%.

46. What is anterior cord syndrome?

Characterized by complete motor deficit with preservation of deep pressure and proprioception resulting from an incomplete spinal cord injury. Fifty percent of patients recover weak motor skills, but only 10% ambulate.

47. What role (if any) do steroids have in the treatment of acute spinal cord injuries?
Bracken et al. (1990) reported significant improvement in motor and sensory deficits in incomplete motor lesions with methylprednisone administered within 8 hours (30 mg/kg then 5.4 mg/kg for 23 hrs). After 8 hours, only sensory deficits improved.

48. Define spinal cord shock.
Spinal cord shock is a temporary physiologic loss of spinal cord activity that results in areflexia.

49. What physical finding signals the end of spinal shock?
The bulbocavernous reflex signals the end of spinal shock.

50. What is the most common pain pattern of herniated cervical disc?
The most common pain pattern for the cervical disc is radiation into the scapular area and down the lateral aspect of the arm in to the forearm and hand.

51. Name the most common methods of conservative treatment of herniated cervical disc.
The most common methods of treating a herniated cervical disc include a cervical collar, physical therapy with cervical traction, epidural steroid blocks, nonsteroidal antiinflammatory drugs (NSAIDs), and tincture of time.

52. What is the most common surgical treatment for a herniated cervical disc?
The most common surgical treatment is anterior cervical discectomy and fusion (ACDF) with an iliac crest allograft or autogenous graft. The second most common is cervical laminectomy with removal of the herniated fragment.

53. What is the rate of success for conservative treatment of herniated cervical discs?
Conservative treatment of herniated cervical discs is highly successful in 50–60% of cases. A minimum of 3 months of conservative care should be given before considering surgical intervention.

BIBLIOGRAPHY

1. Chewning S: Comprehensive Review Course—Cervical Spine Trauma. American Academy of Orthopedic Surgeons, 1998.
2. Clark CR, Ducker T, Dvorak J, et al (eds): The Cervical Spine, 3rd ed. Philadelphia, Lippincott-Raven, 1997.
3. Hoppenfeld S: Orthopaedic Neurology: A Diagnostic Guide to Neurological Levels. Philadelphia, J.B. Lippincott, 1977.
4. Walt RT: Comprehensive Review Course—Rehabilitation of Spinal Cord Injuries. American Academy of Orthopedic Surgeons, 1998.

49. LOW BACK PAIN, LUMBAR DISC DISEASE, SPINAL STENOSIS, AND LUMBAR FUSION

Stephen E. Doran, M.D., and Randall D. Neumann, M.D.

LOW BACK PAIN

1. What is the lifetime incidence of low back pain?
The lifetime incidence of low back pain ranges from 50% to 70%, whereas the incidence of sciatica ranges from 13% to 40%.

2. What risk factors are associated with the development of back pain?

Risk factors include jobs that require heavy and repetitive lifting, use of jackhammers and machine tools, and operation of motor vehicles. Smokers are at greater risk for low back pain, which may be severe. Individuals slightly above normal body weight are more likely to report back pain than those below or at normal weight.

3. Where does acute low back pain originate?

All structures of the lumbar spine can contribute to significant back pain, including the paraspinous muscles, ligaments, facet joints, annulus fibrosus, disc, and nerve roots.

4. What is the differential diagnosis of low back pain?

Multiple entities may produce back pain, ranging from spinal diseases to vascular diseases.

Common Conditions That Cause Low Back Pain

Spinal disorders	Herniated disc	Metabolic disorders	Osteoporosis
	Spondylolisthesis	Osteomalacia	
	Spinal stenosis		Paget's disease
	Osteoarthritis		
		Trauma	Fracture
Rheumatologic	Rheumatoid arthritis		
conditions	Reiter's syndrome	Hemoglobinopathies	Sickle-cell disease
	Psoriatic arthritis	Renal disorders	Stones
	Ankylosing spondylitis		Tumors
			Infection
Tumor	Benign		
	Malignant	Female genital disorders	Ovarian cysts
	Metastatic		Ovarian tumors
Infections	Bacterial	Vascular disease	Aortic aneurysm
	Tuberculosis		
		Gastrointestinal disease	Peptic ulcer
			Pancreatic disease
			Gall bladder

5. What is the treatment for acute low back pain?

The vast majority of patients with low back pain improve within 2 months. Patients should be treated symptomatically with aspirin and nonsteroidal anti-inflammatory drugs (NSAIDs). No drug treatment has proved superior to aspirin alone, although some medications may have fewer side effects. Bedrest should be limited to 1–2 days while spasms subside. No evidence shows that prolonged bed rest is of benefit in patients with acute low back pain. The use of corsets, transcutaneous nerve stimulation (TENS), or conventional traction for the treatment of back pain remains controversial; no studies have proved the efficacy of these treatments. Some evidence suggests that exercise provides some benefit, and patients should begin with general stretching and range-of-motion activities.

6. List the other symptoms that should be evaluated in patients with acute low back pain and their possible etiologies.

Evaluation of Symptoms in Patients with Low Back Pain

SYMPTOM	LABORATORY	DIAGNOSTIC	PROCEDURE	POSSIBLE ETIOLOGY
Fever or weight loss	Culture	Radiograph Bone scan CT scan MRI	Biopsy Surgery	Infection Tumor

Table continued on following page.

Evaluation of Symptoms in Patients with Low Back Pain (Continued)

SYMPTOM	LABORATORY	DIAGNOSTIC	PROCEDURE	POSSIBLE ETIOLOGY
Night pain	Complete blood count Sedimentation rate Chemical profile	Radiograph Bone scan CT scan MRI	Biopsy Surgery	Tumor Spinal cord tumor
Morning stiffness	RA factor ANA Sedimentation rate	Radiographs		RA Ankylosing spondylitis Psoriatic arthritis
Colicky pain	Urinalysis Urine culture & sensitivity Amylase	IVP Gallbladder scan CT scan Aortogram Ultrasound	GI workup Surgery Biopsy Peptic ulcer Pancreas	Kidney Gallbladder Aneurysm

ANA = antinuclear antibody, RA = rheumatoid arthritis, IVP = intravenous pyelography

7. What is the treatment for chronic low back pain?

Chronic low back pain is defined as pain that persists for more than 6 months. Less than 5% of patients with low back pain develop chronic back pain syndrome; these patients, however, account for approximately 85% of the total cost of back pain care. Because chronic back pain is often due to multiple factors, such as pathology of the intervertebral disc, facet joints, and soft tissues, amelioration of symptoms is difficult. Anatomic and psychological factors both contribute to the development and persistence of chronic low back pain. Psychosocial factors such as narcotic dependency, depression, and litigation/compensation issues may perpetuate or intensify the anatomic factors that cause back pain. Successful treatment of chronic low back pain addresses both the anatomic and psychosocial factors. Physical therapy is beneficial for improving flexibility, strength, and endurance. TENS units decrease pain for some patients. Antidepressants and counseling may benefit patients experiencing depression. Some patients successfully return to their occupations via work-hardening/conditioning programs. Injections of local anesthetics or epidural/caudal corticosteroids may reduce pain for a small number of patients with chronic symptoms, but are much more effective in relieving acute symptoms of back and radicular pain. Lumbar fusion may be helpful for a selected group of patients whose symptoms are primarily due to intervertebral disc degeneration.

LUMBAR DISC DISEASE

8. Describe the usual history of patients with lumbar disc herniation.

Most people relate back and leg pain to a traumatic event, but close questioning sometimes reveals that patients have had intermittent episodes of back pain for months or years. The pain may be brought on by heavy exertion, repetitive bending, twisting, or heavy lifting. Pain usually begins in the low back and radiates to the sacroiliac region and buttocks. Radicular pain usually extends below the knee and follows the dermatome of the involved nerve root. When patients have sustained a disc herniation, the pain is generally worse in the leg than in the back. Pain may be intermittent in nature and usually increases with activities, especially sitting in a car for a long period of time. The pain may be relieved by standing or by bed rest. The hallmark is exacerbation of leg pain by straining, sneezing, or coughing. Patients may complain of weakness. The weakness is usually localized to the neurologic level of involvement. Paresthesias are common and follow the nerve root distribution for the sensory areas.

9. What is cauda equina syndrome?

Cauda equina syndrome is a large midline disc herniation that may compress several roots of the cauda equina; it occurs in only 2% of patients with a herniated disc. The L4–L5 disc is the most commonly offending herniation. The mode of onset may be rapid or slowly progressing. Often back pain or perianal pain predominates, and disc symptoms are minimal. Patients complain of difficulty with urination, increased frequency, or overflow incontinence. In men, a recent history of impotence may be elicited. Patients may have leg pain that progresses to severe numbness of the feet and difficulty with walking. Myelography shows a complete block with large disc herniations. Prompt surgical intervention is the treatment of choice.

10. Describe the physical examination for patients with lumbar disc disease.

Patients should be examined in the standing, sitting, and lying positions. A list or limp can be seen with the patient walking. Range of motion of the spine should be examined. Patients with disc herniation frequently complain of leg pain on forward flexion, whereas patients with spinal stenosis often have leg pain on back extension. Muscular atrophy or muscle spasm should be identified with range-of-motion evaluation. Weakness is also determined. A complete neurologic examination is necessary, including testing of motor strengths, reflexes, and sensory deficits. The presence or absence of tension sign is the most important finding in patients suspected of having disc herniation. Evaluation should include examination for hip and knee pathology.

11. What are the physical findings in patients with unilateral disc herniation at the L3–L4 disc?

Unilateral herniation at the L3–L4 disc generally involves compression of the L4 nerve root, with possible sensory deficits in the posterolateral thigh, anterior knee, and medial leg. Motor weakness is variable in the quadriceps and hip adductors. Changes also are apparent in the patellar reflex.

12. What are the physical findings in patients with unilateral disc herniation at the L4–L5 disc?

The L5 nerve root is compressed with disc herniation at L4–L5. Sensory deficit occurs in the anterolateral leg, dorsum of the foot, and great toe. Motor weakness includes the extensor hallucis longus, gluteus medius, and extensor digitorum longus and brevis. Usually no reflex changes are present.

13. What are the physical findings in patients with unilateral disc herniation at the L5–S1 disc?

Disc herniation at L5–S1 signifies compression of the S1 nerve root. Sensory deficits occur in the lateral malleolus, lateral foot, heel, and web of the fourth and fifth toes. Motor weakness involves the peroneus longus and brevis, gastrocnemius-soleus complex, and gluteus maximus. The Achilles reflex is usually diminished.

14. What is a far lateral disc herniation?

A far lateral disc herniation occurs when the disc herniation occurs lateral to the spinal canal and neural foramen, producing pressure on the nerve root cephalad to the disc of origin. For example, a far lateral L4/5 disc herniation produces a L4 radiculopathy as opposed to the expected L5 radiculopathy. Conservative treatment is identical to other disc herniations. Surgical management requires an approach lateral to the spinal canal and facet joints.

15. What are the "tension" signs in lumbar disc herniation?

Tension signs are maneuvers that tighten the sciatic nerve and in doing so further compress an inflamed nerve root against a herniated lumbar disc. Variations of the test include the following:

Lasegue's test. This classic straight-leg raising test is performed with the patient in the supine position and the head flat or on a low pillow. One of the patient's hands is placed on the ilium to stabilize the pelvis. The other hand slowly elevates the leg by the heel, with the knee straight. The patient should be questioned as to whether the maneuver produces leg pain. Only when leg pain or radicular symptoms are produced is the test considered positive; back pain alone is not a positive finding.

The bowstring sign. This variation of the straight-leg raising test is performed as usual until pain is elicited. At this point, the knee is flexed, usually with significant reduction of symptoms. Finger pressure applied to the popliteal space over the terminal aspect of the sciatic nerve reestablishes the painful radicular symptoms.

The sitting root test. With the patient sitting and the cervical spine flexed, the knee is extended while the hip remains flexed to 90°. The patient may complain of leg pain or may attempt to extend the hip, again indicating nerve root compression.

Contralateral straight-leg raising test. This test is performed in the same manner as the straight-leg raising test, except that the nonpainful leg is raised. If this maneuver produces the patient's sciatica in the opposite extremity, the test is considered positive. A positive test is highly suggestive of a herniated disc and usually indicates the location of the extrusion. This test is commonly positive in patients who have disc herniations medial to the nerve root in the axilla.

Reverse straight-leg raising test. This test may be done with the patient in a prone position or in a lateral position with the unaffected side down. The test involves hip extension and knee flexion, exactly opposite to the standard straight-leg raising test. A positive result signifies irritation in the roots of the femoral nerve, commonly the L4 nerve root.

16. What is a list?

A list is produced when patients have herniation of a lumbar disc. Herniation that is lateral to the nerve root produces what is called a list away from the side of the irritated nerve root. Herniation of the disc that is medial to the nerve root, however, in what is called the axillary position, usually produces a list toward the side of the irritated nerve root. When the disc herniation is lateral, patients feel that they must move from the side of the irritated nerve in an attempt to draw the nerve root away from the disc fragment. When the herniation is in the axillary position medial to the nerve root, the patient lists toward the side of the nerve root in an attempt at decompression.

17. What other tests should be done in evaluation for lumbar disc disease?

No back examination is complete without evaluation of the peripheral circulation. The posterior tibial and dorsal pedis artery should be examined. Vascular claudication is an important cause of leg pain and may mimic lumbar disc disease. The hip and knee also should be evaluated. Limitations in range of motion of the hip, particularly in rotation, along with groin discomfort, is indicative of hip disease. Tenderness over the piriformis muscle in external rotation may implicate piriformis syndrome. Rectal tone should be evaluated in patients suspected of having cauda equina syndrome.

18. Are rotine radiographs helpful in evaluation of lumbar spine disease?

Only 1–2% of the spine radiographs in patients with back pain between 20 and 50 years of age have unsuspected findings. Most studies have found some disc space narrowing or osteophyte formation in this age group. Spondylolisthesis and spondylolysis may be seen on radiographs, along with some disc space narrowing at the affected level. Such findings, however, are also present in patients with no back pain and no clinically significant pathology.

19. What imaging techniques are used in evaluation of lumbar disc disease?

Myelography. Indications include suspicion of an intraspinal lesion or questionable diagnosis resulting from conflicting clinical findings in other studies. Myelography has value in previously operated spines and in spinal stenosis, especially in conjunction with CT. Water-soluble contrasts are the most popular contrast agents. Because myelography is an invasive study, reactions may occur, including headache, pain, nausea, vomiting, meningitis, and localized infection.

Computed axial tomography. The advantages of CT over myelography include better visualization of lateral lesions, such as foraminal stenosis and lateral disc herniations, lower radiation dose, and absence of adverse reactions. CT generally allows discrimination between neural compression caused by soft tissue and that caused by bone. CT is extremely useful in the diagnosis of lateral or foraminal herniations of the lumbar disc. The disadvantages are that more radiology centers scan the third lumbar through the sacral disc. Higher lesions may be missed if scanning is limited to the levels.

Magnetic resonance imaging. The advantage of MRI over a CT scan includes the ability to demonstrate intraspinal tumors, to examine the entire spine, and to identify degenerative discs. Anatomic detail of neural elements is much better than CT, but MRI does not demonstrate bone anatomy as well as CT.

Bone scan. Bone scans can be used when physicians suspect diseases other than lumbar disc disease or spinal stenosis. Bone scan confirms neoplastic, infectious, traumatic, or arthritic problems of the spine.

20. Is electromyography useful in patients with lumbar disc disease?

Electromyography is commonly used to help in differentiating radicular symptoms from peripheral neuropathy or upper motor neuron lesions and in determining the presence or absence of generalized myopathy.

21. Compare the natural history of conservative and surgical treatment in patients with lumbar disc herniation.

In a controlled prospective study of 280 patients with lumbar disc herniation, treatment included conservative or surgical treatment. The surgically treated group was doing better at 1-year follow-up. However, comparison of the results at 4 and 10 years revealed no statistically significant difference in outcome. Surgery, therefore, provides more rapid relief of pain, but the ultimate endpoint is approximately the same, regardless of treatment.

22. What conservative treatment modalities can be used for patients with acute lumbar disc herniations?

Nonsurgical treatments include bed rest, NSAIDs, narcotic analgesics, oral or epidural corticosteroids, physical therapy, bracing, traction, manipulation, and techniques such as TENS. Epidural steroids may be beneficial in eliminating acute pain but have limited efffectiveness in relieving chronic pain. Only approximately 10% of patients with symptoms and signs ultimately require surgery. Therefore, physicians may expect a 90% relief rate with conservative treatment for patients with lumbar disc disease.

23. What surgical procedure is used for the treatment of lumbar disc disease?

The traditional surgery is laminectomy and lumbar disc excision by means of a midline incision. The paraspinous muscles are stripped from the lamina of the vertebra on each side of the lesion. The lamina is identified, and the ligamentum flavum is excised. Portions of the superior and inferior lamina may be removed. After the nerve root is retracted, the disc herniation identified and then removed, the disc is dissected free of loose fragments. Closure is routine. Patients are allowed to turn in bed, to walk, and to stand. General exercise is begun within the first 48 hours after surgery. Sitting is generally minimized, whereas lying and walking are progressively increased. Patients should refrain from long trips in a car for approximately 3 months. Exercises for lower extremity strength and rehabilitation are begun 6–8 weeks postoperatively. Patients are returned to sitting jobs within 4–6 weeks. The success rate for relief of leg pain is 93%; for relief of low back pain, 80%.

24. Describe microlumbar disc excision.

Microlumbar discectomy requires an operating microscope. The procedure is performed much like an open disc excision and laminectomy, except the laminae are not removed. Microlumbar discectomy requires less dissection and has the potential of less reactive scar tissue. Surgical results are approximately the same as with open disc surgery.

25. What are the complications of lumbar disc surgery?

Cauda equina syndrome	Dural tears
Thrombophlebitis	Nerve root injury
Pulmonary embolism	Cerebral spinal fluid fistula
Wound infection	Laceration of abdominal vessels
Pyogenic spondylitis	Injury to abdominal viscera
Postoperative discitis	

26. What minimally invasive techniques are available to treat lumbar disc herniations?

Most minimally invasive techniques attempt to treat disc herniations contained by the posterior longitudinal ligament (i.e., subligamentous disc herniations) and are ineffective in treating herniations in which a fragment of disc material has migrated cephalad or caudal to the disc space. Percutaneous injection of **chymopapain** into the intervertebral disc has been used in the past to partially dissolve the disc, reducing pressure on the nerve root. Most spine surgeons no longer use chymopapain because it is not very effective, has a small but significant risk of serious allergic reaction, and accelerates the degeneration of the disc, increasing the risk of chronic back pain. **Percutaneous automated discectomy** involves placing a cannula into the disc and aspirating disc material until the patient reports relief of radicular symptoms. This technique is not used widely because of a relatively high failure rate in relieving symptoms and the need to proceed with open techniques. **Endoscopic techniques** have been developed to treat lumbar disc herniations. An intradiscal approach involves placing a cannula within the disc and then removing disc material using an endoscope. A foraminal approach involves placing a cannula into the foramen of the nerve root and then removing disc material using an endoscope. This technique is most useful for far-lateral disc herniations. The most recently developed minimally invasive technique is **microendoscopic discectomy (MED Sofamor Danek).** Microendoscopic discectomy uses a posterior approach identical to standard lumbar discectomy or microdiscectomy. A cannula is docked onto the lamina under fluoroscopic guidance and a laminotomy; ligament removal and discectomy are then performed using a microscope. Migrated disc fragments are accessible using this technique.

SPINAL STENOSIS

27. What is lumbar spinal stenosis?

Lumbar spinal stenosis is an abnormal narrowing of the osteoligamentous vertebral canal and/or vertebral foramina; the result is compression of the dural sac and/or the nerve roots. Lumbar spinal stenosis specifically excludes disc herniation as a causative agent.

28. What is the most common cause for neurologic leg pain in the older population?

Spinal stenosis.

29. What pathology is involved with spinal stenosis?

Spinal stenosis involves the three-joint complex of the disc facet joint and intervertebral disc. The intervertebral disc usually undergoes significant degenerative changes. Subsequent degeneration leads to collapse of the disc and facet arthritis, which tend to narrow the neural foramina progressively. Soft-tissue impression may result anteriorly from the disc or posteriorly from ligamentum flavum. On a mechanical basis, the neural foramina are then more narrowed with lumbar extension than with lumbar flexion. The site of such compression may either be centrally within the canal or more laterally within the lateral recess or neural foramina. Canal narrowing may be congenital, involving genetic conditions such as achondroplasia, or due to degenerative scoliosis or spondylolisthesis.

30. What is the classification of spinal stenosis?

Congenital	Acquired
Idiopathic	Degenerative
Achondroplastic	Central canal

Acquired *(cont.)*

Peripheral canal, lateral recesses,
  nerve root canals
Degenerative spondylolisthesis
Iatrogenic
  Postlaminectomy
  Postfusion

Postchemonucleolysis
Posttraumatic
Miscellaneous
  Paget's disease
  Diffuse interstitial skeletal hypertrophy

31. What is the most common cause of spinal stenosis?
Acquired degenerative spinal stenosis.

32. What is the differential diagnosis of spinal stenosis?
- Disc herniation
- Cauda equina syndrome
- Spinal cord tumor
- Primary or metastatic vertebral body tumors
- Infections
- Fractures
- Vascular insufficiency
- Peripheral neuropathy

33. Describe the epidemiology of spinal stenosis.
The age at onset of symptons is variable, but the fifth and sixth decades are common. Achondroplasia usually presents in the fourth decade. Degenerative spondylolisthesis is infrequent in patients younger than 50 years. Distribution between men and women is equal. Degenerative spinal stenosis occurs more frequently in workers who have done heavy manual labor.

34. Describe the common history in patients with spinal stenosis.
Low back pain is a common finding but usually is not the reason for referral to an orthopedic surgeon. Patients describe feelings of aching and stiffness that often worsen with weather changes. The back pain is usually insidious rather than acute in onset. Pain is relieved with rest and generally aggravated by overactivity. Patients also describe buttock discomfort, tightness, or burning, induced by walking or standing. Patients complain of limited spine movement and increased amount of pain with extension of the spine. Urinary dysfunction is uncommon but occurs in approximately 3–4% of cases.

35. What presenting symptom is the hallmark of spinal stenosis?
Patients complain of pain that increases with walking or standing, whereas sitting and leaning forward or lying down alleviates the discomfort.

36. Distinguish neurogenic claudication from vascular claudication.
With vascular claudication, the claudication distance is usually fixed. Patients may stand in an erect position for relief of pain, which is brought on by walking uphill or bicycle riding. Pain is described as a cramp or a tightness in the calf. With neurogenic claudication, the claudication distance is generally variable. Patients must sit or get in a flexed position for relief of pain; walking uphill and bicycle riding usually do not induce pain. Patients describe neurogenic claudication as numbness, ache, or sharp pain; cramping is usually not included.

37. What radiographic examinations are important in the diagnosis of spinal stenosis?
Both CT scan and MRI provide excellent delineation of the stenotic areas. True stenosis is considered absolute with a 10–12 mm sagittal diameter. Both studies show the neural foramina, facet joints, ligamentum flavum, and any compression on the spinal canal. Other abnormalities, including posttraumatic deformities, overgrowth of spinal fusions, Paget's disease, vertebral ligament hypertrophy, and intraspinal masses also can be identified.

38. What is the treatment for spinal stenosis?
Nonoperative treatment involves a vigorous physical therapy program emphasizing postural changes, stretching, and strengthening of the tightened lumbar and lower extremity mus-

culature. Biofeedback may be helpful. Transcutaneous electrical nerve stimulator units occasionally have been successful in relieving acute pain. Epidural steroids remain controversial. NSAIDs, particularly aspirin, may reduce leg and back pain. Braces may be used to decrease lumbar lordosis.

39. What are the indications for surgery with spinal stenosis?

Surgery is indicated in patients with severe spinal stenosis and intractable pain and in patients who fail an appropriate nonoperative course. Other causes of pain should be ruled out. Surgery is elective, except in the presence of bowel or bladder dysfunction.

40. What is the surgical treatment for spinal stenosis?

Surgical treatment involves removal of the lamina, ligamentum flava, spinous process, medial facets, and arthritis spurs in the lateral recesses. Attempts should be made to leave portions of the facet joints intact.

41. What complications are seen after decompression for spinal stenosis?

Instability	Arachnoiditis	Nerve root injury
Dural tears	Infection	Epidural scarring

LUMBAR FUSION

42. What are the indications for lumbar fusion?

Lumbar fusion is indicated for unstable fractures, symptomatic spondylolysis and spondylolisthesis, recurrent disc herniations, and disc degeneration (a.k.a. segmental instability). Examples of unstable lumbar fractures include burst fractures with greater than 50% canal compromise, compression fractures with significant angulation ($> 35\%$), or chance fractures.

43. When is fusion indicated for spondylolysis and spondylolisthesis?

Patients who have significant back and/or radicular pain are candidates for decompression and possibly fusion if their symptoms do not respond to appropriate conservative care. Patients with spondylolysis without spondylolisthesis have been treated with decompression alone or with simultaneous fusion. Patients with spondylolysis and spondylolisthesis are usually treated with decompression and fusion. The treatment of patients with spinal stenosis and degenerative spondylolisthesis is controversial. Although some studies have shown improved outcome in patients treated with decompression and fusion, other studies have shown similar results with decompression alone.

44. When is fusion indicated for recurrent lumbar disc herniations?

Recurrent lumbar disc herniations may occur in up to 10–15% of patients. Fusion is usually not indicated for the first recurrent disc herniation. However, after the second recurrent disc herniation, fusion is often recommended, especially if the two recurrences occur soon after the original disc herniation.

45. When is fusion recommended for lumbar disc degeneration?

Fusion for lumbar disc degeneration is indicated for the treatment of low back pain of discogenic origin refractory to extensive conservative care (usually at least 6 months). Determining who may benefit from lumbar fusion for disc degeneration is a difficult decision. The primary challenge is determining whether the back pain originates from the disc or from other sources. Some surgeons rely on the appearance of the disc on MRI and x-ray to determine whether the back pain originates from the disc. A flattened disc with low signal characteristics on T2-weighted images is an indication of disc degeneration. Other surgeons rely on discography to determine whether a disc is the source of back pain. Discography involves the injection of contrast material into the disc space under fluoroscopic guidance. A discogram is considered positive if it provokes the patient's typical back pain or if an anatomic defect such as an annular tear is noted.

46. What are the surgical options available for lumbar fusion?

Lumbar fusion can be performed from a posterior approach with or without the simultaneous use of instrumentation. During a posterolateral fusion, bone graft is placed over the decorticated transverse processes, lateral facet joints, and sacral ala. During a posterior lumbar interbody fusion (PLIF), bone graft is placed into the disc space from a posterior approach. Spinal instrumentation increases fusion rates, especially if instability or spondylolisthesis is present. Posterior instrumentation usually involves placement of pedicle screws connected together with rods.

Lumbar fusion can also be performed from an anterior (either trans- or retroperitoneal) approach. During an anterior lumbar interbody fusion (ALIF), bone graft is placed into the disc space anteriorly and is often accompanied by posterior instrumentation.

More recently, threaded titanium cages have been developed that are placed into the disc space from either an anterior or posterior approach (ALIF or PLIF). Simultaneous pedicle screw instrumentation is usually not necessary because the cages provide adequate stability. Endoscopic techniques have been developed for the anterior placement of cages.

BIBLIOGRAPHY

1. Bridwell KH, DeWald RL, et al (eds): The Textbook of Spinal Surgery, 2nd ed. Philadelphia, Lippincott-Raven, 1997.
2. Frymoyer JW: Back pain and sciatica. N Engl J Med 318:291–300, 1988.
3. Lonstein JE, Winter RB, Bradford DS, Ogilvie JW (eds): Moe's Textbook of Scoliosis and Other Spinal Deformities, 3rd ed. Philadelphia, W.B. Saunders, 1995.
4. Herkowitz HN: Spinal stenosis: Clinical evaluation. In Instructional Course Lectures, vol XLI. Rosemont, IL, American Academy of Orthopedic Surgeons, 1992, pp 183–185.
5. McCowin PR, Borenstein D, Wiesel SW: The current approach to the medical diagnosis of low back pain. Orthop Clin North Am 22:315–325, 1991.
6. Menezes AH, Sonntag VK (eds): Principles of Spinal Surgery. New York, McGraw-Hill, 1996.
7. Tuite GF, et al: Outcome after laminectomy for lumbar spinal stenosis. Part I: Clinical correlations. J Neurosurg 81:699–706, 1994.

50. SCOLIOSIS AND KYPHOSIS

Glen M. Ginsburg, M.D.

1. What two deviations of the spine must be present in order to classify a curvature as scoliosis?

For a spinal deformity to be classified as scoliosis, both lateral (coronal plane) curvature and rotation (transverse plane) must be present.

2. What types of scoliosis are most commonly seen?

- Idiopathic (infantile, juvenile and adolescent)
- Congenital
- Neuromuscular
- Nonstructural

Scoliosis and kyphosis are also seen in other disease processes:

- Neurofibromatosis
- Mesenchymal (Marfan syndrome, Ehlers-Danlos syndrome)
- Tumors
- Osteochondrodystrophy (dwarfism)
- Traumatic (spinal cord) injuries
- Infections
- Metabolic disorders
- Spondylolisthesis
- Degenerative

3. What is the incidence of idiopathic scoliosis?

The incidence of scoliosis has been reported to range from 3% to 5%, with a slightly higher female predominance.

4. What are the three types of idiopathic scoliosis and their respective age groups?

The three types of congenital scoliosis are infantile (birth to 3 years), juvenile (3 years to puberty), and adolescent (at or just after puberty).

5. What is the most common curve pattern seen in infantile idiopathic scoliosis?

The most common curve pattern seen in infantile idiopathic scoliosis is a convex left thoracic curve, unlike adolescent idiopathic scoliosis, in which a left thoracic curve is rare and often is associated with intraspinal pathology.

6. Which radiographic measurement techniques are currently used to determine the prognosis of infantile idiopathic scoliosis?

The rib-vertebral angle difference of Mehta (RVAD) measures the intersection of a line perpendicular to the apical vertebral end plate and a line drawn for the midneck to the midhead of the right and left corresponding ribs A difference > 20° means that curve progression is likely. The rib phase describes the amount of overlap between the rib head and the vertebral body. A phase one rib does not overlap the body, and progression is unlikely. A phase two rib overlaps the vertebral body and means that progression is likely.

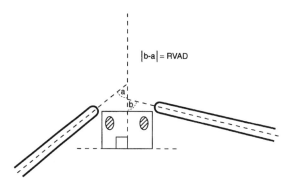

7. What two developmental anomalies of the vertebral angle are responsible for the deformities seen in congenital scoliosis?

Congenital scoliosis results from either a failure of formation or a failure of segmentation of the vertebral anlage. Examples of failure of formation include hemivertebrae and butterfly vertebrae. Examples of failure of segmentation include unilateral bars and block vertebrae.

8. What other congenital anomalies (non-musculoskeletal) are seen in association with congenital scoliosis?

Genitourinary anomalies are seen in up to 33% of children with congenital scoliosis. Klippel-Feil syndrome is seen in 25%. Fifteen percent have intraspinal anomalies, and 10% have congenital heart defects.

9. What studies (in addition to radiographs) should be performed when congenital scoliosis is discovered?

Because of the prevalence of genitourinary anomalies associated with congenital scoliosis, an ultrasound examination of the retroperitoneum may reveal anomalies of the kidneys and the urinary collection system. Because of the incidence of intraspinal anomalies reported in a recent study of magnetic resonance imaging (MRI) evaluations of congenital spine deformities (31%),

MRI should probably be performed as part of the initial evaluation of congenital scoliosis, even in the absence of clinical findings.

10. What does the term *segmentation* mean in reference to hemivertebra?

Segmentation of a hemivertebra means that it is separated from the adjacent vertebral body by a disc (and growth plate). A hemivertebra may be fully segmented (separated by a disc on both sides), semisegmented (a disc on one side only), or nonsegmented (no discs on either side). Obviously, a fully segmented hemivertebra has the greatest potential for growth.

11. What does the term *hemimetameric shift* mean?

Hemimetameric shift is the presence of hemivertebra on opposite sides of the spine that often will balance one another. This combination of deformities is often benign.

12. Which of the vertebral anomalies seen in congenital scoliosis causes the most rapid progression of deformity?

The most rapid progression of deformity seen in congenital scoliosis is a fully segmented hemivertebra with a contralateral unsegmented bar (up to 10°/year).

13. What is the treatment of choice for the anomalies described in questions 8–11?

The treatment of choice for a hemivertebra and a contralateral unsegmented bar is an in situ fusion as soon as the diagnosis is made. The fusion should include a mobile segment above and below the bar. Recent literature offers significant support for excision of fully segmented hemivertebra, either from a combined anterior and posterior approach, or from a posterior approach. This treatment allows immediate correction of the deformity that withstands the effects of growth.

14. According to the Scoliosis Research Society, what is the minimal amount of lateral (coronal) curvature necessary to qualify as scoliosis?

Lateral (coronal) curvatures $< 10°$ are generally not referred to as scoliosis.

15. Name three conditions that may cause lateral (coronal) curvature of the spine not associated with rotation (i.e., not true scoliosis).

Lateral (coronal) curvature of the spine without rotation can be seen with leg length discrepancy, posterior element tumors such as osteoid osteoma and osteoblastomas, and psychiatric conditions such as hysterical scoliosis.

16. What is the most frequently used clinical tool to measure spinal rotation?

The most commonly used clinical tool to measure spinal rotation is the scoliometer, which is drawn over the spinous processes of the patient while he or she bends at the waist with straight knees and dangling arms. The rotations in degrees are recorded at each spinal level.

17. How much spinal rotation should be present in order for a patient to be referred to an orthopaedic surgeon from a school nurse or primary care physician?

Under the guidelines of the Scoliosis Research Society, spinal rotations of greater than 7–8° are appropriate for referral to an orthopaedic surgeon. This amount of rotation corresponds to approximately 20° of coronal curvature on radiographs. At 5° of rotation, the false positive rate for scoliosis referral (curves $< 10°$) was 36%.

18. What spinal radiograph measurement system is currently the most widely used, and how are radiographs measured with this system?

The Cobb method of radiographic measurement is currently the most widely used measurement system. A postero-anterior 3-ft standing radiograph is taken of the entire spine, including the iliac crests from a 6-ft distance. The superior and inferior vertebra of each curve is located. The superior and inferior surfaces of the vertebrae tilt maximally into the concavity of the curve.

The superior and inferior surfaces of these vertebrae tilt maximally into the concavity of the curve. Perpendicular lines are then constructed from the superior end plate of the superior end vertebra and the inferior endplate of the inferior end vertebra. The angle subtended by the intersection of these two lines is the magnitude of the curve.

19. How are the apical and end vertebrae determined?

The vertebra that is maximally rotated and/or the most deviated from the vertical axis of the patient. More than one apical vertebra in a curve may be present if the apex is at a disc space. The superior end vertebra is the most cephalad vertebra of a curve whose superior surface tilts maximally into the concavity of the curve. The inferior end vertebra is the most caudad vertebra of a curve whose inferior surface tilts maximally into the concavity of the curve.

20. What are the neutral and stable vertebrae?

The neutral vertebrae are the first non-rotated vertebrae at the caudal and cranial ends of a curve. The stable vertebra is the vertebra that is bisected by the midsacral line (a vertical line erected from the S1 spinous process).

21. Describe the King classification of adolescent idiopathic scoliosis.

The King classification of thoracic idiopathic curves describes five patterns.

King I: a double thoracic and lumbar curve in which the lumbar curve is larger than the thoracic curve

King II: a structural thoracic curve and a compensatory lumbar curve

King III: a single thoracic curve with either no lumbar curve or a small lumbar curve that does not cross the midline

King IV: a long thoracolumbar curve in which L4 tilts into the curve

King V: represents a double thoracic curve in which T1 tilts into the structural upper curve that is structural on side bending.

22. What is the major deficiency of the King classification system for adolescent idiopathic scoliosis?

The King classification system does not take into account the sagittal profile of the spine, which is an important determinant of the proximal and distal extent of the spinal fusion. The system developed and recently published by Lenke et al. is a two-dimensional system that takes into account both the coronal curvature of the spine as well as the sagittal alignment of the spine. By accounting for the relative hypo- or hyperkyphosis of the thoracic spine in scoliosis, the decision between anterior or posterior spinal fusion is more predictable. This option was not recognized when the King classification was devised. The new system has demonstrated significant inter- and intraobserver reliability.

23. Describe the Nash-Moe classification of vertebral rotation.

The Nash-Moe classification of vertebral rotation is based on the radiographic appearance of the apical vertebral pedicle shadows in reference to the sides of the vertebra. In grade 0 rotation,

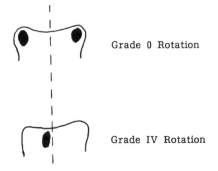

Grade 0 Rotation

Grade IV Rotation

the pedicles of the apical vertebra are equidistant from the sides of the vertebra. In grade IV rotation, one pedicle has crossed the midline.

24. Describe the Risser radiographic classification of skeletal maturity.
The Risser classification of skeletal maturity is based on the ossification pattern of the iliac crest epiphysis. Ossification occurs from the anterior superior iliac spine to the posterior superior iliac spine.
Excursion of ossification is divided into four grades:

Risser 1: 25% excursion   **Risser 4:** 100% (complete) excursion
Risser 2: 50% excursion   **Risser 5:** fusion of the epiphysis to the ilium,
Risser 3: 75% excursion   representing the end of spinal growth

25. What are the risk factors for progression of curvature in adolescent idiopathic scoliosis?
The risk factors for progression of idiopathic scoliosis are curve magnitude (the larger the curve, the greater the risk), growth potential of the patient (the more growth remaining, the greater the risk), and the curve type (double curves have a greater risk of progression). Female sex has not been statistically proved to increase the risk of progression because of the small numbers of males in the large reported series.

26. When is nonsurgical treatment of adolescent idiopathic scoliosis appropriate?
No treatment is generally required for patients with curves measuring $< 20°$. Nonsurgical treatment is indicated for curves measuring between $20°$ and 40–$45°$ in skeletally immature patients.

27. What nonsurgical treatment of adolescent idiopathic scoliosis has been shown to alter the natural history of the disease?
The only nonsurgical treatment of adolescent idiopathic scoliosis that has been shown to alter the natural history is the use of a spinal orthotic (brace). Bracing is indicated in the skeletally immature patient (Risser ≤ 3) who presents with a curve of $25°$–$45°$, or who presents with a curve of $< 25°$ with a history of documented progression. Electrical stimulation, exercises, manipulation, and biofeedback have not been shown to alter the natural history.

28. What are the three most common types of braces used for adolescent idiopathic scoliosis, and how are they most effectively used?
The three most common types of spinal braces are the Milwaukee (apex T8 and above), TLSO or Boston (apex below T8), and the Charleston bending brace (nighttime use only).

29. What are the indications for operative treatment of adolescent idiopathic scoliosis?
Operative treatment of adolescent idiopathic scoliosis is recommended for curves > 40–$45°$ in the skeletally immature patient, curves that progress despite bracing, or curves > 50–$60°$ in the mature adolescent.

30. Describe the crankshaft phenomenon. How is this complication avoided?
The crankshaft phenomenon is the progression of spinal curvature despite solid posterior arthrodesis. It was described by Dubousset in 1973 and is thought to be related to continued anterior spinal growth against a posterior tether. This complication can be avoided by combining the posterior fusion with an anterior arthrodesis and is recommended in premenarchal patients, in patients who are Risser 1 or less, or in patients < 10 years of age with open triradiate cartilage.

31. What is kyphosis?
Kyphosis is a spinal deformity characterized by an increase in the posterior convex angulation in the sagittal plane. The normal posterior convex angulation of the thoracic spine is 20–$40°$ measured by the Cobb method.

32. What types of kyphosis are normally seen?
- Scheuermann's
- Postlaminectomy
- Postural congenital
- Myelomeningocele
- Developmental (achondroplasia)
- Posttraumatic

33. Describe the two congenital defects that are most commonly seen in congenital kyphosis.

The two congenital defects commonly associated with congenital kyphosis are failure of formation (hemivertebra) and failure of segmentation (anterior unsegmented bar).

34. Which type of congenital kyphosis carries the greatest risk for neurologic impairment?

Failure of anterior formation of the vertebral body carries a high risk for paraplegia due to tethering of the cord over the sharp kyphus. Early (between 1 and 3 years of age) posterior fusion is the treatment of choice for this type of congenital kyphosis.

35. What is Scheuermann's kyphosis?

Scheuermann's kyphosis is a disorder of endochondral ossification that affects the vertebral endplates and ring apophyses, resulting in intravertebral disc herniation, anterior wedging of consecutive vertebra ($> 5°$ in three adjacent thoracic vertebrae), and a fixed thoracolumbar kyphosis.

36. What is the prevalence of Scheuermann's kyphosis?

The prevalence of Scheuermann's kyphosis has been estimated to be between 0.4% and 8% of the general population, mainly affecting adolescents at puberty. The male:female ratio is about equal.

37. What is the etiology of Scheuermann's kyphosis?

The exact etiology of Scheuermann's kyphosis is unknown. A familial predilection has been theorized. Increased height and repetitive loading may be inciting factors.

38. What are the most common presenting symptoms of Scheuermann's kyphosis?

The most common presenting symptoms of Scheuermann's kyphosis are spinal deformity and pain at the apex, which is aggravated by prolonged sitting, standing, and activity. This disorder may account for as much at one-third of back pain complaints in pediatric patients.

39. What is the initial treatment of Scheuermann's kyphosis?

The initial treatment of Scheuermann's kyphosis is nonsurgical, consisting of thoracic extension, abdominal strengthening exercises, and avoidance of heavy lifting. Symptoms usually resolve by the end of growth.

40. When is bracing recommended for Schuermann's kyphosis?

Bracing is recommended in Scheuermann's kyphosis when the curve exceeds 70° in the skeletally immature patient. A Milwaukee brace is recommended for the thoracic form of the disease and a TLSO can be used for the atypical lumbar form. According to a recent natural history study, patients treated conservatively may have more pain at the apex of the curve as adults, but their overall quality of life should not be affected.

41. When is surgery recommended for Scheuermann's kyphosis?

Surgery is recommended for Scheuermann's kyphosis if the curve exceeds 75° and the patient is symptomatic or if neurologic signs appear. Restrictive lung disease may be seen if the kyphosis exceeds 100°.

42. What is the surgical treatment of choice for Scheuermann's kyphosis?

The surgical treatment of choice for symptomatic Scheuermann's kyphosis is anterior release and fusion (preferably with anterior column support), followed by a posterior arthrodesis with instrumentation of the entire kyphotic segment.

BIBLIOGRAPHY

1. Bodner RJ, Heyman S, Drummond DS, Gregg JR: The use of single-photon emission computed tomography (SPECT) in the diagnosis of low-back pain in young patients. Spine 13:1155–1160, 1988.
2. Freeman BL: Scoliosis and kyphosis. In Canale ST (ed): Campbell's Operative Orthopaedics, 9th ed. St. Louis, Mosby, 1998, pp 2849–2969.
3. Ginsburg GM, Bassett GS: Back pain in children and adolescents: Evaluation and differential diagnosis. J Am Acad Orthop 5:67–78, 1997.
4. Klemme WR, Polly DW, Orchowski JR: Hemivertebral Excision for congenital scoliosis in very young chlidren. J Pediatr Orthop 21; 761–764, 2001.
5. Lenke LG, Betz RR, Harms J, et al: Adolescent idiopathic scoliosis: A new classification to determine extent of spinal arthrodesis. J. Bone Joint Surg 83A:1169–1181, 2001.
6. Lonstein JE: Idiopathic scoliosis. In Lonstein JE, Winter RB, Bradford DS, Ogilvie TW (eds): Moe's Textbook of Scoliosis and Other Spinal Deformities, 2nd ed. Philadelphia, W.B. Saunders, 1995.
7. McMaster MJ: Congenital scoliosis caused by a unilateral failure of vertebral segmentation with contralateral hemivertebrae. Spine 23:998–1005, 1998.
8. McMaster MJ, Singh H: Natural history of congenital kyphosis and kyphoscoliosis: A study of 112 patients. J Bone Joint Surg 81A:1367–1383, 1999.
9. Murray PM, Weinstein SL, Spratt KF: The natural history and long-term follow-up of Scheuermann's kyphosis. J Bone Joint Surg 75A:236–247, 1993.
10. Suh SW, Sarwark JF, Vora A, Huang BK: Evaluating congenital spine deformities for intraspinal anomalies with magnetic resonance imaging. J Pediatr Orthop 21:525–531, 2001.

51. SPONDYLOLYSIS AND SPONDYLOLISTHESIS

Glen M. Ginsburg, M.D.

1. Define spondylolysis.

Spondylolysis describes a defect in the pars interarticularis, usually affecting the lumbar spine.

2. Define spondylolisthesis.

Spondylolisthesis describes the slipping forward of an upper vertebral segment on the lower segment, usually after a bilateral pars defect (spondylolysis) at the same level.

3. What is the incidence of spondylolisthesis in the general population?

The incidence of spondylolisthesis is 5% for the general population. The incidence in adult Caucasian males is 5–6% and in females is 2–3%. In Eskimos, the incidence has been reported to be 50% and is < 3% in African-Americans. The incidence increases up to the age of 20 years and then remains constant. This lesion is rarely seen in children < 5 years of age.

4. Spondylolysis is strongly associated with what other adolescent spinal condition?

Spondylolysis is seen frequently in association with Scheuermann's kyphosis, in which the excessive lumbar lordosis places the L5–S1 articulation under shear. A study published in 1987 demonstrated a 50% incidence of spondylolysis in 18 patients with Scheuermann's kyphosis. The authors recommend obtaining oblique lumbar spine radiographs for patients with Scheuermann's kyphosis who develop low back pain.

5. Name the five common types of spondylolisthesis.

Dysplastic, isthmic, degenerative, traumatic, and pathologic.

6. Describe the congenital defect associated with dysplastic spondylolisthesis.

The congenital defect associated with dysplastic spondylolisthesis is a deficiency in the inferior facets of L5 and/or the superior facets of S1, along with the elongation of the pars interarticularis. The elongated pars may not have a segmental defect and has been likened to "pulled taffy."

7. What is the most common presenting symptom of spondylolysis or spondylolisthesis?

In both children and adults the most common presenting symptom of spondylolysis and spondylolisthesis is pain. In one study, spondylolisthesis was found in 47% of adolescent athletes complaining of back pain. The pain is usually lumbar in location and mild but may radiate to the posterior thighs with increasing degrees of slip.

8. What repetitive motion has been postulated as the inciting factor in the development of isthmic spondylolisthesis?

The defect in isthmic spondylolisthesis has been attributed to repetitive hyperextension, which causes shear of the posterior elements.

9. Which sports have been linked to the development of isthmic spondylolisthesis?

Sports with cyclic flexion-extension activity have been positively associated with isthmic spondylolisthesis. An increased incidence has been reported in diving, weightlifting, wrestling, and gymnastics.

10. What physical findings have been associated with spondylolisthesis?

Several physical findings are commonly associated with spondylolisthesis. Hamstring tightness is common, causing a stiff-legged gait with a short stride length ("pelvic waddle"). Forward bending is limited. Pain may be found on palpation of the paraspinal muscles. If the slip is severe, a step-off may be seen at the L5–S1 level. The buttocks may appear heart-shaped due to the verticality of the sacrum. The abdomen will protrude, causing the appearance of a transverse abdominal crease.

11. Describe the difference between the Scotty dog sign and the greyhound sign.

The Scotty dog sign is the radiographic appearance of the pars interarticularis defect seen on oblique films in isthmic spondylolisthesis. The actual defect resembles a collar around the Scotty dog's neck. The greyhound sign is the radiographic appearance of the elongated pars interarticularis of L5 seen in dysplastic spondylolisthesis.

12. Define stress reaction.

Stress reaction refers to the phase of spondylolysis before the appearance of the actual bony defect. Radiographically, a stress reaction can be associated with sclerosis or elongation of the pars. It is often seen with on the contralateral side of a unilateral spondylolysis.

13. How long after the onset of symptoms of back pain before a technetium bone scan shows increased uptake at the level of the pars interarticularis?

A technetium bone scan delineates an acute lesion within 5–7 days of the onset of symptoms.

14. What is the best study to diagnose spondylolysis in symptomatic patients with normal radiographs and bone scan?

Single photon emission computed tomography (SPECT) has proved effective in patients with positive symptoms and normal radiographs and bone scans. This test has been shown to be the most sensitive method of diagnosing stress reactions, allowing early diagnosis and treatment before the development of an established lysis.

15. How are the slip percentage and slip angle determined?

Slip percentage is measured by representing the distance between the posterior border of the body of L5 and the posterior border of the body of S1 as a percentage of the anteroposterior di-

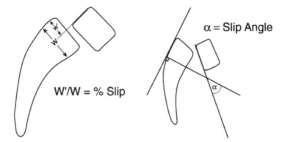

ameter of S1. The **slip angle** is measured by drawing a perpendicular to a line along the posterior border of the sacrum and another line parallel to the inferior endplate of L5. The angle subtended by the intersection of these two lines is the slip angle.

16. How is spondylolisthesis classified?
The commonly accepted classification system for spondylolisthesis was devised by Meyerding. No anterior slip of the upper vertebral body on the lower is grade 0; 1–25% slippage is grade I; 26–50% slippage is grade II; 51–75% is grade III; and 76–100% is grade IV. Complete anterior dislocation of the upper on lower vertebral body is called spondyloptosis.

17. What percentage of spondylolisthesis has occurred at the time of the first radiograph in symptomatic patients?
According to a study of 272 patients by Seitsalo et al, 90% of the slip had occurred by the time that the patient was first seen.

18. Which spinal segments are most commonly affected by spondylolysis/listhesis?
The most common spondylolisthetic level is L5–S1, followed by L4–L5 and then L3–L4. Slips higher than L5 are usually seen in young adults, not in children or adolescents.

19. What is the treatment of choice for spondylolysis and grade I spondylolisthesis?
The treatment of choice for spondylolysis and grade I spondylolisthesis associated with a history of recent injury and short duration of symptoms involves restriction of aggravating activities and a regimen of muscle strengthening for the back and abdomen. Healing may be monitored by the resolution of back pain and hamstring tightness. If symptoms do not resolve and a bone scan shows increased uptake in the area of the pars, a program of rest, nonsteroidal anti-inflammatory medications, and application of a TLSO or cast with a pantaloon extension down one thigh usually alleviates symptoms. The pantaloon portion of the brace may be removed after pain resolves. If symptoms persist despite immobilization and the bone scan becomes "cold," primary repair of small defects (≤ 2 mm) with internal fixation and bone grafting has been successful for L1–L4 defects in patients younger than 25 years of age. (See figure next page.)

20. What is the Gill procedure? What role does it play in the treatment of spondylolysis/listhesis?
The Gill procedure involves complete removal of the loose laminar fragment and fibrocartilagenous pars defect, and has no role in the treatment of spondylolisthesis because it further destabilizes the spine. This procedure should always be combined with arthrodesis in young patients.

21. Define the three columns of the spine as described by Denis.
The posterior column includes the spinous process, lamina, facets, pedicles, and posterior ligamentous structures. The middle column consists of the posterior vertebral body, posterior annulus fibrosus, and posterior longitudinal ligament. The anterior column consists of the anterior vertebral body, anterior annulus fibrosus, and anterior longitudinal ligament.

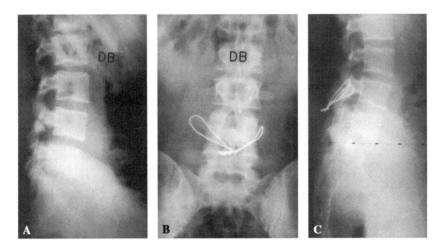

A, L4/L5 spondylolysis. *B*, Anteroposterior (AP) radiograph after fusion with bone graft and fixation. *C*, Lateral radiograph after fusion with bone graft and fixation.

22. What is the treatment of choice for spondylolisthesis of 25–50%?

Grade II slips in asymptomatic patients should be followed every 4–6 months with spot lateral radiographs of the lumbosacral junction until the end of growth. In situ posterolateral fusion of L5–S1 remains the gold standard for patients with progressive slips, persistent back pain, or neurologic deficits.

23. What is the treatment of choice for spondylolisthesis of 50–75%?

In grade III slips, the procedure of choice is in situ posterolateral fusion, including L4 in the arthrodesis. Intertransverse fusion may be performed by either a midline incision with two paraspinal fascial incisions or by two paraspinal skin incisions. Anterior fusion alone, in the absence of posterior column stabilization, is not biomechanically stable and is contraindicated.

24. What are the current indications for reduction of spondylolisthesis?

Reduction of spondylolisthesis is currently reserved for high-grade slips (grade III and IV) with a sagittal imbalance that is functionally debilitating or cosmetically unacceptable or in the presence of a neurologic deficit in which a decompressive laminectomy would jeopardize the fusion. Thorough nerve root decompression should be done before any reduction attempt.

25. What methods are currently used for slip reduction?

Current methods for slip reduction include closed reduction by gradual pelvic extension with or without halo-skin traction, followed by segmental posterior instrumentation and posterolateral bone grafting. The use of anterior column support (either anterior or posterior interbody fusion) may preserve the slip angle correction.

26. What is the most common neurologic injury seen with spondylolisthesis reduction maneuvers?

Injury to the L5 nerve root has been described in several studies reporting the results of high-grade spondylolisthesis reductions. The strain per increment of reduction increased rapidly during the second half of reductions in human cadaveric spines. Partial reduction of high-grade slips may be safer than full reduction, as long as the slip angle is improved.

BIBLIOGRAPHY

1. Askar Z, Wardlaw D, Koti M: Scott wiring for direct repair of lumbar spondylolysis. Spine 15:354–357, 2003.
2. Connolly PJ, Fredrickson, BE: Surgical management of isthmic and dysplastic spondylolisthesis and spondylolysis. In Fardon DF, Garfin SR (eds): Orthopaedic Knowledge Update Spine, 2nd ed. Rosemont IL, American Academy of Orthopaedic Surgeons, 2002.
3. Denis F: Spinal instability as defined by the three-column spine concept in acute spinal trauma. Clin Othop 189:65–76, 1994.
4. Dubousset J: Treatment of spondylolysis and spondylolisthesis in children and adolescents. Clin Orthop 337:77–85, 1997.
5. Freeman BL: Scoliosis and kyphosis. In Canale ST (ed): Campbell's Operative Orthopaedics, 9th ed. St. Louis, Mosby, 1998, pp 2952–2961.
6. Ginsburg GM, Bassett GS: Back pain in children and adolescents: Evaluation and differential diagnosis. J Am Acad Orthop 5:67–78, 1997.
7. Hensinger RN: Current concepts review: Spondylolysis and spondylolisthesis in children and adolescents. J Bone Joint Surg 71A:1098–1107, 1989.
8. Ogilvie JW, Sherman J: Spondylolysis in Scheuermann's disease. Spine 12:251–253, 1987.
9. Omey ML, Michaeli LJ, Gerbino PG: Idiopathic scoliosis and spondylolysis in the female athlete. Tips for treatment. Clin Orthop 372:74–84, 2000.
10. Petraco DM, Spivak JM, Cappadona JG, et al: An anatomic evaluation of L% nerve stretch in spondylolisthesis reduction. Spine 21:1133–1138, 1996.
11. Seitsalo S, Osterman K, Hyvarinen H, et al: Progression of spondylolisthesis in children and adolescents: A long-term follow-up of 272 patients. Spine 16:417–421, 1991.

52. SPINAL TRAUMA

Randall D. Neumann, M.D., and Jonathan Fuller, M.D.

1. Discuss the mechanism of spinal injury.

It is helpful to think of the spine as divided into three columns. The anterior column includes the anterior longitudinal ligament, the anterior portion of the annulus, and the anterior half of the vertebral body. The middle column consists of the posterior longitudinal ligament, the posterior portion of the annulus, and the posterior portion of the vertebral body. The posterior column is made up of the pedicles, facets, lamina, and posterior ligamentous complex, including the interspinal ligaments, ligamentum flavum, and facet joint capsule. These columns may fail individually or in combination as a result of four basic mechanisms of injury: (1) compression, (2) distraction, (3) rotation, and (4) shear forces. These forces result in the most common major types of spinal fractures.

2. What is the conus medullaris?

The conus medullaris is the end of the spinal cord and is usually found at the level of the first or second lumbar vertebra in a vertebral disc.

3. What is the cauda equina?

Below the level of the conus medullaris, the spinal canal is filled with the cauda equina, which consists of the motor and sensory nerve roots. These roots are less likely to be injured because they have more room in the canal and are not tethered to the same degree as the spinal cord.

4. Describe the sensory levels in the lower extremity.

Sensory Levels in the Lower Extremity

SENSORY LEVEL	AREA OF INNERVATION
L2	Anterior thigh
L3	Anterior knee
L4	Anterior lateral ankle
L5	Dorsum of the great and second toe
S1	Lateral side of the foot
S2	Posterior calf
S2–S5	Perianal sensation

5. Describe the muscle groups and their respective nerve root innervations in lower extremity examination.

Muscle Groups and Nerve Root Innervations

NERVE ROOT	MUSCLE GROUP
L1–L2	Hip adductors
L3–L4	Knee extension
L5–S1	Knee flexion
L5	Great toe extension
S1	Great toe flexion

6. What is neurogenic shock?
Neurogenic shock is defined as vascular hypotension with bradycardia as a result of spinal injury. Neurogenic shock is attributed to the traumatic disruption of the sympathetic outflow and unopposed vagal tone.

7. What is spinal shock?
Spinal shock is defined as a dysfunction of the nervous tissue of the spinal cord based on physiologic rather than structural disruption; it occurs after spinal cord injury. Shock is resolved when reflex arcs, including the bulbocavernosus reflex, resume function.

8. What is the bulbocavernosus reflex?
The bulbocavernosus reflex involves the S1, S2, and S3 nerve roots and a spinal cord-mediated reflex arch. Bulbocavernosus reflexes are tested by compressing the glans penis and observing contraction of the anal sphincter. When this reflex returns, spinal shock is resolved.

9. What is sacral sparing?
Sacral sparing means that an incomplete spinal cord lesion is present, with at least partial structural continuity of the white-matter long tracts. Sacral sparing is evidenced by perianal sensation, rectal motor function, and great toe flexor activity.

10. What is complete spinal cord injury?
A complete spinal cord injury is manifested by total motor and sensory loss distal to the injury level. When the bulbocavernosus reflex is positive but no sacral sensation or motor function has returned, the paralysis is permanent and complete in most patients.

11. What is an incomplete spinal cord injury?
In an incomplete spinal cord injury some motor or sensory function is spared distal to the cord injury. Several types of incomplete spinal cord syndromes have been identified:

Brown-Séquard syndrome, an injury to either half of the spinal cord, results either from lamina or pedicle fracture or from penetrating injury. Symptoms include motor weakness on the side of the lesion and contralateral loss of pain and temperature sensation. Prognosis for recovery is good; neurologic improvement often is significant.

Anterior cord syndrome is usually caused by a hyperflexion injury in which bone compresses the anterior spinal artery and cord. Patients have complete motor loss and loss of pain and temperature discrimination below the level of injury. Posterior columns, including deep-touch position sense and vibratory sensation, are spared. Prognosis for recovery is poor.

Posterior cord syndrome, which involves the dorsal columns of the spinal cord, is characterized by loss of proprioceptive vibratory sense with sparing of sensory and motor function. This syndrome is rare.

Central cord syndrome, which is the most common type of incomplete spinal cord injury, involves destruction of the central area of spinal cord. Centrally located arm tracts are most severely affected, whereas the leg tracts are affected to a lesser extent. Sensation is variably spared. Central cord syndromes usually result from hyperextension injury in an older person with preexisting spinal stenosis or from flexion injuries in younger patients.

12. List the classification of thoracolumbar spine fractures.
- Compression
- Burst fracture
- Flexion–distraction injuries
- Extension injuries
- Dislocations

13. Describe a compression fracture.
A compression fracture results in a typical anterior wedging of the vertebral body in the anterior column. The middle and posterior columns generally are not involved. Compression fractures are usually stable and rarely involve a neurologic deficit.

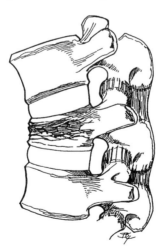

Compression fracture.

14. What is a burst fracture?
A burst fracture is a fracture of the anterior and middle columns; fracture fragments are displaced into the neural canal to a variable extent. Other common findings include spreading of the posterior elements and an increase in interpedicular distance.

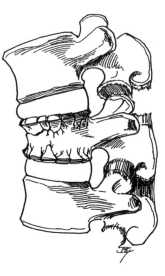

Burst fracture.

15. What is a flexion–distraction injury?

A flexion–distraction injury, also known as a Chance fracture when it occurs through osseous structures, is common in motor vehicle accidents when the victim is wearing only a lap seatbelt. The fracture involves the anterior, middle, and posterior columns or the posterior ligaments. With a true flexion–distraction injury, neurologic compromise is most likely when a dislocation occurs.

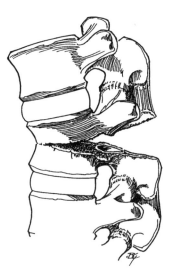

Chance fracture.

16. Describe a fracture–dislocation.

A fracture–dislocation involves disruption of all three columns by a combination of anterior compression with distraction and rotation. On the anteroposterior radiograph, significant translation is seen. This fracture is highly unstable and often associated with significant neurologic deficit, dural tears, and intra-abdominal injuries.

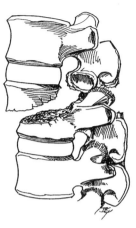

Fracture–dislocation.

17. Describe dislocations.
Dislocations are disruptions of the soft tissue structures of the spine. They are considered to be unstable because all three columns have failed. Usually multiple forces are involved, including rotation, distraction, compression, and shear forces. Dislocations are highly unstable and are often associated with a neurologic deficit.

18. Describe an extension injury to the thoracolumbar spine.
When the lumbar spine is hyperextended, the usual result is an anterior vertebral body avulsion fracture accompanied by fractures of the posterior columns, including the spinous process, lamina, and occasionally pedicles. These fractures are generally stable.

19. What other fractures occur?
   • Transverse process fractures result from blunt trauma, particularly at L5.
   • Spinous process avulsions are stable injuries related to distraction.
   • Facet fractures are uncommon but may occur in patients with prior laminectomies or stress fractures.

20. What radiographic examinations are necessary for patients with spinal cord injury?
Initial assessment consists of anterior and posterior lateral and oblique radiographs of the spine. Computed tomography (CT) demonstrates bony impingement on the neural canal and assesses stability. Sagittal and coronal reconstructions are advantageous in the evaluation of transverse or axially oriented injuries, horizontal lamina fractures, and some facet injuries. Magnetic resonance imaging (MRI) may demonstrate more precisely the status of the intervertebral disc, potential sites of ligamentous injury, epidural hematoma, and extent of spinal cord injury.

21. Describe some of the various MRI findings that may be found with patients with spinal cord injuries.
   • Edema is seen as fusiform enlargement of the cord with increased signal intensity on T2-weighted images.
   • Hematoma is characterized by increased signal intensity on T2 images acutely and is often surrounded by a halo of T2 enhancement from adjacent edema.
   • Extrinsic cord compression by osseous elements, soft tissue, or fluid.
   • Disc herniation
   • Transection

22. How often does noncontiguous, multilevel spinal injury occur?

Multilevel spinal cord injury is now more readily recognized with MRI. Various studies show an incidence between 4.5 and 16% of noncontiguous, multilevel spinal cord injury.

23. Describe the management of compression fractures.

Compression fractures generally are stable and rarely involve neurologic compromise. The patient may be treated effectively by hyperextension brace or casting. Compression > 50% of the vertebral body height or multiple adjacent compression fractures are considered potentially unstable. Some authors recommend open reduction and internal fixation with anterior grafting, posterior instrumentation, and arthrodesis.

24. Describe the treatment for unstable thoracolumbar and lumbar fractures.

An anterior, posterior, or combined approach may be used. Various plates and screw devices are available anteriorly or posteriorly. Pedicle screws with rods or plates are placed posteriorly. For significant anterior decompression with removal of the vertebral body, an iliac strut graft is used.

25. What surgical approaches may be used for spinal fractures and dislocations?

Anterior: commonly used for anterior decompression of the cord by removing portions of the retropulsed vertebral body. Iliac strut grafts and instrumentation are used for stabilization. Used mostly in the thoracolumbar junction and lumbar spine.

Posterior: used in thoracic spine in conjunction with posterior instrumentation and fusion. Laminectomy alone should never be the sole treatment of unstable spine injuries.

Posterior lateral: usually used in the thoracolumbar spine, removing portions of the transverse process and pedicle. Instrumentation and fusion may be difficult through this approach. This approach is hazardous and ineffective and is of historical interest only.

26. Discuss the common posterior instrumentation options for spinal stabilization.

- Pedicle screws.
- Multiple hooks and rod: so-called third-generation instrumentation to increase translational and rotational stability.
- Luque: rod with sublaminar wires.

27. What is meant by the term SCIWORA?

This acronym stands for **s**pinal **c**ord **i**njury **w**ithout **r**adiologic **a**bnormality and describes a phenomenon most commonly observed in pediatric spinal cord injuries. The relative elasticity of the pediatric spine can allow enough elongation under load to injure the neural elements without obvious injury to the bony elements of the spine.

BIBLIOGRAPHY

1. Bohlman HH, Ducker TB, Levine MD: Spine trauma in adults. In Herkowitz HN, Garfin SR, Balderston RA, et al (eds): Rothman-Simeone The Spine, 4th ed. Philadelphia, W.B. Saunders, 1999, pp 889–1070.
2. Bucholz RW, Gill K: Classification of injuries to the thoracolumbar spine. Orthop Clin North Am 17:67–73, 1986.
3. Frymoyer JW (ed): Orthopedic Knowledge Update Four. Rosemont, IL, American Academy of Orthopaedic Surgeons, 1993, pp 461–473.
4. Haher TR: Thoracic and lumbar fractures: Diagnosis and management. In Bridwell KH, DeWald RL, et al (eds): The Textbook of Spinal Surgery, 2nd ed. Philadelphia, J.B. Lippincott, 1996.
5. Leventhal MR: Fractures, dislocations, and fracture dislocations of the spine. In Canale ST (ed): Campbell's Operative Orthopedics, 9th ed. St. Louis, Mosby, 1998, pp 2704–2790.
6. Spivak JM, Vaccaro AR, Cotler JM: Thoracolumbar Spine Trauma: I. Evaluation and classification. J Am Acad Orthop Surg 3:345–352, 1995.
7. Spivak JM, Vaccaro AR, Cotler JM: Thoracolumbar Spine Trauma: II. Principles of management. J Am Acad Orthop Surg 3:353–360, 1995.
8. Stauffer ES: Fractures and dislocations of the spine. In Bucholz RW, Heckman JD (eds): Rockwood and Green's Fractures in Adults, 5th ed. Philadelphia, J.B. Lippincott, 2002.
9. Vaccaro AR, An HS, Betz RR, et al: The management of acute spinal trauma: Pre-hospital and in-hospital emergency care. AAOS Instr Course Lect 46:113–125, 1997.

VII. Hip and Pelvis

53. EVALUATION OF HIP DISEASE

Randall D. Neumann, M.D.

1. What is the normal range of motion for the hip?

Extension	0°
Flexion	120°
Abduction	45°
Adduction	30°
External rotation	45°
Internal rotation	45°

2. What is pelvic obliquity?

Normally the iliac crests are at the same relative level on physical examination. When they are at different levels, the descriptive term is pelvic obliquity. This condition may be due to scoliosis or contractures about the hip. The most common contractures are adduction and flexion contractures.

3. In degenerative arthritis of the hip, where do most patients complain of pain?

Most patients describe pain in the groin area, with possible radiation into the anterior portion of the thigh. Patients rarely describe buttock or posterior pain, and the pain rarely radiates below the knee.

4. Differentiate referred pain from the spine and hip pain.

Most patients with hip pathology describe pain anterior to the hip or along the greater trochanteric region. Spinal pain usually involves the buttocks and posterior thigh.

5. What is the Thomas test?

The Thomas test assesses flexion contracture of the hip. Normal flexion allows the anterior portion of the thigh to rest against the abdomen, almost touching the chest. The patient holds one leg to the abdomen and lowers the other leg until it is flat on the examination table. If the hip does not extend fully, the patient has a fixed flexion contracture or a positive Thomas test.

6. What is a Trendelenburg test?

The Trendelenburg test assesses the gluteus medius muscle and the hip joint. The examiner stands behind the patient and observes the dimples overlying the posterior-superior iliac spine. The patients is asked to stand on one leg. As the patient stands erect, the gluteus medius muscle on the supported side should contract to keep the pelvis level. If the pelvis remains unsupported and the opposite side drops, the gluteus medius muscle is either weak or nonfunctioning, and the test is positive.

7. Describe a patient with a "hip limp."

During midstance the hip is displaced laterally by approximately one inch to the weight-bearing side. With a hip limp, lateral displacement is accentuated and results in an exaggerated limp.

8. What is the most common abnormality of patients with a congenitally dislocated hip?

Patients present with adduction contracture of the hip at 90° of flexion. Unilateral dislocation generally results in shortening of the involved leg.

9. What physical abnormality is seen in patients with slipped capital femoral epiphysis?

Because the femoral head is displaced in a posterior-inferior direction, patients generally have increased external rotation and diminished internal rotation of the leg. As the hip is flexed, it drifts into external rotation with more acute flexion.

10. Which motion is usually the last to be affected in patients with degenerative arthritis of the hip?

Most patients lose internal and external rotation before abduction and adduction. Flexion is usually maintained until severe changes occur.

11. What is the most common contracture in patients with cerebral palsy?

Patients with cerebral palsy generally have an adduction and flexion contracture of the hip. This contracture, along with scoliosis, may lead to the progressive development of dislocation.

12. What is the Ortolani maneuver?

The hip is gently abducted and the thigh is raised with the fingers to reduce the hip. When performing this test, the examiner should use one hand to stabilize the pelvis. The Ortolani maneuver is used to assess dislocation in a congenitally dislocated hip.

13. What is the Barlow test?

With the thumb placed on the inner aspect of the thigh and the hip adducted, longitudinal pressure is exerted on the thigh, pushing it toward the examination table. A dislocatable hip then becomes completely displaced, and when the leg is allowed to abduct, the hip reduces. The Barlow test establishes the diagnosis of a dislocatable hip.

14. What test is used to differentiate hip pathology from spine pathology?

The patient is placed on the examination table in a supine position and asked to perform a straight-leg raise with the heel approximately 12 inches off the table. Patients with hip pathology, such as fracture and degenerative arthritis, are unable to maintain the leg in the straight position. Reproduction of groin pain is common. Patients with spine pathology rarely have difficulty with this maneuver.

15. What physical abnormality is seen in patients with femoral neck or intertrochanteric fractures?

Patients who present with an intertrochanteric or femoral neck fracture have a shortening of the involved leg in external rotation. Generally the patient is unable to move the leg and finds it quite painful to place the hip through a passive range of motion.

16. List areas of tenderness about the hip and possible diagnoses.

Area of Tenderness	Diagnoses
Femoral triangle	Hernia
Trochanter	Trochanteric bursitis, snapping hip
Sciatic notch	Sciatic disorder, radiculopathy
Posterior trochanter	Pyriformis syndrome
Posterior iliac spine	Sacroiliac joint pathology
Sacrum	Insufficiency fracture
Coccyx	Coccydynia

Continues

Area of Tenderness	Diagnoses
Iliac crest	Iliac apophysitis
Anterior-superior iliac spine	Avulsion fracture
Iliac wing	Pelvic fracture, metastatic disease, primary tumors
Pubic rami	Stress fracture, metastatic disease
Proximal femur	Stress fracture, tumor

17. What is the differential diagnosis of patients who have catching in the hip?
- Arthritic conditions, including osteoarthritis and rheumatoid arthritis
- Loose bodies from chondral lesions or osteochondral lesions
- Pigmented villonodular synovitis
- Snapping hip syndrome

18. What range of motion test is a quick test for hip pathology?
The figure-four test is a quick test for hip pathology. The patient is in a supine position. The examiner flexes, externally rotates, and abducts the hip to place the heel across the uninvolved knee. Patients with hip pathology generally have diminished range of motion and are unable to perform the maneuver or do so without significant pain.

19. What are other names for the figure-of-four test?
Patrick's test and FABER test (flexion, abduction, external rotation).

20. What is the FAdIR test?
This apprehension test evaluates the presence of an anterior labral tear. The patient is placed supine. The affected hip is flexed, adducted, and internally rotated. Positive pain may mean anterior labral pathology.

21. How do you test for an iliotibial band contracture?
Ober's test, which is performed with the patient lying on the unaffected side. The examiner assists the patient in abducting the leg with the hip extended and the knee flexed to 90°. The leg is then slowly released from abduction to neutral, and if there is a contracture of the iliotibial band, the thigh remains in an abducted position.

22. What does Ely's test evaluate?
A contracture of the rectus femoris. This test is performed with the patient in the prone position. The examiner then flexes the knee to 90°. If the rectus femoris is contracted, the patient's hip on the same side as the flexed knee will flex spontaneously. Normally, the hip remains flat on the table or in a neutral position.

23. What is the Thomas test?
A test for hip flexion contracture. The patient is placed in the supine position on the exam table with the pelvis square to the trunk. The hips are flexed so that contact is made with the trunk. This position flattens the lumbar lordosis, allowing more accurate assessment of hip contracture. The affected hip is allowed to extend as much as possible. The degree of fixed flexion is measured from the angle of the thigh to the table.

24. How are leg length's measured?
Leg lengths are measured between true bony landmarks. The examiner should measure from the anterior superior iliac supine to the medial malleolus. This approach measures the true leg length. Apparent leg length can be measured from the umbilicus to the medial malleolus. Apparent leg

length discrepancies from the true leg length can be related to pelvic obliquity, flexion, or adduction contractures. As an example, an adduction of 10° can cause a 3.2 cm leg length discrepancy.

25. What radiographs are used to assess patients with hip pathology?

The standard radiographs are anteroposterior views of the pelvis, including the iliac crest, inferior portion of the spine, and hip joints. Cross-table lateral radiographs evaluate the lateral aspect of the hip and can be taken without moving the affected hip. In patients who have sustained trauma, inlet and outlet views of the pelvis, as described by Tile, are also recommended. If fractures involving the acetabulum are suspected, obturator and iliac oblique views of the acetabulum are taken.

26. When is hip aspiration useful?

Hip aspiration is extremely helpful in differentiating septic arthritis and transient synovitis of the hip in children. It may also be used to assess infectious processes after surgery, including hemiarthroplasty and total hip replacement. Hip aspiration for synovial fluid analysis and subsequent injection of steroids may be useful in differentiating hip pathology from spinal pathology.

27. What are the indications for tomography?

Tomography is normally used in victims of trauma. Its use has become limited, however, with the advent of computed tomography (CT). Plain tomography is still indicated in patients with nonunion of femoral neck fractures and internal fixation devices. It also may be helpful after reduction of a hip dislocation to look for loose bony fragments. The configuration of an acetabular fracture may be viewed on tomograms if a CT scan is not available. Tomograms also are helpful in evaluating the extent of stress fractures or femoral neck fractures.

28. Which hip disease processes are evaluated with magnetic resonance imaging (MRI)?

MRI has proved quite successful in evaluating transient osteoporosis of the hip, avascular necrosis, and both benign and malignant processes.

29. What are the indications for bone scan?

Bone scans are indicated for patients with hip disease that is not clearly defined by physical examination or plain radiographs. Examples include questionable infections; stress fractures; benign tumors, such as osteoid osteomas; and nondisplaced femoral neck fractures in the elderly. Bone scans are highly sensitive but generally nonspecific for differentiating disease processes.

30. Which areas are commonly affected with stress fractures about the hip?

Athletes may have stress fractures in the femoral neck and pubic rami, which usually are seen on plain radiographs. Patients with osteomalacia may develop bilateral stress fractures in the subtrochanteric region.

31. Which patients benefit from CT scans of the hip and pelvis?

CT scans are indicated for patients with traumatic conditions; they are highly effective in delineating the extent of fractures involving the acetabulum, iliac crest, and sacrum. Bony fragments in the acetabulum after hip dislocation are readily identified. Three-dimensional reconstructions of computed tomography are indicated preoperatively for difficult revisions of total hip arthroplasties and reconstruction procedures with ill-defined anatomy.

BIBLIOGRAPHY

1. Callaghan, JJ, Rosenberg AG, Rubash HE: The Adult Hip. Philadelphia, Lippincott-Raven 1998.
2. Glick JM:Hip arthroscopy. In McGinty JB, Casper RB, Jackson RW, Poehling GG (eds): Operative Arthroscopy. New York, Raven Press, 1991, pp 663–676.
3. Rockwood CA, Green DP, Bucholz RW, et al (eds): Fractures, 4th ed. Philadelphia, Lippincott-Raven, 1996.

54. HIP ARTHROSCOPY

Randall D. Neumann, M.D.

1. What are the indications for arthroscopy of the hip?
Loose bodies, labral tears, degenerative arthritis, chondral injuries, avascular necrosis, synovial disease, ruptured ligamentum teres, joint sepsis, and unresolved hip pain.

2. What are the contraindications to hip arthroscopy?
Ankylosis, arthrofibrosis, abnormal anatomy, severe obesity, advanced degenerative arthritis.

3. What significant history is the best indicator of a likely successful outcome from hip arthroscopy?
The history of a significant traumatic event is the best indicator of a likely successful outcome. Insidious onset or minor precipitating episodes suggest underlying predisposition or degenerative process and a less than certain prognosis.

4. Where is the classic localizations of symptoms from intra-articular hip pathology?
Classically, anterior groin pain radiating into the medial thigh is the location signifying hip disease. Patients often give a C sign, describing symptoms with the hand gripped above the greater trochanter, the thumb positioned over the posterior aspect of the greater trochanter, and the index finger in the groin. Posterior pain is rarely characteristic of hip joint pathology, even with posterior intra-articular pathology.

5. Describe the physical findings of patients with intra-articular hip pathology.
Rotating the femoral head in relationship to the acetabulum, as in log rolling, is specific for intra-articular pathology. In addition, pain is elicited with a flexion/internal rotation movement producing anterior groin or deep anterolateral symptoms.

6. What are the classic causes of a "snapping hip?"
The iliopsoas tendon may snap and characteristically produces a clunk elicited by bringing the hip from the flexed, externally rotated position to extension with internal rotation. Symptoms then occur in the deep anterior groin with an audible clunk. The iliotibial band may produce a visible and palpable snap. This occurs laterally along with the symptoms located laterally.

7. What two positions can be used in hip arthroplasty?
The patient can be placed in a supine position or a lateral position.

8. Describe the operative procedure.
The patient is placed in the lateral position. A 9-cm peroneal post is placed, and distraction is applied. Twenty-five to 50 pounds of distraction is placed on the limb. Anterior paratrochanteric and posterior paratrochanteric portals are made. The 70° and 30° arthroscopes are used. Image intensification is used for portal placement and placement of the needles.

9. Describe the portal placement.
Anterior portal. This portal allows visualization of the anterior femoral neck, anterior aspect of the joint, and ligamentum teres. The portal is placed at the intersection of perpendicular lines drawn laterally from the superior aspect of the symphysis pubis and inferiorly from the anterior superior iliac spine. A spinal needle is directed from this point medially and superiorly at a 45° angle in each plane.

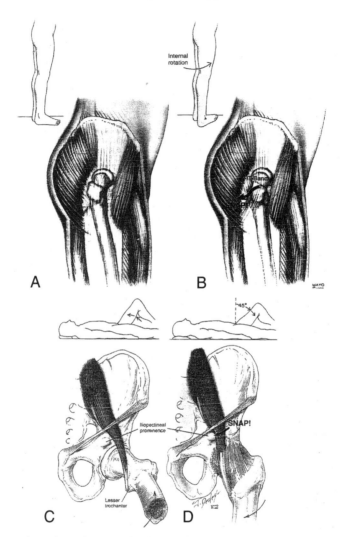

Typical sources of snapping tendons about the hip. Snapping iliotibial band: the iliotibial band subluxates over the greater trochanter causing a snapping sensation over the lateral hip (**A, B**). Snapping iliopsoas tendon: The iliopsoas tendon snaps over the pectineal eminence of the pelvis as the hip is extended causing a snapping sensation in the groin (**C, D**). (From Callaghan JJ, Rosenberg AG, Rubash HE (eds): The Adult Hip, vol 1. Philadelphia, Lippincott-Raven, 1998, with permission.)

Anterior paratrochanteric portal. The anterior paratrochanteric portal is placed 2 cm anterior and 1 cm proximal to the anterosuperior corner of the greater trochanter. Under fluoroscopic examination, the needle is followed to the joint level. This portal allows visualization of the femoral head, anterior neck, and anterior intrinsic capsular folds.

Posterior paratrochanteric portal. The entry site is 2–3 cm posterior to the tip of the greater trochanter at the level of the anterior paratrochanteric portal. Using imaging intensification, the needle is observed going into the joint.

10. What nerves are at risk at each of the portals?

Anterior portal—lateral femoral cutaneous nerve and femoral nerve.
Anterior paratrochanteric portal—femoral
Posterior paratrochanteric portal—sciatic nerve

11. What are the complications of hip arthroscopy?
- Transient neuropraxia to the lateral femoral cutaneous nerve, femoral nerve, pudendal nerve, or sciatic nerve
- Pressure necrosis of the foot, scrotum, or perineum
- Breakage of arthroscopic instrumentation
- Infection
- Enterotopic ossification
- Intraabdominal fluid extravasation

BIBLIOGRAPHY

1. Byrd JWT: Operative Hip Arthroscopy. New York, Thieme, 1998.
2. Byrd JWT: Hip arthroscopy utilizing the supine position. Arthroscopy 10:275–280, 1994.
3. Byrd JWT, Pappas JN, Pedley MJ: Hip arthroscopy: An anatomic study of portal placement and relationship to the extra-articular structures. Arthroscopy 11:418–423, 1995.
4. Glick JM: Hip arthroscopy. In McGinty JB (ed): Operative Arthroscopy. New York, Raven Press, 1991, pp 663–676.
5. Glick JM: Hip arthroscopy using the lateral approach. American Academy of Orthopaedic Surgery Instructional Course Lectures 37:223–231, 1988.

55. PEDIATRIC HIP DISEASE

Walter W. Huurman, M.D.

1. What is developmental dysplasia of the hip?
Developmental dysplasia of the hip is a progressive condition in which the hip structures do not develop adequately. The condition has three characteristic components: (1) varying degrees of abnormality in the slope of the acetabulum; (2) excessive laxity of the hip joint that over time permits the femoral head to slide gradually upward and laterally out of its normal relationship with the acetabulum; and (3) abnormal torsion (rotation) of the upper end of the femoral shaft, which creates an abnormal relationship between the femoral head and the acetabulum. As a consequence, three stages may be identified: (1) the head of the femur is retained within an inadequate acetabulum, with minimal physical findings; (2) the head of the femur has moved slightly away from the acetabular medial wall; and (3) the head of the femur has slipped out of the acetabulum. The first two stages probably should be considered precursors to dislocation. Unfortunately, the examination may be normal in an infant or child at risk for developing a true dislocation.

2. How does developmental dysplasia differ from congenital dislocation of the hip?
The term *congenital* implies a condition present at birth. It has been recognized recently that hip dislocation may develop during the first year of life due to dysplasia of the hip's anatomic components; dysplasia without dislocation is often clinically undetectable at birth. The term *developmental dysplasia* encompasses hip dislocation developing in utero as well as that occurring postnatally.

3. What is subluxation of the hip?
By definition subluxation is a partial dislocation. The head of the femur has not completely lost contact with the articular surface of the acetabulum; therefore, physical findings may be entirely normal or reveal some degree of laxity on physical exam when the examiner attempts to passively dislocate the hip (Barlow test).

4. Describe the dislocated hip.
In a true dislocation of the hip, the head of the femur has completely lost contact with the articular surface of the acetabulum and is most commonly displaced posteriorly and upward out of

the acetabulum. Various external factors may produce dislocation in the presence of a hypoplastic acetabulum. Efforts to bring the hip into extension tend to displace the hip laterally and superiorly due to tightness in the psoas muscle-tendon and ultimately may lead to dislocation. Use of confining swaddling clothes that bring the hip downward into premature extension may explain the high incidence of developmental dislocation in northern Italy around the turn of the century. Risk factors that point to the possibility of developmental dysplasia are now fairly well documented: (1) first child, (2) female sex, (3) breech delivery, and (4) family history. Family history of infantile hip disease in an infant, whether it be dysplasia or dislocation, should raise a red flag. Other coexisting contributory factors include teratologic and neurologic deficits, particularly meningoceles and cerebral palsy. In addition, the physician should be wary when abnormalities are noted in the physical examination of the lower extremity of a newborn infant, particularly the Galeazzi sign, Barlow test, and the Ortolani maneuver (see question 5).

5. Discuss the physical examination of a newborn infant, particularly with reference to the hip.

The examination must be carried out with all clothing removed and the infant placed in a warm, comfortable setting on a flat examining table—**not** in a bassinet or crib. The infant should be checked visually, particularly for neck motion and any abnormalities of the low back, such as dimpling over the distal sacrum or at the sacrococcygeal joint. There are three specific tests for hip abnormality, all of which may be normal in an infant who has only dysplasia when instability has not yet developed.

1. The **Galeazzi sign** is an evaluation of apparent thigh length. The child lies on his or her back, the thighs are held together and raised to a 90° hip and knee flexion position, and the level of the knees evaluated. Any difference in height between the knees should precipitate concern and further examination. Because a positive Galeazzi sign relies upon apparent shortening of one femur in comparison with a normal contralateral femur, it is negative in the presence of bilateral dislocation.

2. **Barlow's test**, which assesses the potential for passive dislocation of a located hip, also is done with the infant supine on an examining table. The hip and knee are flexed 90° and the thigh is held at right angles to the trunk in a slightly adducted position; gentle pressure is applied downward on the knee in an effort to slide the head of the femur out of a normal relationship to the acetabulum. The examiner looks for a piston-type motion, which may or may not be accompanied by a palpable clunk or jerking sensation as the femoral head slides out of the acetabulum.

3. The **Ortolani maneuver** usually is combined with Barlow's test. When the hip is gently abducted from 90° of flexion and adduction, a resistance may be felt. The examiner holds the knee flexed and the fingers gently hold the proximal femur between the thumb on the medial side and the index and long finger laterally at the greater trochanter, pressing upward on the greater trochanter. If abducting the hip with a little pressure over the trochanter produces a clunk that is felt (rather than heard), the Ortolani test is positive. The "clicks" that are frequently felt in a newborn infant when the hips are passively moved are simply the iliopsoas tendon sliding over the crest of the ilium or the iliotibial band sliding across the greater trochanter. Ortolani's test may be negative with a completely dislocated hip; a negative test is simply a sign that the hip is firmly dislocated and cannot be reduced with manipulation in the nonanesthetized child.

If any physical findings are at all suspicious, further evaluation is necessary.

6. Describe the physical findings in a newborn infant with a developmentally dislocated hip.

If unilateral, Galeazzi's sign should be positive; Barlow's test is negative, and Ortolani's test may be positive or negative. Abduction limitation, the classic sign for dislocation, is not reliably present in a newborn infant.

7. Describe the physical findings in a 6-month-old infant with a developmentally dislocated hip.

The findings are usually fairly clear: short thigh and multiple folds in the medial skin on the dislocated side are evidence of proximal migration of the skeletal structures in the thigh. The trochanter is displaced upward in comparison with the normal side. The perineum on the side of the dislocation is broadened, indicating that the femoral head is displaced laterally. Hip abduction may be limited, but relying on this finding alone is dangerous.

8. Describe the physical findings in a 2-year-old child with a developmentally dislocated hip.

The usual presenting complaint is a limp; the limp of a unilateral hip dislocation is classic. The lurching gait has a tendency toward a Trendelenburg sway. This type of sway is not as clear in a young child as in a teenager or an adult, but it is still present in an effort to swing the center of gravity over the unstable hip joint. Parents often complain of unilateral toe walking. This is due to extremity shortening; they also may complain of intoeing or outtoeing. Bilateral hip dislocation often leads to a waddling gait that is frequently overlooked. A detailed examination (similar to that of a 6-month-old infant) of the lower extremity reveals shortening of the thigh, multiple skin folds, broad perineum, prominence of the trochanter, and shortening of the distance between the crest of the ilium and the tip of the trochanter. One of the best ways of measuring this distance is simply to use one's fingertips as a guide and compare the two sides.

9. What is the best radiographic evaluation?

Radiographic evaluation depends entirely on the age at first presentation. Ultrasound studies have changed the imaging evaluation of the hip joint in **newborn** infants. Such studies should be done as a dynamic test by an experienced ultrasonographer. The experienced examiner first visualizes the bony elements of the acetabulum and then identifies the elements that are inadequate. Laxity in the capsule may be noted when an effort is made to displace the femoral head out of the acetabulum or away from the medial wall of the acetabulum. Femoral head subluxation visible during real-time ultrasound scanning is evidence of hip joint laxity, which poses an immediate risk. In its more severe form, the femoral head displaces out of the acetabulum. If any of the findings are positive, anteroposterior radiographs of the pelvis (note: **pelvis**, not hip) should be done for confirmation. Infants older than 3–4 months are best diagnosed using anteroposterior and frog x-rays of the pelvis.

10. Describe the complete diagnosis in a newborn infant with hip abnormalities.

The best approach is to say simply that the hip is dysplastic and then describe the type: shallow acetabulum, hip joint laxity, subluxed hip, or dislocatable hip. A dislocatable hip should be additionally described as either reducible or not reducible.

11. What is the treatment for a newborn with developmental dysplasia of the hip?

At present the treatment of choice is a Pavlik harness, applied by an individual who is knowledgeable in harness fit, desired position, and potential complications. The principal effect of the Pavlik harness is to hold the hips in flexion while permitting a moderate degree of abduction in the horizontal plane. This effect allows both maintenance of a stable position of the hip and a reasonable degree of motion, which is necessary for development of normal joint anatomy. More rigid braces and splints are also used but lack the freedom of motion that a Pavlik harness allows. If the hip is dislocated and not simply dysplastic or subluxable at birth, it is necessary to check the harness fairly frequently; if hip reduction has not been obtained by the time the harness has been worn for 3–4 weeks, additional treatment is necessary.

12. Describe the Pavlik harness.

The Pavlik harness was described first in 1958 by Arnold Pavlik in Czechoslovakia and was introduced into the United States several years later. The harness incorporates a chest component similar to ordinary suspenders with a cerclage strap around the thorax, forming a suspending medium for two stirrup-type boots. The boots are connected to the cerclage component by straps that hold the hips in flexion and control the degree of abduction. The anterior strap acts to flex, whereas the posterior strap maintains abduction. The harness should be worn continuously for the first weeks, depending on the developmental status of the hip. As the hip stabilizes, ultrasound examinations should be repeated at 1, 4, and 8 weeks, and a pelvic x-ray should be obtained at 12 weeks and at the end of treatment. Patients should be followed after conclusion of harness treatment by an x-ray examination at 6 months of age with the hip held in both the "frog" and neutral positions.

13. What complications may occur with use of the Pavlik harness?
Osteonecrosis of the femoral head, failure of reduction, and femoral nerve praxia.

14. What is the treatment for a 6–9-month-old infant with a newly diagnosed hip dislocation?
If a hip dislocation is identified in this age group, two choices of treatment are available. One may use a Pavlik harness with the hope that over a period of 2–3 weeks the hip will reduce and may then be held in a reduced position by a more rigid brace. If this method fails, the second choice is a closed method of treatment. The established routine is to put the infant in traction for a short period of time with the hips flexed about 45°. Occasionally this is done at home, but generally it is done in the hospital. The position of the hip joint is followed sequentially during the traction period with radiographs. The femoral head initially rides high and lateral in relation to the acetabulum. The goal is to pull the femur downward to the point that the femoral head is at station zero, i.e., opposite the triradiate cartilage. Palpation for hip reduction is carried out every day or two during traction, and when treatment has brought the hip downward to an adequate relationship with the acetabulum, the child is examined under anesthesia. An arthrogram will make certain that the hip indeed enters the acetabulum properly, and frequently iliopsoas and adductor tenotomies are performed. The child is then placed in a well molded cast in the "safe" position, i.e., 90° of flexion and abduction of no more than 60° with the hips in a stable, reduced position. Casting is continued for as many months as the child is old, up to a maximum of 6 months.

15. What is the treatment for a 2-year-old child with a newly diagnosed hip dislocation?
A newly diagnosed hip dislocation in a 2-year-old child probably requires surgery. By this time the capsule of the hip and the musculature above the hip joint are shortened enough that a procedure must be performed to permit easy introduction of the femoral head into the acetabulum. The surgery, which is best done by a pediatric orthopedist, consists of femoral shortening, opening the acetabulum and introducing the femoral head, and then augmenting or repositioning the acetabulum and/or proximal femur through reconstruction.

16. What is the indication for open reduction of a developmentally dislocated hip?
The obvious indication is irreducibility by closed means. As a rule, open reduction of the hip joint involves acetabular augmentation if the hip is not stable after reduction. Acetabular modeling without augmentation at the time of operative reduction can be expected to progress only if the hip is well reduced and held in place, but potential improvement is not complete until the child is about 5 years old. If dysplasia persists after this age, augmentation and/or redirection of the acetabular roof is clearly necessary.

17. What is slipped capital femoral epiphysis (SCFE)?
SCFE is a common hip disorder that affects adolescents, most often between 12 and 15 years of age. Clinically, the femoral capital epiphysis of the hip displaces or "slips" off the femoral neck to a variable degree.

18. Describe the clinical features of a patient with SCFE.
The most frequent presenting complaint is a painful hip. Early on pain may be referred to the knee, and knee pain may be the sole presenting complaint. Pain is usually intermittent and gradual in onset. Some patients describe one or more episodes of trauma prior to diagnosis. Boys are affected approximately twice as frequently as girls. Physical examination reveals mild to severe

pain on motion with limited internal rotation and abduction. Flexion of the hip results in obligatory external rotation of the thigh because of the abnormal relationship between the femoral head and neck.

19. What are the early radiographic features of SCFE?

In the earliest "preslip" stage, the only x-ray finding may be a subtle widening of the physis on the involved side when compared with the opposite hip. Hence it is important to obtain a view of the entire pelvis, not just the involved hip.

20. Describe the subsequent radiographic features of SCFE.

On the anteroposterior film the epiphysis displaces posteriorly and inferiorly. A rim of new bone formation is found at the posterior aspect of the neck adjacent to the femoral head. In addition, the femoral neck becomes uncovered by the femoral head anteriorly, producing the characteristic bony bump of the superior neck. A slip of less than one-third the width of the neck is considered grade I; a slip between 33 and 50% is grade II; and a slip > 50% is termed grade III. The severity of the condition may be determined by measuring the percentage of slip.

21. What is the treatment of SCFE?

Treatment is designed to stabilize the epiphysis on the femoral neck and to prevent further slipping, a goal generally achieved by inserting a single strong screw into the center of the epiphysis from the anterior aspect of the greater trochanter or femoral neck. Surgery should be performed without undue delay after diagnosis.

22. What are the complications of treatment for SCFE?

• Chronic and diminished range of motion
• Osteonecrosis
• Chondrolysis
• Degenerative arthritis
• Gait abnormalities

23. What is Legg-Calvé-Perthes (LCP) disease?

LCP disease is temporary interruption of the blood supply to the bony nucleus of the proximal femoral epiphysis with impairment of the epiphyseal growth and subsequent remodeling of revascularized, regenerated bone in the pediatric patient.

24. Describe the clinical presentation of a patient with LCP disease.

LCP disease may occur between the ages of 3 and 12 years, most commonly in children between 5 and 7 years of age. The disorder may be bilateral in up to 20% of patients; boys are affected 3–5 times more often than girls. Patients usually present with a limp accompanied by pain in the hip or referred to the thigh or knee and may report an associated traumatic event. The gait is usually described as Trendelenburg-type. Shortening of the extremity is rare. However, range of motion, especially abduction and internal rotation of the hip, is limited.

25. What is the etiology of LCP disease?

The etiology of the avascular changes in the femoral head of children with LCP disease remains unclear. This condition is different from the avascular necrosis of the femoral head that develops after a fracture or use of steroids. Theories include an endocrine- or trauma-induced loss of interosseous or extraosseous blood supply as well as perhaps a local manifestation of systemic epiphyseal disease.

26. Describe the radiologic findings in LCP disease.

In the early stages standard radiographs may remain normal. Technetium bone scans often provide evidence of disease in the early stages, but it is difficult to quantitate the information.

Magnetic resonance imaging facilitates the early diagnosis and quantification of osteonecrosis and provides a clear picture of the articular cartilage.

27. Describe the classification of LCP disease.
Some confusion surrounds the treatment of LCP disease because of the lack of uniformity in classification systems. The following are currently in use:
1. The **Waldenström classification** is divided into two periods: (1) evolution and (2) healing and growth. The evolutionary period is characterized by (a) an initial stage in which the epiphysis is dense, patchy, and uneven, and (b) a second stage of fragmentation in which the epiphysis appears radiographically to be in pieces. In the period of healing the epiphysis becomes homogenous; the final period is distinguished by normal growth and reossification of the deformed femoral head.
2. The **Catterall classification** identifies four groups:
   (1) 25% of the femoral head in the anterior central region is involved.
   (2) Nearly 50% of the femoral head including the anterior lateral region is involved.
   (3) Approximately 75% of the femoral head is involved with the formation of a large sequestrum; the large medial pillar is usually uninvolved.
   (4) The entire femoral head is involved, with widespread collapse of the epiphysis.
3. The **Salter-Thompson classification** divides LCP disease into two groups on the basis of the extent of the subchondral fracture that defines the limit of underlying osteonecrosis and the presence or absence of an intact viable lateral margin of the femoral epiphysis:
   (1) Group A: a subchondral fracture line involves approximately one-half of the femoral head.
   (2) Group B: more than half of the femoral head involved; the fracture and the underlying avascular segment of the femoral head extend across more than one half the epiphysis.

28. Describe the prognostic factors and natural history in LCP disease.
1. Recovery without residual problems is more likely when the signs and symptoms of the disease develop before the age of 5 years. Patients older than 9 years at presentation almost universally have a poor prognosis.
2. Some question remains whether an increased amount of femoral head involvement correlates with a poorer result, but in general it is believed that this is true.
3. Patients who demonstrate lateral subluxation or extrusion of the femoral head are thought to have less likelihood of an ultimate good or excellent result.
4. Persistent loss of range of motion carries a poor prognosis.
5. Premature closure of the physis leads to poor results.

29. What are the goals of treatment of LCP disease?
The goal of treatment is a spherical, well-covered femoral head with a range of motion in the hip that approaches normal. The principles of treatment include maintenance of range of motion and acetabular containment of the femoral head during the active period of the process.

30. What treatment options are available for patients with LCP disease?
1. Patients should be instructed on range-of-motion exercises and work with a physical therapist.
2. Braces are used to abduct the leg to contain the femoral epiphysis in the acetabulum; they may be either non–weight-bearing or weight-bearing orthoses. They must be used for 18–24 months. Favorable results of brace treatment are limited.
3. Varus osteotomy of the proximal portion of the femur centers the femoral head more deeply within the acetabulum while maintaining the limb in a weight-bearing position.
4. Innominate osteotomy may be used to rotate the acetabulum into a position that better contains the head of the femur.

BIBLIOGRAPHY

1. Carney BT, Weinstein SL, Nuhe J: Long term follow up of slipped capital femoral epiphysis. J Bone Joint Surg 73A:667–674, 1991.
2. Catterall A: The natural history of Perthes' disease. J Bone Joint Surg 53B:37–53, 1971.
3. Coates CK, Paterson JM, Woods KR: Femoral osteotomy in Perthes' disease: Results at maturity. J Bone Joint Surg 72B:581–585, 1990.
4. Evans IK, Deluca PA, Gage JR: A comparative study of ambulator-abductor bracing and varus derotation osteotomy in the treatment of severe Legg-Calvé-Parthes disease in children over 6 years of age. J Pediatr Orthop 8:676–682, 1998.
5. Harding M, Harcke HT, Bowen JR, et al: Management of dislocated hips with Pavlik harness treatment and ultrasound monitoring. J Pediatr Orthop 17:189–198, 1977.
6. Kasser J (ed): Orthopedic Knowledge Update No. 5. Rosemont, IL, American Academy of Orthopedic Surgery, 1996, pp 355–357.
7. Kislic PJ: Congenital dislocation of the hip: A misleading term. J Bone Joint Surg 71B:136, 1989.
8. Salter RB, Thompson GM: Legg-Calvé-Perthes disease. J Bone Joint Surg 66A:479–489, 1984.
9. Wenger DR, Ward WT, Herring JA: Legg-Calvé-Perthes disease. J Bone Surg 73A:778–788, 1991.

56. ARTHRITIS OF THE HIP

Kim J. Chillag, M.D.

1. In the adult patient with chronic symptoms, what are the most common causes of hip arthritis?

The most common causes of chronic arthritic symptoms in the adult can be divided into two broad categories. The first is **osteoarthritis,** which is also called degenerative or idiopathic osteoarthritis. This category includes the majority of patients over the age of 50 years with chronic arthritic pain in the hip. The second broad category is **inflammatory arthritis,** which includes connective tissue diseases such as rheumatoid arthritis, ankylosing spondylitis, systemic lupus erythematosus, and the crystalline-induced arthritides, such as gout and pseudogout.

2. The most common complaint of patients with arthritis of the hip is chronic pain. In the patient who presents with extreme acute pain, what etiologic factors must be considered?

The patient who presents with an acute onset of hip pain and no history of trauma should be assumed to have an infection of the hip until *proven* otherwise. The nature, duration, clinical course, and precipitating factors of the complaint should be considered in evaluation of the patient with acute hip pain. If no other cause is determined, an infection should be considered, and an aspiration of the joint should be performed.

If there is a history of trauma, such as a fall, and routine radiographs are normal, occult femoral neck fracture should be considered. The earliest confirmatory test is an MRI; radionuclide bone scanning is positive after several days.

3. How can the types of hip arthritis be differentiated?

The most common methods of differentiating the types of arthritis are the clinical history, physical examination, and radiographic evaluation. The typical radiographic changes in the common types of arthritis are listed in the table on the next page. If the diagnosis is still in question, serologic tests can be helpful; the common serologic tests are listed in the second table.

Radiographic Changes in Arthritis

DISEASE	FINDINGS
Degenerative joint disease	Joint space narrowing
	Bony sclerosis
	Osteophyte formation
Rheumatoid arthritis	Periarticular osteoporosis
	Joint erosions
	Loss of joint space
	Subluxation
	Ankylosis
Gout	Punched-out bone erosions
Pseudogout	Punctate linear calcification in hyaline and fibrocartilage
Infectious arthritis	No change (early), then osteoporosis
	Cartilage destruction and erosions if untreated (late)

Serologic Tests

DISEASE	TESTS	USUAL FINDINGS
Degenerative joint disease	Erythrocyte sedimentation rate (ESR)	Normal
	C-reactive protein (CRP)	
	Complete blood count (CBC)	
	Antinuclear antibody (ANA)	
	Lupus erythematosus cell preparation (LE prep)	Negative
	Rheumatoid factor (RF)	
Rheumatoid arthritis	ESR	Elevated
	Red blood cell count	Mild anemia
	White blood cell count (WBC)	Mild leukocytosis (40%)
	RF	Positive (80%)
	ANA	Positive (30%)
Gout	ESR	Elevated
	Serum uric acid	Elevated 95%
	CBC	Usually normal, occasionally mild leukocytosis
	ANA, LE prep, RF	Negative
Pseudogout	Same as above	Same as above, except serum uric acid is elevated in 30%
Infectious arthritis	ESR	Elevated
	Blood cultures	Positive
	WBC	Leukocytosis
	ANA, LE prep, RF	Negative

4. What nonsurgical treatments are available for patients with osteoarthritis or rheumatoid arthritis of the hip?

Especially early in the course of the disease, arthritis of the hip can be managed successfully by nonoperative means. Activity modification, weight loss, and walking aids, including canes, may significantly reduce the patient's symptoms. Nonsteroidal antiinflammatory drugs (NSAIDs) are the most frequently used pharmacologic agents for relief of symptoms. Other medications, including corticosteroids, are frequently prescribed for the inflammatory arthritides.

5. What are the common side effects of NSAIDs?

As with any medications, side effects may occur. In the broad category of drugs that includes the common NSAIDs, gastrointestinal (GI) side effects are the most common serious complication. Peptic ulceration and GI bleeding have been reported with all of the NSAIDs. Minor GI problems such as dyspepsia also are common. Actual GI bleeding may occur in as many as 2–4% of patients treated with long-term therapy. The physician and patient should be alert to the symptoms of this complication. Other serious side effects, including hepatic and renal toxicity, may occur, and patients on long-term therapy should be monitored appropriately.

Recently, a new category of NSAIDs termed COX-2 inhibitors has become available. They may have a lower incidence of GI side effects.

6. What is the chief advantage of the newer selective COX-2–inhibiting NSAIDs?

The chief advantage of the selective COX-2 inhibitors is decreased gastrointestinal bleeding when compared to nonselective COX-1 and COX-2 inhibitors.

7. Are there disadvantages of these newer drugs?

The COX-2 inhibitors have been associated with significant increases in systolic blood pressure in 10–17% of patients, as well as fluid retention. These drugs are 5 to 6 times more expensive that the generic NSAIDs.

8. What surgical procedures are used to correct osteoarthritis, the most common cause of hip arthritis?

Through the years many surgical procedures have been advocated for the treatment of osteoarthritis of the hip. As advancements have occurred, most of the procedures have been relegated to historical interest. Currently, arthrodesis, femoral or pelvic osteotomy, and total hip arthroplasty are the three commonly used procedures for treatment of osteoarthritis. The patient's age, activity level, overall health, other joint involvement, and specific radiographic presentation are considered in choosing the best surgical procedure.

9. Why consider alternatives to total hip arthroplasty, which is highly successful?

Alternatives to total joint arthroplasty are most often considered in young patients. Regardless of the advances that have been made in design and technique of total hip replacement, worrisome long-term results in young patients have been reported by numerous authors.

10. How is fixation of the prosthetic components achieved?

Excellent long-term fixation has been achieved using both methylmethacrylate (cement) fixation and porous or bone ingrowth (noncemented) fixation. The surgeon should consider the patient's age, activity level, and bone quality in selecting the type of prosthesis.

11. What is the most common long-term complication of total hip replacement?

Aseptic loosening is the most common long-term complication of total hip replacement and is frequently associated with osteolysis. This was originally thought to be the result of cement failure, but also is seen after noncemented total hip replacement. The body's reaction to polyethylene particulate debris is now thought to be the prime cause of late aseptic loosening and osteolysis. Alternatives to metal on polyethylene bearing surfaces are in use and may eliminate this problem.

12. What is the infection rate following total hip replacement? Which patients are most at risk?

The prevalence of infection after total hip replacement of Medicare patients in the United States is approximately 2.3%. Patient factors associated with increased risk for infection include rheumatoid arthritis, diabetes mellitus, poor nutrition, obesity, oral steroid use, and previous surgery.

BIBLIOGRAPHY

1. Beaule PE, Matta JM, Mast JW: Hip arthrodeisis: Current indications and techniques. J Am Acad Orthop Surg 2002;10:249–258.
2. Callaghan JJ: The clinical results and basic science of total hip arthroplasty with porous coated prosthesis. J Bone Joint Surg 75A:299–310, 1993.
3. Chandler HP, Reineck FT, et al: Total hip replacement in patients younger than thirty years old. J Bone Joint Surg 63A:1426–1434, 1981.
4. Door JD, Takei GK Connly JP: Total hip replacement in patients younger than thirty years old. J Bone Joint Surg 65A:474–479, 1983.
5. Hanssen AD, Rand JA: Evaluation and treatment of infection at the site of a total hip or knee arthroplasty. J Bone Joint Surg 80A:910–922, 1998.
6. Harris WH: The problem is osteolysis. CORR 311:46–53, 1995.
7. Jazrawi LM, Kummer FJ, DiCesare PE: Alternative bearing surfaces for total joint arthroplasty. J Am Acad Orthop Surg 1998;6:198–203.
8. Lane JM: Anti-inflammatory medications: Selective COX-2 inhibitors. J Am Acad Orthop Surg 2002;10:75–78.
9. Masterson EL, Masri BA, Duncan CP: Treatment of infection at the site of total hip replacement. J Bone Joint Surg 79A:1740–1749, 1997.
10. McCarthy GM, McCarty DJ: Intrasynovial corticosteroid therapy. Bull Rheum Dis 43:2–4, 1994.
11. McCoy TH, Salvati EA, Ranawat CS, et al: A fifteen year follow-up study of one hundred Charnley low-friction arthroplasties. Orthop Clin North Am 19:467, 1988.
12. Moreland JR, Gruen TA, Mai L, et al: Aseptic loosening of total hip replacement: Incidence and significance. In The Hip Proceedings of the Eighth Open Scientific Meeting of the Hip Society. St. Louis, Mosby, 1980.
13. Needleman P, Isakson PC: The discovery and function of COX-2. J Rheumatol 24:6–7, 1997.
14. Sells LL, German DC: An update on gout. Bull Rheum Dis 43:4–7, 1994.

57. AVASCULAR NECROSIS OF THE HIP

Kim J. Chillag, M.D.

1. What are other names for avascular necrosis (AVN) of the hip?

ON (osteonecrosis)
Ischemic necrosis of bone
Aseptic necrosis of bone

2. What are the causes of avascular necrosis of the femoral head?

The most common cause of avascular necrosis is disruption of the blood supply to the femoral head from a displaced femoral neck fracture. The most common *nontraumatic* causes are excessive alcohol use and systemic steroid use. Nontraumatic causes include:

Caisson disease	Corticosteroids	Smoking
Sickle cell disease	Alcohol	Pancreatitis
Postirradiation	Lipid disturbances	Kidney disease
Chemotherapy	Connective tissue disease	Liver disease
Arterial disease	Lupus	
Gaucher's disease	Clotting disorders	

3. If one hip has been diagnosed with avascular necrosis, what is the likelihood that the opposite hip is involved?

Whether the opposite hip is symptomatic or asymptomatic, there is at least a 50% chance that is is already involved.

4. What symptoms are caused by avascular necrosis of the hip?

Early in the course of the disease, the patient may be asymptomatic. As the disease progresses, the patient complains of pain in the groin area. Later, severe pain, limp, and loss of hip motion occur.

5. Can other areas of the skeleton be affected by avascular necrosis?

Yes. The humeral head and the distal femur, particularly the medial femoral condyle, may be involved in 10–15% of patients with avascular necrosis of the hip.

6. What tests are most useful in the diagnosis and evaluation of avascular necrosis?

The most important test is routine AP and lateral x-rays of the affected hip. This test is the most cost-effective and may be sufficient alone. Magnetic resonance imaging (MRI) is the most sensitive and specific test to evaluate the femoral head for the presence of avascular necrosis. MRI can detect the lesion before it is apparent on plain x-rays and allows the physician to quantitate the extent of femoral head involvement.

7. What is the original and most common classification system for avascular necrosis of the hip?

The most common classification system is the Ficat system, which is based on radiographic exposure of the femoral head (see table).

Ficat System for Clinical and Radiographic Evaluation and Staging of the Hip in Avascular Necrosis of the Femoral Head

STAGE	SYMPTOMS	RADIOGRAPH	BONE SCAN
0	None	Normal	Decreased uptake
1	None/mild	Normal	Cold spot on femoral head
2	Mild	Density change in femoral head	Increased uptake
2A		Sclerosis or cysts, normal joint line, normal head contour	
2B		Flattening (crescent sign)	
3	Mild to moderate	Loss of sphericity, collapse	Increased uptake
4	Moderate to severe	Joint space, acetabular changes	Increased uptake

8. Has the classification system changed since MRI has become available?

Yes. Classification systems now use MRI of the femoral head to take into account the size of the lesion and amount of articular surface involved. These systems are more accurate and useful in determining prognosis and treatment. The University of Pennsylvania System is the most useful (see table).

University of Pennsylvania System for Staging Osteonecrosis

STAGE	CRITERIA	STAGE	CRITERIA
0	Normal or nondiagnostic x-ray, bone scan, and MRI	IV	Flattening of femoral head A. Moderate (15% of surface and < 2 mm depression) B. Moderate (15–30% if surface or 2–4mm depression) C. Severe (> 30% of surface or > 4 mm depression)
I	Normal x-ray: abnormal bone scan and/or MRI A. Mild (< 15% of femoral head affected) B. Moderate (15–30%) C. Severe (> 30%)	V	Joint narrowing and/or acetabular changes A. Mild ⎫ Average of femoral head B. Moderate ⎬ involvement, as determined in stage IV, and estimated C. Severe ⎭ acetabular involvement
II	"Cystic" and sclerotic changes in femoral head A Mild (< 15% of femoral B. Moderate (15–30%) C. Severe (> 30%)	VI	Advanced degenerative changes
III	Subchondral collapse (crescent sign) without flattening A. Mild (< 15% of articular surface) B. Moderate (15–30%) C. Severe (> 30%)		

9. What surgical procedures are recommended for treatment of avascular necrosis of the hip?

No single surgical procedure has been accepted for treatment of all patients with avascular necrosis of the hip. In the early stages, before collapse of the femoral head, core decompression with or without bone graft and osteotomy may be effective in preserving the femoral head. Variable results have been reported. In the later stages of the disease, when femoral head collapse has progressed, total joint arthroplasty is more frequently recommended.

10. Where can patients and physicians obtain further information about treatment and research?

The National Osteonecrosis Foundation, Inc.
5601 Loch Raven Blvd., Suite 201
Baltimore, MD 21239
Phone: 410.532.5985
Fax: 410.532.5908
Website: http://www.nonf.org

BIBLIOGRAPHY

1. Aaron RK, Ciombor DM: Electrical stimulation, demineralized bone matrix, and bone morphogenic protein. Semin Arthroplasty 9:221–230, 1998.
2. Amstutz HC, Sparling EA, Grigoris P: Surface and hemi-surface replacement arthroplasty. Semin Arthroplasty 9:261–271, 1998.
3. Bauer TW, Plenk H: The pathology of early osteonecrosis of the femoral head. Semin Arthroplasty 9:192–202, 1998.
4. Cabanela ME: Femoral endoprostheses and total hip replacement for avascular necrosis. Semin Arthroplasty 9:253–260, 1998.

5. Calandruccio RA, Hungerford DS, Kenzora JE, et al: Symposium: Osteonecrosis of the femoral head. Contemp Orthop 14:119–162, 1987.
6. Camp JF, Colwell CW Jr: Core decompression of the femoral head for osteonecrosis. J Bone Joint Surg 68A:1313–1319, 1986.
7. Dutkowski JP: Miscellaneous nontraumatic disorders. In Canale ST (ed): Campbell's Operative Orthopaedics, 9th ed., St. Louis, Mosby, 1998, pp 787–855.
8. Hungerford DS: Bone marrow pressure, venography, and core decompression in ischemic necrosis of the femoral head. In The Hip: Proceedings of the Seventh Open Scientific Meeting of the Hip Society. St. Louis, Mosby, 1979, pp 175–181.
9. Jones JP: Etiology and pathogenesis. Semin Arthroplasty 9:184–191, 1998.
10. Santore RF: Intertrochanteric osteotomies for femoral head necrosis. Semin Arthroplasty 9:242–252, 1998.
11. Steinberg ME: Early diagnosis, evaluation, and staging. Semin Arthroplasty 9:203–212, 1998.
12. Steinberg ME: Core decompression. Semin Arthroplasty 9:213–220, 1998.
13. Sutker BD, Urbaniak JR: Grafting procedures. Semin Arthroplasty 9:231–241, 1998.

58. TOTAL HIP REPLACEMENT

Craig R. Mahoney, M.D., and Peter K. Buchert, M.D.

1. What is arthritis?
Arthritis is inflammation of the joint.

2. What are the causes of arthritis?
- **Noninflammatory:** This category includes idiopathic and posttraumatic degeneration of the joint, congenital deformities(e.g., congenital hip dysplasia), and avascular necrosis.
- **Inflammatory:** The most common is rheumatoid arthritis; others include mixed connective tissue disease, lupus erythematosus, and psoriatic arthritis.

3. What are the clinical manifestations of hip arthritis?
Pain is the main symptom, but the patient also may demonstrate decreased walking distance, decreased range of motion, inability to sleep, limp, and inability to actively flex the hip.

4. Why do patients commonly complain of groin pain?
The obturator nerve runs directly by the hip joint; therefore; it is irritated by the arthritis.

5. What are the common radiographic findings?
The most common findings are narrowing of the hip joint space, osteophyte formation, and subchondral cysts.

6. Why do the osteophytes form?
Once the articular cartilage begins to degenerate, the ability of the cartilage to distribute stress begins to fail, and stress on the bone increases. The bone responds to increased stress by laying down increased bone (Wolff's law). Thus, more surface area is produced to cover the increased stress.

7. Why do subchondral cysts form?
In areas of very high stress, stress fractures occur. Because of continued pressure, the frac-

tures cannot heal and cysts form. Once the stress is relieved (i.e., once a total hip replacement [THR] is done), the cysts usually heal and fill in with bone.

8. What conservative approach should be tried before recommending total hip replacement (THR)?

Most authors agree that antiinflammatory agents, cane, decreased activity, and weight loss (if appropriate) should be tried for at least 6 months before surgery is recommended.

9. On which side of the patient should the cane be used?

The cane should be in the hand opposite the involved hip to decrease the reactive force on the joint.

10. Besides THR, what other surgical procedures are sometimes offered?

Femoral osteotomies, while popular outside the United States, have not gained popularity here. Hip arthroscopy has been shown to be of limited benefit.

11. What are the most popular surgical approaches to the hip?

The most popular are posterior, transtrochanteric, and anterolateral approaches. The posterior and anterolateral approaches are now the most popular. The advantages and disadvantages of each are listed in the table below.

Surgical Approaches to the Hip

APPROACH	ADVANTAGE	DISADVANTAGE
Posterior	Easy to do	Harder to see acetabulum
	Easy to see femur	Increased rate of dislocation
	Rarely trouble with limp	
Transtrochanteric	Easy to do	Complication of trochanteric
	Great exposure	nonunion
		Limp
Anterolateral	Easy to do	Limp
	Good exposure	Heterotopic bone
	Low dislocation rate	

12. What characteristics do modern cemented components have in common?

- Made of super alloys (cobalt-chrome or titanium alloys)
- Smooth edges with no sharp corners
- Fill at least one-half of the diameter of the femoral canal

13. Describe the modern femoral cement technique.

Modern cement technique consists of distal femoral plugging, washing and drying of the canal, use of a cement gun to fill the canal from distal to proximal, and pressurization of the cement. In addition, most surgeons recommend either vacuum mixing or centrifugation to decrease porosity of the cement.

14. What are the advantages of cementless stems?

Cementless stems rely on bone, a biologic interface, for fixation. This interface can react to stresses and strengthen itself over time. Cement is a nonbiologic interface that can degrade with time. Theoretically this could lead to loosening of a previously stable femoral stem.

15. What size should the pores be to facilitate bone ingrowth?

Most authors agree that the pore size should be between 100 and 450 microns.

16. How much porous ingrowth typically occurs in well fixed fully porous coated stems?

Autopsy retrieval studies have shown that porous ingrowth occurs over 30–40% of well fixed fully porous coated femoral stems.

17. What design characteristics should a cementless acetabular component have?

The component should be circular in shape, fully porous coated, and placed in a press-fit (tight) fashion. The necessity and advisability of screw reinforcement are under debate.

18. What size head and liner should be used?

Most experts agree that a 26- or 28-mm head minimizes wear while not increasing dislocation risk secondary to small head size. At least 6 mm of polyethylene in the socket should be available.

BIBLIOGRAPHY

1. American Academy of Orthopaedic Surgeons: Orthopaedic Knowledge Update 2, 3, 4, 5, 6. Elk Grove, IL, American Academy of Orthopaedic Surgeons.
2. Harkess JW: Arthroplasty of hip. In Canale ST (ed): Campbell's Operative Orthopaedics, 9th ed. St. Louis, Mosby, 1998, pp 296–381.
3. Maloney WJ and Hartford JM: The cemented femoral component. In Callaghan JJ (ed): The Adult Hip, Philadelphia, Lippincott-Raven, 1998, pp 959–979.
4. Salvati EA: Academy of Orthopaedic Surgeons Instructional Course Lectures: Complications in Primary THR: Avoidance and Management. Elk Grove, IL, American Academy of Orthopaedic Surgeons, 2002.
5. Tullos HS (ed): American Academy of Orthopaedic Surgeons Instructional Course Lectures 40:117–160, 1991.

59. COMPLICATIONS OF TOTAL HIP REPLACEMENT

Craig R. Mahoney, M.D.

INTRAOPERATIVE COMPLICATIONS

1. What is the vascular effect of insertion of the cement?

The cement is a potent vasodilator and thus can cause hypotension (and in severe cases, death). It is important that the patient remain well hydrated or take vasopressors before insertion of the stem into the femoral canal.

2. What nerves can be injured? What are the common mechanisms of injury during total hip replacement (THR)?

The most common nerve injury is to the sciatic nerve (79% of all nerve palsies after THR). Femoral nerve palsies account for 13% of all palsies. Obturator nerve injury is rare. The etiology of nerve injury is unknown in 47% of cases, attributed to traction in 20%, secondary to contusion in 18% and hematoma in 11%.

3. When putting in screws for an acetabular component, what area is to be avoided?

The anterior half of the acetabulum, defined by the area anterior to a line drawn from the anterior superior iliac spine dividing the acetabulum into two equal halves, should be avoided during screw placement. Structures deep to the bony pelvis in this area include the external iliac artery and vein, and the obturator artery, nerve, and vein. Injury to these structures can occur during screw placement.

4. What factors can lead to intraoperative femoral fractures?
The most common factors are (1) failure to ream straight down the canal; (2) attempts to put too large a component down the canal; (3) attempts to pound the component down the canal too rapidly without allowing the viscoelastic nature of the bone to accept the component (bone expands with time); and (4) failure to appreciate preoperative deformities or distal tightness of the canal.

IMMEDIATE POSTOPERATIVE PERIOD (IN THE HOSPITAL)

5. What is the incidence of thrombophlebitis in untreated patients?
The incidence in most studies is around 50%.

6. What is the reported fatal pulmonary embolus rate after THR?
Approximately 0.1–0.2%.

7. What measures are available to decrease the incidence of thrombophlebitis?
- Early mobilization
- Sequential compression stockings and venous compression devices
- Anticoagulation (warfarin, aspirin, heparin, dextran, low–molecular-weight heparin)

8. What positions should the patient avoid to minimize the possibility of dislocation?
The patient should avoid combinations of excessive flexion, internal rotation, and adduction and combinations of excessive extension, external rotation, and adduction.

9. What are the most common organisms causing infections in THR?
Staphylococcus aureus is the most common infecting organism when all orthopedic procedures are examined; however *Staphylococcus epidermidis* is the most common infecting organism in when orthopedic prostheses are present.

10. What known factors decrease the incidence of infection?
Before surgery, the patient should be in satisfactory dental health and free of infection in any other organ system, which later may seed the artificial joint. Patients should also be adequately nourished and free of any skin conditions that may provide a portal for bacterial entrance. Perioperative prophalactic antibiotics effectively reduce the incidence of deep wound infection. Laminar air flow within an enclosed area, combined with total body exhaust-ventilated suits, further decreases exogenous wound contamination. Efficient surgical technique with meticulous hemostasis and closure also contribute to uneventful wound healing.

LONG-TERM COMPLICATIONS

11. What is the most common long-term complication?
Loosening that causes pain is the most common complication.

12. How can one determine if a component is loose on radiographs?
Radiographic evidence of loosening includes (1) migration of the component, (2) fracture of the cement, and (3) a 2-mm lucent line completely surrounding the prosthesis.

13. What is osteolysis?
Osteolysis is a severe absorption of bone around the prosthesis mediated by collagenases, prostaglandins, and proteases.

14. What is thought to be the initiating factor in osteolysis?
Debris from polyethylene wear is thought to be the most common initiating factor. When the polyethylene of the acetabular liner wears, it can travel throughout the effective joint space, which includes all the areas around the hip that are accessed by the synovial fluid of the hip.

15. How can one minimize polyethylene debris?
Factors that can minimize polyethylene debris include (1) proper head; size (26–28 mm); (2) maximal polyethylene thickness (at least 6 mm); (3) alternative bearing surfaces, such as ceramics or metal; and (4) highly cross-linked polyethylene.

16. How can late hematogenous infections be prevented?
Preventive strategies include (1) prophylactic antibiotics for dental work, nonclean operations, and urologic manipulations, and (2) aggressive treatment of systemic infections.

17. How can heterotopic bone be prevented in high-risk patients?
The risk can be decreased intraoperatively by meticulous handling of soft tissues and eliminating the contents of the intrameduallary canal from the wound after reaming. A single dose of 600 rads 2–3 days after surgery is recommended. Indomethacin also may be used.

BIBLIOGRAPHY

1. American Academy of Orthopaedic Surgeons: Orthopaedic Knowledge Update 2, 3, 4, 5, 6. Rosemont, IL, American Academy of Orthopaedic Surgeons.
2. Balderston RA: The Hip. Philadelphia, Lea & Febiger, 1992, pp 393–352.
3. Fitzgerald RH: Infected total hip arthroplasty: Diagnosis and treatment. A comprehensive review. J Am Acad Orthop Surg 3:249–262, 1995.
4. Harkess JW: Arthroplasty of hip. In Canale ST (ed): Campbell's Operative Orthopaedics, 9th ed., St. Louis, Mosby, 1998, pp 381–424.
5. Pritchard DJ (ed): Instructional Course Lecture, vol. 45. American Academy of Orthopaedic Surgeons, 1996, pp 171–198.
6. Salvati EA: Academy of Orthopaedic Surgeons Instructional Course Lectures—Complications in Primary THR: Avoidance and Management, 2002.

60. TOTAL HIP ARTHROPLASTY INFECTIONS

Joshua A. Urban, M.D.

1. What is the deep infection rate after primary total hip arthroplasty?
The deep infection rate after total hip arthroplasty currently averages between 1–2 %. In tertiary centers that specialize in total hip arthroplasty procedures, this infection rate is as low as 0.6%.

2. What are the two most common routes of pathogenic seeding of the periprosthetic environment?
Direct seeding of the prosthetic hip occurs either at the time of surgery or in the early postoperative period. During surgery, before the wound has been closed, the prosthetic hip is vulnerable to seeding as it lies open and exposed to its environment. Bacteria that gain access to the wound via this route of seeding can originate from the patient, the operating room environment, or from operating room personnel. Direct seeding of the joint also can occur in the early postoperative period, most commonly in the setting of delayed wound healing and its accompanying pro-

longed wound drainage. Contiguous infectious processes such as superficial wound infections or suture abscesses can also directly seed the periprosthetic environment during this time period.

Hematogenous seeding refers to the inoculation of the prosthetic joint by a bacteremic event originating at a remote site. This type of seeding can occur at anytime during the life of the prosthesis.

3. What organisms commonly cause total hip arthroplasty infections?

Staphylococci bacteria are the most commonly isolated pathogens from total hip arthroplasty infections. Among the staphylococci, *Staphylococcus epidermidis* is the most common, with *Staphylococcus aureus* representing the second most common bacterial species. Streptococci, enterococci, and gram-positive cocci also are frequent pathogens, while gram-negative bacteria are less common. Fungi and mycobacteria are infrequently encountered in these infections.

4. What is the concept of "the race for the surface"? How does it apply to total hip arthroplasty infections?

The race for the surface describes the competition between host tissue and bacteria for the colonization of the surface of implanted materials. According to this concept, the surface of the prosthetic components are immediately coated with a "conditioning film" when they are implanted into a biologic environment. This film is derived from host tissue and consists of proteins, macromolecules, and cellular elements. It is this "film" that is able to be colonized by either host tissue cells or bacteria. Therefore, the "race" between host tissue cells and bacteria occurs for the dominance of this conditioning film. If the host tissue cells colonize the film prior to bacterial colonization, subsequent bacteria encounter a living integrated cell surface with intact host defense mechanisms that are resistant to secondary bacterial colonization. Conversely, if bacteria are able to colonize the film prior to host cell colonization, it is unlikely that host tissue cells will be able to displace them and an infection will ensue.

The importance of the race for the surface in total hip arthroplasty infections is due to the large amount of foreign body implanted in total hip arthroplasty. Less bacteria has been shown to be necessary to establish an infection in the presence of a foreign body. Furthermore, the specific biomaterials used in total hip arthroplasty may also increase the risk of infection by preferentially attracting certain bacterial species. In *in vitro* retrieval studies, *Staphylococcus epidermidis* was the predominant organism in wounds containing polymers. *Staphylococcus aureus,* on the other hand, was the predominant organism isolated in wounds containing metals. These phenomena have also been tied to studies showing that wear of the polyethylene may release esters that can be metabolized by *Staphylococcus epidermidis*. Also, ions released from corrosion of metal may stabilize the glycocalyx that may lead to increased bacterial adhesion and antagonistic resistance.

5. Describe the signs and symptoms of an infected total hip arthroplasty (THA).

The clinical picture of a periprosthetic total hip infection is highly variable. The majority of patients present with relatively mild signs and symptoms. Often, mild pain is its only symptom. Less frequently do these infections present as fulminant processes with a combination of local signs such as deep throbbing pain, wound drainage, erythema, and swelling about the hip. In these fulminant infections it is not uncommon to have associated fever, chills, and generalized malaise.

6. What diagnostic studies should be ordered in the work-up of a painful total hip arthroplasty that is suspected of being infected?

Plain radiographs, complete blood count with differential, erythrocyte sedimentation rate, and C-reactive protein

7. Describe the findings associated with total hip infections on plain radiographs.

Plain radiographs are rarely diagnostic for a total hip infection, however they should be obtained in each suspected case to rule out other cases of pain and serve as a baseline for future radiographs. A differential diagnosis for total hips with mild pain includes fracture, component failure, and heterotopic ossification. One finding that has shown to be helpful to distinguish septic from aseptic loosening is periosteal new bone formation. This finding is considered by some to pathognomonic for total hip infection. Excluding this finding, all of the radiographic changes consistent with periprosthetic infection can also be found in aseptic loosening.

8. Describe the results of a complete blood count with differential, erythrocyte sedimentation rate, and C-reactive protein associated with total hip arthroplasty infections.

In fulminant infections, the CBC with differential may demonstrate the presence of leukocytosis with an increased percentage of immature white blood cells. Unfortunately, this phenomenon rarely occurs in the indolent presentations, and therefore this test is rarely abnormal in most THA infections.

The ESR is an indirect indicator of a systemic response to an inflammatory process. Unfortunately, the ability of the ESR to be influenced by any inflammatory condition decreases its specificity and predictive value when used independently. For example, in uncomplicated THA the ESR may not return to baseline levels for at least 6 months to a year after surgery making this an especially unreliable test in the early post-operative period. When used alone, the reported sensitivity and specificity of ESR in diagnosing total hip infections are 0.82 and 0.86, respectively.

CRP is also a non-specific indicator for information, infections, and neoplastic processes. In contrast to the ESR, CRP levels return to baseline shortly after surgery as normal values have been demonstrated at an average of three weeks post-operatively (range 1–8 weeks). Elevated CRP levels are greater than 10 mg per liter have been associated with periprosthetic infection. Although the reported sensitivity (0.96) and specificity (0.92) of CRP alone are superior to those reported ESR, its specificity has been shown to increase to 1.00 when used concurrently with the ESR.

9. What are the second-tier diagnostic studies that may be used in the work-up of a suspected infected THA?

Hip aspiration and radionucleotide imagining

10. What is the current recommendation for the use of hip aspiration in the work-up of infected THA?

Although hip aspiration has been previously used as a routine screening tool to rule out infection in all arthroplasty failures, current recommendations discourage this practice. When used for all THA failures, the sensitivity and specificity of hip aspiration have widely varied. Therefore, the use of hip aspiration is currently recommended only in cases that are suspicious for an infection. The addition of a pre-operative hip aspirate to abnormal ESR and CRP values has been shown to increase the probability of infection from 83% to 89%. In addition, in a study of 202 THRs, the possibility of infection was 0 when the hip aspirate, ESR and CRP were all negative.

Various methods have been recommended to increase the accuracy of a single hip aspiration, including: (1) discontinuing any concurrent antibiotic used 2–3 weeks prior to aspiration, (2) limiting the use of local anesthetics during the procedure to just the superficial tissues, as these are bacteriostatic, (3) confirmation of intra-articular position with arthrogram, (4) obtaining multiple samples during the same aspiration, (5) obtaining a fine-needle biopsy of synovial tissue during aspiration.

11. List the intra-operative diagnostic studies used in the diagnosis of THA infection. Describe the accuracy of each study.

Gram stain: This study has been fairly unreliable in the diagnosis of periprosthetic total hip infections. Sensitivities ranging from 0 to 0.23 (average 0.19) have been reported. The gram stain is not to be totally abandoned as positive results could provide early information regarding the offending organism and guide initial antibiotic therapy.

Cultures: Intra-operative cultures remain the standard to which all of the intra-operative diagnostic modalities are compared. As with the other diagnostic tests for this disease process, cultures are not fool-proof as both significant false-positive and false-negative rates have been reported. To avoid inaccurate results, precise technique must be followed:

1. Antibiotics should be withheld until specimens have been obtained.

2. Instruments used to obtain the culture should be prevented from touching the skin of the patient.

3. Samples should be obtained from the environment close to the prosthesis and if possible, from inflamed tissue.

4. A minimum of three specimens should be sent fresh to the laboratory for immediate processing.

5. The specimen should be obtained immediately after the pseudocapsule is opened from an area not previously cauterized before any irrigation has been used. Using this technique, sensitivities and specificities as high as 0.94 and 0.97 have been reported respectively.

Frozen sections: Intra-operative frozen sections of the prosthetic environment are used to diagnosed THA infections by determining the quantity of inflammatory cells. The previous threshold of five polymorphonuclear leucocytes per high powered field (5 PMN/hpf) has been thought to be highly suggestive of infection. Sensitivities and specificities of > 0.80 and 0.90, respectively, have been reported using this 5 PMN/hpf threshold. When 10 PMN/hpf is used as the threshhold, the specificity increases from 0.96 to 0.99 without decreasing the sensitivity (0.84).

Polymerase chain reaction: PCR is a technique that shows promise in diagnosing infection in THA. The PCR technique involves the amplification of nucleic acid extracted from periprosthetic synovial fluid and screening it for the presence of bacterial DNA. This technique has the ability to diagnose periprosthetic infections when only a small quantity of bacteria is present. This ability to detect minute amounts of nucleate acid may result in a high false-positive rates. This hypersensitivity of PCR currently limits this diagnostic test's use to the laboratory but it is anticipated that this technique will provide a useful tool in diagnosing THA infections in the future.

12. List the four types of THA infection according to the Tsukayama classification system.

Positive intraoperative cultures: When at least two intraoperative cultures obtained at the time of revision are positive. Often these results are known only after the revision is performed as many of these of cases typically have no preoperative signs or symptoms suggesting infection.

Early postoperative infection: In these types of infection, symptoms develop within one month after implantation.

Late chronic infection: In these types of infection, symptoms develop one month or more after implantation.

Acute hematogenous infection: Symptoms develop acutely in a previously well-functioning hip.

13. What are the general treatment principles for an infected THA?

The mainstays of treatment are a prolonged course of antibiotics and surgery. Most treatment regimens that incorporate both of these modalities yield fairly consistent eradication rates. When these modalities are used alone, the chance for true eradication diminishes and the likelihood for failure of treatment increases.

14. Describe the typical antibiotic regimen for treatment of THA infections.

Essentially the same antibiotic regimen is used regardless of the choice of surgical treatment for infected THA. Parenteral antibiotics should be initiated immediately after cultures of the periprosthetic environment are obtained. The initial antibiotic should be a broad spectrum agent that is likely to be active against the organisms common to periprosthetic infections. In most cases, a first-generation cephalosporin (cefazolin) or a penicillinase-resistant penicillin (methicillin or oxacillin) will suffice. Once the organism or organisms have been identified, antibiotic treatment is modified in favor of a more specific agent to which the pathogens are sensitive. It is advised that consultation with an infectious disease specialist be obtained to aid in selecting the appropriate antibiotic regimen.

Serum bactericidal titers (SBT) should be obtained during each antibiotic regimen to ensure adequate serum levels of the selected antibiotic. An SBT threshold of 1:8 has been determined to be a sufficient serum concentration in the majority of patients.

15. What is the optimum duration of antibiotic treatment?
The optimum duration of antibiotic treatment is controversial. However, most authors favor an antibiotic course lasting for 4–6 weeks.

16. What are the treatment options available in the management of infected total hip arthroplasty?
- Two-stage reimplantation
- One-stage reimplantation
- Resection arthroplasty
- Debridement with retention of the prosthesis
- Chronic suppressive antibiotics without surgical intervention
- Arthroscopic debridement with retention of the prosthesis
- Hip arthrodesis
- Hip disarticulation

17. What factors are important in determining the optimal treatment method for a particular total hip infection?
The duration of the infection is an important factor and must be considered in determining which surgical option is the best for a particular THA infection. This factor chiefly influences whether the original prosthesis may be retained or removed. Studies have shown that a high rate of success can be achieved with component retention in infections of less than 1-month duration. Component retention is preferable as it is a less extensive procedure and bone stock is preserved. This 1-month threshold is believed to be directly related to the amount of glycocalyx bacteria are able to produce. In bacterial infections of less than one month, it is believed that insufficient amounts of glycocalyx are present which allows local debridement and prosthetic retention to be effective in the majority of cases. On the other hand, infections of greater than one month in duration are thought to have increased amounts of glycocalyx to the point where prosthetic retention is less reliable than removal.

Other factors that influence which treatment options should be chosen include: the virulence of the offending pathogen, the quality of the remaining bone in the periprosthetic environment, the stability of the implant, the patient's overall medical condition and the patient's willingness to undergo additional procedures.

18. Of the available surgical treatment options, which has yielded the highest success rate?
Two-stage reimplantation. This is considered the surgical treatment method of choice in all but a minority of cases. The success rates with two-stage reimplantation have averaged 92%. Less extensive procedures such as debridement with retention of components or one-stage reimplantation may be considered only if their relative indications exist.

19. Define two-stage reimplantation. What are the indications and success rate for this technique?
Two-stage reimplantation involves the removal of the prosthesis and resection of all infected tissue followed by reimplantation of a new prosthesis at a second surgical setting. The interval between surgeries lasts at least six weeks and consists of a regimen of intravenous antibiotics. Once the antibiotic interval is completed, if diagnostic studies indicate the eradication of the infection, components are then reimplanted. Determining whether successful eradication has occurred is imperative prior to reimplantation and, like the diagnosis of infection itself, may be challenging.

The indications for this method of treatment include adequate bone stock, or a bone stock deficiency amenable to reconstruction, minimal serious medical comorbidity, and the patient's willingness to undergo two additional procedures.

Two-stage reimplantation is considered the gold standard in the treatment of periprosthetic hip infections as the highest success rates (average 92%) have been reported with this technique.

20. Define one-stage reimplantation. What are the indications and success rates for this technique?

One-stage reimplantation involves the excision of all prosthetic components and infected tissues and the reimplantation of new components during the same surgical procedure. After surgery, the patient undergoes a parenteral antibiotic regimen of at least 4–6 weeks.

The indications for a one-stage reimplantation include:

- A pathogen sensitive to antibiotics
- Non-glycocalyx producing bacteria
- A patient with few or no risk factors for infection (rheumatoid arthritis, diabetes mellitus, etc)
- A wound in which there is adequate bone and soft tissue to support reconstruction of the hip
- Comorbid medical conditions that place the patient at increased risk with a second major procedure.

The overall experience with one-stage reimplantation has demonstrated inferior success rates in comparison with the two-stage technique. In a recent literature review, a cumulative success rate of 83% has been reported. Recent studies that followed more stringent indications (as listed above), however, have demonstrated success comparable to two-stage reimplantation. The advantages of this technique over a two -stage procedure including decreased cost and morbidity associated with the need for one less procedure.

21. Define resection arthroplasty. What are the indications and success rates for this technique?

Resection arthroplasty involves the removal of all components and involved tissue with no subsequent reimplantation. After the resection, a parenteral antibiotic regimen similar to that used for the reimplantation techniques is begun. Resection arthroplasty is essentially considered a salvage operation for the patient who is not a candidate for one of the reimplantation techniques or for debridement with retention of components.

The accepted indications for this technique include:

- The presence of a highly resistant organism
- Poor quality of bone and soft tissues
- Patient risk factors predisposing to recurring infections (chronic immosuppression, IV drug use, rheumatoid arthritis, etc.)
- The inability or unwillingness of the patient to comply with the post-operative regimens of the reimplantation techniques
- A medically unfit patient

The success of this technique has been reported to be as high as 100% in a small series of patients. The disadvantage of this technique, however, is the resulting function of the patient as an inevitable leg length discrepancy occurs which is manifested as a prominent lurching gait and a corresponding increase in energy expenditure during ambulation. Furthermore, the functional results after resection arthroplasty for infection tend to be inferior compared to resection arthroplasty for other diagnoses. This technique does however result in acceptable success with respect to pain relief and eradication of infection and, most patients are able to function at least satisfactorily but will require ambulatory aides and shoe lifts.

22. What are the indications and success rates associated with a hip arthrodesis?

Limited experience exists in the literature regarding the use of hip arthrodesis for the treatment of total hip infections. Much like resection arthroplasty, hip arthrodesis is considered to be a salvage operation. Hip arthrodesis is actually preferable to resection arthroplasty as the functional results from hip fusion are considerably better compared to resection arthroplasty. In contrast to resection arthroplasty, arthrodesis patients can stand unaided, do not have difficulties performing household duties, do not require the security of external support, and are more likely to be able to perform heavy occupational activities. In those cases in which the reimplantation techniques or debridement with potential components is not indicated, this procedure represents the most attractive salvage option.

The success rates with this technique with respect to eradication of infection are quite high and often reach 100%. Most of this reported series deal with a small number of patients however, and the potential risk of recurrent infection associated with retained hardware implanted at the time of fusion must be considered.

23. Define debridement with retention of components. What are the indications and success rates associated with this technique?

This technique involves the debridement of the involved soft tissues, exchange of the polyethylene insert, and retention of the remaining components combined with a post-operative course of parenteral antibiotics lasting 4–6 weeks.

Generally accepted criteria for the use of this technique include:

- Duration of infection of less than 1 month
- A pathogen sensitive to antibiotics
- The absence of extensive scar tissue
- Minimal and no risk factors for infection
- A well-fixed prosthesis

The results of this technique have been variable with success rates reported between 0–80 %. As with the one-stage reimplantation technique, adherence to specific criteria has been shown to be necessary to optimize the results when using debridement and retention.

24. Of the aforementioned indications for debridement with retention of components, which factor is considered to be the most crucial?

Of all the indications for debridement with retention of components, the factor that is considered most crucial is the *duration of infection* (less than 1 month). The difficulty for the treating surgeon lies in determining the true onset of infection. The onset of infection in the early postoperative period is relatively straightforward as these infections are presumed to be the result of seeding of the hip at, or shortly after, the time of surgery. Likewise, it is usually not difficult to determine that the onset of infection in late chronic infections is greater than 1 month as these are usually characterized by several months of gradually increasing symptoms. The difficulty occurs in attempting to accurately determine the onset of infection in acute hematogenous infections.

In the acute hematogenous infection, the treating surgeon is dependent upon the duration of symptoms as an indicator of the duration of infection. Unfortunately, it can be difficult to determine whether the development of symptoms is from an acute infection that has just begun or from a subacute indolent infection that has just become symptomatic despite being present for several weeks or months. Those patients in whom this distinction cannot be made should be managed as if they had a chronic infection and should undergo two-stage reimplantation.

25. Define chronic suppressive therapy. What are the indications and success rates associated with this technique?

This method of treatment entails long-term antibiotic therapy without any adjunctive surgical intervention. The goal of this technique is to control the infection by inhibiting the growth and proliferation of the offending bacteria.

This form of therapy should not be considered as a first-line modality and is only appropriate when the following indications exist:

- Patients with serious comorbid medical conditions associated with an unacceptable surgical risk
- Patients who refuse surgery
- The infecting organism must be identified.

- The infecting organism must be sensitive to an oral antibiotic.
- The oral antibiotic should have the potential for minimal side effects when given long term.

Chronic suppressive therapy has demonstrated inferior success rates (between 47–67%) compared to the combination of antibiotic and surgical techniques. The unanswered question with respect to this therapy is, how long should the patient receive the antibiotics. Many studies suggest life-long antibiotics while other studies suggest shorter regimens (6 months). Unfortunately, prolonged suppressive antibiotic therapy does risk the emergence of resistant organisms which may necessitate one of the salvage procedures.

26. Define arthroscopic debridement with component retention. What are the indications and success rates with this technique?

Arthroscopic debridement with component retention, as its name implies, involves the debridement and lavage via arthroscopy of the prosthetic hip. No components are exchanged with the use of this technique. A standard antibiotic regimen is begun after surgery lasting approximately 4–6 weeks. To our knowledge, only one study has reported the use of this technique. The result was 100% success at a mean of 70 months in eight THA infections.

The indications for this type of intervention are the same as that for chronic suppressive therapy. In fact, this treatment alternative should be considered a variant of chronic suppressive therapy, as long-term oral suppression was used in the only study describing this technique once the antibiotic regimen had been completed. Further studies are needed to investigate the role of this technique in the treatment of THA infections.

27. What are the indications and success rates for hip disarticulation in the treatment of THA infections?

Hip disarticulation should only be entertained when life threatening infections or severe loss of soft tissue and bone stock are present. In one of the few studies describing this technique, 10 of 11 (91%) patients with chronically infected THA were treated successfully.

28. What prophylactic technique has been shown to be most effective in reducing the incidence of THA infection?

The most effective prophylactic measure in the prevention in THA infections has been the administration of systemic antibiotics immediately prior to surgery and in the immediate post-operative period.

29. When should prophylactic antibiotics be given in relation to the surgical procedure?

Pre-operative systemic antibiotics have been shown to be more effective if given shortly before the skin incision. It is currently recommended that the antibiotic be given 50–60 minutes prior to the skin incision to allow adequate tissue levels to be obtained. Arthroplasties that require a tourniquet (total knee arthroplasties) should receive antibiotic prophylaxis at least 5–10 minutes prior to inflation. Administration of antibiotics one or more days pre-operatively provides no additional protection and may alter the patients natural skin flora.

30. What is the optimal duration of antibiotic prophylaxis?

The optimal duration of antibiotic prophylaxis is controversial. Several studies have investigated one-day, three-day, and seven-day regimens. The current consensus on the duration of systemic antibiotic prophylaxis for a routine primary THA is for a single pre-operative dose followed by 2–3 post-operative doses. Shorter regimens are thought to minimize the expense, toxicity, and potential for the development of resistant organisms while still providing adequate antimicrobial activity.

31. What are the current recommendations with respect to the use of antibiotics in the cement of primary THAs as a means of preventing periprosthetic infection?

Currently, no standards or clinical guidelines have been established with respect to the routine use of antibiotics in bone cement. Concerns over the potential for the emergence of resistant organisms, toxic reactions to the antibiotics, whether any additional protective effect is gained when used in combination with system antibiotics, and the mechanical effects of adding antibiotics have tempered its use to less than 20% of primary THAs. In our center, we reserve prophylactic antibiotic impregnated cement for THA revisions, as there seems to be an additional benefit to the use in preventing infection in this population.

32. Define "clean air technology." What are the current recommendations for clean air technology in the prophylaxis of total hip infections?
Clean air technology refers to the various techniques used to minimize the number of airborne bacteria in the operating room during surgery. Clean air technology is a common term referring to the use of laminar airflow within operating room suites, full body exhaust suits, and the reduction of operating room traffic.

Although clean air technology has been shown to reduce the number of bacteria-containing particles within the operating room suite, its use is controversial in the setting of concurrent prophylactic systemic antibiotics. In a study that compared the efficacy of prophylactic antibiotics versus clean air technology, both techniques resulted in a decrease in total hip infections. Systemic prophylactic antibiotics resulted in a greater degree of reduction than clean air technology. When the techniques were used together, further reduction of infection was noted, but this difference was not significant. Proponents of clean air technology point to the trend of lower infection rates seen in this study and the need to provide additional prophylaxis in an era of the increasing antibiotic resistance. Critics point to the lack of significant differences in infection rates in the setting of concomitant use of prophylactic antibiotics, and the increased expense of installing and maintaining laminar air flow systems.

REFERENCES

1. Callaghan JJ, RP Katz, RC Johnston: One-stage revision surgery of the infected hip: A minimum 10-year follow-up study. Clin Orthop 1999; 369:139–143.
2. Garvin KL, AD Hanssen: Current concepts review: Infection after total hip arthroplasty. J Bone Joint Surg 1995; 77-A:1576–1588.
3. Hanssen AD, Osmon DR, Nelson CL: Prevention of deep periprosthetic joint infection. J Bone Joint Surg 1996; 78-A:458–471.
4. Tsukayama DT, R Estrada, RB Gustilo: Infection after total hip arthroplasty. A study of the treatment of 106 infections. J Bone Joint Surg 1996; 78-A:512–523.
5. Urban JA Garvin KL: Infected total hip arthroplasty. In Fitzgerald R, Kaufer H, Malkani A (eds): Orthopaedics. Philadelphia, Mosby, 2002 pp 755–768.

61. REVISION OF TOTAL HIP REPLACEMENT

Randall Neumann, M.D.

1. What are the mechanisms of failure of total hip replacement?
Aseptic loosening is due to poor patient selection, modulous mismatch between implant and bone, generation of wear debris, or fixation failure.

Infection may be decreased by the use of prophylactic antibiotics, laminar flow, ultraviolet lights, and exhaust systems. The incidence varies from 0.4–1.5%.

Dislocation is caused by component malposition, component impingement, sepsis, and patient factors such as senility, noncompliance, alcoholism, and revisional surgery. The surgical approach is also important; a posterior approach is associated with a higher dislocation rate than an anterior approach. The incidence of dislocation is 1–10%.

Heterotopic ossification is usually associated with revision operations. The incidence is higher in patients with previous heterotopic ossification, ankylosing spondylitiis, diffuse idiopathic skeletal hyperostosis (DISH syndrome), and Paget's disease. Current prophylactic treatment favors single-dose radiation therapy. Indomethacin has been used, but diphosphonates usually do not work.

Unstable fractures about the total hip replacement should undergo internal fixation if the implant is not loose. If the implant is loose, revision arthroplasty should be performed.

Component breakage is not a contemporary problem, because components are now made of superstrength metals and with stronger designs.

Particle generation has caused concern about dissimilar metals and corrosion at the interface of modular head-neck components, which may result in component fracture.

Osteolysis is focal endosteal erosion due to wear debris or particle disease (polyethylene, metal, or cement). It may occur in both cemented and noncemented forms.

2. What are the current problems with wear?

Wear in total hip arthroplasty may occur at any interface: the articulating surface, modular connections, and fixation interfaces. All biomaterials can wear: methacrylate, polyethylene, metallic alloys, and bone. Accumulation of wear debris in periarticular tissues results in a foreign-body reaction that is linked to bone resorption. Migration may occur with gross wear. Systemic accumulation also may occur, but the consequences are unknown. Factors affecting wear include polyethylene thickness (early designs with less than 6 mm of polyethylene show increased wear), head diameter (a large head in a small metal-backed acetabulum leads to increased polyethylene wear), and properties of the polyethylene. Metal backing of the acetabular component causes thinning of the acetabular polyethylene. In addition, hemispherical polyethylene liners fit the metal shell better than cylindrical designs. The locking mechanism is also important to prevent polyethylene wear within the metal shell. Recently, more wear problems have been reported secondary to heightened awareness and longer service of the implant.

3. Describe the symptoms of patients with failed total hip arthroplasty.

Patients frequently complain of pain. Start-up pain results when the patient must stand and place weight on the prosthesis before beginning to walk. Patients feel that they must seat the prosthesis into a stable position so that it will bear their full weight during stance phase. Patients sometimes have night pain. Those with infection have pain daily and certainly complain of night pain. Deformity may be noted, especially external rotation and shortening of the lower extremity. Dislocations may be the first sign of polyethylene wear.

4. What common surgical approaches can be used for revision total hip arthroplasty?

- **Posterior**—common approach for uncomplicated revisions.
- **Direct lateral**—used if index procedure was a direct lateral. Can be extended posteriorly distally to elevate the vastus lateralis and expose the proximal femur.
- **Transtrochanteric**—removes the trochanter with gluteus medius and minimus intact. High nonunion rates.
- **Trochanteric slide**—keeps vastus lateralis intact with exposure of the shaft.
- **Extended trochanteric osteotomy**—popularized by Paprosky, this technique involves trochanteric osteotomy extended down the shaft.
- **Triiraiate**—for complex reconstructions.

5. What is an extended trochanteric osteotomy?

The femur is osteotomized during the surgical approach to the hip. The vastus lateralis is first elevated off the shaft. A high speed burr is used to make multiple perforations from the base of the trochanter distally along the shaft. These perforations are just anterior to the linea aspera. These holes should also extend to the anterolateral cortex, which should include approximately one-third of the circumference of the femoral shaft between them. Wide osteotomes are used to open the previously perforated cortices. The vastus, gluteus medius, and minimus remain attached to the trochanter and shaft as a single unit.

6. What is the technique of component removal?

Acetabular component removal. The strategy for component removal should include the selection of an appropriate surgical approach to maximize visualization and access, while minimizing risk to the adjacent neurovascular structures of the hip joint. Thin, curved osteotomes may be used to disrupt the cement prosthesis interface. Extraction devices may be embedded into the polyethylene. Levering against the thin, attenuated bony columns should be avoided, because a fracture may occur. High-speed burs may be used to divide well-fixed cups. Cement may be removed from the acetabulum by fragmenting the cement with sharp osteotomes or a high-speed bur. Special caution is required when the cement and the anchor hole protrude into the acetabulum and pelvis, because vascular structures may be entrapped; in such cases, a preoperative arteriogram or contrast CT should be considered.

Femoral component removal. Cement overhanging the bone should be removed. A slap hammer, vice grips, or bone tamps may be used to remove the cement in a retrograde fashion. Broken stems must be removed by creating an anterior perforation hole, removing the proximal portion, and using the controlled perforation for retrograde removal of the distal portion. The femoral cement is removed with hand instruments for fragmentation, such as high-speed drills or ultrasonic equipment. The cement fails under tension. Ultrasonic instruments may be used at all levels of the femur. Precoated or fully porous coated stems require special caution. Use of the extended trochanteric osteotomy has reduced the need for perforations and lessened the risk of fractures of the shaft.

7. Describe the classification of acetabular defects developed by the American Academy of Orthopaedic Surgeons.

1. Segmental defects
    - Peripheral (rim)
    - Central (medial)
2. Cavitary defects
    - Superior
    - Anterior
    - Posterior
    - Medial (protrusio)
3. Combined defects (cavitary and segmental), which are the most common
4. Pelvic discontinuity
5. Arthrodesis

8. Describe the principles of acetabular reconstruction.

Restore the center of rotation.
Restore bony continuity and integrity of the acetabulum.
Contain the prosthesis.
Contain the graft.
Use rigid graft fixation.
Secure prosthetic fixation.

9. Describe acetabular reconstruction.

Preoperative planning includes templating to determine the size and to find the center of rotation. The contralateral hip should be used, if normal. Special studies may be required, such as an arthrogram to rule out sepsis, arteriography, or contrast CT to study vascular structures in cases of protruded components or cement. An attempt should be made to classify the deficiencies postoperatively.

Bone grafting may be used to feel the defect. The graft depends on the type of deficiency. Bulk graft may be used for segmental and large cavitary defects, whereas particulate graft is preferred for cavitary defects. Small defects may heal spontaneously. The sources of bone include autograft from the iliac crest, allograft femoral heads, femoral condyles, or acetabula. The defect also may be filled with a custom prosthesis or oblong cups. Cement may be used to fill smaller defects. Pelvic discontinuity needs to be repaired with reconstruction plates.

For **severe deficiencies**, trochanteric osteotomy or plating may be performed in patients with an anteroposterior column defect, as necessary. Triradiate exposure may be used for anterior column disruption or whole acetabular allograft. Anterior, trochanteric slide, direct lateral, extended trochanteric osteotomy, or posterior approaches may be used, depending on the preoperative defect.

Pelvic discontinuity may be treated with antiprotrusio reconstruction rings. These provide screw fixation to the distant periacetabular bone of the ilium and ishium. Bone graft is used behind the ring, and a polyethelene acetabular component is cemented into position. Failure rates vary from 2% to 30% due to migration, fracture, malposition, and component loosening.

With **segmental and large cavitary defects**, the component may be unstable in the host bone. In this case, structural graft is required. Allograft using femoral heads or distal femoral condyles are fixated with K-wires or Steinmann pins. The defect is reamed, as well as the allograft, to size the acetabulum. Fixation is performed with screws and/or plates directed along the weight-bearing forces. The graft is then prepared for the acetabular component, which is usually placed in a noncemented mode. The goals of acetabular grafting are to restore hip mechanics and bone stock. Many studies of hip revision indicate that failed grafts were performed with poor graft preparation, poor bed preparation, and poor internal fixation.

10. What are the options for reconstruction of the femur?

Cemented reconstruction: Indications include an intact cortex and intact intramedullary content, advanced age (75 years or older), metabolic bone disease, low activity level, and limited life expectancy.

Cementless reconstruction: Indicated for patients who have lost the intramedullary content of the femur but have an intact cortex, or in whom the proximal femur is destroyed. Cementless fixation is used for younger, active patients with no significant medical history, medium or high activity expectations, and an absence of significant metabolic bone disease. Porous coating is used to achieve a "scratch fit," stabilizing the construct in axial and rotatory fashion.

Reconstruction with impaction grafting and a cemented prosthesis: Indicated for patients with mechanical femoral failure and proximal bone loss. An "intact femoral tube" is reconstructed with struts, wire, and mesh. Cancellous allograft is impacted into the canal, using sized femoral broaches as a tamp to compact the bone. A smooth prosthesis is then cemented into the canal using modern cement techniques.

11. Outline the incidence of fracture associated with total hip arthroplasty.

Intraoperative Fractures	Incidence (%)
Cemented primary arthroplasty	1–3.2
Cemented revision	3–12
Uncemented primary arthroplasty	3–28
Uncemented revision	3–46
Postoperative Fractures	
Primary cemented arthroplasty	0.6
Uncemented primary arthroplasty	0.4
Cemented revision	2.8
Uncemented revision	1.5

12. How are femoral fractures classified?

Type 1: proximal to stem tip
Type 2: spiral, proximal, and distal to stem tip
Type 3: distal to stem tip

13. What factors contribute to femoral fractures?
- Osteoporosis
- Need for removal of cement and implant
- Bone preparation mistakes
- Oversizing the implant
- Overzealous insertion

14. What measures can be taken to prevent femoral fractures?

Prevention includes preoperative planning and radiographs to avoid femoral perforation; prophylactic cerclage wires when fracture is possible; cleaning of the canal of residual cement to avoid fracture during reaming; and bypassing cortical defects or stress fractures by two femoral canal diameters.

15. Discuss the treatment of femoral fractures.

Most **intraoperative fractures** are proximal and minor. A routine cerclage is advisable for treatment.

Postoperative fractures have high complication rates. Closed treatment gives variable results with a higher nonunion rate. The malunion rate is lower with revision or open reduction and internal fixation. Treatment options include cerclage wire, Ogden plates, bone grafts or struts, long-stemmed prosthesis, and cement. Postoperative fracture management includes partial non–weight-bearing strategies and casting. Most patients require open reduction and internal fixation or revision of the prosthesis if it is loose or if the fracture is unstable.

16. Describe the management of infected total hip arthroplasty.

The incidence of infection is approximately 1%. Prophylactic antibiotics are the most important factor in reducing the rate of deep sepsis. The organism is usually gram-positive; 90% are staphylococci. Organisms with increased virulence include the methicillin-resistant *Staphylococcus aureus*, gram-negative bacilli, group D streptococci, and enterococci. The incidence is increased in patients who have had previous hip surgery, including fracture or total hip arthroplasty. Treatment options include:
- Surgical debridement in acute infections (less than 2–3 weeks after arthroplasty)
- Antibiotic suppression in patients with limited life span
- Prosthetic removal, organism-specific antibiotics, and reimplantation of the prosthesis
- Resection arthroplasty or arthrodesis

One-stage reimplantation has a 77% success rate with antibiotic-impregnated cement. Delayed reimplantation, which is more common, involves removal of the prosthesis and cement followed by a period of parenteral antibiotics. Reimplantation delayed from 3 months to 1 year has been shown to have a success rate of approximately 88%. If the reconstruction is delayed longer than 1 year, the rate of recurrence is 7.1%. If the reimplantation is done within the first year, the rate of recurrence is 26%. In patients infected with an organism of increased virulence the time frame between debridement and reimplantation should be prolonged. The Hospital for Special Surgery in New York reports that a 6-week time frame is adequate for eradication of infection and improves the functional outcome. The success rate of this protocol is 92%.

17. What are the results of revision hip total arthroplasty?

With acetabular revision, cementless, ingrown sockets are useful in all types of deficiencies. Results show re-revision of 2.5–8% during a 2–7 year follow-up. With massive acetabular allografts, 17% of the porous cups migrated within 2 years. Although bipolar acetabular components have high early rates of migration and failure, they may be indicated in the elderly or inactive patient with a nonstable ingrowth socket. Cemented revision of the socket acetabular component shows a re-revision ranging from 0–30% during a follow-up for 2–10 years. The loosening in patients with allografts has been reported as 0–62%. Radiolucent lines may be seen in the cemented component but do not necessarily indicate failure.

Cemented femoral components have high radiolucent rates and loosening compared with most cementless revisions. A re-revision rate of 4.5–10% was observed in patients followed for 4–10 years; loosening was apparent on radiographs in 12–64%. The results of cementless femoral components depend greatly on prosthetic stability, bone stock deficiency, prevention of interoperative fracture, and type of implant chosen for a specific deficiency. Re-revision rates of 3–10% were observed in patients followed for 2–8 years. Radiographic lucency is as high as 37%. Studies of the cortical strut allograft for femoral bone grafting report a rate of 80–90% union during an average of 2–5 year follow-up. Rigid fixation and maximal host–graft contact have been shown to increase union. In patients who have had an entire proximal femoral allograft, union at the graft–host junction has been shown to be 77%, but the incidence of infection approaches 5%.

Improved results may be seen with careful preoperative planning, proper prosthetic selection, provision of necessary equipment and inventory with back-up, and use of long stems (both cementless and cemented). Surgical technique should show wide exposure, preserve proximal bone, avoid fracture and perforation, expose defects, and ensure implant stability.

BIBLIOGRAPHY

1. Archibeck MJ, Rosenber AG, Berger RA, Silverton CD: Trochanteric osteotomy and fixation during total hip arthroplasty. J Am Acad Orthop Surg 11:163–173, 2003.
2. Dennis DA: Management of massive acetabular defects in revision total hip arthroplasty. J Arthroplasty 18(3) Supplement 1: 121–125, 2003.
3. Hall RM: Wear of polyethylene acetabular components in total hip arthroplasty. An analysis of one hundred and twenty-eight components retrieved at autopsy or revision operations. J Bone Joint Surg 80A:764–765, 1998.
4. Masri BA, Campbell DG, Garbuz DS, Duncan CP: Seven specialized exposure for revision hip and knee replacement. Orthop Clin North Am 29:229–240, 1998.
5. Masterson EL, Masrie BA, Duncan CP. Surgical approaches in revision hip replacement. J Am Acad Orthop Surg 6:84–92, 1998.
6. Mikhail WEM, Ling R, Weidenhielm LA, Gie GA: Revision of the femoral component: Impaction grafting. In Calaghan JJ, Rosenberg AG, Rubash HE (eds): The Adult Hip. Philadelphia, Lippincott Raven Publishers, 1998.
7. Paprosky WG, Burnett RS: Extensively porous-coated femoral stems in revision hip arthroplasty: Rationale and results. Am J Orthop (US) 31(8):471–474, 2002.
8. Paprosky WG, Sporer, SM: Controlled femoral fracture. J Arthroplasty 18(3) Supplement 1: 91–93, 2003.
9. Rubash HE, Sinha RK, Shanbhag AS, Kim SY: Pathogenesis of bone loss after total hip arthroplasty. Orthop Clin North Am 29:173–186, 1998.
10. Weeden SH, Paprosky WG: Minimal 11-year follow-up of extensively porous-coated stems in femoral revision total hip arthroplasty. J Arthroplasty (US) 17(4) Suppl 1: 134–137, 2002.
11. Younger TI, Bradford MS, Magnus RE, Paprosky WG: Extended proximal femoral osteotomy. A new technique for femoral revision arthroplasty. J Arthroplasty 10:329, 1995.

62. ALTERNATIVES TO TOTAL HIP ARTHROPLASTY: OSTEOTOMY

Joseph Yao, M.D.

1. What are the goals of hip osteotomy?

In prevention of osteoarthritis, the goal of osteotomy is to restore anatomy to as normal a state as possible and thereby to eliminate excessive load to the joint caused by abnormal joint mechanics. In the case of limited joint damage (e.g., osteonecrosis with partial femoral head involvement), the goal is to direct a more normal part of the joint into the weight-bearing area. Such goals may be accomplished by osteotomy of the pelvis, femur, or both.

2. What common conditions may be treated by hip osteotomy?

Hip osteotomy is used for treatment of osteoarthritis, osteonecrosis, slipped capital femoral epiphysis, Legg-Calvé-Perthes disease, and congenital hip dysplasia (CHD). The first four entities involve the femoral head and are treated by femoral osteotomy. CHD involves acetabular deformity and is treated with pelvic osteotomy; concurrent femoral deformity is treated with femoral osteotomy. CHD rarely involves primary femoral deformity; hence, it is generally not treated by isolated femoral osteotomy.

3. List the desirable clinical characteristics for hip osteotomy.

- Young age with life expectancy greater than the expected survivorship of a primary total hip replacement (e.g., generally less than 50 years old)
- Lack of obesity
- Occupation other than heavy labor
- Good joint range of motion
- Mild degree of symptoms

4. What are the desirable radiographic characteristics for hip osteotomy?

- Good cartilage space
- Correctable malalignment
- Impingement and joint incongruity that can be improved by altering acetabular or femoral alignment
- Preoperative radiographs showing hip joint capable of being positioned in the desired postoperative alignment (e.g., radiograph taken with the hip abducted that demonstrates improved joint congruity and joint space)

5. What part of the femur is usually osteotomized in hip osteotomy?

Intertrochanteric region.

6. What are the major disadvantages of osteotomy in the femoral neck area?

Avascular necrosis of the femoral head and chondrolysis.

7. List the major types of femoral osteotomy.

- Flexion
- Extension
- Varus
- Valgus
- Rotational (e.g., Sugioka osteotomy)
- Combinations of the above

8. What are the indications for flexion osteotomy?

Indications for flexion osteotomy include hip extension contracture, osteonecrosis with anterior involvement and posterior sparing of the femoral head, and full range of hip extension pre-operatively. The apex of the osteotomy is located posteriorly so that the shaft of the femur is flexed and the proximal femur is extended.

9. What are the indications for extension osteotomy?

Indications for extension osteotomy include hip flexion contracture and deficient anterior ac-etabular coverage (e.g., as seen frequently with CHD). The apex of the osteotomy is located an-teriorly so that the shaft of the femur is extended and the proximal femur is flexed.

10. What are the indications for varus osteotomy?

Indications for varus osteotomy include relative valgus neck–shaft angle (i.e., $> 135°$), lateral joint space disease, and an enlarged and congruent joint space with the leg abducted on preoperative radiographs. Results are best if the femoral head is spherical and acetabular dysplasia is minimal.

11. What are the indications for valgus osteotomy?

Indications for valgus osteotomy include relative varus neck–shaft angle, medial joint space disease, and and enlarged and congruent joint space with the leg adducted on preoperative radi-ographs. The medial femoral head osteophyte is rotated superiorly to a weight-bearing location.

12. What are the indications for rotational osteotomy?

CHD is often associated with increased femoral neck anteversion. Derotation of the femoral neck into a more normal degree of anteversion may be combined with angular osteotomy. Rota-tional osteotomy also assists in moving osteonecrotic segments of femoral head away from the weight-bearing aspect of the joint.

13. Describe the role of medial or lateral displacement of the femoral shaft in combination with varus or valgus osteotomy.

Varus and valgus osteotomies change the center of femoral head rotation and hence alter the mechanical alignment of the lower extremity. Varus osteotomy displaces the center of hip rota-tion medially and should be combined with medial displacement of the femoral shaft to maintain the lower extremity mechanical axis; this technique avoids overloading the medial compartment of the ipsilateral knee. Valgus osteotomy displaces the center of hip rotation laterally and should be combined with lateral displacement of the femoral shaft; this technique avoids overloading the lateral compartment of the ipsilateral knee.

14. What is the effect of osteotomy on leg lengths?

Varus osteotomy usually shortens the limb at least 1 cm, whereas valgus osteotomy gener-ally lengthens the limb. However, valgus osteotomy may shorten the limb by as much as 2 cm if a closing wedge is used.

15. Describe preoperative planning for femoral osteotomy.

Fluoroscopy and radiographs are used to assess whether a limb can be placed in a position that will improve hip joint space and congruity. The appropriate degree of angular and rotational correction can then be determined. Tracings are used to determine optimal locations for the os-teotomy and hardware, the size of wedge resection, and the possible need for femoral shaft dis-placement. Radiographs can determine the degree of femoral head involvement in cases of os-teonecrosis. Femoral angular osteotomy may be appropriate when $< 33\%$ of the femoral head is involved on the anteroposterior (AP) radiograph or when the necrotic angle is $< 200°$.

16. What is the most common indication for pelvic osteotomy?

CHD, which involves deficient coverage of the femoral head laterally and often anteriorly.

17. What is the goal of pelvic osteotomy?

The goal is to improve femoral head coverage by the acetabulum.

18. Describe preoperative planning for pelvic osteotomies.

Radiographs should include an AP view of the pelvis and a false-profile (faux-profil) view taken with 20° of rotation while the patient is standing. Some patients have nearly normal-appearing hips on AP pelvis radiographs, whereas the false-profile view demonstrates anterior subluxation of the femoral head. AP and lateral center-edge (CE) angles are measured to assess femoral containment. Lateralization of the femoral head can be assessed. Computed tomographic (CT) scans provide three-dimensional reconstructions to help in visualizing acetabular deficiencies and the results of different osteotomies.

19. What is the role of pelvic osteotomy in a young patient (second or third decade) with a congruent hip joint and deficient femoral head coverage?

Pelvic osteotomy can be used to redirect the acetabulum without altering its shape or capacity. Improved femoral head coverage is then achieved. Osteotomy should be done early before significant arthritis develops.

20. Give examples of redirection osteotomies.

The Salter osteotomy can increase the CE angle by 20–30° in children, but only about 10° of improvement can be expected in patients older than 10 years. The Salter osteotomy allows correction in only one direction. Double osteotomy (Sutherland and Greenfield) and triple osteotomy (Steel) can be used in patients with preoperative CE angles of 0–15°. However, such osteotomies essentially create an unstable setting similar to a pelvic fracture. The dial osteotomy involves separating the acetabulum from the pelvis and rotating it in the appropriate direction; it can accomplish almost any degree of correction, but it is a technically difficult operation. The periacetabular osteotomy (Ganz) also corrects any degree of acetabular coverage deficiency and also allows the acetabulum to be medialized. The periacetabular osteotomy is done from inside the pelvis and is slightly easier to perform than the dial osteotomy.

21. Does pelvic osteotomy have a role in patients in whom hip arthritis has already developed?

Yes. A simple shelf procedure that consists of bone-grafting the superior-lateral acetabulum may be used in cases of congruous acetabular hypoplasia. The Chiari osteotomy may be considered as a salvage procedure in patients with deficient femoral head coverage and arthritis. This osteotomy should be considered only if there is no congruous portion of acetabulum to rotate superiorly; often an intact portion of acetabulum, located posteriorly and inferiorly, can be rotated superiorly.

22. What is the Chiari osteotomy?

An osteotomy is created just cephalad to the superior hip joint capsule. The osteotomy is angled from the distal anterolateral to the proximal posteromedial aspect. The acetabular (distal) fragment is abducted and medialized. An iliac crest bone graft is placed just cephalad to the hip capsule over the uncovered femoral head. The interposed superior-lateral joint capsule assumes a weight-bearing role. A triangular bony defect is created anteriorly by the osteotomy. Iliac crest bone graft is placed into the bony defect to serve as a buttress and to prevent anterior instability.

CONTROVERSIES

23. How does hip osteotomy influence subsequent total hip arthroplasty (THA)?

Pelvic osteotomy may simplify later THA by allowing the acetabulum to be reconstructed in a more normal position and by reducing the need for acetabular bone-grafting. Femoral osteotomy is generally done at the intertrochanteric level and consequently may make femoral preparation for THA more difficult. Therefore, angular corrections accomplished by femoral osteotomy should be limited to 15–20°. A custom-made femoral prosthesis or intraoperative femoral osteotomy may be necessary for successful THA in cases of severe alteration of proximal femoral anatomy due to previous reconstructive femoral osteotomy.

24. Is pelvic osteotomy warranted in young patients in view of the fact that later THA will probably be more difficult as a result of the altered anatomy?

Osteotomy has an important role, especially in young patients. Although excellent clinical results can be expected after THA, there are long-term problems, such as component wear and stress-shielding. Osteotomy is a particularly desirable alternative in young patients with early arthritis. In appropriate cases, osteotomy can alter the mechanisms of the hip joint and thereby arrest or reverse a degenerative process that would progress if left untreated. A major benefit of osteotomy is to delay the need for THA until the patient is older.

BIBLIOGRAPHY

 1. Aronson J:Osteoarthritis of the young adult hip:Etiology and treatment. Instr Course Lect 35:119. St. Louis, Mosby, 1986.
 2. Atsumi T, Kuroki Y: Modified Sugioka's osteotomy: More than 130 degrees posterior rotation for osteonecrosis of the femoral head with large lesion. Clin Orthop 334:98, 1997.
 3. Bombelli R:Osteoarthritis of the Hip, 2nd ed. Berlin, Springer-Verlag, 1989.
 4. Boos N, Krushell R, Ganz R, Muller M: Total hip arthroplasty after previous proximal femoral osteotomy. J Bone Joint Surg 79B:247, 1997.
 5. Chiari K:Medial displacement osteotomy of the pelvis. Clin Orthop 98:55, 1974.
 6. Gotuh E, Inao S, Okamoto T, Ando M: Valgus-extension osteotomy for advanced osteoarthritis in dysplastic hips. Results at 12 to 18 years. J Bone Joint Surg 79B:609, 1997.
 7. Marti RK, Chadecott LR, Kloen P: Intertrochanteric osteotomy for posttraumatic arthritis after acetabular fractures. J Orthop Trauma 15:384, 2001.
 8. Matsuno T, et al: Modified Chiari osteotomy: A long term followup study. J Bone Joint Surg 74A:470, 1992.
 9. Millis MB, Poss R, Murphy SB: Osteotomies of the hip in the prevention and treatment of osteoarthritis. Inst Course Lec 41:145. Park Ridge, IL, American Academy of Orthopedic Surgeons, 1992.
10. Morgensen BA, Zoega H, Marinko P: Late results of intertrochanteric osteotomy for advanced osteoarthritis of the hip. Acta Orthop Scand 51:85, 1980.
11. Morita S, Yamamoto H, Hasegarwa S, et al: Long-term results of valgus-extension femoral osteotomy for advanced osteoarthritis of the hip. J Bone Joint Surg 82B:824, 2000.
12. Mount MA, Fairbank AC, Krackow KA, Hungerford DS: Corrective osteotomy for osteonecrosis of the femoral head: The results of a long-term follow-up study. J Bone Joint Surg 78A:1032, 1996.
13. Pauwels F:Biomechanics of the Normal and Diseased Hip. Berlin, Springer-Verlag, 1976.
14. Poss R:Current concepts review:The role of osteotomy in the treatment of osteoarthritis of the hip. JBone Joint Surg 66A:144, 1984.
15. Poss R:Intertrochanteric osteotomy in osteoarthritis of the hip. Instr Course Lec 35:129. St. Louis, Mosby, 1986.
16. Schatzker J:The intertrochanteric osteotomy. Berlin, Springer-Verlag, 1984.

63. ALTERNATIVES TO TOTAL HIP ARTHROPLASTY: ARTHRODESIS

Joseph Yao, M.D.

1. What are common indications for hip arthrodesis?

The ideal clinical setting for hip arthrodesis is a unilaterally painful hip with greatly restricted range of motion in older adolescents or young adults, particularly if their occupation involves heavy labor.

2. What common hip problems may require treatment with hip arthrodesis?

- Osteonecrosis of the femoral head
- Osteoarthritis secondary to congenital hip dysplasia (CHD)
- Joint destruction due to tuberculosis and pyogenic septic arthritis
- Posttraumatic arthritis
- Previously failed total hip replacement, especially after infection by a highly virulent organism

3. What is the most common indication for hip arthrodesis in children?

Infection of the hip.

4. Name the major prerequisites to hip fusion.

The patient must have a normal lumbosacral spine, contralateral hip, and ipsilateral knee. These joints should be checked by examination and radiographs. Because an immobile hip that has undergone arthrodesis places increased stresses on these joints, the clinical results of hip arthrodesis are compromised if they are diseased.

5. Describe the optional position in which to perform arthrodesis on a hip.

Flexion of 30–40°, adduction of 0–5°, and external rotation of 0–7°.

6. What are the consequences of performing arthrodesis on a hip in an abducted position?

- Increased incidence of pain in the back and knee
- More degenerative changes on radiographs of the knee
- More pronounced limp

7. What is the advantage of using internal fixation?

Internal fixation helps to ensure maintenance of the arthrodesis position obtained at surgery and decreases the duration of immobilization in a spica cast after surgery. In some cases, it eliminates the need for postoperative spica cast immobilization and permits earlier mobilization of the patient.

8. Describe the common methods for hip arthrodesis.

One of the most common methods of hip arthrodesis uses an AO cobra head plate spanning the pelvis and the proximal femur. Another method uses screws or pins passing through the femoral head and neck into the pelvis. The use of intramedullary nails transfixing the pelvis to the intramedullary canal of the femur also has been described. External fixation has also been used for hip arthrodesis.

9. What is the role of osteotomy in hip arthrodesis?

Pelvic and femoral osteotomies have been used by some surgeons in an attempt to maximize contact at the site of arthrodesis. Schneider described a pelvic osteotomy that allowed the femoral head to be medialized. He believed that the osteotomy increased bony contact between pelvis and femur. Subsequent cadaver studies did not confirm the increased bony contact that Schneider hypothesized. Charnley described central dislocation of the femoral head through the acetabulum to increase bony contact. Charnley's osteotomy had the advantages of avoiding distortion of the pelvis and reducing blood loss compared with Schneider's pelvic osteotomy. Others have used proximal femoral osteotomies to enhance bone contact at the arthrodesis site. Subtrochanteric osteotomy with adduction of the femoral shaft has the effect of abducting the hip and thus provides a larger contact area for arthrodesis.

10. Describe the role of bone grafts in hip arthrodesis.
Bone grafts have been used to improve the chances of successful arthrodesis. Iliac crest bone grafts can be packed into the arthrodesis site. Various techniques of transferring vascularized bone grafts to the arthrodesis site have been described. Davis transferred a portion of the anterior ilium along with the attachments of the tensor fascia lata and the anterior portions of the gluteus medius and minimus muscles to the arthrodesis site. Ranawat transferred a larger piece of anterior ilium with attachments of the tensor fascia lata, anterior portions of the gluteus medius and minimus, rectus femoris, and sartorius muscles. Kostuik transferred the greater trochanter with its attached gluteal muscles to the posterior aspect of the arthrodesis site.

11. Describe a relatively simple method to maintain the desired portion of the hip before use of internal fixation in hip arthrodesis.
Blasier et al. described a technique that uses a vacuum-splint beanbag to support the lower extremity. The patient is placed in the lateral decubitus position with the involved hip facing the ceiling. One beanbag is placed beneath the patient to maintain the body in the lateral position. A second beanbag is placed between the legs. After the involved leg is placed in the desired arthrodesis position, the beanbag between the legs is evacuated of air, thereby maintaining the desired position. The patient is then prepared and draped, and the arthrodesis procedure is completed.

12. What long-term results should a patient expect after hip arthrodesis?
Preoperative hip pain is generally relieved. About 70% of patients can walk more than 1 mile and sit comfortably for 2 hours after hip arthrodesis. Patients also should be able to drive an automatic transmission car. They generally cannot run or jog.

13. What are the effects of hip arthrodesis on other joints?
About 60% of patients have pain in the ipsilateral knee, 75% have anteroposterior laxity, and 80% have mediolateral laxity of the ipsilateral knee. About 60% of patients experience back pain, and 25% have pain in the contralateral hip.

14. What effect does hip arthrodesis have on contralateral total hip replacement?
Mechanical loosening of a total hip replacement probably occurs at a higher rate when the opposite hip has undergone arthrodesis.

15. What effect does hip arthrodesis have on an ipsilateral total knee replacement?
Loosening rates for the total knee replacement are not increased. However, there is an increased incidence of knee stiffness and the need for postoperative manipulation of the total knee replacement.

16. What are the major potential complications associated with hip arthrodesis?
Injury to blood vessels and nerves can occur during surgical exposure or during insertion of internal fixation. The internal fixation devices may loosen or fracture. Rates of pseudarthrosis range from 0% to 50%, with reported figures most commonly between 15% and 25%. Femur fractures occur in 5–15% of patients. Variable amounts of leg length shortening may occur, necessitating the use of a shoe lift. Accelerated degenerative changes may occur in the back, contralateral hip, and ipsilateral knee.

17. What are the major indications for converting a hip arthrodesis to a total hip arthroplasty?
- Low back pain
- Pain in the ipsilateral or contralateral knee or in the contralateral hip
- Severe gait abnormality secondary to bilateral hip arthroplasty

18. How does conversion of a hip arthrodesis to a total hip arthroplasty affect pain in adjacent joints?
Pain is improved in the back (76% of patients), knee (35% of patients), and contralateral hip (12% of patients).

19. What is one of the most important determinants of a successful conversion of a hip arthrodesis to a total hip arthroplasty?
The condition of the gluteus medius muscle.

20. How does the anticipated future conversion to a total hip arthroplasty affect the choice of hip arthrodesis technique?
The surgical technique should minimize injury to the gluteus medius muscle. The use of a cobra head plate requires greater soft-tissue dissection and hence involves the potential for greater disruption of the gluteus medius muscle than the use of screws placed through the femoral neck and head into the pelvis. It is best to avoid altering pelvic or femoral anatomy, if possible, as well as creating pelvic or femoral osteotomies.

21. What are the clinical results of total hip arthroplasty after hip arthrodesis?
The postoperative flexion arc averaged 87° in the review by Kilgus et al. Leg-length discrepancy improved by an average of 2.5 cm. The need for supportive walking devices decreased after surgery. Patients regained strength slowly, sometimes for as long as 5 years postoperatively. Patients who have spontaneous hip arthrodesis and no subsequent surgeries until total hip arthroplasty may have results comparable to those in patients who have primary total hip arthroplasty for more common causes of hip arthrosis. Failure of total hip arthroplasty after hip arthrodesis is more common in patients ≤ 50 years of age at the time of conversion, patients with two or more previous hip operations, and patients with an injury to the hip.

CONTROVERSY

22. Is it better to offer hip arthrodesis or total hip replacement to a young patient with isolated arthritis of one hip?
The treatment of isolated hip arthritis in a young patient is a difficult problem. Hip arthrodesis generally provides a painless and stable joint for many years. The patient can bear weight on the arthrodesed limb without concern about limiting the degree of activity. A hip arthrodesis can be converted to a total hip arthroplasty in the future when the patient is older and less active. The disadvantages of arthrodesis include leg-length discrepancy, an immobile joint, and pain in adjacent joints with long-term follow-up. Total hip arthroplasty relieves pain associated with an arthritic joint and preserves joint motion. Usually leg lengths can be restored to almost normal after total hip arthroplasty. The major problem with total hip arthroplasty in a young patient is the generation of prosthetic wear debris over time. Wear rates may be accelerated in young patients because they have higher activity levels than older patients. Significant osteolysis may result from wear debris in joints. Osteolysis makes future reconstruction much more difficult and also may lead to fracture. Stress-shielding of bone by stiffer metal femoral prostheses leads to bone loss over time. Subsequent revision total hip arthroplasties are associated with a greater incidence of complications and poorer clinical results. Both hip arthrodesis and total hip arthroplasty have advantages and disadvantages. Hip arthrodesis still has a role in the treatment of arthritis in young patients despite the improving technology associated with hip arthroplasty. However, as more pa-

tients become familiar with hip arthroplasty, it is often difficult to convince them to choose hip arthrodesis.

BIBLIOGRAPHY

1. Amstutz HC, Sakai DN: Total joint replacement for ankylosed hips. J Bone Joint Surg 57A:619, 1975.
2. Barnhardt T, Stiehl JB: Hip fusion in young adults. Orthopedics 19:303, 1996.
3. Blasier RB, Holmes RH: Intraoperative positioning for arthrodesis of the hip with the double beanbag technique. J Bone Joint Surg 72A:766, 1990.
4. Callaghan JJ, Brand RA, Pedersen DR: Hip arthrodesis: A long-term follow-up. J Bone Joint Surg 67A:1328, 1985.
5. Charnley J: Stabilization of the hip by central dislocation. J Bone Joint Surg 37A:514, 1955.
6. Duncan CP, Spangehl M, Beauchamp C, McGraw R: Hip arthrodesis: An important option for advanced disease in the young adult. Can J Surg 38(Suppl 1):539, 1995.
7. Endo N, Takahashi HE, Toyama H, et al: Arthrodesis of the hip joint using an external fixator. Orthop Sci 4:342, 1999.
8. Garvin KL, Pellicci PL, Windsor RE, et al: Contralateral total hip arthroplasty or ipsilateral total knee arthroplasty in patients who have a long-standing fusion of the hip. J Bone Joint Surg 71A:1355, 1989.
9. Kilgus DJ, Amstutz HC, Wolgin MA, Dorey FJ: Joint replacement for ankylosed hips. J Bone Joint Surg 72A:45, 1990.
10. Kostuik JP: Arthrodesis of the hip. In Amstutz HC (ed): Hip Arthroplasty. New York, Churchill Livingstone, 1991.
11. Murrell GA, Fitch RD: Hip fusion in young adults using a medial displacement osteotomy and cobra plate. Clin Orthop 300:147, 1994.
12. Schneider R:Hip arthrodesis with the cobra head plate and pelvic osteotomy. Reconstr Surg Traumatol 14:1, 1974.
13. Sofue M, Kono S, Kawaii W, Homma M: Long-term results of arthrodesis for severe osteoarthritis of the hip in young adults. Int Orthop 13:129, 1989.
14. Strathy GM, Fitzgerald RH: Total hip arthroplasty in the ankylosed hip. J Bone Joint Surg 70A:963, 1988.

64. PELVIC FRACTURES

Donald J. Walla, M.D.

1. What are the most common causes of pelvic fractures?
The automobile is responsible for most fractures of the pelvis in all age groups except for people over 60 years of age, for whom falls at home lead to the majority of pelvic fractures.

2. What clinical findings are present in a patient with a fractured pelvis?
A patient with a fractured pelvis may present with pain, tenderness, difficulty with ambulation, crepitus, ecchymosis, and swelling of the pelvis or perineum. Exerting posterior pressure on the iliac crests of a supine patient produces pain at the fracture site, because the pelvic ring is opened. Compressing the pelvic ring in a side-to-side direction by pressure on the iliac wings may be painful. Pain also may be elicited by downward pressure on the symphysis pubis.

3. On what does the stability of the pelvic ring depend?
The stability of the pelvic ring depends on both bony and ligamentous structures. The anterior portion of the pelvic ring does not participate in normal weight bearing, nor is it essential for maintenance of pelvic stability. The posterior arch (consisting of the sacrum, sacroiliac (SI) joints and ilia) serves as the weight-bearing portion of the pelvis. The posterosuperior SI ligaments connecting the iliac tuberosities to the sacrum provide most of the ligamentous stability to the SI joints.

4. What is meant by a stable pelvic fracture?

Pelvic fractures that do not involve the pelvic ring or that have minimal displacement of the pelvic ring are considered stable.

5. Name and describe the most commonly used mechanical classification scheme for pelvic fractures.

Pennal and Tile's classification of pelvic disruptions into three separate patterns is based on the presumptive injurious force primarily responsible for the disruption.

1. The **anteroposterior compression (open book)** injury hinges the pelvis open on the intact posterosuperior SI ligaments. It is not grossly unstable.

2. The **lateral compression injury** occurs as a result of a direct force to the iliac crests. It may be stable or unstable, depending on the magnitude of force and the degree of disruption of the posterior pelvic arch.

3. **Vertical shear injuries** result from forces through the femur directed perpendicularly to the pelvic ring and cause disruption of the SI joint or unimpacted fractures through the sacrum or ilium. The hemipelvis is unstable both rotationally and vertically. Displacements of 1 cm of the SI joint or 0.5 cm vertically of the hemipelvis are signs of instability.

6. What radiographic studies are useful in evaluating a patient with a pelvic fracture?

A complete baseline radiographic evaluation would include anteroposterior, 40° cephalad (outlet), 40° caudad (inlet), and 45° oblique projections of the pelvis. Further radiographic studies include computed tomographic (CT) scans and possible three-dimensional imaging. Push-pull or stress radiographs may be used to predict stability of a fractured pelvis.

7. What are the basic treatment principles for stable pelvic fractures?

The basic principles or treatment of pelvic fractures include fracture healing and rapid rehabilitation. Most pelvic fractures are stable and treated nonoperatively, initially with bed rest and protected ambulation.

8. What are the basic treatment principles for unstable fractures?

All pelvic fractures should be assessed for instability and displacement. Complications of unstable fractures may lead to later instability and nonunion, which in turn may lead to complaints of sacroiliac pain, leg-length discrepancy, painful sitting, and functional impairment. Women may have problems with parturition and dyspareunia. When instability is defined, the preferred treatment is surgical stabilization.

9. What is the indication for provisional stabilization of pelvic fractures?

Provisional fixation is indicated for patients with lesions that increase the pelvic volume and all unstable fractures. Application of a pelvic clamp or external fixator frame plus a supracondylar femoral traction pin reduces the pelvic volume, partially stabilizes the bones and soft tissues, and reduces the amount of bleeding and pain from the pelvis and facilitates nursing care.

10. What is the role of an external fixator in the treatment of pelvic fractures?

The traditional external fixator uses two or three pins in each iliac crest. The pins are joined by an anterior frame. The pelvic clamp and external skeletal fixator may restore adequate stability to a partially stable open book fracture; however, neither can restore adequate stability to the unstable pelvic fracture.

11. Define definitive internal fixation treatment of unstable pelvic fractures.

Definitive internal fixation should be done only by surgeons experienced with these techniques. The timing of surgery is dependent on the general state of the patient, but as a general rule it should be done as early as safety allows (usually within the first 5–7 days). Neurologic monitoring is desirable, as is use of a cell saver device; hemorrhage in open pelvic surgery can be massive. Prophylactic antibiotics are essential. It is important to avoid operating through crushed or contused skin or soft tissues, which helps to determine the choice of surgical approach. The specific incisional site should be based on the soft tissue injury and pelvic fracture pattern.

12. What is a Malgaigne fracture?

Malgaigne fractures usually refer to unstable fracture-dislocations of the pelvis. A simple definition includes all pubic fractures of both the superior and inferior pubic rami or pubic symphysis dislocation in conjunction with an ipsilateral posterior disruption that involves a sacral fracture, an iliac fracture, or a sacroiliac dislocation. Such injuries may lead to cephalad migration of the fragment containing the hip joint and thus to a leg-length discrepancy. Current treatment options favor surgical stabilization, including open reduction and internal fixation (ORIF) of the disrupted segments. Stabilization with external fixation in combination with ORIF is also an option.

13. Discuss the initial measures in management of a patient who has sustained a high-energy pelvic fracture.

Emergency resuscitative protocols are frequently involved, including control of intrapelvic bleeding, which can lead to shock and ultimately to death. Volume replacement by intravenous crystalloid solutions and whole blood, use of MAST suits, angiography, transarterial embolization, vascular repair, and surgical stabilization of unstable pelvic fractures are other considerations.

14. What potential injuries are associated with high-energy pelvic fractures?

High-energy pelvic trauma carries a significant risk of associated injury to the neurologic, urologic, gynecologic, gastrointestinal, and vascular systems as well as to the skin and subcutaneous tissues.

15. What common urologic and gynecologic injuries are associated with pelvic fractures?

Pelvic fractures may lead to disruption of the urethra and bladder by direct laceration or by tension stresses. Intravenous pyelograms, transurethral cystograms, and retrograde urograms are specialized radiographic exams useful in evaluating the extent of genitourinary injuries.

16. What types of gastrointestinal injuries are associated with high-energy pelvic fractures?

Perforations of the large and/or small bowel and lacerations of the rectum may occur. When a rectal laceration is present, a diverting colostomy should be considered.

17. What types of neurologic injuries are associated with severe pelvic fractures?

Fractures of the sacrum may lead directly to neurologic injury, whereas pelvic fracture or displacement may lead indirectly to nerve root and peripheral nerve-stretch injuries. A complete baseline neurologic exam, including a rectal evaluation, is necessary.

18. What treatment is necessary for uncontrolled hemorrhage in the patient with a pelvic fracture?

Management of uncontrolled hemorrhage from a pelvic fracture requires both general surgical and orthopedic approaches. Abdominal injuries are associated with 22–45% of pelvic fractures. Peritoneal lavage is useful in evaluating the presence or absence of intraabdominal bleeding. Laparotomy is usually required in the hemodynamically unstable patient who exhibits unstable pelvic fracture or dislocation. Immediate pelvic stabilization by either internal or external fixation may stabilize the retroperitoneal hemorrhage. If bleeding is not controlled, one must consider the possibility of a coagulopathy, disseminated intravascular coagulation (DIC), or hemorrhage from a major vessel. If hemorrhage from a major vessel is suspected, pelvic angiography is the next step.

19. What is the overall mortality rate associated with pelvic fractures?

The mortality rate for open pelvic fractures is 30–50% compared with 10–30% for closed pelvic fractures. Major causes of death related to open pelvic fractures are (1) hemorrhage and (2) sepsis and/or renal failure.

20. What complications are associated with pelvic fractures in children?
Several unique features are associated with pelvic fractures in children, including displacement of the pelvic ring through the triradiate cartilage with lateral compression injury; undergrowth of the hemipelvis in association with SI joint injury and subsequent fusion; and pelvic deformity with leg-length discrepancy in unreduced vertical shear fractures.

BIBLIOGRAPHY

1. Chapman MW: Fractures of the pelvic ring and acetabulum in patients with severe polytrauma. Instr Course Lect 3:591–593, 1990.
2. Guyton JL: Fractures of hip, acetabulum, and pelvis. In Canale ST (ed): Campbell's Operative Orthopaedics, 9th ed., St. Louis, Mosby, 1998, pp 2252–2279.
3. Helfet DL: Open reduction internal fixation of the pelvis. Techn Orthop 4:67–78, 1990.
4. Perry JF: Pelvic open fractures. Clin Orthop 151:41–45, 1980.
5. Peters PC Jr, Bucholz RW: The assessment of pelvic stability following pelvic ring disruptions. Techn Orthop 4:52–59, 1990.

65. ACETABULAR FRACTURES

Donald J. Walla, M.D.

1. What radiographs are best suited for evaluation of acetabular fractures?
The acetabular fracture is best evaluated on anteroposterior (AP) views of the pelvis and hip and 45-degree oblique views of the pelvis. CT scans are also useful in most patients.

2. What is meant by the anterior and posterior columns of the acetabulum?
The anterior or iliopubic column runs obliquely downward, inward, and anteriorly from the anterior part of the superior iliac crest to the pubic symphysis. The posterior of ilioischial column descents downward from the level of the angle of the greater sciatic notch to the ischial tuberosity.

3. What is meant by a transverse acetabular fracture?
Transverse fractures involve both the anterior and posterior columns and divide the innominate bone into a superior segment that contains the acetabular roof and intact ilium and an inferior segment that consists of the ischiopubic bone.

4. How are acetabular fractures classified?
The Letournel classification includes ten types of fracture. In the five elementary or simple fractures, a part or all of one column of the acetabulum has been detached. Elementary fractures include (1) posterior column fractures, (2) anterior column fractures, (3) anterior wall fractures, (4) posterior wall fractures, and (5) transverse fractures.
The five complex associated fractures include at least two of the simple fractures: (1) fractures of the posterior column and posterior wall, (2) associated transverse and posterior wall fractures, (3) T-shaped fractures, (4) associated anterior and posterior hemitransverse fractures, and (5) fractures of both columns.

5. What are the goals of acetabular fracture management?
The goals are to restore motion of the hip, to mobilize the patient, and to avoid posttraumatic

arthritis. An imperfect reduction with as little as 1–2 mm of displacement may lead to osteoarthritis. Bony fragments within the hip joint and injury of articular cartilage may lead to early posttraumatic arthritis.

6. What are the basic treatment principles of acetabular fractures?

As with any articular injury, the goal is to restore function and prevent late osteoarthritis, the most common long-term complication. Most osteoarthritis is caused by imperfect reduction, and residual displacements as small as 1–2 mm, particularly in weight-bearing surfaces, may lead to degenerative changes. Other common causes are incarcerated bony fragments or articular surface damage that is not evident radiographically.

7. Can acetabular fractures be life-threatening?

An acetabular fracture is usually not life-threatening. Massive pelvic hemorrhage occurs usually from associated pelvic injuries and rarely from displaced acetabular fragments.

8. What types of treatment are used to manage acetabular fractures?

Nonoperative treatment is a consideration for nondisplaced acetabular fractures as well as transverse fractures and minimally displaced two-column fractures. Traction of the affected leg should be maintained for 4–8 weeks to obtain fracture healing. Open reduction and internal fixation (ORIF) of displaced fractures of the acetabulum have become the standard of care.

9. Does timing of surgical treatment of acetabular fractures make a difference?

Urgent surgical treatment is necessary when a patient has an anterior or posterior dislocation that cannot be reduced by closed means. A delay of 2–3 days with the patient maintained in distal femoral traction is appropriate for all other fractures. A delay longer than 10 days makes reduction more difficult, and by 3 weeks callus formation significantly complicates reduction.

If such delays are unavoidable, open reduction and internal fixation should be undertaken in younger patients. In older patients, particularly those with complex fractures, surgery may be deferred with the anticipation that total joint replacement may be required later.

10. How are acetabular fractures stabilized surgically?

Various surgical exposures are available, depending on the location of the fractures. One should select an approach that allows the complete operation to be performed and stabilization of the fractures with a combination of screws and plates. The exposure also should allow exploration of the joint surface when necessary. The most common surgical exposures are (1) the Kocher-Langenbeck, (2) the ilioinguinal, (3) the extended iliofemoral, and (4) the triradiate incisions.

11. What complications are associated with operative management of acetabular fractures?

Infection	Heterotopic bone formation
Sciatic nerve palsy	Posttraumatic arthritis
Thrombophlebitis	Avascular necrosis of the femoral head

12. What are the principles of postoperative management of open reduction and internal fixation of acetabular fractures?

Closed suction drainage and antibiotic therapy is used for 48 hours. Passive motion of the hip is initiated after drain removal and crutch walking with limited weightbearing starts as soon as pain is diminished. Eight weeks after internal fixation, weightbearing is increased progressively as long as the fracture shows evidence of healing.

13. What are the causes of sciatic nerve palsy?

The sciatic nerve may be injured by initial trauma or by retraction of the nerve during a posterior surgical approach to the acetabulum.

14. What are the causes of heterotopic bone formation or myositis ossificans?
Ectopic bone formation usually occurs after an extended iliofemoral approach, which provides lateral exposure of the innominate bone. This complications can be minimized by use of Indocin or postoperative low-dose irradiation.

15. How can the risks of postoperative infections be minimized?
The incidence of wound infection can be reduced by careful manipulation of the soft tissues, use of profuse antibiotic irrigation, perioperative intravenous antibiotics, hemostasis, and suction drains.

16. How can the risk of thrombophlebitis be minimized?
A patient may be fitted with compression stockings and sequential compression devices. Heparin or Coumadin may be used for anticoagulation.

17. What is the significance of the superior gluteal artery?
The superior gluteal artery may be incarcerated in fractures that communicate with the greater sciatic notch. It also may be injured during a surgical approach, resulting in massive bleeding and possibly ischemic necrosis of the gluteal musculature.

18. What is the treatment for heterotopic ossification?
Removal of established ectopic bone may be considered if it inhibits motion of the hip joint. The removal is usually done 12–18 months after the initial surgery when there is less likelihood of recurrent ectopic bone formation.

19. What should be done if a bony fragment is evident on radiographs after ORIF of an acetabular fracture?
The fragment(s) should be removed.

20. What is the infection rate after ORIF of displaced acetabular fractures?
The infection rate is 2–4%.

BIBLIOGRAPHY

1. Frymoyer JW (ed): Orthopaedic Knowledge Update 4. Rosemont IL, American Academy of Orthopedic Surgeons, 1993.
2. Guyton JL: Fractures of hip, acetabulum, and pelvis. In Canale ST (ed): Campbell's Operative Orthopaedics, 9th ed., St. Louis, Mosby, 1998, pp 2234–2252.
3. Letournel E: Classification and evaluation of acetabular fractures. Techn Orthop 4(4)5–23, 1990.
4. Mears DC, Gordon RG: Internal fixation of acetabular fractures. Techn Orthop 4(4):36–51, 1990.
5. Pennal GF, et al: Results of treatment of acetabular fractures. Clin Orthop 151:115–124, 1980.
6. Bucholz RW, Heckman JD, Beaty JH, Kasser JR: Rockwood, Green, and Wilkins' Fractures, 5th ed. Philadelphia, J.B. Lippincott, 2001.

66. HIP DISLOCATIONS AND FEMORAL HEAD FRACTURES

Samar K. Ray, M.D., FRCS

1. What is a hip dislocation?
The hip joint is a ball-and-socket type of joint: the acetabulum is the socket and the head of the femur is the ball. It is one of most stable joints in the body because of the deep acetabular

cavity, the spherical concentric head of the femur, strong capsular ligaments, and massive surrounding muscles. The head of the femur may get displaced in relation to the acetabulum from severe trauma, causing dislocation.

2. Why is a hip dislocation so important?
Hip dislocation causes immediate, profound disability and, if not treated properly, may cause life-long disability due to complications such as as avascular necrosis and early degenerative arthritis in the joint.

3. What important features must be remembered in the initial evaluation of a patient with hip dislocation?
Because hip dislocation occurs from high-energy trauma, such as motor vehicle or pedestrian accidents, patients may have other life-threatening injuries. In 35–40% of cases, other severe injuries occur, including craniofacial, chest, abdominal, and other musculoskeletal injuries. An estimated 50% of patients have fractures in other parts of the body.

4. What are the principles of treatment?
- Careful evaluation of the patient for associated injury
- Immediate closed reduction with assessment of stability and reduction
- Careful radiographic evaluations, including postreduction computed tomography (CT), if necessary, for evaluation of congruency of reduction and associated fractures of the femoral head or acetabulum.

5. Discuss the classification of hip dislocations.
Hip dislocations are divided into three types: anterior, posterior, or central dislocation. Classification depends on the position of the femoral head in relationship to the acetabulum. In anterior dislocation, the femoral head rests anterior to the coronal plane of the acetabulum, perhaps with associated fractures of the acetabulum or femoral head. In posterior dislocations, the femoral head rests posteriorly to the coronal plane of the acetabulum. Posterior dislocations may occur with fracture of the posterior acetabular rim, the acetabular floor, or the femoral head. In central of fracture dislocation, a fracture is present on the inner wall of the acetabulum with inward displacement of the femoral head.

6. What is the most common dislocation?
Only 10–15% of all hip dislocations are anterior. Posterior dislocations occur in 85–90% of cases.

7. How are posterior and anterior dislocations differentiated clinically?
In a posterior dislocation, the lower extremity is flexed, adducted, and internally rotated at the hip. In anterior dislocations, the extremity is slightly shortened, abducted, and externally rotated.

8. What types of anterior dislocations are seen?
Anterior dislocations may be classified as superior or inferior. Both types result from abduction and external rotation. Superior dislocations occur in extension, whereas inferior dislocations occur in flexion.

9. What neurovascular structures are in jeopardy with anterior dislocations?
Trauma to the femoral artery, vein, and nerve has been reported in superior and open anterior dislocations.

10. Describe the treatment for anterior dislocations of the hip.
Early diagnosis with prompt closed reduction under general anesthesia is the treatment of choice. If multiple attempts at closed reduction fail, open reduction is necessary.

11. What maneuvers must be done to reduce anterior dislocations of the hip?

Most clinicians believe that elements of longitudinal traction, adduction of the hip, and internal rotation are needed. Stimson's gravity method has sometimes been used for reduction. The patient lies in a prone position with the affected leg placed in a downward position. Traction is placed longitudinally, and the pelvis is stabilized. Internal and external rotation and abduction are then used to reduce the dislocation.

12. What are the complications of anterior dislocations?

Early complications include neurovascular compromise of the femoral artery, vein, or nerve, which occur mainly with the superior anterior dislocation. Inferior dislocations do not have a high incidence of compromise. Anterior hip dislocations may be irreducible by closed means. Obstructions to closed reduction include fractures and iliopsoas and rectus muscles. Late complications include posttraumatic arthritis, aseptic necrosis, and recurrent dislocations.

13. What is the incidence of aseptic necrosis after anterior dislocation of the hip?

Aseptic necrosis, which is less common in anterior than in posterior dislocation, is reported in approximately 5–8% of the cases. Aseptic necrosis may appear from 2–5 years after dislocation.

14. What is the mechanism of injury of posterior dislocation?

Posterior dislocation is usually related to high-energy trauma. The mechanism of injury is usually force applied to the flexed knee in an abducted position, as often occurs when the knee strikes the dashboard in an automobile accident.

15. Describe the clinical findings in posterior dislocation.

The limb is shortened, internally rotated, and adducted. Sciatic nerve injury may be seen in 10–14% of patients. Associated fractures of the femoral head and femoral shaft are common. Knee ligament injuries also are seen because of the high-energy trauma.

16. What anatomic areas should be carefully scrutinized on the radiographs?
- The femoral head for fracture.
- The acetabulum for fracture.
- The femoral neck for nondisplaced fractures that may displace when closed reduction is attempted.

17. With posterior dislocation and associated acetabular fractures, is stability of the joint an issue?

Studies have shown that fragments < 20–25% of the acetabular wall usually do not affect hip stability, whereas those > 40% result in instability and recurrent dislocations.

18. What radiographs should be taken in patients with suspected dislocations?
- Anteroposterior (AP) radiograph
- Oblique lateral view of the pelvis
- Posterior oblique view of the pelvis
- Lateral film of the hip to show the position of the fragments

19. What other radiographic studies are indicated?

Radiographs must be taken postoperatively to show the adequacy of reduction, the presence or absence of fragments in the joint, and the accuracy of reduction of associated femoral head and acetabular fracture fragments. CT scans may be helpful in patients suspected of having loose fragments in the joint, incomplete reduction of the fractured femoral head fragment, or soft-tissue interposition.

20. What is the method of treatment for posterior dislocations without fractures?

The Allis reduction maneuver involves traction at the level of the knee at 90° with internal and external rotation of the extremity and progressive extension.

21. What is the postoperative treatment for dislocation of the hip?

Postoperative treatment involves gentle traction until the hip is pain-free, usually from several days to 2 weeks. General passive range of motion is begun. Spica cast and immobilization after reduction are not used. Controversy exists as to when the hip can safely bear weight. Opinions range from 2 weeks to 12 months after reduction. Most authors state that weightbearing may resume with crutches when pain and spasm disappear.

22. What are the indications for open reduction in posterior dislocations of the hip?

- To remove loose fragments from the joint.
- To restore joint stability and joint congruity by open reduction and internal fixation of large fragments.
- To ensure the accuracy of the reduction.

23. What complications may occur in posterior fracture dislocations of the hip?

Approximately 10% of patients have **sciatic nerve palsy,** usually involving the peroneal component. In patients with simple dislocations, reduction removes the pressure on the nerve, and recovery usually is complete. If sciatic nerve deficit occurs after reduction, surgical exploration is indicated.

Irreducible posterior dislocations occur in 3–16% of patients with simple dislocations usually because of buttonholing of the femoral head through the hip capsule or interposition of the piriformis muscle and tendon. Nonconcentric reductions are usually caused by fracture fragments; surgical removal is necessary.

Approximately 20% of patients have significant **knee injuries,** involving collateral or cruciate ligaments. Most often the posterior cruciate ligament is injured. Because the injury is related to an anterior blow to the tibia, posterior lateral instabilities are found.

Recurrent dislocations usually occur in patients with a posterior fracture; they also may be associated with paralysis and sepsis.

Myositis ossificans, which develops in approximately 2% of patients, is related to muscle damage and hematoma formation.

The incidence of **aseptic necrosis** may be diminished significantly by reduction within 6 hours. Delay greater than 12 hours results in a high incidence of avascular necrosis.

Posttraumatic degenerative arthritis develops in approximately 35% of patients with posterior fracture dislocation of the hip. The severity of the initial trauma is usually the major factor in determining the development of posttraumatic arthritis. Posttraumatic arthritis is found approximately twice as often in fracture dislocations as in simple dislocations.

24. Describe the femoral head fractures that are seen with dislocations.

Femoral head fractures were classified by Pipkin in four categories:

Type 1: Femoral head fracture caudad to the fovea centralis, which is the most inferior portion of the femoral head.

Type 2: Femoral head fracture from inferior to superior to the fovea centralis.

Type 3: Type 1 or 2 with associated femoral neck fracture.

Type 4: Type 1, 2, or 3 with associated acetabular fracture.

25. List the treatment options for central fracture dislocation at the acetabulum.

- Traction with or without closed reduction of the femoral head
- Open reduction and internal fixation
- Primary arthroplasty
- Primary arthrodesis

BIBLIOGRAPHY

1. Guyton JL: Fractures of the hip, acetabulum, and pelvis. In Canale ST (ed): Campbell's Operative Orthopaedics, 9th ed. St. Louis, Mosby, 1998, pp 2224–2234.
2. Rockwood CA, Green DP, Bucholz RW (eds): Rockwood and Green's Fractures in Adults, vol. II, 9th ed. Philadelphia, J.B. Lippincott, 1996, pp 1756–1803.

67. FEMORAL NECK FRACTURES

Michael J. Schmidt, M.D., and Randall D. Neumann, M.D.

1. What are the major risk factors contributing to the occurrence of hip fractures?
Individuals at risk include urban Caucasian women who are of slight build and physically inactive. Other significant risk factors include a history of excessive alcohol intake, use of psychotropic medications, senile dementia, and history of previous hip fracture.

2. What is osteoporosis?
Osteoporosis is a disease process associated with aging and inactivity; it is characterized by decreased bone mass with normal mineralization and results in loss of bone strength.

3. Does osteoporosis contribute to the incidence of hip fractures?
By decreasing bone strength, osteoporosis increases the likelihood of fracture from minor trauma such as falls.

4. What is the effect of hip fractures on mortality rates?
In general, the mortality rate increases during the first year after a hip fracture. After 1 year, the mortality rate returns to normal for age- and sex-matched controls.

5. What are the two major types of femoral neck fractures?
The two major types of neck fractures are **nondisplaced/impacted** and **displaced.**

6. What are the signs and symptoms of an impacted femoral neck fracture?
- Groin pain referred down the medial thigh, sometimes to the level of the knee
- Antalgic gait
- Limitation of hip motion

7. What are the signs and symptoms of displaced femoral neck fractures?
Generalized pain occurs in the hip region with the thigh in external rotation and abduction. Slight shortening of the extremity is often present.

8. What major medical complications may result from femoral neck fractures and subsequent surgical management?
Deep venous thrombosis, pulmonary embolism, and infection.

9. What is the major cause of hip fractures in young adults?
High-energy trauma resulting from motor vehicle accidents or falls from heights.

10. Do femoral neck and femoral shaft fractures occur together?
Ipsilateral (same side) femoral neck and femoral shaft fractures occur in about 2.5–6% of all femoral shaft fractures.

11. What is the recommended treatment for nondisplaced/impacted femoral neck fractures?
The recommended treatment is usually surgical, consisting of internal fixation with 3 or 4 parallel, cannulated lag screws. The procedure can be performed through a small incision or percutaneously.

12. What is the recommended treatment for displaced femoral neck fractures?

In general, prompt closed or open reduction with internal fixation is recommended in the younger, active patient. Hemiarthroplasty or total hip arthroplasty is generally recommended for the older, less active patient whose physiologic age is > 70 years. Younger patients with Parkinson's disease, dementia, or psychosis also are candidates for hemiarthroplasty.

13. What are the major bony complications after internal fixation of displaced femoral neck fractures?
- Nonunion (10–30% of patients)
- Avascular necrosis (15–33%)
- Late segmental collapse (7–27%)

14. What are the major bony complications after treatment of displaced femoral neck fractures with hemiarthroplasty?
- Hip pain secondary to acetabular erosion and prosthetic loosening
- Hip dislocation
- Femur fractures
- Heterotopic ossification

15. What is avascular necrosis?

Avascular necrosis is a phenomenon that occurs early after femoral neck fracture and results in the actual death of bone in the femoral head secondary to ischemia.

16. What is late segmental collapse?

It refers to the collapse of subchondral bone and articular cartilage overlying avascular necrotic bone resulting in joint incongruity, subsequent degenerative joint disease, and pain.

17. Do all patients who develop avascular necrosis after femoral neck fracture later develop late segmental collapse?

No. After adequate reduction and internal fixation, portions of the femoral head that develop avascular necrosis may revascularize and repair before stresses on the hip joint result in collapse of the necrotic area.

18. What are the two most important factors in decreasing the occurrence of nonunion or avascular necrosis after femoral neck fracture?

The two most important factors are prompt, anatomic fracture reduction and stable internal fixation. Acceptable reduction may include up to 15° of valgus angulation (valgus impacted fracture) and < 10° of anterior or posterior angulation.

19. What is the treatment for ipsilateral femoral neck and shaft fractures?

The femoral neck fracture takes precedence. Treatment should include anatomic reduction with stable internal fixation. Avascular necrosis occurs in up to 20% of cases.

20. What are the indications for performing a total hip arthroplasty after a femoral neck fracture?

Indications include displaced femoral neck fractures in patients > 60 years old with rheumatoid arthritis, preexisting osteoarthritis or degenerative joint disease, and Paget's disease or pathologic fractures with associated acetabular involvement.

21. What problems arise with the patient when performing a total hip arthroplasty after femoral neck fracture?

In one study, 21% had perioperative medical complications, which included an extremely high incidence (10%) of dislocation. Both complication rates are higher than for patients undergoing total hip arthroplasty for arthritis, who showed good long-term function and survival.

22. Which of the four ascending cervical arteries (anterior, medial, posterior, and lateral) provide the major source of blood supply to the femoral head and neck?

The lateral ascending branches arising from the lateral femoral circumflex artery.

23. What prophylactic measures are useful in preventing thromboembolic disease after hip fractures?

Prophylactic measures include aspirin (particularly in male patients), warfarin, and dextran alone or in combination with dihydroergotamine. Low-dose intravenous heparin alone or in combinations with dihydroergotamine and intermittent pneumatic compression stockings also have proved useful in reducing the incidence of thromboembolic disease.

24. What diagnostic tools are useful in evaluating patients with suspected nondisplaced stress fractures or impacted fractures of the femoral neck?

Useful diagnostic tools include anteroposterior pelvic and lateral radiographs, bone scans, and tomograms. If a fracture is not confirmed by these methods, radiographs should be repeated in 10–14 days.

25. Can fractures of the femoral neck occur in younger patients without significant trauma?

Yes. The most common patients are amenorrheic female athletes, especially runners, who develop pain and subsequent stress fractures. Such fractures also may occur bilaterally.

BIBLIOGRAPHY

 1. Canale ST (ed): Campbell's Operative Orthopaedics, 9th ed. St. Louis, Mosby, 1998.
 2. Frymoyer JW: Orthopaedic Knowledge Update-4. Rosemont, IL, American Academy of Orthopaedic Surgeons, 1993.
 3. Koval KJ, Zuckerman JD: Hip fractures: I. Evaluation and treatment of intertrochanteric fractures. J Am Acad Orthop Surg 2:150–156, 1994.
 4. Koval KJ, Zuckerman JD: Hip fractures: I. Overview and evaluation and treatment of femoral neck fractures. J Am Acad Orthop Surg 2:141–149, 1994.
 5. Lee BP, Berry DJ, Harmsen WS, Sim FH: Total hip arthroplasty for the treatment of an acute fracture of the femoral neck: Long-term results. J Bone Joint Surg Am 80:70–75, 1998.
 6. Peljovich AE, Patterson BM: Ipsilateral femoral neck and shaft fractures. J Am Acad Orthop Surg 6:106–113, 1998.
 7. Poss R: Orthopaedic Knowledge Update-3. Rosemont, IL, American Academy of Orthopaedic Surgeons, 1990.
 8. Rockwood CA, Green DP, Bucholz RW, Heckman JD (eds): Rockwood and Green's Fractures in Adults, Vols. 1 and 2, 4th ed. Philadelphia, J.B. Lippincott, 1996.
 9. Voss L, DaSilva M, Trafton PG: Bilateral femoral neck stress fractures in an amenorrheic athlete. Am J Orthop 26:789–792, 1997.
10. Wosinsky PR, Johnson KD: Ipsilateral femoral neck and shaft fractures. Clin Orthop 92:81–90, 1995.

68. INTERTROCHANTERIC FRACTURES

Randall D. Neumann, M.D.

1. What is an intertrochanteric fracture of the hip?
An intertrochanteric fracture of the hip is an extracapsular fracture that occurs along a line between the greater and lesser trochanters with variable comminution.

2. Which is more common in the elderly: intertrochanteric fracture, subtrochanteric fracture, or femoral neck fractures?
In one study, 47% were intertrochanteric, 23% were subtrochanteric, and 37% were femoral neck fractures.

3. What clinical signs and symptoms and physical findings are associated with an intertrochanteric fracture of the hip?
- Swelling and pain in the hip region
- Ecchymosis over the greater trochanter
- Tenderness over the greater trochanter
- Severe pain when testing range of motion
- Range of motion loss
- Marked shortening of the extremity with as much as 90° of external rotation deformity

4. What other fractures are common in patients sustaining intertrochanteric fracture?
- Vertebral compression fractures
- Distal radius Fractures
- Proximal humers fractures

5. What diagnostic tools are necessary to evaluate an intertrochanteric fracture?
An anteroposterior radiograph, preferably in internal rotation, and a lateral radiograph. Bone scans may take 48 hours to become positive. An MRI is likely a better alternative to bone scan.

6. Evans' classification divides intertrochanteric fractures into two main types, depending on the direction of the fracture. What are the characteristics of a type I fracture?
The type I fracture extends upward and outward from the lesser trochanter. Fracture stability is obtained by anatomic medial-cortical reduction.

7. What are the characteristics of type II fractures?
The fracture line is in reversed obliquity or extends downward from the lesser trochanter. Type II fractures retain a degree of istability secondary to a tendency of the distal segment or femoral shaft to displace medially.

8. What is a four-part intertrochanteric fracture?
A four-part intertrochanteric fracture is composed of four major fracture fragments, including the femoral head neck, greater trochanter, lesser trochanter, and femoral shaft.

9. Which major muscle groups create indirect forces that contribute to the formation of a four-part intertrochanteric fracture?
The iliopsoas muscle on the lesser trochanter and the abductor muscles on the greater trochanter.

10. Describe the Orthopaedic Trauma Association (OTA) alphanumeric fracture classification.

31-A. Femur, proximal trochanteric

- 31-A1. Pertrochanteric simple

    31-A1.1 Along intertrochanteric line

    31-A1.2 Through greater trochanter

    31-A1.3 Below lesser trochanter

- 31-A2. Pertrochanteric multifragmentary

    31-A2.1 With one intermediate fragment

    31-A2.2 With several intermediate fragments

    31-A2.3 Extending more than 1 cm. below lesser trochanter

- 31-A3. Intertrochanteric

    31-A3.1 Simple oblique

    31-A3.2 Simple transverse

    31-A3.3 Multifragmentary

11. What is the Singh index?

The Singh index is a classification system that measures the degree of osteoporosis in the proximal femur based on radiographic evaluation of the trabecular patterns.

12. Are intertrochanteric fractures stable?

Not always. Unstable intertrochanteric fractures result from comminution of the posteromedial cortical buttress of the distal fragment, fracture extension into the subtrochanteric area, and reverse oblique fractures. Unstable fractures may account for 50–65% of all intertrochanteric fractures.

13. What is the recommended treatment for intertrochanteric fractures?

Most intertrochanteric fractures are treated with sliding hip compression screws after closed reduction. Calcar replacement prostheses are used in selective cases involving severe comminution.

14. How is closed reduction of intertrochanteric fractures achieved before internal fixation?

The patient is positioned supine on a fracture table, and the physician applies longitudinal traction, slight abduction, and usually slight external rotation to the hip under anesthesia.

15. What are the implant choices for treatment of intertrochanteric fractures?

- Sliding hip screw—the implant of choice for most fractures
- Intramedullary hip screw—patients who have an intertrochanteric fracture with subtrochanteric extension.
- Ender nails—patients who have proximal soft tissue compromise
- Alta nail
- Medoff plate—reverse oblique fractures

16. What are the advantages of a sliding hip compression screw for fixation of an intertrochanteric fracture?

The sliding hip compression screw may be used to treat both stable and unstable intertrochanteric fractures, because it provides secure fixation of the head and neck fragment to the distal fragment and allows controlled impaction at the fracture site. Therefore, its use decreases the risk of fixation failure compared with rigid nail-plate devices and allows earlier mobilization and weightbearing.

17. What is medial displacement osteotomy?

Medial displacement osteotomy is a reduction technique for unstable intertrochanteric fractures involving medial displacement of the distal segment or femoral shaft in hopes of achieving better mediocortical stability. This technique was commonly used in conjunction with rigid nail-plate fixation devices.

18. Is medial displacement osteotomy useful in conjunction with sliding screw compression devices?

In general, anatomic reduction of unstable intertrochanteric fractures results in less shortening and better stability and is preferred over medial displacement osteotomy.

19. What position within the femoral head and neck of the lag screw portion of the sliding hip screw is the most secure fixation?

Central position of the lag screw within the femoral head and neck to within 1 cm of subchondral bone is usually recommended. The tip apex distance is the sum of the distance from the tip of the lag screw to the apex of the femoral head on both the AP and lateral views. If this is greater than 25 mm, screw cut-out is more likely. Short of this position, a posteroinferior position is acceptable.

20. The strength of the fracture-implant combination is determined by which five variables?
- Degree of osteoporosis
- Fragment geometry
- Adequacy of reduction
- Implant design
- Placement of the implant

21. What complications are seen with the internal fixation of intertrochanteric fractures?
- Device failure, including plate fatigue fracture and lag screw cutting-out of the femoral head posteriorly and superiorly
- Malunion with shortening and rotation
- Nonunion
- Avascular necrosis
- Infection

22. How are calcar replacement prostheses used in the treatment of intertrochanteric fractures?

Calcar replacement prostheses are used primarily to salvage fixation failure of an intertrochanteric fracture when repeat open reduction and internal fixation are not possible. Their use as a primary prosthetic replacement for treatment of unstable intertrochanteric fractures is controversial; they should be confined to patients with severe osteoporosis that renders proximal fixation with any device questionable.

23. Complications of unstable intertrochanteric fractures can be significantly decreased by what two measures?

Stronger implants and restoration of the posteromedial cortical buttress.

24. Are nonunions of intertrochanteric fractures common?

No. Because intertrochanteric fractures occur in cancellous bone with good blood supply, the actual incidence of nonunion is reported to be < 2%.

25. Does avascular necrosis occur in association with intertrochanteric fractures?

Rarely. The actual incidence is ~ 0.8%.

BIBLIOGRAPHY

1. Canale ST (ed): Campbell's Operative Orthopaedics, 9th ed. St. Louis, Mosby, 1998.
2. Frymoyer JW: Orthopedic Knowledge Update-4. Rosemonth, IL, American Academy of Orthopaedic Surgeons, 1993.
3. Koval KJ, Zuckerman JD: Hip fractures: I. Evaluation and treatment of intertrochanteric fractures. J Am Acad Orthop Surg 2:150–156, 1994.
4. Michelson JD, Myers A, Jinnah R, et al: Epidemiology of hip fractures among the elderly. Risk factors for fracture type. Clin Orthop 311:129–135, 1995.
5. Poss R: Orthopaedic Knowledge Update-3. Rosemont, IL, American Academy of Orthopaedic Surgeons, 1990.
6. Rockwood CA, Green DP, Bucholz RW, Heckman JD (eds): Rockwood and Green's Fractures in Adults, Vols. 1 and 2, 4th ed. Philadelphia, J.B. Lippincott, 1996.

69. SUBTROCHANTERIC FEMUR FRACTURES AND FEMORAL SHAFT FRACTURES

Steven G. Kumagai, M.D.

SUBTROCHANTERIC FEMUR FRACTURES

1. What is a subtrochanteric fracture?

A subtrochanteric fracture occurs between the lesser trochanter and a point 5 cm distal to the lesser trochanter.

2. Who is most susceptible to hip fractures?

Three distinct categories of people are susceptible to hip fractures:
- The elderly population (especially white women > 50 years of age, who account for approximately 80% of all hip fractures);
- Patients (usually young, with normal bones) who have sustained high-energy trauma such as motor vehicle accidents, falls from a height, or gunshot wounds; and
- Older patients with impending pathologic fracture due, for example, to multiple myeloma or metastatic cancer.

3. What percentage of falls in the elderly result in proximal femur fractures?

One percent of falls in the elderly result in hip fractures. However, such falls make up 40% of nursing home admissions, and more than 90% of hip fractures are caused by falls.

4. What work-up is appropriate for a recent fall and proximal femur fracture?

The work-up should include electrocardiogram, x-rays of the pelvis, hip, proximal femur, and chest. Complete blood count, electrolytes, blood urea nitrogen, serum creatinine and blood glucose, liver function analysis, and stool guiac are usual laboratory tests.

5. What underlying medical conditions may a history of falls indicate?

The differential diagnosis should include dehydration, urinary tract infection, malnutrition, orthostatic hypotension, neoplasm, and cardiac and neurologic disease.

6. Which measures may prevent falls in the elderly?

- Encouraging patients to report falls
- Rubberized mats on bathroom floors and slippers with nonslip soles
- Grab bars near bathtubs and toilets
- An obstacle-free path to the bathroom at night
- Night-lights for better visibility
- An external hip protector for dissipation of energy may reduce the risk of hip fractures in the nursing home population
- Evaluation for adequate nutrition

7. What are the main causes of proximal femur fracture in young populations?

The quality of a young person's bone requires a much more violent injury, such as a motor vehicle accident or a fall from a height, to sustain a fracture. The bone is able to absorb more energy; therefore, the fracture tends to be more severe and difficult to treat.

8. What associated medical problems contribute to proximal femur fractures in the elderly?

Associated medical problems such as coronary artery disease, cardiac arrhythmias, and diabetes may cause dizziness and syncope that result in falls and associated proximal femur fractures. Osteoporosis, which is probably the most important factor in development of a hip fracture, places white elderly women at highest risk.

9. What factors are responsible for a slower rate of union and a higher rate of nonunion in subtrochanteric fractures?

The subtrochanteric area of the femur is composed mainly of cortical bone, which is often comminuted in fractures. Less vascularity and fracture surface are available for healing in cortical bone than in cancellous bone (e.g., intertrochanteric fractures). The large mechanical stresses in the subtrochanteric area may result in failure of internal fixation devices before bony union occurs.

10. How are subtrochanteric fractures classified?

Several classification systems are based on the area of the fracture. Fielding bases his system on distance at or below the lesser trochanter. The incidence of complications after treatment increases as the fracture becomes more distal. Seinsheimer's classification is based on the number of major fragments and the location and shape of fracture lines. The higher grade fractures extend into the intertrochanteric region and have a high level of comminution. Others categorize subtrochanteric fractures as stable or unstable. In stable subtrochanteric fractures it is possible to reestablish bone-to-bone contact in the medial and posterior cortexes. In unstable fractures the medial cortical apposition is not attainable because of comminution or fracture obliquity.

11. Describe the treatment options for subtrochanteric fractures.

Patients may be treated operatively or nonoperatively. In the past nonoperative treatment resulted in high rates of morbidity and mortality. Nonoperative treatment includes traction, hip spica cast, and a cast-bracing technique. Operative treatment includes the use of plate and sliding hip screws or intramedullary devices.

12. What operative treatment is used for treatment of subtrochanteric fractures?

Many devices are available. The most common are a plate and screw assembly, intramedullary devices, and sliding hip screws. Sliding compression hip screws and plates have difficulty withstanding the stresses placed at the subtrochanteric region with weightbearing. In the past they have had a higher incidence of plate fracture and nonunion at the fracture site. When feasible, intramedullary devices are generally the treatment of choice; they are usually done with image intensification and essentially closed treatment of the fracture with a proximal incision.

13. What is an intramedullary device? What are its advantages?

The center of the proximal femur is hollow and filled with cancellous bone and fat. An intramedullary nail acts as an internal splint. The nail is generally completely circular, or it may be slotted. A proximal incision in the trochanteric region gives access to the medullary canal. The nail is driven proximally to distally and holds the fracture fragments in place until the fracture heals. Often early weightbearing is allowed. Intramedullary rods, the most stable form of fixation, are the treatment of choice in pathologic fracture.

14. What is the most common cause for nonunion of a subtrochanteric fracture?

Lack of stability at the fracture site and comminution. The proximal medial cortex normally sustains high compressive forces, whereas the lateral cortex sustains high tensile forces. The goal of treatment is to attempt exact reduction of the fracture fragments (particularly the posterior medial cortex). When this goal cannot be accomplished because of comminution, the fracture must heal by secondary healing and callus formation. Bone grafting is indicated in the presence of significant medial comminution.

15. What are the mechanical advantages of intramedullary fixation over hip screws and sideplates?

The screw and sideplate configuration results in high tensile forces laterally on the plate. An intramedullary nail and sliding hip screw has the advantage of moving the shaft fixation medially lessening the tensile force on the intramedullary rod.

16. What are the most common early complications of proximal femur fractures?

Acute blood loss and hypovolemia are initial considerations, especially in younger patients who experience more violent trauma. Third space blood loss may account for a significant drop in blood volume. Other significant injuries in young patients include knee ligament disruption, associated spinal or pelvic fractures, and nerve or vessel damage. Complications associated with trauma and requiring subsequent bed rest may include deep venous thrombosis, pneumonia, and urinary tract infection if a Foley catheter is in place.

FEMORAL SHAFT FRACTURES

17. What is the mechanism for femoral shaft fractures?

Most femoral shaft fractures require major trauma, including motor vehicle and motorcycle accidents, falls from heights, and gunshot wounds. Patients who have pathologic bone due to osteoporosis, tumor, or osteomyelitis may sustain a fracture. Stress fractures rarely occur.

18. Why is a femoral shaft fracture considered an emergency?

Femoral shaft fractures result from significant trauma and often are associated with multiple injuries. Early treatment may prevent medical as well as orthopedic complications.

19. What is the appropriate mechanism of transportation of a patient with proximal femur fracture, either from the accident scene or from an initial emergency room visit?

The patient should be transported by ambulance; intravenous access is crucial because of the possibility of initial blood loss. A form of longitudinal traction and/or strapping is appropriate for comfort and prevention of additional injury.

20. How are femoral shaft fractures classified?

No classification is universally accepted. Femoral shaft fractures generally are categorized by the amount of soft-tissue injury, geographic location, fracture geometry, fracture comminution, and associated injury. Geographic classification includes three categories: proximal third, midshaft, and distal third. Categories based on geometric shape with a major fracture line include transverse, oblique, spiral, and segmental. Classification as an open or closed injury depends on whether the bone has broken through the skin. Distinction should be made between minimal and moderate comminution at the fracture site.

21. What is the incidence of ligamentous injuries with ipsilateral femoral shaft fractures?

The incidence of ligamentous injuries about the knee is as high as 5%. It is easy to miss a ligamentous injury, because the patient is in a great deal of pain. Deformity of the leg is common, and there may be no easy way to test the stability until the fracture is internally reduced or has healed.

22. What is the incidence of ipsilateral femoral neck and femoral shaft fractures? How are they treated?

The incidence is 5%. The most common area is the femoral neck, but other sites are also possible. Pelvic radiographs should be routine in patients with a femoral shaft fracture to rule out femoral neck and intertrochanteric fracture, hip dislocation, and acetabular or pelvic fracture. Ipsilateral femoral neck and shaft fractures should be treated with internal fixation. Several devices allow internal fixation of the femoral shaft with intramedullary nail and proximal screw fixation through the nail or around the nail. Alternatively, standard fixation of the neck fracture with retrograde intramedullary nailing of the shaft facture.

23. What are the common immediate complications associated with femoral shaft fractures?

Vascular injuries occur in 2% of patients with femoral shaft fractures. Even without an arterial injury, bleeding may be significant and lead to hypovolemia. Arteriograms are indicated for any fracture related to penetrating trauma and in patients with suspected arterial injury. Because ligamentous injuries are associated with femoral shaft fractures, careful palpation of collateral ligaments and joint spaces is necessary. Nerves escape injury with most fractures of the femoral shaft, although the incidence of nerve injury is higher with penetrating trauma, such as stab wound or gunshot wounds.

24. What types of treatment are available for femoral shaft fractures?

Treatment may be either non-operative with casting or operative with internal fixation. Balanced skeletal traction is a good option in pediatric patients, followed by treatment with spica cast and immobilization. In adults internal fixation is the treatment of choice; intramedullary nails are preferred for subtrochanteric femoral shaft fractures. Traction followed by a cast brace is not as commonly used as in the past. External fixation is used in open, contaminated femoral shaft fractures.

25. What is the initial treatment of choice for an open femur fracture?

An open femur fracture should be treated as an emergency with initial debridement and irrigation of the fracture site, appropriate antibiotic coverage, and initial cultures. Primary internal fixation continues to be controversial.

26. Can internal fixation be used with an open fracture of the femur?

Two options are available with an open shaft fracture. The first consists of debridement, irrigation, delayed wound closure, and skeletal traction, followed by fracture stabilization in 7–10 days. Multiple injuries dictate the necessity for stabilization. The severity of the wound also dictates the appropriateness of internal fixation. Wounds with minimal contamination may be treated with internal fixation with no significant increase in risk of wound infection after debridement. Patients with grossly contaminated wounds and vascular injuries should be treated on an individual basis.

27. What is a Kirchner wire traction pin? How is balanced skeletal traction used?

The Kirchner wire traction pin is a small pin that is inserted under sterile techniques through the distal femur or proximal tibia with care to avoid the neurovascular structures. This technique allows application of longitudinal skeletal traction, which extends the bone fragments to full length, and helps to control pain and to diminish bleeding. An intramedullary device should not be inserted unless the bone fragments are extended to length or the fracture is acute. Balance suspension is any form of sling below the leg to align the fracture fragments and to prevent undue pressure on any one area of the leg. When the fracture fragments show evidence of callus or new bone formation, a cast brace or hip spica cast is applied.

28. Describe the technique for closed intramedullary rodding of the femur.

The patient is placed on the fracture table with image intensification for proximal and distal visualization. An incision is made over the greater trochanter, and dissection is taken down to the piriformis tendon, which is the entrance into the canal. A guidewire is placed through the proximal fragment and across the fracture site into the distal fragment, which is then reamed until cortical bone is exposed on both sides of the fracture site. The rod is then driven across the fracture site until it is level with the proximal bone.

29. What surgical techniques are used when the femur is highly comminuted?

One option is longitudinal traction, which has the disadvantages of prolonged bed rest and the need for a hip spica cast. Longitudinal traction is no longer used frequently. Also available are intramedullary rods with screws that lock above and below the fracture site, allowing the fracture fragments to life in near-anatomic position. Plate and screw techniques are less satisfying for severely comminuted fractures; reduction of the involved comminuted fragments is difficult.

30. What are the complications from intramedullary rod reduction of femur fractures?

Intraoperative nerve damage may result from either a stretch injury due to excessive traction or direct compression due to poor positioning of the patient. A sciatic nerve is the most frequently stretched. Incidence of infection is approximately 1% in closed femoral nailings. Open wounds treated with intramedullary nailing have a higher incidence of infection. Vascular injury generally does not occur during intramedullary nailing but may be found in 2% of acute femoral shaft fractures. Any fracture of the femoral shaft that has not healed by 6 months clearly qualifies as a delayed union. A union rate of 95% is generally obtained within 20 weeks. Nonunion may occur, especially when the intramedullary device fails.

31. What is the role of external fixation of femoral shaft fractures?
The most appropriate indication for an external fixator is a highly comminuted, open fracture of the midshaft of the femur. An external fixator allows repeated debridement of the leg to facilitate soft-tissue coverage as well as early mobilization; it also can be applied quickly in a limited open procedure. External fixation is often complicated by knee stiffness, pin tract infection, and delayed union.

32. What are the indications for retrograde intramedullary nailing of femur fractures?
Polytrauma with an ipsilateral femoral neck fracture or unstable pelvis fractures and associated ipsilateral tibia fracture (floating knee), which is amenable to retrograde nailing of the femur and antegrade nailing of the tibia through the same incision. Another relative indication is morbid obesity, which may make access the the poximal femur difficult.

BIBLIOGRAPHY

1. Canale ST (ed): Campbell's Operative Orthopaedics, 9th ed. St. Louis, Mosby, 1998.
2. McElbinney J, Lauritzen JB, Petersen MM, Lund B: Falls and the elderly. Arch Am Acad Orthop Surg 2:1998.
3. Lauritzen JB, Petersen MM, Lund B: Defective external hip protectors on hip fractures. Lancet 341: 11–13, 1993.
4. Orthopaedic Knowledge Update 1, Home Study Syllabus. Rosemont, IL, American Academy of Orthopaedic Surgeons, 1984.
5. Orthopaedic Knowledge Update 3, Home Study Syllabus. Rosemont, IL, American Academy of Orthopaedic Surgeons, 1990.
6. Orthopaedic Knowledge Update 4, Home Study Syllabus. Rosemont, IL, American Academy of Orthopaedic Surgeons, 1993.

VIII. The Knee

---

70. EVALUATION OF THE INJURED KNEE

Brett W. Fischer, M.D.

HISTORY AND PHYSICAL EXAM

1. The evaluation of the injured knee begins with a detailed history. What are the important aspects of the history?
- Mechanism of injury—the position of the knee at the time of injury, the weight-supporting status, varus or valgus load, contact versus noncontact injury
- Noncontact injury with an audible "pop"—associated with anterior cruciate ligament (ACL) injury
- Contact injury with an audible "pop" more likely a collateral ligament injury, meniscal tear, or fracture
- Swelling—intraarticular swelling or effusion within the first 2 hours after trauma suggests hemarthrosis, whereas swelling that occurs overnight is an indication of acute traumatic synovitis.
- Pain—location, severity, type
- Instability—was there a sensation of the knee slipping out of joint, giving way, or deforming with weight bearing?
- Past history—previous injury or problems before current injury

2. What are the four most common causes of an acute hemarthrosis?
- ACL or posterior cruciate ligament (PCL) tear
- Peripheral tear of the medial or lateral meniscus
- Osteochondral fracture
- Capsular tear

3. What are the general principles of a knee examination?
The physical exam should be complete, precise, systematic, and carried out as soon after the injury as possible. Both lower extremities should be completely undressed to allow comparison. Always examine the uninjured knee first to obtain a baseline for comparison.

4. What are the three grades of ligamentous injuries according to O'Donoghue?
Grade I: mild sprain—a tearing of a few fibers, no instability, localized pain
Grade II: moderate sprain—incomplete tears with fibers still opposed, no pathologic laxity
Grade III: severe sprain—complete loss of integrity of the ligament with pathologic laxity.

5. Describe the three grades of pathologic laxity when assessing a ligament injury.
- I (0–4 mm of opening)
- II (5–9 mm)
- III (10–15 mm)

6. What is the terrible triad of O'Donoghue?
Medial meniscus tear

Rupture of the ACL
Rupture of the medial collateral ligament (MCL)

7. The general overview of the patient should include what points?
- Height
- Weight
- Body build
- Muscular tone
- Overall alignment of both knees (varus or valgus)
- Amount of disability estimated by observing the patient walking and making transfers
- Alignment of adjacent joints, such as the tibia, foot, and hip (e.g., presence of external or internal tibial torsion, pes planus, pelvic obliquity)

8. What general evaluations of the lower extremity must be recorded?
- Circumferential measurements of the thigh, vastus medialis obliquus area, midpatellar area, and midcalf
- Active range of motion and passive range of motion of both knees
- Hamstring, quadriceps, and heel cord tightness
- Hip and ankle of both sides
- Note pain caused by forced extension, flexion, or varus or valgus motion
- Neurovascular status of the lower extremity

9. What details of swelling should be noted?
- Whether it is intraarticular or extraarticular*
- Location of extraarticular swelling
- Degree of swelling—mild, moderate, severe
- Acute versus subacute onset of swelling

*Severe injuries often present with little intraarticular swelling, because the blood escapes from the joint and into the soft tissues.

10. What is the KT-2000 arthrometer?
It is the most common instrumented knee laxity measurement or device.

11. What is the significance of the manual maximal test with the KT-2000?
It is the most common reported value, and side-to-side comparison > 3 mm difference is significant for anterior instability or ACL deficiency.

12. List the radiographic studies that should be obtained for all knee injuries.
AP, lateral, notch view, and patellofemoral view

13. What radiographic finding may indicate a medial collateral ligament injury?
Pellegrini-Stieda lesion

14. What is the significance of a Segund sign (fracture)?
This represents an avulsion of the capsule from the lateral tibia. It is pathognomonic for an ACL injury.

15. What are the important points in evaluation of the extensor mechanism?
1. Inspect the quadriceps femoris muscles for atrophy, tenderness, and tone. Note dysplasia of the VMO.
2. Palpate the quadriceps and patellar tendons for integrity and tenderness.
3. Identify the position of the patella (midline, subluxed, or dislocated).
4. Note the height of the patella. Patella alta (high-riding) is associated with subluxation and patella baja (low-riding) with chondromalacia.

5. Note the mobility of the patella and presence or absence of the apprehension test.

6. Note retropatellar grating, which may or may not be associated with pain.

7. The medial joint line and lateral joint lines, patellar tendon, anterior fat pad, and tibial tubercle are examined for tenderness and size.

16. How do I check for an apprehension sign? What is its significance?

The patient's leg is supported at 30° of flexion by the examiner's leg, thus guaranteeing the appropriate amount of flexion, muscle relaxation, and reassurance of the patient. A firm, laterally directed force is applied to the medial border of the patella, subluxating it laterally, while applying a small amount of passive flexion to the knee. The test is positive if the patient experiences acute apprehension, as if the patella were about to dislocate. A positive test is associated with acute and subacute subluxation or dislocation of the patella.

17. How do you measure the Q angle? What is its significance?

The quadriceps angle is formed by two lines, one projecting from the anterosuperior iliac spine to the midpatella and the second from the midpatella to the tibial tubercle. The angle is measured while the quadriceps is contracted. The average Q angle in men is 10°; in women, 15°. The Q angle is not diagnostic of any particular patellofemoral disorder; however, an increased angle should be viewed as an indication of a potential force that may act to subluxate or dislocate the patella.

ONE-PLANE INSTABILITY

18. How do I perform abduction or valgus stress tests at 30° and 0°? What is their significance?

With the patient supine on the examining table, the knee to be examined is placed on the side of the table and flexed to 30°. One hand is placed about the lateral aspect of the knee, and the other supports the ankle. Abduction or valgus stress is applied gently to the knee while the hand at the ankle externally rotates the leg slightly. Note stability with the knee flexed to 30°. Bring the knee into full extension and repeat the gentle rocking or valgus stressing with a gentle swinging motion.

Instability at 30° of flexion indicates injury limited to the medial compartment ligaments (tibial collateral ligament, medial collateral ligament, medial capsule, or any combination of the above).

Instability to valgus stress at 0° indicates injury to the posterior structures of the knee (posterior capsule and/or posterior cruciate ligament) and medial structures.

19. How do I perform adduction or varus stress tests at 30° and 0°? What is their significance?

The adduction or varus stress test is carried out in a manner similar to the valgus stress test after examining the normal knee. Adduction or varus stress is applied by changing the hand to the medial side of the knee and applying an adduction or varus force. Examination should be done both in full extension and in 30° of flexion. In addition, with the patient's hip abducted and externally rotated and the knee flexed, the heel of the injured leg is placed on the opposite knee (figure-of-four position), and the lateral aspect of the knee is palpated for a taut narrow band consisting of the fibular collateral ligament (FCL). When the FCL is torn, it is not as prominent as on the uninjured knee.

Varus instability at 30° suggests injury to the lateral compartment ligaments (lateral [fibular] collateral ligament, iliotibial tract, and lateral capsule).

One-plane lateral instability with the knee in extension is apparent on the adduction or varus stress testing when the knee opens on the lateral side. This indicates disruption of the lateral capsular ligament, the lateral collateral ligament, the biceps tendon, the iliotibial band, the arcuate-popliteus complex, the popliteofibular ligament, the anterior cruciate ligament, and, often, the posterior cruciate ligament.

20. What structure is at risk for injury with any varus or adduction injury to the knee?

The peroneal nerve is at risk for injury in any lateral or varus knee injury. It should be assessed in all varus knee injuries.

ANTERIOR CRUCIATE LIGAMENT

21. Which test is the most sensitive for evaluation of the anterior cruciate ligament? How is it performed?

The Lachman test. The Lachman test is performed with the patient supine. The leg is positioned in 30 degrees of flexion. The femur is stabilized with one hand, while the other hand directs an anterior force to the proximal tibia from behind. Anterior translation of the tibia associated with a soft or no endpoint is a positive test.

22. What is the pivot-shift exam?

This is a test for injury to the ACL. It is most commonly performed during the exam under anesthesia at the time of surgery. The leg is held in extension and brought into flexion. Internal rotation and a valgus moment are applied to the knee during flexion. A positive test is seen when the anteriorly subluxed tibia "shifts" or reduces to its anatomic position.

23. Which bundle of the ACL is tight in flexion?

The anterior medial bundle.

24. Why is the anterior drawer test least reliable for anterior cruciate ligament tears?

If the posterior horn of the medial meniscus is torn or displaced, it may block anterior translation of the tibia on the femur.

POSTERIOR CRUCIATE LIGAMENT

25. How is PCL injury tested?

A posterior drawer test is performed in a similar fashion to the anterior drawer test, except that a posterior force is applied on the proximal tibia, again in neutral position as well as internal and external rotation. Posterior movement of the tibia on the femur demonstrates posterior instability when compared with the normal knee. It is sometimes difficult to interpret whether the tibia is abnormally moving too far anteriorly or too far posteriorly. Careful attention to the neutral position or unstressed reduction point avoids misinterpretation. This misinterpretation can be prevented by carefully palpating the relationship between the femur and tibia of both knees simultaneously. Place both knees in the position for a posterior drawer test with the patient supine and the hips flexed 45° and the knees flexed 90°. Place a thumb on the anteromedial joint line of each knee. Normally the anterior aspect of the tibia can be palpated as a 10-mm anterior step-off in relation to the anterior aspect of the medial femoral condyle. A posterior drop back with decreased prominence of the tibial margin compared to the opposite knee indicates injury to the posterior cruciate ligament. When posterior instability is present, the tibia, as sighted across the horizon of the flexed knee, visibly sags posteriorly from the effects of gravity, producing the "gravity sign," "posterior sag," or "drop-back sign."

One-plane posterior instability is apparent when the tibia moves posteriorly on the femur during the posterior drawer test. Such instability indicates disruption of the PCL, the arcuate ligament complex (partial or complete), and the posterior oblique ligament complex (partial or complete).

The posterior cruciate ligament can also be evaluated by the quadriceps active test. With the patient supine, support the relaxed limb with the knee flexed to 90° in the drawer test position. It is important to adequately support the thigh so that the patient's muscles are completely relaxed. Have the patient execute a gentle quadriceps contraction to shift the tibia without extending the knee. At this 90° angle the patellar ligament in the normal knee is oriented slightly posterior, and contraction of the quadriceps does not result in an anterior shift. If the posterior cruciate has

ruptured, the tibia sags into posterior subluxation and the patellar ligament is then directed anteriorly. Contraction of the quadriceps muscle in a knee with a posterior or cruciate ligament deficiency results in an anterior shift of the tibia of = 2 mm.

From such abnormal anatomic findings one can see that severe grades of instability—that is,
severe varus, valgus anterior, or posterior instability—are accompanied by additional central or peripheral ligamentous deficiencies. Most, therefore, are accompanied by rotary instabilities as well.

26. With the knee in full extension, why is one-plane varus or valgus instability important?

It is a sign of significant knee injury that includes not only the medial or lateral structures
(MCL or LCL), but also the cruciate ligaments.

ROTARY INSTABILITIES

**27. Rotary instabilities result when the PCL remains intact to serve as the axis about which
the tibial plateaus rotate under the femur. Anteromedial rotary instability (AMRI) is apparent when stress testing produces anterior and external rotation of the medial plateau of
the tibia as the joint opens on the medial side. Which tests are positive in AMRI? Which
structures are likely to be disrupted?**

Positive tests include the anterior drawer at 90° with the leg externally rotated and the abduction stress test at 30°. Positive tests imply disruption of the medial capsular ligament, the tibial collateral ligament, the posterior oblique ligament, and the anterior cruciate ligament.

**28. In anterolateral rotary instability (ALRI), the lateral tibial plateau subluxates forward
on the femur as the knee approaches extension. This implies disruption of the ACL and lateral capsular ligament. Which tests for ALRI are positive? How are they performed?**

Jerk test (Hughston and Losee): Perform the test with the patient supine and the examiner supporting the lower extremity, flexing the knee to 90°, and internally rotating the tibia. When the right
knee is examined, grasp the foot with the right hand and internally rotate the tibia while exerting a
valgus stress with the left hand over the proximal end of the tibia and fibula. Then extend the knee
gradually, maintaining the internal rotation and valgus stress. When the test is positive, subluxation
of the lateral femorotibial articulation becomes maximal at about 30° of flexion; then, as the knee extends further, spontaneous relocation occurs. The relocation takes the form of a sudden jerk.

Lateral pivot shift test (Macintosh): Lift the foot with the knee extended, internally rotate
the leg, and apply a valgus stress to the lateral side of the leg in the region of the fibular neck with
the opposite hand. Slowly flex the knee while valgus and internal rotation are maintained. If the
test is positive, a subluxation will occur at 30–40° of flexion as the iliotibial band passes posterior to the center of rotation of the knee and provides the force that reduces the lateral tibial plateau
on the lateral femoral condyle.

Flexion rotation drawer test (Noyes): With the patient supine and the knee at 0° (not hyperextended), lift the leg upward, allowing the femur to fall back and rotate externally. This results in anterolateral tibial subluxation as the starting position for the test. While the knee is flexed,
the tibia moves backward and the femur rotates internally, causing the joint to reduce when the
test is positive.

Anterolateral drawer test: With the patient supine, the knee flexed at 90°, and the foot resting on the table, apply an anterior and internal rotation stress to the proximal tibia. The test is positive if the lateral tibial plateau subluxates anteriorly and internally.

**29. Posterolateral rotary instability (PLRI) is apparent when stress testing produces pos-
terior rotation of the lateral tibial plateau in relation to the femur with lateral opening of
the joint. This implies disruption of the popliteus tendon, the arcuate ligament complex
(partial or complete), the lateral capsular ligament, and at times stretching or loss of integrity of the PCL. Which tests are useful in diagnosing PLRI? How are they performed?**

External rotation recurvatum test: Perform this test with the patient supine and compare
it with the normal knee. Lift the affected extremity by the large toe and evaluate any external ro-

tation of the tibia, posterior displacement of the tibia, or recurvatum. Check for peroneal nerve injury.

Reverse pivot shift (Jacob): The lateral tibial plateau shifts from a position of posterior subluxation to a position of reduction as the knee is extended under valgus stress with the foot held in external rotation. The plateau subluxates again as the knee is flexed in the opposite manner. Position the patient supine on the examining table. To test the right knee, face the patient and lift the foot and ankle with your right hand, resting it on the right side of your pelvis. Support the lateral side of the calf with the palm of your left hand on the proximal fibula. Bend the knee to 70–80° of flexion. At this position, externally rotate the foot and the leg to cause the lateral tibial plateau to subluxate posteriorly in relation to the lateral femoral condyle. This position is seen as a posterior sag of the proximal tibia. Now allow the knee to straighten, using nothing more than the weight of the leg. Lean slightly against the foot and transmit an axial load through the leg. Apply a valgus stress to the knee, using your iliac crest as a fulcrum. As the knee approaches 20° short of full extension, feel and observe the lateral tibial plateau moving anteriorly in a jerklike shift from a position of posterior subluxation and external rotation into a position of reduction and neutral rotation.

Posterolateral drawer test: The posterolateral drawer test is performed with the patient supine and the hip flexed 45°, the knee flexed 80°, and the tibia in 15° external rotation. With the foot flexed, perform posterior drawer testing.

Tibial external rotation test: When an injured knee is tested for posterolateral instability, external rotation of the tibia on the femur is measured at both 30° and 90° of knee flexion. The test can be performed with the patient supine or prone. The medial border of the foot in its neutral position is used as a reference point for external rotation. At the chosen knee flexion angle, forcefully externally rotate the foot. Measure the degree of external rotation of the foot relative to the axis of the femur and compare it with the opposite leg. Measure external rotation by the foot-thigh angle. Additionally palpate the tibial plateaus to determine whether the external rotation is caused by the lateral medial tibial plateau moving anteriorly (AMRI). A 10° difference between knees is pathologic.

30. How is posteromedial rotary instability diagnosed?

Posteromedial rotary instability is present when, with stress testing, the medial tibial plateau rotates posteriorly in reference to the femur, with medial opening of the joint.This implies disruption of the medial collateral ligaments, the medial capsular ligament, the posterior oblique ligament, the posterior cruciate ligament, and the medial portion of the posterior capsule, plus stretching or major injury to the semimembranosus insertions. The anterior cruciate ligament also may be injured.

BIBLIOGRAPHY

1. Carson WG:Diagnosis of extension mechanism disorders. Clin Sports Med 4:231–245, 1985.
2. Hughston JC, Andrews JR, Cross MJ, et al: Classification of knee ligament instabilities. Part I. The medial compartment and cruciate ligaments. J Bone Joint Surg 58A:159, 1976.
3. Hughston JC, Andrews JR, Cross MJ, et al: Classification of knee ligament instabilities. Part II. The lateral compartment. J Bone Joint Surg 58A:173, 1976.
4. Jenson JE, Conn RR, Hazelrigg G, Hewett JE: Systematic evaluation of acute knee injuries. Clin Sports Med 4:295–312, 1985.
5. Miller RH: Knee injuries. In Canale ST (ed): Campbell's Operative Orthopedics, 9th ed. St. Louis, Mosby, 1998, pp 1113–1299.
6. Bucholz RW, Heckman JD (eds): Rockwood and Green's Fractures in Adults, vol. II, 5th ed. Philadelphia, J.B. Lippincott, 2002.
7. O'Donoghue DH: Treatment of acute ligamentous injuries of the knee. Orthop Clin North Am 4:617–645, 1973
8. Linton RC, Indelicato PA, Medial ligament injuries. In DeLee JE, Drez D, Miller M (eds): Orthopaedic Sports Medicine 2nd ed. Philadelphia, WB Saunders, 2003.
9. Daniel DM, et al (eds): Knee Ligaments: Structure, Function, Injury and Repair. New York, Raven Press, 1990, pp 427–447.

71. MENISCAL INJURIES

Brett W. Fischer, M.D.

ANATOMY/BIOMECHANICS

1. Describe the shape of the medial meniscus.

It is semilunar in shape and has a larger anterior-posterior dimension than width. It covers roughly two-thirds of the peripheral articular surface of the tibial plateau. It has a thick convex outer edge, that tapers to a thin inner edge; this yields its familiar triangular cross-section.

2. Describe the shape of the lateral meniscus.

It is more circular in shape than the medial meniscus, with approximately the same anterior-posterior dimension as width. It covers more tibial surface area than the medial meniscus.

3. What are the menisci composed of?

Fibrocartilage

4. Describe the tibial attachments of the medial and lateral menisci.

The meniscal insertion into the bone is called the *enthesis,* and it represents a transition from uncalcified to calcified fibrocartilage. These attachments occur at the horns of meniscus.

Medial meniscus—The entire periphery of the medial meniscus is attached to the capsule by the coronary ligaments. This accounts for the medial meniscus being less mobile than the lateral meniscus.

Lateral meniscus—The lateral meniscus also has capsular attachments but is not as developed or organized as the medial meniscus. There is no fixation to the lateral collateral ligament.

5. Describe the microstructure of the meniscus and its relation to injury.

The menisci are composed of dense, tightly woven collagen fibers arranged in a pattern that is highly elastic and able to withstand compression. The major orientation of collagen fibers in the meniscus is circumferential; radial and perforating fibers are also present. The arrangement of the collagen fibers determines to some extent the characteristic patterns of meniscal tears. Collagen fibers function primarily to resist tensible forces along the directions of the fibers. The normal tensile stresses on the menisci are in the longitudinal axis. Because the predominant fiber pattern is in this plane, tears are not unusual. The small number of peripheral radial collagen bundles is inadequate to prevent longitudinal tears when the force is substantial. Likewise, horizontal cleavage tears occur because of the paucity of vertically oriented fibers.

6. Discuss the composition of the menisci.

Collagen makes up 60–70 % of the dry weight of the meniscus. Type I collagen accounts for 90% of the collagen fibers. There are also small amounts of type II, III, IV, V, and VI.

7. What is the role of proteoglycans in the menisci?

They have a high content of carbohydrates that are able to trap approximately 50 times their weight in water, which accounts for much of the physical properties of the menisci.

8. What is the vascular supply to the meniscus?

Superior and inferior branches of the medial and lateral geniculate arteries arborize to form the perimeniscal capillary plexus. Approximately 10–30% of the periphery of the medial meniscus and 10–25% of the lateral meniscus are vascularized in adulthood. There are additional vessels from the middle geniculate artery that supply the horns of the menisci.

9. **Describe the three vascular zones of the menisci.**
   - Red on red zone: This represents the outer or peripheral one-third of the meniscus. This is the vascular zone.
   - Red on white zone: This is the middle one-third that represents a transitional zone between the vascular and avascular sections of the meniscus.
   - White on white zone: This is the inner one-third of the meniscus which is completely avascular in adults.

10. **Name several functions of the menisci.**
    The menisci, which have reached their highest level of development in humans, are essential to the normal function of the knee joint. Their specific contributions include joint filler, joint lubrication by helping to distribute synovial fluid and aiding the nutrition of articular cartilage, joint stability (especially rotary), absorption of shock and energy (load transmission), and sparing the articular cartilage from compressive loads.

11. **What happens to load transmission and shock absorption if a meniscectomy is performed?**
    The menisci transmit approximately 50% of the load in extension and up to 85% of the load with the knee flexed 90 degrees. With removal of the medial meniscus there is a 50–70% reduction in femoral contact area and a 100% increase in contact stress. With lateral meniscectomy, that contact stress can increase to 200–300% of normal.

EPIDEMIOLOGY

12. **What is the rate or incidence of meniscal tears?**
    60–70 per 100,000 persons

13. **In which gender is a meniscal tear more likely?**
    Males. The male to female radio is reported to range from 2.5:1 to 4:1.

14. **Which meniscus is most commonly torn?**
    Medial. This may be in part due to the difference in excursion between the medial and lateral meniscus. The average excursion of the medial meniscus is 5 mm and for the lateral is 11 mm.

15. **Which meniscus is more likely injured with an acute ACL injury? Chronic ACL injury?**
    - Acute injury—lateral meniscus.
    - Chronic injury—medial meniscus, may help define the meniscus' role as a secondary restraint

IMAGING

16. **Describe the appearance of the meniscus on MRI.**
    It is a uniformly low-signal structure on both T1 and T2 images.

17. **How is the meniscus signal "graded" on MRI?**
    Grade 0—Normal meniscus
    Grade I—Stellate intrameniscal signal that does not extend to a free articular surface
    Grade II—Linear intrameniscal signal that also does not extend to the articular surface
    Grade III—Signal change in the meniscus that does extend to the articular surface represents a torn meniscus
    The accuracy of the MRI in detection of a meniscal tear is estimated at 95% or better.

MENISCAL TEARS

18. What is the usual mechanism of injury for meniscal tear?

Tears are thought of occurring from excessive loads on a normal meniscus. This is usually a rotational force as a flexed knee comes into extension. Tears also occur from normal forces acting on a degenerative meniscus.

19. What is the most common meniscal tear?

Longitudinal tear of the posterior horn of the medial meniscus is the most common tear. However, increased use of the arthroscope has made more thorough inspection of both menisci possible; medial and lateral meniscus tears are believed to occur with almost equal frequency.

20. Name common symptoms of a torn meniscus.

Pain	Locking	Swelling
Catching	Giving away	Popping

21. List signs and tests that help diagnose a meniscal tear.

Joint line tenderness	Quadriceps atrophy
Effusion	Positive McMurray test
Lack of complete knee extension	Positive Apley grind test

22. How do I perform a McMurray test?

With the patient supine and the knee acutely and forcibly flexed, the examiner checks the medial meniscus by palpating the posteromedial margin of the joint with one hand while grasping the foot with the other hand. Keeping the knee completely flexed, the leg is externally rotated as far as possible; then the knee is slowly extended. As the femur passes over a tear in the meniscus, a painful click or pop is felt or heard if the test is positive. The lateral meniscus is checked by palpating the posterolateral margin of the joint, internally rotating the leg as far as possible, and slowly extending the knee while listening and feeling for a click. A negative McMurray test does not rule out a tear.

23. How is the grinding test as described by Apley performed?

With the patient prone the knee is flexed to 90°, and the anterior thigh is fixed against the examining table. The foot and leg are then pulled upward to distract the joint and rotated to place rotational strain on the ligaments; when ligaments are torn, this part of the test is usually painful. Next, with the knee in the same position, the foot and leg are pressed downward and rotated as the joint is slowly flexed and extended; when a meniscus is torn, popping and pain localized to the joint line may be noted.

DECISION MAKING

24. What are the indications for operative management of a meniscal injury?

- Typical symptoms of a tear including joint line pain, intra-articular effusion, and mechanical symptoms
- Positive physical including palpable joint line pain, effusion, loss or limitation of motion and positive provocative signs
- Absence of other sources of knee pain that may mimic a meniscal tear
- Failure to respond to nonoperative treatments
- A locked knee secondary to a displaced meniscal fragment

25. Does nonsurgical treatment have a place in the management of meniscal tears?

Yes. An incomplete meniscal tear or a small (5 mm) stable peripheral tear with no other pathologic condition, such as a torn anterior cruciate ligament, can be treated non-surgically with predictably good results. Meniscal tears that cause infrequent and minimal symptoms can be treated with rehabilitation and restricted activity.

26. What are some of the most commonly accepted criteria for meniscal repair?
- A complete longitudinal tear > 10 mm long
- A tear in the Red-red or Red-white zone or within 3–4 mm of the meniscocapsular junction
- A tear that can be displaced by probing
- A tear without secondary degeneration or deformity
- A tear in a young active patient
- A tear associated with an ACL stabilization procedure

MANAGEMENT

27. Outline the seven general guidelines for partial meniscectomy.
1. Remove all mobile fragments.
2. Smooth the remaining meniscal rim of any sudden changes in contour.
3. A perfectly smooth rim is not necessary. The rim smooths and remodels for 6–9 months after surgery.
4. Use meniscal probe repeatedly to check for rim stability.
5. Maintain the meniscocapsular junction and rim. This maintains the circumferential fibers for load transmission.
6. Use both manual and mechanized instrument.
7. If uncertain leave more rather than less rim to avoid segmental resection.

28. What management options for repair of a torn meniscus are available?
- Open suture repair
- Biologic repair with fibrin glue
- Non-fixation healing enhancement such as synovial abrasion or meniscal trephination
- Arthroscopic inside-out repair
- Arthroscopic outside-in repair
- Arthroscopic all-inside repair
- Arthroscopic non-suture repair

29. During medial meniscal repair, what structure is most commonly injured?
Branches of the saphenous nerve

30. Describe the medial approach to the knee for meniscal repairs.
A 3- to 4-cm incision is made with the knee flexed at 90 degrees just posterior to the MCL. The sartorial fascia is opened with care to protect the saphenous vein and nerve. They are retracted posteriorly and plane is developed between the sartorious and capsule.

31. During lateral meniscal repair, what structures are at risk for the injury?
The peroneal nerve is at greatest risk, as well as the popliteal artery and vein and the tibial nerve.

32. Describe the lateral approach to the knee for meniscal repairs.
A 3- to 4-cm incision is made posterior to the LCL with the knee flexed to 90 degrees to relax the biceps femoris and peroneal nerve. The interval between the biceps femoris and iliotibial band is developed. The biceps tendon is retracted posteriorly to protect the peroneal nerve. The lateral head of the gastrocnemius must be swept off the capsule for visualization.

33. Describe the suture placement for meniscal repairs.
Evenly spaced 2 to 3 mm apart in a vertical mattress fashion, which is stronger than a horizontal placement. Either absorbable or nonabsorbable 2.0 sutures can be used.

34. What are the reported healing rates of meniscal repairs?
Seventy-five to 90%. With associated ACL reconstruction, the reported results have exceeded 90% clinical healing.

35. What clinical factors may positively influence meniscal repairs?
Repairs done in association with ACL surgery, tears with rim widths less than 3 mm, acute tears, and lateral meniscus tears

36. List criteria used to assess healing of a meniscal repair.
Second-look arthroscopy is the gold standard, but is impractical. MRI has been shown to be unreliable. Therefore, clinical criteria such as return of motion, decrease in symptoms, and physical examination are most commonly used.

37. At present, who is an ideal candidate for meniscal allograft transplantation?
A patient who has previously undergone a total or near total meniscectomy and has joint line pain, early or minimal chondral changes, normal limb alignment, and a stable knee.

BIBLIOGRAPHY

1. Lee J, Fu FH: The meniscus: Basic science and clinical applications. Oper Tech Orthop 2000; 10 (3): 162–168.
2. Renstrom P, Johnson RJ.: Anatomy and biomechanics of the menisci. Clin Sports Med 1990; 9: 523–538.
3. Johnson DL, et al: Insertion-site anatomy of the human aenisci: Gross, arthroscopic and topographic anatomy as a basis for meniscal transplantation. Arthroscopy 1995; 11: 386–394.
4. McDevitt CA, Webber RJ: The ultrastructure and biochemistry of meniscal cartilage. Clin Orthop 1990; 252: 8–18
5. Arnoczky SP, Warren RF: Microvasclarture of the human meniscus. Am J Sports Med 1982; 10: 90–95.
6. Duncan JB, Hunter R, Purnell M, Freeman J: Meniscal injuries associated with acute anterior cruciate ligament tears in alpine skiers. Am J Sports Med 1995; 23: 170–172.
7. Sanders TG, Fults-Ganey KA: Magnetic resonance imaging of knee menisci: Diagnostic interpretation and pitfalls. Oper Tech in Orthop 2000; 10 (3): 169–182.
8. Metcalf RW, et al: Arthroscopic meniscectomy. In McGinty JB, et al (eds): Operative Arthroscopy, 2nd ed. Philadelphia, Lippincott- Raven, 1996, pp 263–297.
9. Shelbourne KD, et al: Rehabilitation after meniscal repair. Clin Sports Med 1996; 15: 595–612.
10. Post WR, Akers SR, Kish V: Load to failure of common meniscal repair techniques: Effects of suture technique and suture material. Arthroscopy 1997; 13: 731–736.
11. Jackson DW, et al: Meniscal transplantation using fresh and cryo-preserved allografts: An experimental study in goats. Am J Sports Med 1992; 20: 644–656.

72. ANTERIOR CRUCIATE LIGAMENT INJURIES

Randall D. Neumann, M.D., and David E. Brown, M.D.

1. Describe the anatomy of the anterior cruciate ligament.
The anterior cruciate ligament (ACL) is an intraarticular structure that traverses the joint attaching the tibia and the femur. It consists of multiple longitudinal fascicles that insert proximally on the medial aspect of the lateral femoral condyle and distally on the anterior tibial plateau. These fascicles are described as fanning out as they approach the tibial insertion. The ACL provides the primary restraint to anterior displacement of the tibia. The intact ACL is a secondary stabilizer to varus and valgus stress.

2. Describe the different mechanisms for ACL injuries in contact sports.

- Clipping injury. The most common injury to the ACL is associated with a valgus load and external rotation of the tibia on the femur. The mechanism of injury is often associated with damage to the medial collateral ligament and a medial meniscus.
- Hyperextension. The second most common injury pattern is associated with meniscal tears in approximately 30% of the patients. Contact hyperextension injuries also may damage the posterior cruciate ligament (PCL) and posterior capsule.
- Direct blow. In this pattern of injury, the knee is flexed, as often seen in dashboard and turf injuries. A direct blow to the anterior portion of the knee results in tear of the PCL and possible tear of the ACL.
- Varus load on the flexed knee. This pattern may injure the ACL along with the posterior lateral complex, resulting in anterior instability with posterior lateral instability.

3. Describe the mechanism of ACL injuries in noncontact sports.

- Skiing injuries. The classic cause of knee injury in downhill skiers is a forward fall in which the inside edge of the ski is caught in the snow, placing the knee in external rotation and valgus stress. A second injury mechanism is the so-called "boot-induced" injury, resulting from a backward fall. With the skier's center of gravity posterior to the boot, the back of the boot causes an anteriorly directed force onto the tibia. When coupled with significant quadriceps contraction (the skier attempts to right himself), the ACL undergoes tension failure.
- Deceleration injuries with increased quadriceps contraction. Anterior force on the proximal tibia is caused by tremendous quadriceps contraction. Such injuries may be seen in basketball and football players who suddenly decelerate to change direction.
- Hyperextension. Noncontact ACL injuries also are seen with hyperextension injury in basketball players (e.g., in rebounding) and in gymnasts during the dismount.

4. What percent of patients with acute knee injuries and hemarthrosis have an ACL tear?
70%.

5. What is the ratio of ACL to PCL injuries?
There are approximately 20 ACL injuries for every PCL injury in sports. However, because many isolated PCL injuries go undetected, the exact ratio is unknown.

6. Describe the history given by the patient who sustains an acute disruption in the ACL.
Most patients claim that the knee "gave way," "buckled," or "popped out" at the time of injury. The mechanism of injury includes clipping, hyperextension, and direct blows. Noncontact injuries may be due to twisting and cutting. Swelling is usually immediate in onset and maximizes within the first 2–3 hours after injury. Most patients have immediate and profound disability with guarded or painful range of motion and the inability to ambulate.

7. What is the significance of hearing or feeling a "pop"?
The pop results from a tear of a ligament, tendon, or meniscus. It is often heard by fellow athletes.

8. Describe the physical examination in a patient with suspected tear of the ACL.
The examination should start with evaluating the normal knee for comparison. Some patients have excessive hypermobility or generalized ligamentous laxity that must be taken into account in evaluating knee laxity. The knee should be inspected for areas of ecchymosis, swelling, effusion, or tenderness. Range of motion should be evaluated. Flexion and extension are frequently compromised because of the large amount of effusion following injury. Ligament stability testing is performed and should include a minimum of the Lachman test, anterior drawer, pivot shift, posterior drawer, external rotation measurement, and varus and valgus stability testing.

9. What is the most reliable test during physical examination for an anterior cruciate ligament injury?
The Lachman test.

10. How is the Lachman test performed?
The Lachman test is performed in approximately 15–30° of flexion. The femur is stabilized with the examiner's hand. The opposite hand is used to apply an anteriorly directed force to the posterior tibia while stabilizing the femur. The examiner senses any tibial displacement and compares it with the uninvolved knee. The endpoint may be graded as either firm, marginal, or soft. The Lachman test may be graded as negative, 1+ (3–5 mm displacement), 2+ (5–10 mm displacement), or 3+ (> 10 mm displacement). Excessive anterior displacement compared with the normal side, especially when coupled with a marginal or soft endpoint, usually signifies a torn ACL.

11. What is the anterior drawer test?
The anterior drawer test is performed with the patient's knee at 90° of flexion with muscular relaxation. The hip is flexed at 45°. A smooth, steady pull is placed in an anterior direction on the posterior portion of the tibia. The test is generally done with the foot in neutral position, 15° of external rotation, and 15° of internal rotation. In a positive test, increased anterior step-off occurs between the femoral condyle and tibial plateau.

12. What is the pivot shift test?
The pivot shift describes the anterior subluxation of the lateral tibial plateau on the femoral condyle. With the patient in the supine position and relaxed, the knee is examined in full extension. The tibia is rotated internally, with one hand grasping the foot and the other hand applying a mild valgus stress at the level of the knee joint. Then, with flexion in the knee to approximately 20–30°, a jerk is suddenly experienced at the anterolateral corner of the proximal tibia. The patient also may feel the anterior subluxation and comment that it is the same feeling that occurred when the knee was injured or, in chronic cases, when it is continually injured. The result is graded as 0 (absent), 1+ (mild), 2+ (moderate), or 3+ (severe).

13. What is the differential diagnosis for an acute hemarthrosis?

Ligament tear (ACL, PCL)	Peripheral meniscal tear
Osteochondral fracture	Capsular tear
Patellar dislocation	

14. Describe the radiographic findings in an acute ACL injury.
Anteroposterior, lateral, intercondylar notch, and patellofemoral (sunrise) views are recommended for initial evaluation of acute knee injuries. In the isolated ACL tear, such studies are generally interpreted as normal.

15. What is a Segond fracture?
A Segond fracture is an avulsion fracture of the inferior lateral capsule adjacent to the tibia. It is highly suggestive of an injury to the ACL but is seen in only about 6% of the cases.

16. Describe the radiographic appearance of a chronic ACL tear.
In most cases of chronic ACL tear, degenerative changes with narrowing of the medial and lateral joint space are seen. Osteophytes may be present along the intercondylar portion of the femur, on the tibial spines, and along the medial or lateral joint margins. Femoral osteochondral lesions or loose bodies are often present.

17. What is the best diagnostic radiographic test for ACL tears?
Magnetic resonance imaging (MRI) is the best diagnostic test. The advantages of an MRI include its noninvasive nature, lack of radiation, and ability to image in any plane and to detect

nonosseus injuries such as ligament, meniscal, or articular damage. A complete tear is visualized on both T1- and T2-weighted images as a discontinuity in the ligament, with fluid filling the defect. MRI is also helpful in assessing fractures, medial and lateral collateral ligament injuries, PCL injuries, and meniscal injuries.

18. What is a KT-1000?

The KT-1000 (MedMetric, San Diego, CA) is a measuring system that documents antero-posterior tibial displacement by tracking the tibial tubercle in relation to the patella. Studies using the KT-1000 have shown that a side-to-side difference > 3 mm of anterior displacement at 20 lbs predicts an ACL deficiency with 94% accuracy.

19. What treatment options are available for acute isolated ACL tears?

Conservative nonoperative treatment, repair, repair and augmentation, extraarticular reconstruction, and intraarticular reconstruction.

20. What factors should be considered when discussing treatment for patients with an ACL injury?

Presence or absence of other pathology involving the knee

Degree of instability

Age of the patient

Level of activity

Associated ligamentous injuries

21. Can ACL injuries be left untreated?

Yes. Many physiologically older patients with a low activity level, no associated injuries, and only mild symptoms may be treated conservatively and nonoperatively.

22. What type of patient generally requires reconstruction of the ACL?

Physiologically young patients with high demands on the knee generally require reconstruction. Demands include the ability to cut, jump, accelerate, and decelerate. Patients with associated meniscal lesions, who often continue to be symptomatic, also may require reconstruction.

23. Is surgical repair of the ACL a treatment option?

No. Studies have indicated that primary repair of the injured ACL results in persistent laxity and instability of the knee.

24. Describe an intraarticular vs. extraarticular reconstruction for ACL loss.

Intraarticular reconstruction tries to reproduce the anatomic ACL. The donor tendon spans the intercondylar notch from the anatomic insertion and origin of the ACL. An extraarticular reconstruction uses structures on the lateral side of the knee to simulate the ACL. Typical extra articular reconstructions include those of Andrews, Steadman, and Arnold. The goal of an extra-articular procedure is to correct anterolateral rotatory instability or to prevent anterior subluxation of the lateral tibial plateau in relation to the lateral femoral condyle. Such procedures surgically stabilize the iliotibial tract so that the excessive lateral excursion of the tibia is halted. Their success has been limited. With the advent of arthroscopically assisted ACL intraarticular reconstructions, the extraarticular procedures are performed less often; however, they may be indicated for the unstable, skeletally immature patient.

25. What appropriate autografts are used for substitution and reconstruction of the ACL?

Central one-third patellar tendon

Semitendinosus tendon (hamstring)

Quadriceps tendon

26. What are the advantages and disadvantages of using the central one-third patellar tendon graft for ACL reconstruction?

Advantages of the central one-third patellar tendon graft are high initial tensile strength, stiffness, and fixation strength. Disadvantages include patellofemoral pain, patellar tendinitis, fracture, and patellar tendon rupture.

27. What are the advantages and disadvantages of using hamstring tendons for ACL reconstruction?

The major advantages of harvesting the semitendinosus tendon grafts are lower surgical morbidity during graft harvest and lower incidence of donor risk complications. The disadvantages are lower tensile strength, stiffness, and less optimal fixation strength compared with the patellar tendon graft, as well as a tendency for failure in women.

28. What associated surgical procedures may be done at the same time as ACL reconstruction?

Meniscus repair or excision and removal or fixation of osteochondral loose bodies are the most common concomitant procedures performed at the time of ACL reconstruction. If associated ligament pathology is present, appropriate repair or reconstruction is indicated. Generally, medial collateral ligament injuries are allowed to heal before arthroscopic ACL reconstruction.

Meniscal repair or excision may need to be performed before the ACL reconstruction if the meniscus is causing a mechanical block to regaining full extension after injury. This type of staged surgical reconstruction has led to a dramatically lower rate of flexion contracture following reconstruction.

29. Describe the procedure for an ACL reconstruction using the central one-third patellar tendon autograft.

1. Diagnostic arthroscopy.
2. Meniscus repair or excision.
3. ACL stump excision.
4. Lateral superior expansion notchplasty.
5. Graft harvest and preparation (some surgeons prefer to perform this at the beginning of the procedure).
6. Placement of appropriately sized tibial tunnel centered 7 mm in front of the posterior cruciate ligament. This center point is usually at, or slightly posterior to, the anterior horn of the lateral meniscus.
7. Placement of an appropriately sized tibial bone tunnel centered 6–7 mm in front of the "over-the-top" position, high and posterior in the intercondylar notch (this position would be at 1:00 in a left knee).
8. Secure fixation of the graft in both bone tunnels. Usually performed with interference screw fixation. Acceptable alternatives include many other types of soft-tissue fixation methods.
9. Careful evaluation of graft fixation, stability, and impingement-free range of motion.
10. Standard wound closure over drains.

30. What are the complications of ACL reconstruction?

Complications include infection, thrombophlebitis, skin necrosis, hemarthrosis, sensory nerve damage, reflex sympathetic dystrophy, and arthrofibrosis. The most common problems include failure to regain full extension or flexion, patellofemoral complications (e.g., chondromalacia and fracture), graft impingement, and graft failure.

31. Does a narrow notch increase the risk for ACL injury?

Yes. Patients who had a narrow notch (< 15 mm) measured during ACL reconstruction have a significantly higher risk for contralateral ACL injury.

32. **What are the reasons for loss of full extension after cruciate surgery?**
   - Lack of full preoperative extension. Patients should regain complete extension before reconstruction. This may be achieved with physical therapy time or arthroscopic removal of mechanical blocks to extension.
   - Anterior tibial placement of the graft causing roof impingement.
   - Cyclops lesion. This nodular abundance of fibrous tissue lying anterior to the tibial portion of the graft impinges on the anterior notch, which may be caused by roof impingement.
   - Infrapatellar contracture syndrome.

33. **What is arthrofibrosis?**
   Arthrofibrosis is a complication of cruciate surgery. This syndrome involves contracture of the retropatellar fat pad and patellar tendon. Patients present with severe postoperative pain, diminished patellar mobility, and failure to gain extension and flexion. The best initial treatment is aggressive physical therapy. Attempts at surgical intervention have met with limited success.

34. **Describe the natural history of the ACL-deficient knee.**
   Patients may report pain related to activity or giving-way episodes, described as either buckling or feeling as if the knee would not hold the patient's weight. Giving-way episodes occur in 17–65% of patients, often in association with strenuous activities; they may not be present during activities of daily living. Recurrent swelling is common after strenuous or prolonged activity; it also may be an early sign of developing osteoarthritis.

35. **In patients with chronic ACL insufficiency, what percentage develop meniscal tears?**
   Between 65 and 91%, with approximately 20% of tears involving both the medial and lateral menisci.

36. **What should be done for the patient who ruptures an anterior cruciate ligament graft?**
   If the individual desires to remain active, revision reconstruction may be performed. Appropriate graft choices include all forms of autogenous graft not previously used, including contralateral knee autografts. Patellar tendon, achilles, and tibialis anterior allografts are also acceptable grafts. Reconstruction with synthetic tissue such as Gortex, Dacron, or Xenografts has largely been abandoned because of high failure rates.

CONTROVERSIES

37. **What is the best graft choice for ACL reconstruction?**
   This issue remains mildly contested. As noted in questions 26 and 27, each major graft choice has advantages and disadvantages. There appears to be little difference in outcome regardless of the graft choice. The graft choice is frequently made in accordance with the surgeon's particular preference or training.

38. **Should continuous passive motion (CPM) be used after ACL reconstruction?**
   The use of CPM seems limited to situations in which individuals are at high risk for restriction of range of motion after surgery, including associated surgical procedures such as meniscus or ligament repairs. In uncomplicated anterior cruciate ligament reconstruction, postoperative CPM use allows an earlier return of range of motion. One month after surgery, there is no statistically significant difference between groups who either did or did not use CPM.

39. **Are cryotherapy devices indicated after ACL reconstruction?**
   Yes. Cryotherapy devices, whether manual or mechanical, reduce pain and swelling in the knee after surgery. Patients use less postoperative pain medicine and have fewer side effects (e.g., narcotic-related nausea).

40. **Can ACL reconstruction be safely performed in an outpatient setting?**
   Yes. Patients who are educated and prepared for the immediate postoperative period can safely be managed at home after ACL reconstruction. This results in cost savings to both the patient and the payer.

41. How should you treat the pediatric patient with a torn ACL?

If the pediatric ACL injury is a tibial spine avulsion fracture, reduction and fixation are performed by either open or arthroscopic methods.

A controversy occurs when a midsubstance ACL disruption occurs in a pediatric patient with widely open physes. Options include activity restriction and bracing until physes are closed, extraarticular reconstructions, standard intraarticular reconstruction, or modified intraarticular reconstruction methods. If the physes are nearly closed (the patient is usually at Tanner stage 3 or greater), standard intraarticular reconstruction methods may be employed.

Extraarticular reconstructions eventually fail in pediatric patients as they do in the adult. However, this may be a compromise for the very young athlete who insists on remaining athletically active. A better alternative may be a modified intraarticular reconstruction in which a smaller groove is made in the anterior tibia for tibial ACL placement and the femoral "over-the-top" method is used for femoral positioning and fixation.

42. In a severe knee injury in which both the ACLs and PCLs are torn in midsubstance and require reconstruction, should both be reconstructed at the same time?

Generally not. PCL reconstruction coupled with appropriate capsular and collateral ligament repairs are performed at the index procedure. After knee range of motion, stability, and muscle control is achieved, an arthroscopic ACL reconstruction is performed.

BIBLIOGRAPHY

1. Clancy WG, Nelson DA, Reider B, et al: Anterior cruciate ligament reconstruction using one-third of the patellar ligament, augmented by extraarticular tendon transfers. J Bone Joint Surg 64A:352, 1982.
2. Corry IS, Webb JM, Clingeleffer AJ, et.al: Arthroscopic reconstruction of the anteior cruciate ligament. Am J Sports Med 27:444–454, 1999.
3. DeHaven KE: Diagnosis of acute knee injuries with hemarthrosis. Am J Sports Med 8:9–14, 1980.
4. Fu FH, Shulte KR: Anterior cruciate ligament surgery 1996. State of the art? Clin Orthop 325:19–24, 1996.
5. Giurea M, Zorilla P, Amis AA, et. al: Comparative pull-out and cyclic loading strength tests of anchorage of hamstring tendon grafts in anterior cruciate ligament reconstruction. Am J Sports Med 27:621–625. 1999.
6. Kaborn DN, Johnson BM: The natural history of the anterior cruciate ligament-deficient knee. Clin Sports Med 12:625–636, 1993.
7. Kartus J, Stener S, Lindahl S, et al: Ipsilateral or contralateral patellar tendon graft in anterior cruciate ligament revision surgery. A comparison of two methods. Am J Sports Med 26:449–504, 1998.
8. Noojin FK, Barrett GR, Hartzog CW, et. al: Clinical comparison of intra-articular anterior cruciate reconstruction using autogenous semitendisosus and gracilis tendons in men versus women. Am J Sports Med 28:783–789,2000.
9. Noyes FR, Mooar PA, Matthews DS, et al: The symptomatic anterior cruciate deficient knee. I: The long-term functional disability in athletically active individuals. J Bone Joint Surg 65A:154–162, 1983.
10. Pressman AE, Letts RM, Jarvis JG: Anterior cruciate ligament tears in children: An analysis of operative versus non-operative treatment. J Pediatr Orthop 17:505–511, 1997.
11. Scarson WG: The role of lateral extra-articular procedures for anterolateral rotatory instability. Clin Sports Med 7:751–772, 1988.
12. Schaefer RK, Jackson DW: Arthroscopic management of the cruciate ligaments. In McGinty JB, et al (eds): Operative Arthroscopy. New York, Raven Press, 1991, pp 389–416.
13. Shelbourne KD, Davis TJ, Klootwyk TE: The relationship between intercondylar notch width of the femur and the incidence of anterior cruciate ligament tears. A prospective study. Am J Sports Med 26:402–408, 1998.
14. Shelbourne KD, Nitz PA: The O'Donoghue triad revisited: Combined knee injuries involving anterior cruciate and medial collateral ligament tears. Am J Sports Med 19:474–477, 1991.
15. Shelbourne KD, Wilckens JH, Mollabashy A, et al: Arthrofibrosis in acute anterior cruciate ligament reconstruction. The effect of timing of reconstruction and rehabilitation. Am J Sports Med 19:332, 1991.
16. Swenson TM, Fu FH: Anterior cruciate ligament reconstruction: Long-term results using autograft tissue. Clin Sports Med 12:709–722, 1993.

73. POSTERIOR CRUCIATE LIGAMENT INJURIES

David E. Brown, M.D.

1. Describe and discuss the anatomy of the posterior cruciate ligament.

The posterior cruciate ligament (PCL) does not have as discrete a bundle arrangement as the anterior cruciate ligament (ACL). Many authors, however, describe an anterolateral (largest) bundle and a posteromedial bundle. The presence of the ligament of Humphrey (45% of individuals) and ligament of Wrisberg (35% of individuals) is variable; if present, however, they may account for up to one-third of the diameter of the PCL.

The femoral attachment area resembles a half circle, thus causing differential bundle tightening with knee motion. The anterolateral bundle tightens with flexion, whereas the posteromedial bundle tightens in extension. The femoral attachment of the PCL is approximately 25 mm in length and 8 mm in width from anterior to posterior, with the center point of the anterolateral bundle 7–10 mm from the articular edge when the knee is flexed. The posteromedial bundle is centered a further 5 mm proximal and 5 mm posterior to the anterolateral bundle The tibial attachment site, which is nearly circular, is 12 mm in width and takes up most of the central sulcus on the posterior aspect of the tibial plateau.

2. What are the relative size and diameter of the PCL?

The PCL previously was thought to be twice the size and strength of the ACL. Recent studies, however, have demonstrated that the PCL is only 40–50% larger than the ACL.

3. What is the incidence of PCL tears?

Injury to the PCL is thought to occur in approximately 3–5% of all knee ligament injuries. The incidence appears to be rising slightly because of improved imaging techniques (MRI), improved techniques of physical examination, and greater knowledge of PCL injuries.

4. What common mechanisms of injury may cause a PCL tear?

- Fall on flexed knee with the foot in plantar flexion
- Dashboard knee (motor vehicle accident with the knee flexed and the tibia forced posteriorly on impact)
- Hyperflexion
- Hyperextension (usually in combination with other ligament injuries)

5. What is the most important test for evaluating PCL injuries?

The 90° posterior drawer test is the most important. The patient is supine, the hip is flexed 45°, and the knee is flexed 90°. Force is applied from anterior to posterior on the proximal tibia. Excessive motion in an anterior to posterior direction is a positive test indicative of PCL injury. A grade I posterior drawer reflects 5 mm of movement. At maximal posterior displacement, the tibial condyles are still anterior to the femoral condyles. A grade II posterior drawer reflects 5- to 10-mm posterior displacement, in which the tibial condyles are flush with the femoral condyles. A grade III posterior drawer reflects > 10-mm posterior displacement. In a grade III posterior drawer, the tibial condyles are displaced posterior to the femoral condyles.

6. What is the primary restraint to the 90° posterior drawer test?

The PCL provides 90% of the posterior restraint to the posterior drawer test at 90° of knee flexion. It contributes relatively little to varus, valgus, and internal and external rotation restraint.

7. What is posterolateral rotatory instability?

Posterolateral rotatory instability is laxity or incompetence of the structures of the posterolateral corner of the knee, including the lateral collateral ligament and the arcuate ligament complex (arcuate ligament, popliteus tendon, fabellofibular ligament, and posterolateral capsule).

Selective ligament-cutting experiments reveal that sectioning all of the structures of the posterolateral corner produces only small amounts of posterior translation of the knee. However, sectioning of the posterolateral ligaments results in markedly increased varus rotation and external tibial rotation with stress testing.

8. What is the posterior sag test?

The posterior sag test is similar to the posterior drawer test. It essentially detects the amount of posterior displacement caused by gravity when the knee and hip are flexed to 90°. When compared with the opposite side, the PCL-injured knee reveals a posterior sag of the tibial condyles relative to the femoral condyles. A positive test reflects absence of the PCL.

9. What is the quadriceps active test?

This test is also useful in evaluating PCL tear. The patient is placed in the same position as for a posterior drawer test. In the PCL-deficient knee, the tibia sags as in the posterior sag test. Quadriceps contraction at this position produces anterior translation of the tibia, verifying PCL injury.

10. What is the natural history of the isolated PCL tear?

Most patients do not have symptomatic instability of the knee. Several studies have demonstrated that > 80% of patients return to preinjury sport level. Quadriceps rehabilitation to a level equal to that of the opposite side correlates with satisfactory activity level. Associated meniscus tears are uncommon.

The PCL-deficient knee appears to be at risk for medial compartment and patellofemoral compartment arthritis. It is not clear whether the risk is related to activity level, but it does appear related to advancing time from injury. PCL-deficient cadaver knees have increased medial and patellofemoral compartment contact pressures, which may lead to articular surface degeneration.

11. What is the recommended treatment for isolated posterior tears?

Because most patients with isolated PCL tears function well, nonoperative treatment is generally recommended. Maximal quadriceps rehabilitation is required. It is unclear whether functional bracing affords any benefit.

12. If the PCL is avulsed from the tibia rather than torn in midsubstance, are the treatment recommendations any different?

Repair of the PCL bone avulsions from the tibia is generally advised. The ligament itself is intact. A simple posteromedial surgical approach affords easy reduction and fixation of the bone fragment. Results are uniformly good, in contrast to the midsubstance PCL tear described in question 11.

13. What are the principles of rehabilitation of the isolated PCL-deficient knee?

Nonoperative rehabilitation treatment emphasizes closed kinetic chain extension exercises, including squats, leg press, bicycling, and stair-stepper exercises. Open kinetic chain extension exercises, which are performed with the foot free, are avoided. Examples include seated or standing knee extension exercises.

In general, before beginning rehabilitation, the patient is evaluated by MRI. Any associated meniscus pathology is treated arthroscopically. Athletes commonly return to their sport within 3–6 weeks after injury. We generally prescribe a posterior cruciate functional brace for athletes involved in contact sports.

14. When should the isolated PCL-deficient knee be reconstructed?

Some clinicians believe that an acute knee injury with a grade III posterior drawer should be acutely reconstructed. Most, however, still recommend conservative treatment. If conservative treatment fails, resulting in persistent pain or functional instability, surgical reconstruction may still be performed.

15. What graft options are available for PCL reconstruction?

- Central one-third patella tendon autograft
- Tibialis anterior allograft
- Quadriceps tendon autograft
- Patella tendon allograft
- Achilles tendon allograft
- Semitendinosus/gracilis autograft

Graft selection depends on the preference of surgeon and patient, availability of graft sources, and whether additional ligament reconstructions are required. Patella tendon autografts appear to result in better success rates (similar to ACL reconstructions). However, many knees undergoing PCL reconstruction have multiple ligament injuries. The morbidity of multiple autogenous graft harvests leads many surgeons to use allograft sources in such cases.

16. What is the best position for postoperative immobilization after PCL reconstruction?

If posterior capsule is intact, the best position is full extension. The posterior capsule limits gravity-induced posterior sag. If the posterior capsule has been injured or if other extraarticular repairs or reconstructions are performed, the position of postoperative immobilization depends more on those repairs than on the PCL.

17. In what position is the PCL graft tensioned and fixated?

Warren advises tensioning and fixation in full extension if the posterior capsule is intact. Paulos performs tensioning and fixation in 70° of knee flexion, which is the quadriceps neutral position. If a two-bundle femoral technique is used, the anterolateral bundle is tightened at 70° of knee flexion and the posteromedial bundle is tightened in either full extension or 30° knee flexion. The tibial side should be secured prior to the femoral side.

18. What are the surgical technique options for posterior cruciate ligament reconstruction?

- Tibial transosseus tunnel — single femoral transosseus tunnel
- Tibial transosseus tunnel — double femoral transosseus femoral tunnel.
- Tibial inlay — single femoral transosseus femoral tunnel
- Tibial inlay — double femoral transosseus tunnel

19. What are the principal techniques involved in PCL tibial transosseus tunnel preparation?

- Reconstruction can be performed by either open or arthroscopic techniques, depending on degree of associated injury and the preference and skill of the surgeon.
- Placement of the tibial guidepin should be directed by intraoperative radiographic evaluation. It is imperative that the tibial guidepin be in the central low position of the tibial attachment of the PCL.
- A miniposterior incision should be used to allow digital evaluation of guidepin placement at the tibial attachment. This incision also allows better control of reamer penetration of the posterior tibial cortex during tunnel preparation.
- Tibial tunnel orientation and placement are possible through multiple methods. Some advocate beginning the tibial tunnel on the medial tibial metaphysis, whereas others begin the tibial tunnel on the lateral side. Some surgeons avoid the tibial tunnel altogether, preferring to fix the bone portion of the graft construct to the posterior tibial cortex at the site of PCL attachment.

20. Describe the technique of tibial inlay graft placement.

1. The patient is placed either in the prone or lateral decubitus position.

2. Use the posteromedial approach described by Burks. The interval between the medial head of the gastrocnemius and the semitendinosis leads to the posterior proximal tibia.

3. Make a unicortical window at the PCL insertion.

4. Secure the tibial side of the PCL graft into the window with a cancellous screw.

21. Describe the placement of the femoral tunnel(s) in PCL reconstruction.

The anterolateral bundle tunnel is placed just below the roof of the notch, 1–2 mm posterior to the articular surface. Care must be taken to orient the tunnel so that the subcortical bone and articular surface are protected from injury. The posteromedial bundle tunnel is placed 5–7 mm proximal and posterior to the anterolateral tunnel margin. Two-tunnel reconstructions are gaining in popularity. Biomechanical data demonstrates that two-tunnel PCL reconstructions most closely resembles the native PCL strain.

22. Describe the clinical examination of the knee with combined PCL and posterolateral ligament instability.

The knee is markedly lax to posterior drawer at both 30° and 90°, usually with a grade III posterior drawer at 90°. The prone external rotation test and varus stress test at 30° are markedly positive. There may be varus opening in 90° of knee flexion. The patient may walk with a varus thrust gait.

23. What is the treatment of combined PCL/posterolateral rotatory instability injuries?

Surgical repair and reconstruction are required. Patients generally are markedly symptomatic, with both pain and instability, if untreated. The rate of medial compartment arthritis is significant.

If the patient has a varus knee or walks with a varus thrust gait, valgus high tibial osteotomy placing is performed first. Some patients are so dramatically improved by this procedure alone that later ligament reconstruction is not required. Most of the time, however, the PCL and posterolateral corner must be reconstructed. The PCL is reconstructed by one of the techniques described above. The posterolateral corner is reconstructed by either ligament advancement, biceps tenodesis, or anatomic reconstruction of the posterolateral corner. Posterolateral corner injuries and reconstruction are further described in the chapter on lateral ligament injury.

24. What is the treatment of an acute PCL tear combined with a medial side injury?

In a patient with an acute grade III medial collateral injury, open primary repair and approximation of the medial structures combined with acute PCL reconstruction is indicated. Patients with grade I or grade II MCL injuries may be treated nonoperatively if they are not athletes. The MCL and PCL injuries are both treated conservatively. Athletes with such an injury may be considered for subacute PCL reconstruction after allowing the partial MCL injury to heal.

25. In patients with knee dislocations or near knee dislocations with multiple ligament injuries, what surgical treatment should be considered?

If the PCL is avulsed, direct repair of the PCL combined with reconstruction of the ACL at the index procedure is an acceptable option. When both the ACL and PCL are torn in midsubstance and thus each requires reconstruction, the cruciates should be reconstructed in stages. At the initial surgery, PCL reconstruction combined with collateral and capsular repair is performed. Once the patient has satisfactorily recovered from the initial surgery, late ACL reconstruction is performed. Staged reconstruction is preferred because these individuals often develop postoperative knee stiffness after the operation if all structures are surgically repaired and reconstructed at the same time.

BIBLIOGRAPHY

1. Burks RT, Schaffer JJ: A simplified approach to the tibial attachment of the posterior cruciate ligament. Clin Orthop 254:216–219, 1990.

2. Clancy WG Jr, Shelbourne KD, Zoellner GB, et al: Treatment of knee joint instability secondary to rupture of the posterior cruciate ligament. Report of a new procedure. J Bone Joint Surg 65A:310–322, 1983.
3. Cosgarea AJ, Jay PR: Posterior cruciate ligament injuries: Evaluation and management. J Am Acad Orthop Surg 9:297–307, 2001.
4. Daniel DM, Stone ML, Barnett P, et al: Use of the quadriceps active test to diagnose posterior cruciate-ligament disruption and measure posterior laxity of the knee. J Bone Joint Surg 70A:386–391, 1988.
5. Fowler PJ, Messieh SS: Isolated posterior cruciate ligament injuries in athletes. Am J Sports Med 15:553–557, 1987.
6. Galloway MT, Grood ES, Mehalik MS, et al: Posterior cruciate ligament reconstruction. An in vitro study of femoral and tibial graft placement. Am J Sports Med 24:437–445, 1996.
7. Gollehon DL, Torzilli PA, Warren RF: The role of the posterolateral and cruciate ligaments in the stability of the human knee: A biomechanical study. J Bone Joint Surg 69A:233–242, 1987.
8. Harner CD, Janaushek MA, Kanamori A, et al: Biomechanical analysis of a double-bundle posterior cruciate ligament reconstruction. Am J Sports Medicine 28:144–151, 2000.
9. Miller RH: Knee injuries. In Canale ST (ed): Campbell's Operative Orthopaedics, 9th ed. St. Louis, Mosby, 1998, pp 1190–1195.
10. Parolie JM, Bergfeld JA: Long-term results of non-operative treatment of isolated posterior cruciate ligament injuries in the athlete. Am J Sports Med 14:35–38, 1986.
11. Shelbourne,KD, Davis,TJ , Patel DV: The natural history of acute, isolated,nonoperatively treated posterior cruciate ligament injuries: A prospective study. Am J Sports Med 27:276–283, 1999.
12. Skyhar MJ, Warren RF, Ortiz GJ, et al: The effects of sectioning of the posterior cruciate ligament and the posterolateral complex on the articular contact pressures within the knee. J Bone Joint Surg 74A:594–699, 1993.
13. Torg JS, Barton TM, Pavlov H, et al: Natural history of the posterior cruciate ligament-deficient knee. Clin Orthop 246:208–216, 1989.
14. Veltri DM, Warren RF: Isolated and combined posterior cruciate ligament injuries. J Am Acad Orthop Surg 1:67, 1993.

74. MEDIAL COLLATERAL LIGAMENT INJURIES

Randall D. Neumann, M.D.

1. What is the medial collateral ligament?

The medial collateral ligament (MCL) complex is a supporting structure on the medial side of the knee. It is a sleeve of tissue extending from the midline anteriorly to the midline posteriorly.

2. What are the components of the MCL?

The important static structures are the superficial MCL, the posterior oblique ligament, and the middle third or deep capsular ligaments. The dynamic supporting structures include the semimembranosus complex and the vastus medialis.

3. What is the superficial MCL?

The superficial MCL, also called the tibia collateral ligament, attaches from the medial femoral epicondyle at the adductor tubercle and inserts distally 5–7 cm below the joint line under the pes anserinus.

4. What is the posterior oblique ligament?

The posterior oblique ligament is the thickened triangular capsular ligament originating posterior to the superficial MCL and inserting below the joint line. This ligament is important in maintaining medial stability and resists anterior medial tibial subluxation.

5. What is the deep capsular ligament?

The middle one-third of the capsular ligament or deep MCL is a short structure attached to the meniscus immediately beneath the superficial MCL. It is divided into meniscotibial and meniscofemoral fibers.

6. What is the function of the MCL?

The main function of the MCL is to resist valgus and external rotation forces of the tibia in relation to the femur.

7. Describe the clinical classification of MCL injuries.

Sprains of the MCL are classified as mild, moderate, or severe. Mild or grade I sprains have few torn fibers with no loss of ligamentous integrity. Moderate or grade II sprains are incomplete tears with no pathologic laxity; the fibers are still opposed. In severe or grade III sprains, the integrity of the ligament is completely disrupted.

8. What is the typical history obtained from a patient with an MCL injury?

Usually the patient discusses the mechanism. Lower-grade MCL injuries may occur with noncontact valgus and external rotation injuries, such as seen in skiing. Moderate-to-severe MCL injuries usually result from a lateral blow to the lower thigh or upper leg that causes valgus stress to be placed on the knee. This mechanism of injury commonly occurs in contact sports such as football, soccer, and rugby. Patients may or may not have the ability to ambulate. Some patients describe the sensation of a "pop" or a tearing of tissue. Usually no deformity exists.

9. Do most patients with a grade III sprain have severe hemarthrosis?

Because patients with a grade III sprain have complete tearing of the capsule, fluid from inside the joint may escape into the soft tissues. Therefore, patients may have only minimal joint space effusion.

10. Do patients with grade III injuries have severe pain and inability to walk?

Hughston et al. found that 50% of athletes with grade III injuries could walk into the office unaided by external support. They also found that some grade I and grade II sprains are actually more painful than grade III. Therefore, the absence of severe pain does not rule out a severe injury.

11. What other ligament is commonly injured along with the MCL?

The anterior cruciate ligament (ACL).

12. Describe the grading system for pathologic laxity of the MCL.

With abduction stress testing, joint opening may occur, displacing the tibia on the femur. Grade 0 is considered normal. Grade I has 1–4 mm of laxity; grade II, 5–9 mm of laxity; and grade III, 10–15 mm of laxity.

13. Where is maximal tenderness located in MCL injuries?

On physical examination palpation reveals that most patients have tenderness over the adductor tubercle. Such tenderness may signify that the posterior oblique ligament and deep fibers of the collateral ligament are torn. Other areas of tenderness occur over the joint line and distally over the insertion of the tibial collateral ligament.

14. What percentage of patients have injury to the extensor mechanism?

Approximately 10–20% of patients damage the extensor mechanism (usually the vastus medialis with patellar dislocation) in association with MCL injuries.

15. What tests on physical examination signify MCL injury?

The **abduction stress test** is done with the patient's knee flexed at 30°. It is best to have the thigh resting on the edge of the table, with the foot supported by the examiner. Abduction stress testing is done with a valgus load to open the medial compartment of the knee. The test should be done with the foot in the same degree of external rotation, because an extra grade of instability may be perceived if the examination allows the tibia to move externally. The test is considered positive when medial instability is present at 30° of flexion.

The **anterior drawer test** checks for anterior medial instability. With the foot in external rotation and the knee flexed at 90°, an anterior pull on the proximal calf is used to palpate laxity. It is best that the examiner sit on the patient's foot and relax the hamstrings before testing. Perceivable anterior rotational instability is seen if the MCL with its posterior oblique portion is torn. Both tests should be done when MCL injury is suspected.

The **Lachman test** should be done for evaluation of the ACL. Instability in full extension suggests that the posterior capsule is disrupted and possibly the posterior cruciate ligament (PCL). Some patients with patellar apprehension also have dislocated the patella.

16. Differentiate the location of tenderness in medial meniscus injuries and medial collateral ligament injuries.

The tenderness with medial meniscus injuries is limited to the medial joint line. MCL injuries occur along the length of the ligament, from the adductor tubercle to the proximal tibia. Tenderness above or below the joint line is indicative of a MCL injury.

17. When should the knee with a medial collateral ligament tear be non-tender?

It takes approximately 3 weeks for most tenderness from a MCL injury to subside. Suspect a medial meniscus injury if pain persists longer that 3 weeks.

18. What diagnostic tests are available for evaluation of MCL injuries?

Stress radiography. This test is done using abduction stress testing at 15–20°. Radiographs are then taken to assess the opening on the medial side of the joint.

Magnetic resonance imaging (MRI). MRI is helpful in assessing the location of the MCL tear and associated meniscal and cruciate pathology.

Arthrograms. Arthrograms are an invasive examination that may show meniscal pathology or contrast extravasation as evidence of capsular tearing; they also may be negative, because the capsule seals in 2–4 days. Arthrograms are generally not indicated at this time, because noninvasive tests are more accurate.

Arthroscopy. Examination under anesthesia and arthroscopy may be helpful in assessing meniscal pathology, ligamentous injury, and cruciate pathology. This invasive test is reserved for patients who are undergoing operative treatment.

19. What is a Pellegrini-Steida lesion?

The Pellegrini-Steida lesion is seen on the anteroposterior radiograph. Calcification adjacent to the adductor tubercle signifies an old collateral ligament injury of longer than 6 weeks.

20. Why are stress radiographs of the knee needed for adolescents?

Adolescents with open epiphyseal lines may have physeal injuries that are mistaken for medial instability because of the appearance of medial laxity. Physeal fractures generally require reduction and casting or internal fixation.

21. What are the treatments for grades I and II isolated MCL injuries?

Grades I and II isolated MCL injuries are treated conservatively. Icing is applied for 20 minutes 2–3 times/day. An elastic wrap may be used. Non–weight-bearing crutches are used. Isometric quadriceps contractures usually can be done within the first 2–3 days of injury. The knee is immobilized to block full extension for 7–10 days. Progressive ambulation and range-of-motion and strengthening exercises are done as the swelling subsides, pain diminishes, and the patient regains the ability to ambulate. Most patients can return to full activities and contact sports within 3–6 weeks.

22. How are isolated grade III MCL injuries treated?
Most patients are now treated nonoperatively. Historically, such patients underwent operative repair of the MCL. Multiple studies have shown that repair in an isolated MCL injury occurs without surgery. Treatment consists of crutches, cast, or bracing. Bracing can continue for 3–6 weeks, depending on healing.

CONTROVERSIES

23. When can patients return to sports after medial collateral ligament injuries?
All patients should be without pain, have normal range of motion, have no swelling or effusion, and have 80–90% strength before returning to sports.
> **Grade I:** 2–3 weeks
> **Grade II:** 3–4 weeks
> **Grade III:** 6 weeks.

24. Describe the treatment for ACL tears combined with MCL lesions.
Controversy exists about the approaches to MCL treatment in association with ACL treatment. Some authors believe that treatment of the MCL with protective weightbearing and bracing should restore full motion and stability before ACL ligament surgery is performed. At approximately 4–6 weeks, the ACL is reconstructed with patellar tendon graft, allograft, or hamstring tendons. If at that time instability continues, the posterior oblique and the superficial MCL are reconstructed. Other authors believe that the isolated MCL injuries should be treated surgically with open repair within 5–7 days after injury. The ACL is reconstructed at that time. Some evidence suggests that increased scarring and arthrofibrosis occur with a higher reoperation rate, when the surgery is done acutely during the first 7–10 days.

BIBLIOGRAPHY

1. Hughston JC, Andrews JR, Cross MJ, Moschi A: Classification of knee ligament instabilities:Part I. The medial compartment in cruciate ligaments. JBone Joint Surg 58A:159–172, 1976.
2. Hughston JC, Barret GR:Acute anterior medial rotatory instability:Long term results of surgical repair. J Bone Joint Surg 65A:145–153, 1983.
3. Indelicato PA: Medial and lateral ligament injuries of the knee. In Insall J, Scott N (eds): Surgery of the Knee. New York, Churchill Livingstone, 2001, pp 651–656.
4. Indelicato PA, Hermansdorfer J, Huegel M:The nonoperative management of complete tears of the medial collateral ligament of the knee in intercollegiate football players. Clin Orthop 256:174–177, 1990.
5. Linton RC, Indelicato PA:Medial ligament injuries. In DeLee JC, Drez D (eds): Orthopedic Sports Medicine:Principles and Practice, vol. 1. Philadelphia, W.B. Saunders, 1994, pp 1261–1274.
6. Neumann RD:Traumatic knee injuries. In Mellion MB(ed): Sports Medicine Secrets, 2nd ed. Philadelphia, Hanley & Belfus, 1999, pp 307–311.
7. O'Donoghue DH:Treatment of acute ligamentous injuries at the knee. Orthop Clin North Am 4:617–645, 1973.
8. Tria AJ: Clinical examination of the knee. In Insall J, Scott N (eds): Surgery of the Knee. New York, Churchill Livingstone, 2001, pp 161–174.
9. Warren LF, Marshall JL:The supporting structures and layers of the medial side of the knee. An anatomical analysis. JBone Joint Surg 61A:56–62, 1979.
10. Warren LF, Marshall JL, Girgis F:The primary static stabilizer of the medial side of the knee. J Bone Joint Surg 56A:665–674, 1974.

75. LATERAL LIGAMENT AND POSTERAL CORNER INJURIES

David E. Brown, M.D., and Brian Konowalchuk, M.D.

1. What is the incidence of isolated fibular collateral ligament tear?

The true incidence is unknown. However, an isolated ligament injury is quite uncommon. Many patients who are given a diagnosis of fibular collateral ligament (FCL) strain (often by inexperienced examiners) have anterior cruciate ligament (ACL) injuries.

2. What is the mechanism of an isolated FCL injury?

Such injuries are thought to result from either a contact or noncontact hyperextension varus stress. Perhaps the incidence is low because varus stress generally has to be applied from the medial side of the knee, a mechanism that is quite uncommon. Because the contralateral knee is likely to be "in the way," the injured knee is more likely to sustain a valgus stress to its lateral side.

3. Describe the examination of isolated FCL injuries.

Examination should show tenderness along the FCL, which is best palpated with the knee in a figure-four position with varus stress applied. There is generally little effusion, because the FCL is extraarticular. The presence of an effusion should arouse suspicion for a cruciate ligament tear. Selective ligament-cutting experiments in cadavers have demonstrated only **slight** varus laxity in knees with sectioned FCLs. **Moderate** varus laxity occurs only with additional sectioning of the posterolateral corner ligaments. **Severe** varus laxity should arouse suspicion of combined FCL, posterolateral corner, and cruciate ligament injuries.

4. Describe the treatment of isolated FCL injuries.

Treatment includes elastic wrapping, ice application, functional bracing, and protection from repeat varus stress for a period of 4–6 weeks. Some authors advocate surgical repair of isolated FCL injuries. However, no study has scientifically evaluated the treatment of isolated FCL injuries.

5. Describe the anatomy of the posterolateral corner.

The principal ligaments of the posterolateral corner include:

- FCL
- Arcuate ligament
- Posterolateral deep capsule
- Short lateral ligament
- Fabellofibular ligament
- Popliteofibular ligament

The tendons of the posterolateral corner are:

- Iliotibial band
- Biceps femoris — short and long head
- Lateral head of gastrocnemius
- Popliteus

Baker has described the arcuate ligament complex as the arcuate ligament, FCL, popliteus tendon, and lateral head of the gastrocnemius. Rupture of the popliteofibular ligament is now believed to be an important cause of posterolateral rotatory instability. The fabellofibular ligament is present in approximately two-thirds of specimens. If the fabella is present, the fabellofibular ligament is present. If the fabellofibular ligament is not present, then the short lateral ligament is generally present.

6. What is posterolateral rotatory instability?

Posterolateral rotatory instability is laxity or incompetence of the structures of the posterolateral corner of the knee, including the lateral collateral ligament and the posterolateral ligaments. Selective ligament-cutting experiments reveal that sectioning of all of the structures of the posterolateral corner produces only small amounts of posterior translation of the knee. However, sectioning the posterolateral ligaments resulted in markedly increased varus rotation and external tibial rotation with stress testing.

7. What is the mechanism of injury to the posterolateral corner?
- Posterolaterally directed blow to the medial part of the tibia
- Hyperextension and external rotation
- Pure hyperextension

8. What symptoms are associated with posterolateral instability of the knee?
The major symptom is pain in the posterolateral aspect of the knee. Up to 25% of patients may have dysesthesias and weakness of the foot and leg muscles due to associated injury of the peroneal nerve. Patients may complain of instability with the knee in full extension, thus leading to a gait pattern that emphasizes knee flexion to avoid instability. With greater laxity, the gait may demonstrate a varus thrust.

9. What is the external rotation recurvatum test?
The external rotation recurvatum test may reflect posterolateral rotatory instability. With the patient supine, the great toe is grasped and the foot is raised from the table. The test is positive if the knee falls into hyperextension, external rotation, and varus.

10. How does one test for varus instability of the knee? Why is such testing important?
With the patient relaxed and supine on the examination table, the distal femur is stabilized manually. The lower leg is grasped with the opposite hand, and varus stress is placed on the knee. The test should be performed at 0°, 30°, 60°, and 90° of knee flexion.
Isolated FCL injury causes minimal varus laxity. When combined with posterolateral corner injury, the varus laxity is moderate to severe. Large degrees of varus instability in full extension should arouse suspicion for combined injuries of the posterolateral corner and one of the cruciate ligaments. An isolated cruciate ligament injury does not affect varus or valgus stability. The presence of varus laxity in full extension is primarily indicative of a posterolateral corner injury.

11. How do you test for external rotation of the tibia? Why is such testing important?
The patient is placed prone on the examining table with the hips and knees resting on the table. The knees are flexed at 30°, and the feet are rotated externally. If external rotation on the injured side is 10° more than on the normal side, the test is considered positive. A positive test is usually consistent with a tear of the posterolateral corner. This is considered the most specific test for posterolateral rotatory instability.

12. Describe the clinical examination of the knee with combined posterior cruciate and posterolateral ligament instability.
The knee is markedly lax to posterior drawer at both 30° and 90°. At 90° there is usually a grade IIIposterior drawer. The prone external rotation test and varus stress test at 30° are markedly positive. Varus opening may be present in 0° of knee flexion. The patient may walk with a varus thrust gait.

13. What is the role of MRI in the evaluation of posterolateral corner injuries?
MRI accurately depicts the extent of injury to the posterolateral ligaments. A bone contusion on the anterior medial femoral condyle is invariably present with complete posterolateral ligament injuries.

14. What are the treatment options in patients with posterolateral rotatory instability?
If tears of the posterolateral corner are recognized acutely, primary repair of all injured structures is recommended. If there is insufficient tissue for primary repair, augmentation is indicated

but depends on what healthy tissues remain in severe posterolateral corner injuries. For example, if the knee has been laterally dislocated, it is common for the iliotibial band and biceps tendon to be disrupted. If the biceps tendon and iliotibial band are intact, they can be used as augmentation sources.

Clancy described biceps tenodesis. The entire distal portion of the tendon is advanced and secured to the lateral femoral epicondyle with a soft-tissue screw and washer. This procedure augments the FCL and theoretically advances part of the posterolateral corner through intertendinous attachments between the biceps tendon and the posterolateral corner.

Warren devised procedures to augment the popliteus tendon with central slips of either the biceps or iliotibial band.

Chronic posterolateral corner injuries also may be reconstructed with either the Clancy or Warren techniques. If the biceps tendon and iliotibial band are insufficient because of chronic stretching laxity or previous tear, Warren has described reconstruction of the popliteus and popliteofibular ligament with a bone-tendon-bone patellar ligament graft. The graft is split on one end to allow reconstruction of both structures. A soft tissue graft, such as allograft anterior tibialis tendon or Achilles tendon, are excellent for this procedure.

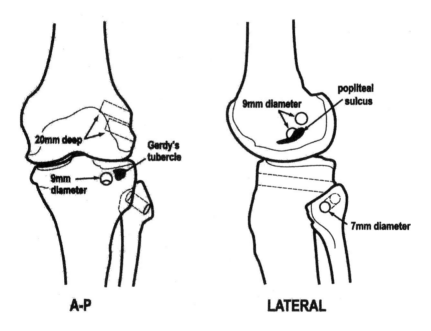

15. What is the surgical approach to repair or reconstruct the posterolateral corner structures?

A single lateral hockey stick incision is made. Longitudinal incisions are made in the iliotibial band, in the interval between the iliotibial band and biceps femoris tendon and along the posterior border of the biceps. The peroneal nerve must be isolated and protected in the latter incision. The reader is referred to Terry and LaPrade for a complete description.

16. Describe the rationale for and technique of anatomic reconstruction of the posterolateral corner.

Previously described reconstructions have not reconstructed all three of the primary contributors to posterolateral corner stability (FCL, popliteus tendon, and popliteofibular ligament). Laprade and colleagues have devised a double-bundle two-graft technique for reconstruction of these primary stabilizers. A split Achilles tendon allograft is used. The popliteus is reconstructed with the first bundle. The femoral tunnel is at the proximal popliteal sulcus. The free end of the tendon is routed through the popliteus hiatus, then through a tibial tunnel that begins at the posterior popliteus sulcus and exits at Gerdy's tubercle. (See figure at left.)

The second graft reconstructs both the FCL and popliteo-fibular ligament. The femoral tunnel is just proximal and posterior to the lateral femoral epicondyle. The free end is now passed through a fibular tunnel (directed lateral to postero-medial) and then through the same tibial tunnel, passed from posterior to anterior. Both grafts are secured anteriorly. (See figure below.)

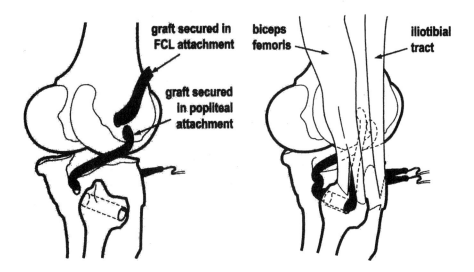

BIBLIOGRAPHY

1. Baker CL Jr, Norwood LA, Hughston JC: Acute posterolateral rotatory instability of the knee. J Bone Joint Surg 65A:614–618, 1983.
2. Baker CL Jr, Norwood LA, Hughston JC: Acute combined posterior cruciate and posterolateral instability of the knee. Am J Sports Med 12:204–208, 1984.
3. Chen FS, Rokito AS, Pitman MI: Acute and chronic posterolateral rotatory instability of the knee. J Am Acad Orthop Surg 8:97–110,2000.
4. Clancy WG Jr: Repair and reconstruction of the posterior cruciate ligament. In Chapman MW (ed): Operative Orthopedics, vol. 3. Philadelphia, J.B. Lippincott, 1988, pp 1651–1665.
5. DeLee JC, Riley MB, Rockwood CA: Acute straight lateral instability of the knee. Am J Sports Med 11:404, 1983.
6. Gollehon DL, Torzilli PA, Warren RF: The role of the posterolateral and cruciate ligaments in the stability of the human knee. A biomechanical study. J Bone Joint Surg 69A:233–242, 1992.
7. Maynard MJ, Deng,X, Wickeiwicz TL,el al: The popliteofibular ligament: Rediscovery of a key element in posterolateral stability. Am J Sports Med 24:311–316,1996.
8. Ross G, Chapman AW, Newberg AR, et al: Magnetic resonance imaging for the evaluation of acute posterolateral complex injuries of the knee. Am J Sports Med 25:444–448, 1997.
9. Terry, GC, LaPrade RF: The posterolateral corner of the knee. Anatomy and surgical approach. Am J Sports Med 24:732–739, 1996.
10. Veltri DM, Warren RF:Posterolateral instability of the knee. JBone Joint Surg 76A:460–472, 1994.
11. Wascher DC, Grauer JD, Markoff KL:Biceps tendon tenodesis for posterolateral instability of the knee:An in vitro study. Am J Sports Med 21:400–406, 1993.

76. PATELLOFEMORAL JOINT DISORDERS

*Michele Helzer-Julin, PA-C, M.S., W. Michael Walsh, M.D.,
and Jeremy J. Vanicek, PA-C*

1. How common are disorders of the patellofemoral joint?
Problems related to the patellofemoral joint are likely to be the most common knee problems encountered in clinical practice. Most are related to overuse, but some will be brought to light by a specific trauma.

2. List some of the many general labels and specific clinical entities related to disorders of the patellofemoral joint.

General Labels	Clinical Entities
Extensor mechanism malalignment	Patellar tendinitis (jumpers' knee)
Patellofemoral pain syndrome	Quadriceps tendinitis
Runner's knee	Osgood-Schlatter disease
Chondromalacia	Plica
Patellar subluxation/dislocation	Fat pad impingement
	Bipartite patella

3. Is there a characteristic somatotype for the patient with patellofemoral problems?
No. Early discussion popularized the concept that patellar problems affect only chubby, knock-kneed, teenage girls—certainly not the vigorous male athlete. It is now clear that the patellofemoral joint is a major source of pain and dysfunction for both males and females in sedentary and athletic populations alike.

4. What anatomic predispositions contribute to patellofemoral disorders?
The many anatomic factors include both bony and soft-tissue abnormalities:

Bony Abnormalities	Soft-tissue Abnormalities
Patella alta	Vastus medialis obliquus dysplasia
Lateral tilting and subluxation of the patella	Tight lateral retinaculum
Shallow trochlear groove	Patellar hypermobility
Genu valgum	Generalized ligamentous laxity
External tibial torsion	Hamstring tightness
Femoral anteversion	Weak ankle dorsiflexors
Pes planus, pronation, forefoot supination	Increased lateral deviation of patellar tendon

5. Does the presence of any or all of the above predispositions guarantee that an individual will have problems?
No. Predispositions are merely that. Anatomic variations are widespread in the general population and may lie dormant, leaving affected individuals asymptomatic for years, decades, or even their entire life. Symptoms are usually provoked by overuse but also may be triggered by a single traumatic event that creates clinical complaints in a previously asymptomatic individual.

6. What are typical patellofemoral complaints?
Most symptoms and complaints relate to either pain, instability, or both:
Anterior knee pain, the most frequent complaint, may be aggravated by any physical activity, but most commonly by repetitive stair climbing or sitting with the knee flexed at 90° for a prolonged period (e.g., sitting in an airplane, car, or theater).
Swelling is not routine and, if present, is only minimal. Many patients have a general puffy appearance to their knees, although no effusion within the joint itself is detectable.

Catching or slipping sensations are common. Catching may occur when underlying inflamed tissue is caught on bony prominences, or it may be due to roughness on the patellar surface or an inflamed synovial plica. Even minor instability episodes may be interpreted by the patient as catching. Feelings of lateral patellar slipping range from a mild catching sensation to a feeling that the patella has completely left the trochlear groove, resulting in the knee giving way.

7. What activities typically aggravate the patellofemoral joint?

Activities that load the patellofemoral joint or create high compressive forces, such as ascending and descending stairs, squatting, and sitting with the knee flexed to 90° for prolonged periods of time, cause significant patellofemoral pain. Many patients also are bothered by running, jumping, cutting, and twisting activities.

8. Describe the typical physical findings.

The most common physical findings are the anatomic predispositions listed in question 4. In addition, there may be pain with compression of the patella, crepitation of the patellofemoral joint with knee range of motion, and apprehension with lateral displacement of the patella.

9. What radiographic techniques are useful?

For routine problems of the patellofemoral joint, radiographs may lend add little additional information to a detailed history and physical examination. Routine anteroposterior and lateral views can rule out other pathologic processes. The lateral view assesses patellar height. The most significant view in dealing with the patellofemoral joint is the infrapatellar view, which assesses lateral tilting and subluxation of the patella. Because the patellofemoral joint is dynamically affected, static radiographs may appear normal in a patient with severe patellofemoral disability.

10. What are the current recommendations for initial treatment of patellofemoral problems?

Physical therapy with a rehabilitative exercise routine is the mainstay of treatment. Techniques that emphasize patellar control rather than pure strength are essential. Flexibility is important, especially of the hamstrings, posterior calf muscles and iliotibial band. Knee extension exercises should be avoided. External support such as patellofemoral bracing or McConnell patellofemoral taping may be helpful. Nonsteroidal antiinflammatory medication, modalities, activity modification and correction of foot alignment abnormalities by orthotics may be appropriate in select patients. More recently, the concepts of total limb rehabilitation with an emphasis on hip rotator strengthening and proprioceptive exercises have come into common use.

11. Do the above techniques cure the problem?

No. Anatomic predisposition is still present. The goal should be a return to a normal, pain-free, functional status. Nonsurgical means control symptoms in 80–90% of individuals. It is human nature to stop rehabilitative efforts once symptoms subside, despite the recurrent nature of patellofemoral problems. Therefore, patients must be made aware that this is a potentially life-long problem with which they need to cope. The patient should be reminded to reintroduce rehabilitative efforts if symptoms return.

12. What surgical options are available for patients in whom conservative treatment fails?

Various surgical options are designed to realign the patella. The simplest is an arthroscopic lateral release, which, unfortunately, does not help in all cases. Currently, this procedure is considered appropriate only for cases of patellofemoral pain with excessive lateral patellar tilt. A more extensive open procedure uses not only a lateral release, but also reattachment or reconstruction of the medial patellofemoral ligament and vastus medialis obliquus muscle along with transfer of the patellar tendon attachment medially. Currently this is the procedure more applicable to the unstable patella. Other less common surgical options include anterior advancement of the tibial tuberosity to decompress the patellofemoral joint, derotational osteotomy of the limb, and patellectomy.

13. At what point during conservative treatment should surgical options be considered?
There is no specific length of time. Routinely, patients have tried conservative treatment and lifestyle modification for months to years. Surgical intervention should occur when the patient feels symptoms are at an unacceptable functional level and when the patient and surgeon agree that there is no trend toward improvement.

14. Can the patient expect a normal knee after surgery?
No. Although surgery may help considerably and allow for further improvement with postoperative physical therapy, the patient will still have anatomic variations that may continue to cause problems in the future.

15. How does treatment change when the patient sustains an acute lateral patellar dislocation?
The acute injury, of course, must be treated in and of itself, including the usual measures for control of swelling and possibly a brief period of immobilization. Current trends replace a strict 6 weeks of immobilization with modest immobilization for symptom control and early return to functional rehabilitation. As the acute phase resolves, treatment options are similar.

16. What findings prompt early surgical intervention after an acute patellar dislocation?
- An osteochondral fracture of the patella, trochlea, or lateral femoral condyle may occur as the patella either leaves or reenters the femoral trochlea. Some large fractures can be reattached with internal fixation, whereas other smaller fractures need to be removed because of mechanical locking episodes.
- If the vastus medialis obliquus and medial patellofemoral ligament have been ruptured at their insertion, and a defect is palpable along the superior medial edge of the patella, then early surgical repair is the best option.

BIBLIOGRAPHY

1. Arroll B, Ellis-Pegler E, Edwards A, et al: Patellofemoral pain syndrome. Am J Sports Med 25(2):207–212, 1997.
2. Conlon T, Garth WP, Lemons JE: Evaluation of the medial soft-tissue restraints of the extensor mechanism of the knee. J Bone Joint Surg 75A(5):682–693, 1993.
3. DeLee JC, Drez D (eds): Orthopedic Sports Medicine: Principles and Practice. Philadelphia, W.B. Saunders, 1994, pp 1163–1248.
4. Desio SM, Burks RT, Bachus KN: soft tissue restraints to lateral patellar translation in the human knee. Am J Sports Med 26(1):59–65, 1998.
5. Dutkowsky JP: Miscellaneous nontraumatic disorders. In Canale ST (ed): Campbell's Operative Orthopaedics, 9th ed. St. Louis, Mosby, 1998, pp 787–855.
6. Dye SF: Patellofemoral pain: A current perspective. J Musculoskel Med 18(9):440–446, 2001.
7. Franz WB III: Overuse syndromes in runners. In Mellion MB, Walsh WM, Shelton GL (eds): Sports Injuries and Athletic Problems. Philadelphia, Hanley & Belfus, 1990, pp 289–309.
8. Fulkerson JP: Diagnosis and treatment of patients with patellofemoral pain. Am J Sports Med 30(3):447–456, 2002.
9. Gigante A, Pasquinelli FM, Paladini P, et al: The effects of patellar taping on patellofemoral incongruence: A computed tomography study. Am J Sports Med 29:88–92, 2001.
10. Galland O, Walch G, Dejour H, Carret JP: An anatomical and radiological study of the femoropatellar articulation. Surg Radiol Anat 12:119–125, 1990.
11. Gilleard W, McConnell J, Parsons D: The effect of patellar taping on the onset of vastus medialis obliquus and vastus lateralis muscle activity in persons with patellofemoral pain. Phys Therapy 78:25–32, 1998.
12. Hautamaa PV, Fithian DC, Kaufman KR, et al: Medial soft tissue restraints in lateral patellar instability and repair. Clin Orthop 349:174–182, 1998.
13. Hughston JC: Knee Ligaments. Injury and Repair. St. Louis, Mosby, 1993.
14. Hughston JC, Flandry F, Brinuer MR, et al: Surgical correction of medial subluxation of the patella. Am J Sports Med 24:486–491, 1996.
15. Kasim N and Fulkerson JP: Resection of clinically localized segments of painful retinaculum in the treatment of selected patients with anterior knee pain. Am J Sports Med 28(6):811–814, 2000.

16. Kowall MG, Kolk G, Nuber GW, et al: Patellar taping in the treatment of patellofemoral pain. Am J Sports Med 24(1):61–66, 1996.
17. Larsen B, Andreasen E, Urfer A, et al: Patellar taping: A radiographic examination of the medial glide technique. Am J Sports Med 23(4):465–471, 1995.
18. Maenpaa H, Lehto Mu: Patellar dislocation: The long-term results of nonoperative management in 100 patients. Am J Sports Med 25:213–217, 1997.
19. McConnell J: The management of chondromalacia patellae: A long-term solution. Aust J Physiother 2:215–223, 1986.
20. Minkoff J, Fein L: The role of radiography in the evaluation and treatment of common anarthrotic disorders of the patellofemoral joint. Clin Sports Med 8:203–260, 1989.
21. Shelton GL, Thigpen LK: Rehabilitation of patellofemoral dysfunction: A review of literature. J Orthop Sports Phys Ther 14:243–249, 1991.
22. Walsh WM, Helzer-Julin MJ: Patellar tracking problems in athletes. Prim Care 19:303–330, 1992.
23. Walsh WM: Patellofemoral joint. In DeLee JC, Drez D (eds): Orthopaedic Sports Medicine, Principles and Practice. Philadelphia, WB Saunders Co., 1994, pp 1163–1248.

77. SURGICAL TREATMENT OF PATELLOFEMORAL DISEASE

W. Michael Walsh, M.D., and Jeremy J. Vanicek, PA-C

1. How often is surgical treatment needed for patellofemoral disorders?

Compared with other orthopedic problems, not frequently. Although the number of patients with patellofemoral disease is high, most can be handled with nonsurgical means. Currently, 10–20% of our patients with a patellofemoral disorder need surgical intervention.

2. What surgical procedures are generally used?

As a general concept, surgery should alter the forces working on the patella and attempt to make patellofemoral tracking as normal as possible. The most commonly used procedures are isolated lateral retinacular release, done as either an arthroscopic or open procedure, and open reconstruction of the extensor mechanism. Occasionally, arthroscopic debridement of painful soft tissues such as synovial plica or infrapatellar fat pad may be done in addition to the other procedures.

3. How does the lateral retinacular release (LRR) procedure work?

With respect to the abnormal forces at work on the patella, a predominance of laterally directed forces is usually quite significant. Such lateral forces may come from both the static structures (lateral retinaculum, lateral patellofemoral ligament, lateral patellotibial ligament) and dynamic structures (oblique portion of the vastus lateralis muscle). An LRR attempts to decrease the lateral forces by dividing the lateral retinaculum and a small portion of the vastus lateralis. Theoretically the patient may be able to control patellar tracking better through rehabilitation of the vastus medialis obliquus. LRR can be done through arthroscopic techniques or a small open incision.

4. Which patients should have an LRR?

In the past, LRR has had a somewhat poor reputation because of its unpredictable results and high complication rate. Therefore, it should not be done unless proved absolutely necessary after failure of nonsurgical treatment, including extensive rehabilitative exercise techniques, external support, and activity modification. If the patient continues to have significant disability (pain, swelling, limitation of function), LRR may be considered. Usually nonsurgical treatment is carried out for at least several months. The surgeon then looks for the specific anatomic finding, either on preoperative computed tomographic (CT) scan or by arthroscopic examination of the patellofemoral joint, that indicate the appropriateness of LR. Such findings include tightness in the lateral retinaculum and lateral tilting of the patella, with or without lateral malposition.

5. Since LRR is an arthroscopic procedure, is it simple to do and followed by quick recovery?

In many instances, no. In addition to possible complications that slow recovery, patients still need to rehabilitate the quadriceps and perhaps to use other forms of nonsurgical treatment (e.g., bracing, orthotics) before returning to normal activity. Routinely 3–6 months may be required for full return of function. This time frame should be emphasized to the patient preoperatively as well as the fact that the surgery is not a total substitute for continued nonsurgical efforts in the future.

6. What complications are seen with LRR?

In studies carried out by the Arthroscopy Association of North America, arthroscopic LRR was the procedure most commonly associated with significant complications, the majority of which involved postoperative development of hemarthrosis. Occasionally, this complication requires return to the operating room for drainage and coagulation of bleeding points. For this reason some surgeons prefer to do LRR as a small open procedure rather than arthroscopically. The open procedure allows identification and coagulation of the large vessels at the time the release is done. Other complications include profound quadriceps disability and medial subluxation of the patella, both of which come from overreleasing the vastus lateralis, and rupture of the quadriceps tendon, which results from releasing too far around the superior edge of the patella.

7. How does an open reconstruction of the extensor mechanism work?

There are three basic components: lateral release, medial advancement or stabilization, and transposition of the patellar tendon insertion. Lateral release is done as described above for the isolated LRR. Various authors have described different techniques for medial advancement or stabilization. The important structures to stabilize are the vastus medialis obliquus muscle and the medial patellofemoral ligament. In some cases, the medial patellofemoral ligament may require allograft augmentation. The distal part of the reconstruction is a transfer of the patellar tendon insertion on the tibial tuberosity to a more medial and distal position. The goal is to correct an excessive Q angle as well as excessive patella alta. Many variations on this basic theme have been described over the years, but most still include the same three elements.

8. Which patients should have an extensor mechanism reconstruction?

In general, the decision to proceed with surgery follows the same line of reasoning mentioned above for LRR. However, most open extensor mechanism reconstructions are done for the unstable patella, not just for patellofemoral pain syndromes. Some may be done in patellofemoral pain patients if an isolated LRR has been unsuccessful. For some authors, the presence of lateral malposition of the patella rather than simple lateral tilt on radiographic studies indicates the need for open reconstruction rather than lateral release. No well-done, long-term studies substantiate one view point over the other.

9. What is involved in recovery from an extensor mechanism reconstruction?

When the patellar tendon insertion is repositioned, some internal fixation with hardware is usually necessary. Traditionally internal fixation has led to a period of immobilization after reconstruction. Most surgeons limit the period of absolute immobilization to 3 or 4 weeks. At that point protected motion can be started with an adjustable hinge brace. Part-time immobilization may be continued for 6 weeks. Crutches are used until ambulation is normal. Extensive quadriceps rehabilitation is necessary postoperatively. Overall functional recovery may easily take 6–9 months after surgery.

10. What specific complications may occur after open reconstruction of the extensor mechanism?

The most frequent complications are related to overzealous repositioning of the patella. If an excessive release is done laterally, along with excessive advancement of the medial structures, medial subluxation or even dislocation may be created. Extreme distal positioning of the patella by excessive transfer of the patellar tendon insertion creates a pathologically low-lying patella, often with abutment of the patella against the proximal tibia. This complication is terribly painful.

11. Do the above surgical procedures cure the problem?

No surgical procedure completely cures patellofemoral disorders. The predisposition is anatomic. The factors are many and varied. Even after surgery, patients must continue with re-habilitative efforts and other adjunctive means, such as bracing and foot orthotics. In the best of cases, patients often have residual symptoms during such high patellar stress activities as walking stairs. These points should be absolutely clear to patients before they undergo surgery.

12. Can other surgical procedures be done?

Yes. Many other surgical procedures have been applied to the patellofemoral joint. Some are now of historical interest only. Simpler procedures that may still be appropriate include excision of areas of chondromalacia (although not as an isolated procedure), removal of osteochondral fractures, synovectomy for pathologic synovial plica, and excision of painful accessory ossification centers of the patella. More complicated as well as controversial is the concept of anteriorization of the tibial tuberosity to decompress the patellofemoral joint. This procedure has enjoyed mixed reviews and somewhat unpredictable results in the past. It should probably be viewed as a salvage procedure. Patellectomy likewise may be used as a salvage procedure when marked deterioration of the patellar articular surface has occurred. In patients who have a severe rotational component to limb malalignment, derotational osteotomies of the femur and tibia may be appealing. However, the sheer magnitude of the undertaking has prevented practical application.

13. Should early surgery be done for an acute patellar dislocation?

It seems sensible that an acute patellar dislocation should be treated like other acute disruptions of soft tissue (e.g., torn ligaments). If this analogy were to hold true, then early, direct suture repair may hold promise of decreasing the incidence of recurrent dislocation. This concept has been promoted by some researchers in the past and may be gaining in popularity. Studies have shown the particular importance of the medial patellofemoral ligament. An acute dislocation rupture of this ligament may be demonstrated by MRI. If documented, early repair would make perfect sense. However, considering the facts that one-half of patients with patellar dislocation may not experience recurrence and that reconstructive techniques work reasonably well, early surgical intervention is not used by most orthopedists.

BIBLIOGRAPHY

1. Aglietti P, Buzzi R, DeBiase P: Surgical treatment of recurrent dislocation of the patella. Clin Orthop Related Research 308:8–17, 1992.
2. Ahmad CS, Stein BE, Matuz D, et al: Immediate surgical repair of the medial patellar stabilizers for acute patellar dislocation. Am J Sports Med 28: 804–810, 2000.
3. Boden BP, Pearsall AW, Garrett WE, et al: Patellofemoral instability: Evaluation and management. J Am Acad Orthop Surg 5(1): 47–57, 1997.
4. Burks RT, Desio SM, Bachus KN, et al: Biomechanical evaluation of lateral patellar dislocations. Am J Knee Surg 11: 24–30, 1998.
5. Canale ST (ed): Campbell's Operative Orthopaedics, 9th ed. St. Louis, Mosby, 1998.
6. Conlon T, Garth WP, Lemons JE: Evaluation of the medial soft-tissue restraints of the extensor mechanism of the knee. J Bone Joint Surg 75A(5:682–693, 1993.
7. Evans IK, Paulos LE: Complications of patellofemoral joint surgery. Orthop Clin 23:697–710, 1992.
8. Flandry F, Hughston JC: Complications of extensor mechanism surgery for patellar malalignment. Am J Orthop 24:534–543, 1995.
9. Fox J: The Patellofemoral Joint. New York, McGraw-Hill, 1993.
10. Fulkerson JP (ed): Disorders of the Patellofemoral Joint, 3rd ed. Baltimore, Williams & Wilkins, 1996.
11. Fulkerson JP: Patellofemoral pain disorders: Evaluation and management. J Am Acad Orthop Surg 2:124–132, 1994.

12. Hautamaa PV, Fithian DC, Kaufman KR, et al: Medial soft tissue restraints in lateral patellar instability and repair. Clin Orthop 349, 174–182, 1998.
13. Kolowich PA, Paulos LE, Rosenberg TD, et al: Lateral release of the patella: Indications and contraindications. Am J Sports Med 18:4, 359–365, 1990.
14. Koskinen SK, Kujala UM: Patellofemoral relationships and distal insertion of the vastus medialis muscle: A magnetic resonance imaging study in nonsymptomatic subjects and in patients with patellar dislocation. Arthroscopy 8: 465–468, 1992.
15. Maenpaa H, Lehto M: Patellofemoral osteoarthritis after patellar dislocation. Clin Orthop 339:156–162, 1997.
16. Muhle C, Brinkman G, Skaf A, et al: Effect of a patellar realignment brace on patients with patellar subluxation and dislocation. Am J Sports Med 27: 350–353, 1999.
17. Sallay PI, Poggi J, Speer KP, Garrett WE: Acute dislocation of the patella. Am J Sports Med 24:52–60, 1996.
18. Shea KP, Fulkerson JP: Preoperative computed tomography scanning and arthroscopy in predicting outcome after lateral retinacular release. Arthroscopy 8: 327–334, 1992.
19. Teitge RA: Treatment of complications of patellofemoral joint surgery. Op Tech Sports Med 2: 317–334, 1994.
20. Vainionpaa S, Laasonen E, Silvennoinen T, et al: Acute dislocation of the patella. J Bone Joint Surg 72(B):366–369, 1990.
21. Walsh WM: Patellofemoral joint. In DeLee JC, Drez D Jr (eds): Orthopaedic Sports Medicine: Principles and Practice. Philadelphia, W.B. Saunders, 1994, pp 1163–1260.

78. ARTICULAR CARTILAGE INJURY AND REPAIR AND MENISCUS TRANSPLANTATION

David E. Brown, M.D.

1. Of what is articular cartilage composed?

Articular cartilage is composed of 70% water. Type II collagen makes up 50% of the dry weight of articular cartilage. Proteoglycans comprise 12%, and chondrocytes are less than 5% of the dry weight.

The collagen provides the tensile strength of the cartilage. The superficial layer provides resistance to shear stress. The glycosaminoglycans have negatively charged ends that have a high affinity for water. This water component provides the resistance to compressive loads. Articular cartilage injury or wear leads to water leakage from the extracellular matrix.

2. What is the incidence of articular cartilage lesions?

Grade IV articular cartilage lesions of the femoral condyles are present in 5–10% of knees in patients who are less than 40 years of age. These lesions are presently the lesions that are most amenable to advanced articular cartilage reconstruction.

3. Why can't articular cartilage repair itself?

Articular cartilage does not have pluripotential cells, which have the ability to migrate and proliferate. Chondrocytes have only a limited capability to participate in a repair process including an increase in the formation of the extracellular matrix components that might repair articular cartilage defects. The subchondral bone acts as a barrier to the pluripotential cells present in the bone. However, if an osteochondral injury occurs, the bone marrow cells migrate to the defect, a fibrin clot forms which matures into type I fibrocartilage.

4. How does initial damage to the articular cartilage lead to osteoarthritis?

Damage to the articular cartilage leads to increased permeability in the superficial layers which allows escape of water during compressive loading. More stress is then transmitted to the subchondral bone. Gradually the subchondral bone becomes stiffer and thus more damage occurs to the articular cartilage.

5. How do articular cartilage lesions cause pain since the cartilage has no nerve endings?
- Mechanical irritation of loose flaps of cartilage
- Cytokines released by inflamed synovium
- Subchondral bone sclerosis causing irritation of peri-articular nerve endings

6. What are the surgical treatment options for articular cartilage defects?
- Arthroscopic lavage and debridement
- Fibrocartilage stimulation techniques: drilling, abrasion arthroplasty, microfracture
- Correction of malalignment by osteotomy
- Cell transplantation (autologous chondrocyte implantation)
- Osteochondral plug implantation: autograft, allograft
- Partial or total knee arthroplasty

7. Why are fibrocartilage stimulation techniques suboptimal in the long term?
These techniques generally result in partial or complete filling of the defect. However, fibrocartilage is principally type I cartilage that has diminished stiffness and is prone to early wear. This results in deterioration of results over time. These techniques are easily performed and less expensive than true reconstructive techniques, thus leading to their popularity.

8. What is autologous chondrocyte implantation?
This procedure (CARTICEL) involves harvesting autologous articular cartilage from the non-weightbearing area of the knee, followed by expansion of the chondrocyte cell number in a sterile tissue culture. The chondrocyte cell suspension that results is then implanted into the defect area under a flap of periosteum. These cells are capable of adhering to the subchondral bone and forming the extracellular matrix, a process which occurs over the ensuing 12 months.

9. What are the indications for autologous chondrocyte implantation?
- Femoral condyle lesion at least 2 cm^2 in size that has failed at least one surgical treatment (see question 6)
- Age less than 50 years
- Absence of kissing lesion on the adjacent tibia
- Stable or reconstructed ligaments
- Neutral or corrected knee alignment
- Absence of synovial based inflammatory disease

10. What are the disadvantages of autologous chondrocyte implantation?
- Cost
- Necessity for two surgical procedures
- Extended postoperative rehabilitation

11. What are the results of autologous chondrocyte implantation?
CARTICEL has 85% good or excellent results when implanted in the femoral condyles. When there is a concomitant anterior cruciate ligament tear (and reconstruction) the rate of satisfactory results drops to 75%. Patella and tibial lesions generally do not have good results with CARTICEL implantation. Patients who have satisfactory results at 2 years have been shown to have similar results for as long as 11 years.

12. What is osteochondral plug implantation?
Osteochondral plug implantation goes by the trade names of Mosaicplasty or Osteochondral Autograft Transfer System (OATS). These techniques differ basically in the size of plugs that are

used, OATS using larger plugs. The technique involves excision of all damaged articular tissue and creating various sized cylindrical holes in the base of the defect. The holes are then filled with autologous matched cylinders of articular cartilage and its underlying bone. This techniques are suitable for confined defects of small to medium size. The limiting factor is the amount of autologous donor tissue available without excessive donor site morbidity.

13. What are the disadvantages of osteochondral plug implantation?
- Donor site morbidity
- Potential for joint incongruity due to non-level plugs (technique faults, settlingof implants)
- 30% of defect (spaces between plugs) becomes fibrocartilage

14. In what circumstances would an allograft osteochondral plug be the preferred graft source?
- Larger than 4 cm^2 defect (excessive autologous donor site morbidity)
- Ability to better restore the articular surface contour
- Noncontained defect
- A defect that can be restored with a single allograft plug of 10- to 20-mm (single plugs of this size are available commercially, thus eliminating the need for an entire hemicondyle)

15. What are the indications for meniscus transplantation?
- Painful meniscus deficient compartment
- Concomitant with articular cartilage reconstruction (with meniscus deficiency)
- Meniscus deficiency in conjunction with anterior cruciate ligament reconstruction

An important challenge in transplantation is the early recognition of the compartment that is symptomatic. It is hoped that earlier recognition and transplantation in young patients will prevent or defer joint degeneration.

16. What are the contra-indications for meniscus transplantation?
- Grade IV articular cartilage lesion
- Stage III and IV Fairbanks changes
- Post infectious disease
- Rheumatoid disease
- Gout
- Obesity
- Unreconstructed ligament instability
- Axial malalignment

17. How is meniscus transplantation performed?
Meniscus transplantation is performed using either double bone block or "keyhole" techniques. The medial meniscus is usually transplanted with the double bone block technique (bone blocks at each of the anterior and posterior horns). The lateral meniscus is reconstructed with the "keyhole" technique. In this technique, the graft contains a bone bridge (shaped like a keyhole) connecting both the anterior and posterior horns.

The knee is arthroscoped, exposure of the posterior horn is achieved, debridement of the remaining rim is performed, bone tunnels or slots are made and posterior passing suture or needle are placed. A mini-arthrotomy allows passage of the graft and additional peripheral sutures are placed and secured.

18. What type of meniscus allograft is used?
Fresh frozen, cryopreserved, nonirradiated allografts are the best graft source. Cell viability and survival are optimized, and the risk of graft-host reaction is reduced.

19. How are grafts sized?
Appropriate sizing of meniscus allografts is essential. Anteroposterior and lateral radiographs

of the affected knee are obtained using a standard radiographic marker. Alternatively, MRI scans can be utilized to measure the dimensions of the recipient tibial plateau.

20. What are the results of meniscus transplantation?

The results of meniscus transplantation vary widely. Patients who have isolated meniscus transplantation and who do not have significant degeneration of the articular cartilage can expect to have good results in 85% of cases. Pain is consistantly reduced while functional improvement varies. Transplantation with bone plugs affords better results. Cadaveric data demmonstrate that intra-articular contact area is improved by the use of bone plugs at the meniscus horns. The improvement is lost when the attachments are released.

BIBLIOGRAPHY

1. Alhalki MM, Howell SM and Hull ML: How three methods for fixing a medial meniscal qutograft affect tibial contact mechanics. Am J Sports Med 27: 320–328, 1999.
2. Browne JE and Branch TP: Surgical alternatives for treatment of articular cartilage lesions. J Am Acad Orthop Surg 8:180–189, 2000.
3. Buckwalter JA, Mankin HJ: Articular cartilage. Part II: Degeneration and osteoarthrosis, repair, regeneration, and transplantation. J Bone Joint Surg 79A: 612–632, 1997.
4. Brittberg M, Lindahl A, Nilsson A, et.al.: Treatment of deep cartilage defects in the knee with autologous chondrocyte transplantation. N Engl J Med 331: 889–895, 1994.
5. Carter TR: Meniscus allograft transplantation. Sports Med Arthros Rev 7:51–62, 1999.
6. Curl WW, Krome J, Gordon ES, et al: Cartilage injuries: A review of 31,516 knee arthroscopies. Arthroscopy 13:456–460, 1997.
7. Hangody L, Kish G, Karpati Z, et al: Mosaicplasty for the treatment of articular cartilage defects: Application inclinical practice. Orthopedics 21:751–756,1998.
8. Jackson DW, Scheer MJ, Simon TM: Cartilage substitutes: Overview of basic science and treatment options. J Am Acad Orthop Surg 9:37–52,2000.
9. Paletta GA Jr, Manning T, Snell E, et al: The effect of allograft meniscal replacement on intraarticular contact area and pressures in the human knee: A biomechanical study. Am J Sports Med 25: 692–698, 1997.
10. Peterson L, Brittberg M, Kiviranta I, et al: Autologous chondrocyte transplantation: Biomechanics and long-term durability. Am J Sports Med 30:2–12, 2002.
11. Rath E, Richmond JC, Yassir W, et al: Meniscal allograft transplantation. Am J Sports Med 29:410–414, 2001.
12. Rodeo SA: Meniscal allografts—Where do we stand? Am J Sports Med 29: 246–261, 2001.
13. Salter RB: The biological concept of continous passive motion of synovial joints: The first 18 years of basic research and its clinical application. Clin Orthop 242:12–25,1989.
14. van Arkel ERA, deBoer HH: Human meniscal transplantation. J Bone Joint Surg 77B:589–596, 1995.

79. KNEE ARTHRITIS

Randall D. Neumann, M.D.

1. What are the three compartments of the knee?

Patellofemoral, medial, and lateral.

2. Which compartments are generally affected in degenerative osteoarthritis of the knee?

The medial compartment is the most commonly affected, followed by the lateral compartment and then the patellofemoral compartment.

3. What is the mechanical axis of the lower extremity?

The mechanical axis goes directly through the femoral head, through the intercondylar notch of the knee to the midportion of the ankle.

4. What is a varus deformity?

In patients with osteoarthritis who have primarily medial compartment disease, collapse of the medial joint space causes medial angulation of the tibia. The clinical appearance is bow-leggedness, which causes the mechanical axis to go through or inside the medial compartment of the knee. This condition is considered varus of the knee.

5. What is valgus of the knee?

When lateral compartment arthritis predominates, joint space collapse occurs in the lateral compartment and causes the weight-bearing axis to fall outside the lateral compartment of the knee. The patient appears knock-kneed. This condition represents a valgus deformity of the knee.

6. What is a flexion contracture?

Patients with degenerative arthritis of the knee commonly have a flexion contracture. Minimal flexion contracture may be 1–2°, whereas other contractures may be as high as 45°. Flexion contracture is commonly caused by posterior osteophytes on the femur, tibial plateau deformities, fracture, or loose bodies. Contractures of the ligaments may occur, especially with the posterior cruciate and posterior capsule.

7. What is the most common symptom in patients with osteoarthritis of the knee?

Pain.

8. Describe the clinical history of patients with degenerative arthritis of the knee.

Most patients report an insidious onset, perhaps with a history of trauma or repetitive trauma that patients may describe as minor or major. The pain is usually described as aching to sharp and is likely to present after excessive activity. With severe stages of arthritis, night pain may occur. Patients describe stiffness on waking in the morning, which gradually diminishes with activity. If the patient is sitting or riding in a car, pain and stiffness occur upon standing or walking. Pain is located at the site of the most affected compartment of the knee. The patient has diminished function, including inability to climb stairs, especially without the help of a railing. Walking may be limited to several blocks or several miles. Some patients lose the ability to do their own grocery shopping or must use the shopping cart as a mandatory aid. Patients commonly notice deformity with swelling, osteophyte function, and varus or valgus deformity.

9. Describe the physical findings in osteoarthritis of the knee.

Patients generally lack some degree of motion. Commonly they will lack 5–10° of full extension and will not be able to lay the leg with the knee flat. Most patients lose flexion because of posterior osteophytes and contracture of the posterior capsule. Tenderness is palpable along the joint line. Effusion may be mild to moderate. Crepitation is generally felt in the affected compartment. Clinical varus or valgus may be present.

10. What other joints should be examined in elderly patients complaining of knee pain?

Elderly patients commonly have degenerative changes in other joints. Patients with spinal stenosis may have referred pain to the knee that increases with walking and is relieved with rest. The referred pain may be due to spinal claudication rather than knee arthritis. Patients with degenerative arthritis of the hip have referred pain through the obturator nerve to the medial side of the knee. It is not uncommon for patients to present with complaints of knee arthritis when the pathology is related to the hip joint.

11. What are the radiographic findings in patients with osteoarthritis of the knee?

Patients have narrowing of the joint space in either the medial, lateral, or patellofemoral compartment. Axial alignment may show varus or valgus deformity on weight-bearing views. Osteophytes are commonly seen in the intercondylar notch area and along the most severely affected joints. Loose bodies from fragmentation of articular cartilage may be seen along the posterior femoral condyles. Destruction of the posterior condyles or posterior portions of the medial and lateral tibia plateau may be seen. On the sunrise view, subluxation of the patella or frank dislocation is noted. Lateral subluxation of the tibial plateau on the femur may be seen on the anterior radiographs.

12. Which disease processes with arthritis may have loose bodies in the knee?
- Osteochondritis dissecans
- Osteonecrosis
- Chondromalacia of the patella
- Degenerative arthritis
- Neuropathic joints

13. Discuss the synovial fluid analysis in patients with noninflammatory arthritis.
The white blood cell count is generally < 2000 mm^3, with $< 25\%$ neutrophils. Cultures are negative. No crystals are seen on light microscopy.

14. What other disease entities should be ruled out before treatment for knee arthritis?
- Spinal stenosis
- Degenerative changes in the hips
- Tumors
- Neuropathy
- Vascular insufficiency
- Vascular insufficiency
- Systemic arthritis, such as rheumatoid arthritis
- Osteonecrosis

15. What conservative treatments should be tried in patients with osteoarthritis of the knee?
Patients should be placed on a trial of nonsteroidal anti-inflammatory drugs (NSAIDs). NSAIDs with COX-2 inhibition include celecoxib and rofecoxib, which have fewer GI side effects. Patients may respond to icing of an overly inflamed joint. Protective weightbearing, such as occasional use of crutches or cane, may be beneficial. Generalized exercise may include walking, swimming, or bicycling. Range-of-motion exercises should be done on a daily basis. Knee braces or neoprene sleeves may be used for comfort and control of swelling. The occasional and cautious use of intraarticular steroids is permitted; overuse of corticosteroids has been known to lead to progression of disease. Viscosupplementation with hyaluronan can be used to replace the diseased synovial fluid.

16. What arthroscopic treatment can be used for degenerative arthritis?
Some success has been gained with arthroscopic debridement. Candidates include patients without contracture or subluxation and patients with mechanical symptoms, including catching or locking, and localized disease. Arthroscopic treatment includes removal of spurs in the intercondylar notch along the anterior cruciate, medial, and lateral gutters. The articular cartilage can be shaved. Loose bodies are removed, commonly from behind the medial and lateral condyles posteriorly, the intercondylar notch area, and beneath the medial and lateral menisci posteriorly.

17. Describe the synovial fluid analysis in patients with inflammatory arthritis such as rheumatoid arthritis.
The inflammatory fluid is usually translucid or opaque. Newspaper cannot be read through the tube.The color ranges from yellowish to yellow-green. The white blood cell count is generally 2000–50,000 mm^3. Gram stain and cultures are negative. White blood cells may include greater than 50% neutrophils.

18. Describe the radiologic findings of rheumatoid arthritis of the knee.
Soft-tissue swelling due to joint effusion synovitis and periarticular edema is usually easily detectable, along with uniform narrowing of the patellofemoral, medial, and lateral compartments. Juxtaarticular osteoporosis is evident. Erosions, if present, are usually sharply marginated. Severe bone destruction may be seen in the advanced stage with considerable angulation, resulting in a varus or valgus knee. Marginal osteophytes and sclerosis are generally lacking.

19. What treatments are available for rheumatoid arthritis of the knee?
Conservative treatment should include nonsteroidal antiinflammatory drugs, interarticular steroids, and aspiration. Joint splinting may be helpful in patients who have tense effusions and synovitis. If synovitis persists, arthroscopic synovectomy may temporarily arrest the disease.

20. Describe the hallmark of calcium pyrophosphate dihydrate deposition (CPPD) disease.
The hallmark of CPPD is calcium deposition on fibrocartilage, particularly the menisci of the knee, which is readily seen on radiographs. Cysts, which may be quite large, are generally found next to the joint margin and may mimic a neuropathic joint.

21. What tests should be done on the synovial fluid in crystalline arthropathies?
Routine microscopy and polarization should be done. The calcium pyrophosphate dihydrate crystals are seen on nonpolarized light microscopy and the uric acid crystals on polarized light microscopy.

22. What are the radiographic findings in patients with hemophilic arthropathy of the knee?
Overgrowth of the distal femur and tibial epiphysis may result in metaphyses that fit the diaphyses poorly. The intercondylar notch of the femur is commonly widened. Squaring of the inferior pole of the patella has been recognized by many investigators. Because flexion contractures are common, patients may have posterior lateral displacement of the tibia on the femur. The patella may be dislocated. Subchondral cysts are seen, along with narrowing of the joint space and sometimes complete loss of joint space.

23. Describe the arthritis in neuropathic joint disease.
Neuropathic joints are commonly seen in diabetes mellitus, tabes dorsalis, and meningomyelocele. The earliest manifestations are soft-tissue swelling that may be massive. Generally pain is minimal despite the massive joint destruction. Typically the joint shows gross disorganization. Subluxation of the tibia on the femur is common, along with complete laxity of the entire joint and dislocation of the patella. Intraarticular fractures and loose bodies are also common. Calcification and bone fragments are seen within the soft tissues adjacent to the joint. The arthropathy is progressive, and severe destruction may take place over several months.

24. What is the differential diagnosis of a neuropathic joint?
- Diabetes mellitus
- Syphilis
- Syringomyelia
- Leprosy
- Amyloidosis
- Charcot-Marie-Tooth disease
- Multiple sclerosis
- Gigantism
- Alcoholism
- Chronic demyelinating polyradiculopathy

25. What is the differential diagnosis for hemarthrosis found on synovial fluid aspiration?
- Anterior cruciate ligament tears
- Peripheral meniscal tears
- Medial or collateral ligament injuries
- Osteochondral fractures
- Hemophilia
- Pigmented villonodular synovitis
- Sickle-cell disease
- Degenerative arthritis
- Other bleeding disorders

BIBLIOGRAPHY

1. Alpert SW, Koval KJ, Zuckerman JD: Neuropathic arthropathy: Review of current knowledge. J Am Acad Orthop Surg 4:100–108, 1996.
2. McCarty DJ: Synovial fluid. In McCarty DJ, Koopman WJ (eds): Arthritis and Allied Conditions. Philadelphia, Lea & Febiger, 1993.
3. Resnick DA: Degenerative diseases of extra spinal location. In Resnick D (ed): Diagnosis of Bone and Joint Disorders. Philadelphia, W.B. Saunders, 1991, pp 1270–1368.
4. Silver RM (ed): Primer on the Rheumatic Diseases, 11th ed. Atlanta, Arthritis Foundation, 1997.

80. OSTEOCHONDRITIS DISSECANS OF THE KNEE

Jason A. Browdy, M.D., and Randall D. Neumann, M.D.

1. What is osteochondritis dissecans?

Osteochondritis dissecans (OCD) is a disorder of one or more ossification centers with sequential degeneration and/or aseptic necrosis and recalcification. Osteochondritis refers to inflammation of the joint surface and dissecans comes from the Latin *dissecare,* which means to separate. Although inflammation is not present, the name has persisted.

2. What are the different types of OCD?

There are two types: juvenile and adult forms. Juvenile OCD occurs in skelletaly immature patients. The two forms have very different natural histories. Overall, prognosis is better in the juvenile form.

3. Describe the epidemiology of OCD.

The male-to-female ratio is about 2–3:1. It is rare in patients younger than 10 and older than 50 years. The average age at presentation is 11–13 years.

4. Describe the theories of the etiology for OCD.

Exogenous trauma. Significant knee trauma is found in approximately 50% of patients with OCD. The trauma may be minor or include falls and twisting injuries.

Endogenous trauma. Patellar dislocations, meniscus tears, and instability syndromes have been associated with OCD.

Repetitive stress. For example, patellar impingement on the medial femoral condyle in extension or impingement of the medial femoral condyle by the tibial spine.

Ischemia. The obstruction of blood supply to the femoral condyle at the site of involvement has been theorized to precipitate cartilage and bone separation.

Abnormal ossification within the epiphysis. Accessory centers of ossification are known to occur. In children this process often is exhibited by a rough or irregular epiphyseal outline. It has been suggested that this accessory bony nucleus separates in childhood and partially reattaches with time.

5. Describe the pathophysiology of OCD.

There is no consensus on the exact etiology. The pathologic process begins in the subchondral bone. A portion of cartilage with subcondral bone partially seperates from underlying bone. Failure of revascularization may lead to fibrous tissue formation at the defect site. There is a spectrum of pathology. At the end of the spectrum is loose body formation, as the fragment completely seperates from the underlying bone.

6. What is the natural history of OCD?

Conservative estimates predict that about 50% of skeletally immature patients with OCD of the knee spontaneously heal without surgery. In this population, it may take 10–18 months to heal. Skeletally mature patients have a worse prognosis. Patients with intact articular cartilage may have only intermittent symptoms, primarily when they are vigorously active. Once the articular cartilage fractures, symptoms increase and swelling ensues. Patients who have sloughed the articular cartilage and bone have symptoms due to loose bodies, including catching, locking, and pain. Defects larger than 1 cm tend to cause degenerative arthritis as the edges of the defect gradually delaminate and fall away.

7. List the common sites of OCD in the body.
- Knee. Overall, 75% of OCD occurs in the knee. It is bilateral in up to 30% of patients.
- Capitellum of the distal humerus
- Talus

8. Where does OCD occur in the knee?
Approximately 85% of cases found on the medial femoral condyle, with 15% on the lateral condyle. The classic presentation is on the medial femoral condyle, immediately adjacent to the intercondylar notch. Affected areas may extend over the weight-bearing surface. On the lateral condyle, they are generally on the weight-bearing surface but may occur anteriorly. Lesions are usually 2–4 cm^2 on the medial side of the joint and contain a 5- to 10-mm thick rim of subchondral bone. Lateral lesions tend to be larger (3–4 cm^2) and usually have a thin rim of bone that makes them more prone to fragmentation. As a result, multiple small fragments may exist.

9. What is the typical history in patients with OCD?
Symptoms usually associated with OCD are often vague and poorly localized. Symptoms include pain, stiffness, and swelling. Loose bodies may cause locking, catching, or giving way. Pain may be severe if the defect is large.

10. Describe the physical findings in the patient with OCD.
Most patients are only mildly uncomfortable. The range of motion is usually within normal limits. Some patients have a small lack of extension, slight quadriceps atrophy, and weakness. Patients with articular surface defects may have recurrent episodes of swelling, and effusion is likely. Tenderness may be present along the medial or lateral joint lines. Loose bodies may be present, and some patients are able to move them around in their knee. Wilson's sign is elicited by flexing the knee to 90°, internally rotating the tibia, and extending the knee slowly. Pain at approximately 30° of flexion is a positive sign that signifies impingement of the tibial spine on the medial femoral condyle OCD.

11. What radiographic studies are obtained to determine if OCD is present?
The standard films are the anteroposterior, lateral, tunnel, and sunrise views. The most useful view is the tunnel view. Lesions on the posterior portion of the medial femoral condyle are commonly missed on standard anteroposterior views. Therefore, when OCD is suspected, an intercondylar notch or tunnel view is mandatory.

12. Describe the classic radiographic appearance of OCD.
The classic radiographic appearance is a well-circumscribed area of subchondral bone, separated from the remaining femoral condyle by a crescent-shaped radiolucent line. OCD is located on the posterior lateral aspect of the medial femoral condyle or the central portion of the lateral femoral condyle. The typical position is seen on the lateral photograph. Seventy-five percent of cases of OCD in the medial femoral condyle.are present in the area between Blumensaat's line (a line along the top of the intercondylar notch and the line drawn distally from the posterior margin of the femoral shaft . The lateral femoral condyle lesions are seen on the lateral radiograph and are located posterior to the line drawn distally from the posterior femoral cortex.

13. What other radiographic techniques are used for evaluating OCD?
Computed tomography (CT) and magnetic resonance imaging (MRI) have been found to be more frequently helpful in the evaluation of OCD. MRI is capable of detecting focal defects in articular cartilage as small as 2 mm. MRI can differentiate in situ versus unstable fragments. MRI without contrast is adequate if the patient has an effusion. In the absence of an effusion, MRI with contrast should be considered.

14. Is bone scan helpful in the diagnosis of OCD?

Bone scan is used for diagnostic purposes and for following the healing and pathologic processes. Some studies suggest that bone scans may be more sensitive and more specific in determining the mechanical stability of the lesions.

15. What is the difference between static and dynamic bone scans?

Both static and dynamic bone scans may be useful. Serial static bone scans are useful to follow disease progression. In a dynamic study, the rate of radioactive uptake per unit time is compared between the normal and pathologic knees. Assuming that uptake is a reflection of blood flow, one can compare the local perfusion of the two knees.

16. What invasive diagnostic test is used in patients with OCD?

Arthroscopy directly visualizes the involved area and allows the examiner to probe the zone of involvement and to determine the degree of articular cartilage separation. Loose bodies are also removed during arthroscopy if it is indeed determined that they are loose. After surgical procedures, arthroscopy can be used to assess the articular surface for healing, degeneration, and mechanical stability.

17. What are the five stages of OCD as described by Cahill and Berg?

Stage 0 has normal bone scan and plain films. Stages 1–4 have abnormal radiographic findings characteristic for OCD, but the bone scans are different for each stage. Stage 1 shows no activity on bone scan. Stage 2 has focal activity at the site of the OCD defect. Stage 3 has focal activity at the OCD defect and increased activity in the femoral condyle supporting the OCD lesion; stage 4 is similar to stage 3 with the addition of activity on the tibia plateau. In regard to healing, Cahill and Berg observed that the OCD with a stage 2 or greater scan has the highest probability of healing. This level of activity indicates potential for repair. Because stage 1 lesions have a poor potential for healing with conservative therapy, surgical intervention may be necessary.

18. Are other classifcation systems available?

There are many systems. The systems are generally based on surgical findings and appearance on radiographs or bone scans. Cahill and Berg created a useful classification system based on anteroposterior and lateral radiographs.

19. Can you describe any arthroscopic staging systems?

Clanton and DeLee described the following system:

Grade 1: Depressed OCD
Grade 2: OCD fragment attached by an osseous bridge
Grade 3: Detached, nondisplaced fragment
Grade 4: Displaced fragment

Ewing and Voto described the following stages:

Stage 1: Intact cartilage
Stage 2: Early cartilage seperation
Stage 3: Partially attached lesion
Stage 4: Crater with loose body

20. What factors affect prognosis?

Age of patient. Skeletally immature patients may heal spontaneously. Most adults do not.

Size of defect. Contained lesions less than 2 square cm may stay asymptomatic for a long time. Poorly contained lesions (those that do not have intact cartilage surrounding the entire lesion) that are larger than 2 cm^2 are more likely to cause symptoms.

Location of defect. Lesions in the classic location clearly have a better prognosis. Medial lesions also tend to be more anterior and access to these lesions is thus better than the more posterior lateral lesions. Lateral lesions also tend to be larger and more prone to fragmentation.

Displacement of fragment. In a skeletally immature patient, a nondisplaced fragment may heal. Signs of fragment dissection at presentation herald a worse prognosis, regardless of treatment. However, a partially displaced or recently displaced fragment may be replaceable. There are many means of fixation. If a fragment has been displaced for a long period of time, it usually cannot be replaced into the defect. Treatment options for this situation are more complex.

Associated meniscus pathology

Associated knee malalignment

21. What is the incidence of osteoarthritis among adult patients with OCD?

Degenerative changes usually begin at age 40 years, with highly progressive deterioration. Approximately 70% of patients at age 50 and 80% at age 60 have osteoarthritis.

22. Describe a conservative treatment plan.

In general, conservative treatment consists of activity modification. Crutches may be required for a short period of time until symptoms improve. Some have advocated prolonged immobilization, but this has proven to be deleterious. The goal is to reduce activity until activities of daily living do not cause pain.

23. What are operative indications in a skeletally immature patient?

1. Detachment or displacement of the fragment
2. Persistant pain in a compliant patient
3. Persistant or progressive bone scan findings
4. Approaching skeletal maturity

Number 1 is an absolute indication. Otherwise a combination of the 2–4 is required.

24. What are the goals of surgical treatment?

- Reestablish the joint surface
- Improve blood supply to the fragment
- Rigid fixation to allow early motion until bony union
- Prevent late arthritis. This is the ultimate goal.

25. What is stem cell stimulation?

Techniques such as microfracture are used to breach subchondral bone in a defect, allowing marrow contents such as stem cells to spill into the defect. These cells later differentiate and produce healing tissue. The problem is that the tissue is type I cartilage which has inferior long term wear characteristics. The literature generally does not support use of this technique for lesions larger than 2 cm in diameter.

26. Should the loose articular portion be removed arthroscopically with no other treatment?

Results of excision of adult or juvenile defects are poor. Therefore, attempts should be made to retain the full-thickness osteochondral defect. If this is not possible, bone grafting or allograft should be used.

27. How should the OCD lesion be prepared for arthroscopic treatment?

Arthroscopy includes the removal of the fibrous membrane, curretting of the necrotic base, and retrograde or antegrade drilling to allow ingrowth of vascular tissue and bone grafting. Fixation of the fragment is mandatory.

28. What lesions are difficult to treat arthroscopically?

Lesions in the anterior and posterior areas of the femoral condyle.

29. What are the advantages of antegrade drilling?

Ease. It is technically easier than retrograde drilling.

30. What are the disadvantages of antegrade drilling?
Creation of defects in articular cartilage that later heal with fibrocartilage.

31. List the various means of fixation of a fragment.
- K-wires
- Herbert screws
- Bioabsorbable pins or screws
- Bone pegs
- Osteochondral plugs

32. What new treatments are available for articular cartilage defects?
Fresh-frozen osteochondral allografts are prepared by removing the diseased area with a section of bone. A fresh-frozen allograft is then matched for size, depth, and radii and held in position by screws.

Mosaicplasty autograft. Osteochondral plugs are taken from the peripheral area of the anteromedial or anterolateral femoral condyle. Corresponding holes that match the size and depth of the plugs are drilled, which are then inserted into the defect. Differing plug size creates a mosaic look.

Chondrocyte transplantation. Articular cartilage is harvested via arthroscopy from the knee. Chondrocytes are cultured and then placed in a defect. With the cells present, a periosteal flap is then sutured over the defect. Weightbearing is not allowed for 3 months. See Chapter 77 for more information.

33. Outline a treatment algorithm.
Conservative management is used for nondisplaced fragments. In juveniles, healing may take 10–18 months. If healing fails to occur and the fragment remains attached, antegrade or retrograde drilling are options to stimulate healing. If the fragment is partially but not totally displaced, internal fixation can be attempted. Fixation choices include Herbert screws, Kirschner wires, corticocancellous bone pegs, osteochondral autograft, osteochondral allograft, and bioabsorbable screws and pins. If the fragment has been detached for a long period, replacement and fixation are not recommended. Long-term results with simple excision are generally poor. Stem cell stimulation is an option, but long-term results are also suboptimal. Thus, for a detached lesion that cannot be replaced, osteochondral autograft, allograft or chondrocyte transplantation should be considered.

34. What should be considered with knee malalignment?
Varus knees with medial leions and degenerative changes may respond to high tibial osteotomy.

OSTEONECROSIS

35. What is osteonecrosis?
Osteonecrosis is a clinical syndrome in which a segment of bone in the weight-bearing portion of the femoral condyle loses its blood supply; later it is associated with subchondral bone collapse and degenerative arthritis.

36. What is the etiology of osteonecrosis?
An occlusion in the blood supply to the femoral condyle interferes with microcirculation in the bone. The diminished microcirculation produces edema in a nonexpandable compartment and leads to increased pressure in the bone marrow, further diminishing the blood supply and resulting in osseous ischemia.

37. In what disease processes is osteonecrosis of the knee seen?
Steroid therapy
Renal transplantation
Gaucher's disease
Idiopathic spontaneous osteonecrosis
Hemoglobinopathies
Caisson's disease
Systemic lupus erythematosus

38. Describe the clinical presentation of patients with osteonecrosis of the femoral condyle.

The typical patient is a woman over 60 years of age who has sudden onset of severe pain on the medial side of the knee that may or may not be associated with trauma. Women are affected approximately three times more commonly than men. The pain is present frequently at night. It may be severe for 6–8 weeks and then gradually subsides.

39. Can osteonecrosis occur in the tibia?

Osteonecrosis of the tibia usually occurs in the medial compartment. It is not nearly as common as its counterpart on the femoral side.

40. Describe the physical findings in patients with osteonecrosis.

Depending on the stage, examination may reveal minimal clinical signs. Mild synovitis and effusion are commonly present. Stability and overall range of motion are generally not affected. Tenderness is localized over the compartment with the disease process and ranges from mild to severe. Loss of range of motion is common when significant degenerative changes occur.

41. Describe the radiographic classification of osteonecrosis of the knee.

In stage I the radiographic appearance is normal. Stage 2 is characterized by slight flattening of the convexity of the condyle, which may be subtle and is easily missed. In stage 3 the typical lesion of osteonecrosis is evident. A radiolucent area of variable size surrounds a sclerotic area in the subchondral bone. In stage 4 the radiolucency is surrounded by a definitive sclerotic halo. In stage 5 secondary changes develop, including narrowing of the joint space, sclerosis, formation of osteophytes, and destructive changes on the tibial side of the joint.

42. What other radiographic abnormalities are seen with osteonecrosis?

Technetium 99-m is the scanning agent of choice. An osteonecrotic lesion appears as a focally intense area of uptake over the affected condyle. If uptake is increased on both sides of the joint, concomitant arthritis may be present. MRI shows an area of low signal intensity in the central lesion on T2-weighted image, with a high-intensity signal about the margin.

43. Which is better for diagnosing osteonecrosis:arthroscopy or MRI?

MRI is better. Arthroscopy cannot visualize the bone changes of necrosis, because the articular cartilage overlying the lesion is usually normal. MRI identifies the area and extent of the lesion.

44. What laboratory studies are significant in osteonecrosis?

Routine laboratory studies are not helpful. The sedimentation rate may be mildly elevated. All other laboratory tests are within normal limits, except those associated with other medical problems.

45. What risk factors affect the clinical course and prognosis in osteonecrosis?

Patients who are in stage 1 or who have a small lesion that is < 45% of the condylar width have a favorable prognosis. Patients who have a large lesion (> 50%of the width of the condyle) generally become disabled with increasing pain, deformity, and eventually secondary joint destruction. Patients with stage 1 or small lesions generally have intense symptoms initially, but they slowly resolve over a period of 9–15 months. Pain may resolve completely.

46. What is the treatment for osteonecrosis?

Conservative treatment consists of nonsteroidal antiinflammatory medications, analgesics for night pain, and protected weight bearing. Most small lesions heal without surgical treatment.

47. What surgical treatments are available for patients with osteonecrosis?

Proximal tibial osteotomy may be beneficial in association with bone grafting by preventing collapse of the lesion and encouraging healing.

Drilling or burring of the lesion involves drilling into the subchondral bone to stimulate new vascularity. This treatment has not been very successful.

Allograft bone involves removal of diseased bone and replacement with matched femoral allograft.

Joint replacement. In reality, patients with ostenoecrosis are usually elderly and prosthetic replacement should be considered for most patients who need surgical intervention.

BIBLIOGRAPHY

1. Anderson AF, Lipscomb B, Coulam C: Antegrade curettement, bone grafting and pinning of osteochondritis dissecans in the skeletally mature knee. Am J Sports Med 18:254–261, 1990.
2. Anderson AF, Pagnani MJ: Osteochondritis dissecans of the femoral condyles: Long-term results of excision of the fragment. Am J Sports Med 24: 830–834, 1997.
3. Anderson AF, Richards D, Pagnani M, Hovis D: Antegrade drilling for osteochondritis dissecans of the Knee. Arthroscopy 13:319–324, 1997.
4. Berlet GC, Mascia A, Miniaci A: Treatment of unstable osteochondritis dissecans lesions of the knee using autogenous osteochondral grafts (mosaicplasty). Arthroscopy 15:312–316, 1999.
5. Cahill BR: Osteochondritis dissecans of the knee: Treatment of juvenile and adult forms. J Am Acad Orthop Surg 3:237–247, 1995.
6. Cahill B, Berg B: 99-M Technetium phosphate compound joint scintigraphy in the management of juvenile osteochondritis dissecans of the femoral condyle. Am J Sports Med 11:329–335, 1983.
7. Ecker ML, Lotke PA: Spontaneous osteonecrosis of the knee. J Am Acad Orthop Surg 2:173–178, 1994.
8. Ewing JW, Voto SJ: Arthroscopic surgical management of osteochondritis dissecans of the knee. Arthroscopy 4:37–40, 1988.
9. Federico DJ, Lynch JK, Jokl P: Osteochondritis dissecans of the knee: A historical review of etiology and treatment. Arthroscopy 6:190–197, 1990.
10. Friederichs MG, Greis PE, Burks RT: Pitfalls associated with fixation of osteochondritis dissecans fragments using bioabsorbable screws. Arthroscopy 17:542–545, 2001.
11. Garrett JC: Fresh osteochondral allografts for treatment of articular defects in osteochondritis dissecans of the lateral femoral condyle in adults. CORR 303:33–37, 1994.
12. Garret JC: Osteochondritis dissecans. Clin Orthop Sports Med 10:569–593, 1991.
13. Hefti F, Beguiristain J, Krauspe R, et al: Osteochondritis dissecans: A multicenter study of the European Pediatric Orthopedic Society. J Pediatr Orthop B 8:231–245, 1999.
14. Mandelbaum B, Browne JE, Fu F, et al: Articular cartilage lesions of the knee. Am J Sports Med 26:853–861, 1998.
15. Matava MJ, Brown C: Technical note: Osteochondritis dissecans of the patella: Arthroscopic fixation with bioabsorbable pins. Arthroscopy 13:124–128, 1997.
16. Mitsuoka T, Shino K, Hamada M, Horibe S: Osteochondritis dissecans of the lateral femoral condyle of the knee joint. Arthroscopy 15:20–26, 1999.
17. Outerbridge HK, Outerbridge RE, Smith DE: Osteochondral defects in the knee. CORR 377:145–151, 2000.
18. Paletta, Jr GA, Bednarz PA, Stanitski CL, et al: The prognostic value of quantitative bone scan in knee osteochondritis dissecans: A preliminary experience. Am J Sports Med 26:7–13, 1988.
19. Peterson L, Minas T, Brittberg M, et al: Two- to 9-year outcome after autologous chondrocyte transplantation of the knee. CORR 374: 212–234, 2000.
20. Schenck RC, Goodnight HM: Current concepts review: Osteochondritis Dissecans. J Bone Joint Surg 78A:439–456, 1996.
21. Slawski DP: High tibial osteotomy in the treatment of adult osteochondritis dissecans. CORR 341:155–161, 1997.
22. Twyman RS, Desai K, Aichroth PM: Osteochondritis dissecans of the knee: A long-term study J Bone Joint Surg 73B:461–464, 1991.
23. Victoroff BN, Marcus RE, Deutsch A: Arthroscopic bone peg fixation in the treatment of osteochondritis dissecans in the knee. Arthroscopy 12:506–509, 1996.

81. TOTAL KNEE ARTHROPLASTY

Adolph V. Lombardi, Jr., M.D., FACS

1. What are the major indications for total knee arthroplasty (TKA)?

TKA is indicated for end-stage degenerative joint disease of the knee, which may result from primary or secondary osteoarthritis, avascular necrosis, and inflammatory arthropathies, such as rheumatoid arthritis.

2. What are the nonoperative treatment modalities of degenerative joint disease of the knee?

1. Limited periods of rest
2. Orthoses, such as elastic knee supports, or valgus unloading braces
3. Nonsteroidal antiinflammatory agents (NSAIDs)
4. Corticosteroid injections
5. Viscosupplementation
6. Ambulatory aids, such as a cane, crutches, or walker

3. What is viscosupplementation?

Viscosupplementation is the use of an injectable viscoelastic preparation containing hyaluron or hylan (crosslinked hyaluron), which has been reported to provide extra joint protection. The preparations are available in various molecular weights. Treatment consists of a series of injections, which may be repeated at 6 month intervals. Since hyaluronic acid is a naturally occurring material, the body absorbs it over a 4-week period. Despite the absorption of the preparation, it has been reported to work for periods ranging from 6 months to 2 years.

4. Describe the ideal candidate for a valgus unloading brace.

A valgus unloading brace is a brace that induces a valgus thrust and therefore decompresses the medial compartment. A patient presenting with moderate degenerative joint disease involving the medial compartment is an acceptable candidate for a valgus unloading brace. These braces are typically used in members of the younger patient population who wish to maintain a high-activity lifestyle. The use of valgus unloading braces has been justified in several reports to date.

5. What are the operative treatments of degenerative joint disease of the knee?

1. Arthroscopic debridement
2. Osteotomy
   High tibial osteotomy for treatment of varus deformity
   Distal femoral osteotomy for treatment of valgus deformity
3. Unicompartmental knee arthroplasty
   Medial
   Lateral
4. Patellofemoral arthroplasty
5. Total knee arthroplasty

6. Describe the ideal candidate for arthroscopic treatment of osteoarthritis of the knee.

- Symptoms of < 1 year duration
- Nontraumatic etiology
- Normal limb alignment
- Mechanical symptoms, such as clicking and catching
- No history of previous knee surgery

7. What are the major indications for high tibial osteotomy in the treatment of degenerative joint disease of the knee?

1. Isolated medial compartment arthritis demonstrated by history, physical examination, and radiograph
2. Young, active patients with a strong desire to continue a vigorous lifestyle
3. Overweight patients
4. Patients with a range of motion $> 90°$ and $< 15°$ of flexion contracture
5. Varus deformity $< 15°$

8. What are the major indications for distal femoral osteotomy in the treatment of degenerative joint disease of the knee?

The indications for distal femoral osteotomy in treatment of degenerative joint disease of the knee are the same as the above indications for high tibial osteotomy with the following exceptions:

1. Isolated lateral compartment arthritis (rather than medial compartment arthritis)
2. Valgus deformity $< 15°$

9. Describe the ideal candidate for unicompartmental knee arthroplasty.

- Physiologic age > 60 years
- Relatively sedentary lifestyle
- Primary diagnosis of osteoarthritis
- Preoperative range of motion $\geq 90°$
- $< 10°$ of flexion contracture
- Angular deformity $< 15°$ that is correctable to neutral

10. What are the absolute contraindications to unicompartmental knee arthroplasty?

Inflammatory arthropathy and infection.

11. What is the difference between unicompartmental knee arthroplasty and TKA?

Unicompartmental knee arthroplasty involves replacement of a singular compartment of the knee, either medial or lateral, whereas TKA involves replacement of all three compartments of the knee: the medial and lateral compartments and most of the patellofemoral compartment.

12. Describe the ideal candidate for patellofemoral arthroplasty.

No ideal candidate can be described; results of this procedure have been less than ideal. The nonsurgical, conservative modalities of treatment for patellofemoral arthrosis include physical therapy, NSAIDs, and intraarticular injections of hyaluronic acids or corticosteroids. Surgical treatments include arthroscopic debridement with or without a lateral retinacular release, Maquet osteotomy (elevation of the tibial tubercle to facilitate a reduction in patellofemoral contact stresses), and, in the case of the elderly patient, TKA.

13. What are the primary goals of TKA?

- Relief of pain
- Restoration of function
- Achievement of intrinsic stability
- Creation of a durable reconstruction

14. What are the major contraindications to TKA?

Infection represents the major contraindication to TKA. Relative contraindications include young age; active, physical lifestyle; and obesity.

15. Should the patella always be resurfaced in TKA?

The answer to this question is twofold. For the treatment of inflammatory arthritis, it is universally agreed that the patella should be resurfaced. Resurfacing of the patella in patients with osteoarthritis, however, is controversial. Close review of the literature reveals that patients without patellofemoral resurfacing experience discomfort during activities associated with patellofemoral compression, such as ascending and descending stairs and rising from a chair.

16. What is the standard surgical approach to TKA? What is the rationale for its use?

The standard surgical approach for TKA involves a straight midline incision followed by a standard medial parapatellar capsular arthrotomy. Despite the fact that a standard medial parapatellar skin incision follows more adequately the lines of Langers, a straight midline skin incision is used with a subsequent medial parapatellar arthrotomy so that the skin and subcutaneous incision are not directly over the capsular incision. This slight mismatch of the capsular and skin incision provides an overlap that allows a better seal and therefore effectively reduces postoperative drainage and subsequent possibility of related infection.

17. Have any approaches other than the straight midline skin incision and the medial parapatellar capsular arthrotomy been popularized?

The midline skin incision remains the standard approach. However, several alternative capsular arthrotomies have been described: the subvastus approach, the vastus medialis splitting approach, the trivector approach, and lateral parapatellar approach.

18. What is the advantage of the subvastus, or southern, approach?

The subvastus approach spares the quadriceps tendon. From proximal to distal aspect, it involves elevation of the vastus medialis obliquus with a medial capsular arthrotomy that begins at the superior medial pole of the patella. Therefore, no incision is made into the quadriceps tendon. Advocates of this approach have noted a quicker return of quadriceps function, but no long-term advantages are seen over the more popular medial parapatellar arthrotomy. Limiting this approach to primary TKA in thin patients is advised.

19. Describe the vastus medialis splitting approach.

The vastus medialis splitting approach begins with a division of the vastus medialis along its fibers at the proximal two-thirds and distal one-third junction. The muscle division ends at the superior medial pole of the patella and the capsular arthrotomy is then carried distally along the medial aspect of the patella. It was initially reported that this approach yielded a diminution in the number of lateral retinacular releases. However, when the study was repeated in a randomized fashion, no difference in lateral retinacular release rates was noted between the medial parapatellar arthrotomy and vastus medialis splitting approach.

20. Describe the trivector approach.

The trivector approach involves an incision of the body of the vastus medialis obliquus, which begins approximately 5 cm proximal to the superior pole of the patella and extends distally along the medial aspect of the patella. Instead of splitting the quadriceps tendon, the muscle belly is divided. The term *trivector* arose as a result of the description of three vectors of pull on the patella: the vastus lateralis, the rectus femoris, and the vastus medialis obliquus. Proponents report that all three vectors are maintained with this approach. Original literature described early benefit with respect to the diminution of the number of lateral retinacular releases and an earlier recovery of the quadriceps function. However, a recent prospective study shows no difference between a standard medial parapatellar arthrotomy and the trivector approach.

21. What is the indication for use of the lateral parapatellar approach?

A straight midline skin incision followed by the lateral parapatellar arthrotomy has become the exposure of choice for the severe valgus deformity. Patients with a valgus deformity often have an associated lateral subluxation of the patella and require a lateral retinacular release at the time of surgical intervention. When a surgeon performs a medial parapatellar arthrotomy and a subsequent lateral retinacular release for a valgus knee deformity, the vasculature to the patella may be somewhat compromised. In an effort to reduce compromise of the patellar vasculature, some surgeons advocate the performance of a lateral parapatellar arthrotomy.

22. If the surgeon experiences difficulty in everting the patella during the standard medial parapatellar approach, what maneuvers can be performed to facilitate eversion?
1. Extending the incision proximally into the quadriceps tendon
2. Releasing adhesions in the lateral retinaculum and patellofemoral ligament
3. Removing the peripheral osteophytes about the patella
4. Tethering the medial portion of the insertion of the patellar ligament
5. Performing a lateral retinacular release

23. Define the mechanical axis of the knee.
The mechanical axis is defined as a line that intersects the center of the femoral head, the center of the knee, and the ankle. The goal of TKA is to reconstruct the mechanical axis with appropriate resection of the tibia and distal femur while carefully balancing the ligamentous structures.

24. What is the normal alignment of the distal femoral condyles with respect to the femoral axis and of the tibial plateau with respect to the tibial axis?
The normal alignment of the distal femoral condyles with respect to the femoral axis is approximately 9° of valgus, whereas the normal alignment of the tibial plateau with respect to the tibial axis is approximately 3° of varus. Therefore, a resultant 6° of valgus facilitates creation of the mechanical axis.

25. How should the proximal tibia be cut with respect to the tibial axis?
This question has a twofold response. Surgeons who follow the teaching of Insall et al. believe that the tibial resection should be created at 90° to the tibial axis in the coronal plane. They stress that varus malalignment leads to early failure. To reconstruct the mechanical axis, the distal femur must be resected at 6° of valgus. Hungerford et al., however, proposed that the proximal tibia be cut in 3° of varus and the distal femur in 9° of valgus. Hungerford argues that such resections place the joint line in the coronal plane parallel to the ground during gait. The majority of physicians, however, continue to resect the proximal tibia at 90° to the axis. As noted above, when the surgeon aims for 3° of varus, the margin is within several degrees; thus a 5° or 6° varus resection may inadvertently be performed. Because such varus malalignment is associated with accelerated loosening, it is safer to aim for a 90° resection and to accept a 2–3° variance in either varus or valgus.

26. What is the normal alignment of the proximal tibia in the sagittal plane?
In the sagittal plane the proximal tibia generally has a posterior slope of approximately 7–10°. Therefore, in resecting the proximal tibia two options exist: (1) resection perpendicular to the axis, in which case the implant should have posterior slope built into the articulation, and (2) resection of the proximal tibia with 5–7° of posterior slope. Reconstruction of the posterior slope is especially important in cruciate-retaining total knee arthroplasty.

27. What are the palpable landmarks used to assist the placement of the extramedullary tibial alignment jigs?
The palpable landmarks used to place the extramedullary tibial alignment jigs are the tibial tubercle, tibial spine, and medial and lateral malleolus. The jigs should be positioned over the tibial tubercle and aligned parallel with the tibial spine while intersecting the medial and middle thirds of the intermalleolar distance; thus, the jigs line up between the first and second ray.

28. Should intramedullary or extramedullary alignment jigs be used in performing the distal femoral and proximal tibial resections?
The literature with respect to distal femoral resection is quite convincing. Intramedullary alignment jigs offer a more reliable, accurate, and reproducible distal femoral resection. The literature with respect to the tibial resection, however, is controversial. The palpability of the land-

marks identified above allows accurate placement of extramedullary alignment jigs and, therefore, reproducible resections. Furthermore, there is debate with respect to bowing of the tibia, which may make it difficult to appropriately place an intramedullary guide and may result in a slight valgus or varus malalignment.

29. Describe the anatomic considerations of the distal femur and proximal tibia that assist in determining rotation of the femoral component.

Rotation of the femoral component is determined by evaluating four distinct anatomic features of the distal femur and proximal tibia: (1) The transepicondylar axis, which intersects the medial and lateral epicondyle, represents the true axis of rotation of the distal femur: (2) the anterior/posterior axis of the femur has been described as a line from the center of the trochlear groove to the center of the intercondylar notch. This axis is reported to be 90° to the transepicondylar axis; (3) the posterior femoral condyles have been identified to be 3° internally rotated to the transepicondylar axis. Therefore, by using a guide that references the posterior condyles with 3° of external rotation the femoral component will be placed in line with the neutral transepicondylar axis; finally (4) the tibial shaft axis has been identified as being 90° to the transepicondylar axis. Therefore, at the time of surgical intervention, the surgeon may incorporate all four of the above anatomic references to assist in determining rotation of the femoral component.

30. What surgical maneuvers can be performed to facilitate patellofemoral tracking?
   1. Appropriate resection and resurfacing of the patella to restore preoperative thickness
   2. Slight medial displacement of the patellar component
   3. Placement of the femoral component in neutral rotation or slight external rotation
   4. Lateral deviation of the femoral component
   5. Appropriate rotation of the tibial component
   6. Release of the patellofemoral ligament and any adhesions within the lateral retinaculum
   7. Lateral retinacular release with preservation of the superior geniculate vessel
   8. Advancement and reefing of the vastus medialis obliquus

31. Outline the steps for correction of varus malalignment at the time of TKA.

In the varus arthritis knee, the medial ligamentous structures are contracted. The object of TKA is to restore alignment and to reestablish the mechanical axis. In addition to the appropriate bony resections, release of the contracted soft tissues with proper ligamentous balance must be performed. The first step in correction of the contracture is removal of peripheral osteophytes from the distal femur and proximal tibia. Next, the deep medial collateral and capsular attachment to the proximal tibia are released. If correction is not afforded at this time, subsequent release of the superficial medial collateral ligament should be performed, followed by release of the pes anserinus. These releases are performed off the proximal tibia and should create a continuous sleeve of soft tissues.

32. Which bony landmarks on the distal femur represent the most reproducible guides in determining the rotation of the femoral component?

Rotation of the femoral component is best determined by locating the transepicondylar axis, which intersects the medial and lateral epicondyles. The axis of the posterior condyles is internally rotated with respect to the transepicondylar axis and, therefore, should not be used as a guide to determine rotation.

33. Describe the steps in correction of a valgus deformity.

The valgus arthritic knee presents with contractures of the lateral soft-tissue structures. The goal of TKA is to restore the mechanical axis with proper soft-tissue balance. Therefore, in addition to the bony resections in the valgus knee, the lateral contracted soft-tissue structures must be released. All authorities agree that peripheral osteophytes should be removed first. The sequence and technique of releasing the various lateral structures, however, is debatable. Contracture of the iliotibial band is generally noted with the knee in full extension. The iliotibial band can be released using a variety of techniques: (1) release from Gerdy's tubercle versus; (2) fractional lengthening with multiple stab wounds; or (3) transection of the iliotibial band at the joint line. The posterior lateral capsule/arcuate complex can be transected with the knee in full extension, taking care to avoid the neurovascular structures. Alternatively, the posterior lateral capsule/arcuate complex can be released from the distal femur with the knee in flexion with a curved osteotome. If the knee remains unbalanced and further release is deemed necessary, gradual release of the popliteus tendon and the lateral collateral ligament from the distal femur is required. The release of these structures should be performed only to the degree deemed necessary, since partial attachment of such structures will allow for the use of a nonconstrained posterior cruciate retaining or posterior stabilized device. However, if full release of the popliteus tendon and lateral collateral ligament is required, a posterior stabilized constrained device is advised to achieve stability. Note that rarely the biceps femoris may require release. Also note that a lateral retinacular release is frequently required in a valgus knee to facilitate tracking of the patellofemoral articulation.

34. What are the steps in release of flexion contracture in TKA?
The type of implant that should be used in patients with degenerative disease and associated flexion contracture is controversial. The literature supports posterior-stabilized arthroplasty in this group of patients, because the posterior cruciate ligament (PCL) is part of the deforming force and, therefore, must be released at the time of surgical intervention to correct the flexion contracture. Proponents of posterior cruciate–retaining arthroplasty advise that posterior cruciate–retaining devices can be used with special attention to the tension within the PCL. They suggest that controlled release of the ligament should be performed as opposed to total excision and substitution of a posterior-stabilized device.

Whichever type of implant is selected, it is imperative to remove all of the posterior condylar osteophytes to assist in reconstruction of the posterior process. In posterior-stabilized arthroplasty, contracture of the PCL can be dealt with by excision and use of an implant that substitutes for the PCL. When a posterior cruciate–retaining system is used, the ligament may need to be tethered from its insertion either in the proximal tibia or distal femur. When the flexion contracture is excessive, the capsule should be released from the posterior femur; ultimately, the medial and lateral heads of the gastrocnemius also may need to be released to enhance extension. Increased distal femoral resection increases the extension space and therefore facilitates correction of the flexion contracture; this resection, however, also elevates the joint line. This effect is not as significant in a posterior-stabilized system. However, in posterior cruciate–retaining arthroplasty, retention of the joint line is crucial to function of the PCL.

BIBLIOGRAPHY

1. Archibeck MJ, White RE Jr: What's new in adult reconstructive knee surgery. J Bone Joint Surg Am 84:1719–1726, 2002.
2. Engh GA, Parks NL, Ammeen DJ: Influence of surgical approach on lateral retinacular releases in total knee arthroplasty. Clin Orthop 331:56–63, 1996.
3. Fisher DA, Trimble SM, Breedlove K: The medial trivector approach in total knee arthroplasty. Orthopedics 21:53–56, 1998.
4. Hewett TE, Noyes FR, Barber-Westin SD, Heckman TP: Decrease in knee joint pain and increase in function in patients with medial compartment arthrosis: A prospective analysis of valgus bracing. Orthopedics 21:131–138, 1998.
5. Lombardi AV, Mallory TH, et al: An algorithm for the posterior cruciate in total knee arthroplasty. Clin Orthop 382:75–87, 2001.
6. Lotke PA, Garino JP (eds): Revision Total Knee Arthroplasty. Baltimore, Lippincott-Williams, Wilkins, 1999.
7. Lotke PA, Lonner JH (eds): Master Techniques in Orthopaedic Surgery: Knee Arthroplasty 2nd ed. Baltimore, Lippincott-Williams, Wilkins, 2002.
8. Mont MA, Booth RE Jr, Laskin RS, et al: The spectrum of prosthesis design for primary total knee arthroplasty. Inst Course Lect 52:397–407, 2003.
9. Scuderi GR, Tria A (eds): Surgical Techniques in Total Knee Arthroplasty. Heidelberg, Springer-Verlag, 2002.
10. Sculco TP, Martucci EA (eds): Knee Arthroplasty, Heidelberg, Springer-Verlag, 2002.
11. Vertullo CJ, Easley ME, Scott WN, Insall JN: Mobile bearings in primary knee arthroplasty. J Am Acad Orthop Surg 9(6):355–364, 2001.

82. COMPLICATIONS IN TOTAL KNEE ARTHROPLASTY

Adolph V. Lombardi, Jr., M.D., FACS

1. What is the most frequent complication following total knee arthroplasty (TKA)?

Complications with respect to the extensor mechanism represent the most frequently reported complications of TKA, with some centers reporting as high as 1.5–12% patellofemoral complications.

2. When minimal patellar resections are performed and a standard patellar component of approximately 8–9 mm is placed, "overstuffing" of the patellofemoral articulation may occur. What are the potential complications from overstuffing of the patellofemoral articulation?

Overstuffing of the patellofemoral articulation has both mechanical and functional implications. Increases in the contact stresses, as well as the shear stresses, that may be applied to the patellar implant may cause early loosening. A caliper should be used at the time of patellar resection to measure the anterior-posterior dimension of the patella (average thickness 23–25 mm); the appropriate amount of the patella should be resected, followed by proper reconstruction of patellofemoral articulation. Caution to avoid over-resection of the patella is also advised, because over-resection may lead to patellar fracture. A minimal postresection patellar thickness of 12–15 mm is required to avoid this complication. The postsurgical patellar composite should equal the presurgical patellar thickness.

3. What is lateral subluxation of the patella and how is it best treated?

Obtaining satisfactory tracking of the patellofemoral articulation is a difficult and multivariant task. It involves proper positioning of the femoral, tibial, and patellar components. To determine the appropriate surgical intervention requires addressing the cause for the subluxation. Radiographic evaluation of the implant may assist in determining proper alignment of the components but is not conclusive. Intraoperative inspection of all three components is required to rule out implant malalignment as the causative factor. Improper positioning of the components would necessitate revision of the implant. If it is determined that all components are in proper alignment, correction may be achieved with a lateral retinacular release, and in some cases a distal and lateral advancement of the vastus medialis obliquus.

4. If the femoral component rotation in the sagittal plane is placed along the axis of the posterior femoral condyles, what error and subsequent complication may result?

If the surgeon places the femoral component in line with the posterior femoral condylar axis, the femoral component will be placed in internal rotation with respect to the transepicondylar axis or true axis of the femur. This placement not only causes ligamentous imbalance but also increases the stresses across the patellofemoral articulation and leads to subluxation and perhaps dislocation of the patella.

5. What is the potential complication from intramedullary jigging of the femur and tibia for TKA?

The potential complication from intramedullary (IM) jigging of the femur and tibia is the generation of fat emboli. Literature stresses that the IM rod should be approximately 8 mm in diameter and should be fluted to allow drainage of fat from the femoral and tibial canals. In addition, the pilot holes should be 12 mm in diameter or approximately 4 mm larger than the intramedullary rod.

6. Describe the preoperative deformity more commonly associated with a postoperative peroneal palsy.

Postoperative peroneal palsy is a rare occurrence with TKA. However, it is more commonly seen in knees that present with significant combined valgus and flexion contracture deformities. Correction of such deformities may cause a stretching type injury to the peroneal nerve resulting in a postoperative neuropraxia. If this is identified in the early postoperative period, all dressings should be removed and the knee should be flexed. Some authors advocate exploration of the peroneal nerve.

7. Describe the patellar clunk syndrome and its treatment.

The patellar clunk syndrome has been described as an audible sound in conjunction with a visual displacement of the patella as the knee moves from a flexed position to an extended position. The clunk is caused by a fibrous nodule that is formed at the superior pole of the patella. Its definitive pathogenesis is debatable; however, it has been identified when there is superior overhand of the patellar component. Treatment generally requires surgical excision of the fibrous nodule and correction of the overhand of the patellar component.

8. What potential complication may result from notching of the anterior femoral cortex in TKA?

Although the significance of notching of the anterior femoral cortex in TKA is somewhat controversial, most of the literature suggests that notching should be avoided, because it may represent an etiologic mechanism for supracondylar fracture. Notching of the anterior femoral cortex is currently avoided by use of sophisticated instrumentation with appropriate sizing guides. Despite this sophisticated instrumentation, however, the surgeon must clear the suprapatellar fat and synovium and carefully monitor the anterior femoral resection.

9. Describe the etiology of an intercondylar distal femoral fracture in posterior stabilized TKA. What can be done to prevent it?

Intercondylar distal femoral fracture is a rare occurrence, exclusive to posterior stabilized arthroplasty (e.g., an intercondylar distal femoral resection for posterior stabilized arthroplasty). This complication occurs when the intercondylar femoral resection is slightly narrower than the intercondylar box of the femoral component or when the femoral component is inserted or extracted in slight varus or valgus malalignment. It may be avoided by accurate intercondylar resection. An intercondylar sizing guide should be used for measuring the intercondylar resection, and great care should be taken in inserting and extracting the trial and final components.

10. Describe the types of intercondylar distal femoral bone fractures that may occur in TKA and the appropriate management of each.

Two types of intercondylar distal femoral fractures may occur in posterior stabilized TKA: nondisplaced and displaced. Nondisplaced fractures are generally recognized on postoperative roentgenographs and require no further treatment. Patients should be placed in a routine physical therapy and rehabilitation program. A displaced intercondylar distal femoral fracture, however, is noted at the time of the surgical intervention and should be stabilized with screws and/or stemmed components. After stabilization of the fracture, no change in the postoperative physical therapy and rehabilitation routine is required.

11. What neurologic complication may arise in correction of the arthritic knee with a valgus malalignment and an associated flexion contracture?

Correction of the arthritic knee with a valgus deformity and associated flexion contracture sometimes leads to peroneal palsy, which is attributed to stretching of the peroneal nerve. If this complication is noted postoperatively, all compressive dressings should be removed immediately and the knee should be flexed. Surgical decompression of the peroneal nerve remains controversial, but recent literature cites the benefit of decompression if nerve function does not spontaneously recover.

12. Describe the major factors in proximal tibial resection that may lead to failure of TKA.
Critical to successful TKA is the technique of proximal tibial resection. The first and foremost factor is the level of proximal tibial resection. Overresection of the proximal tibia should be avoided, because the strength of the proximal tibia decreases with the level of resection. Underresection of the proximal tibia, however, also may be detrimental, because the joint line is elevated. An accurate level of resection is especially critical in a posterior cruciate-retaining arthroplasty. As a rule of thumb, the level of the proximal tibial resection should be approximately 8–10 mm from the lateral tibial plateau with a corresponding resection 3–5 mm from the medial plateau. The proximal tibia normally has approximately 7–10° of posterior slope; thus, resection of the proximal tibia to neutral or reverse angulation affects the flexion gap and may subsequently alter range of motion. This rule must be noted when using a posterior cruciate-retaining knee in which the articulating mechanism does not incorporate posterior slope.

13. What potential error may occur if the intramedullary guide, used for distal femoral preparation, is placed in the center of the intercondylar notch?
Anatomic studies have demonstrated that the femoral axis exits the distal femur at the lateral border of the medial femoral condyle. Therefore, if the intermedullary guide is inserted into the center of the intercondylar notch, it is placed in a slight valgus orientation of approximately 2°; therefore, if one is aiming for 6° valgus resection, the guide should be placed at 4° of valgus.

14. What are the advantages and disadvantages of screw fixation in cementless TKA?
The literature recommends the use of 4 screws to augment fixation of the cementless tibial component. Screws have been shown to enhance stability, to decrease micromotion, and, therefore, to potentiate osseous integration into the tibial component. Several recent articles, however, have revealed osteolytic lesions about the screws; thus the term "screw osteolysis" has been coined. It is postulated that polyethylene debris invades the screw holes and tracks along the body of the screw. Removal of the screws and replacement with morsellized bone grafting has been shown to be an effective treatment of osteolytic lesions.

BIBLIOGRAPHY

1. Favorito PJ, Mihalko WM, Krackow KA: Total knee arthroplasty in the valgus knee. J Am Acad Orthop Surg, 10(1):16–24, 2002.
2. Guyton JL: Arthroplasty of ankle and knee. In Canale ST (ed): Campbell's Operative Orthopaedics, 9th ed. St. Louis, Mosby, 1998, pp 232–295.
3. Kelly MA. Ligament Instability in Total Knee Arthroplasty. Instr Course Lect, 50:399–401, 2001.
4. Kelly MA. Patellofemoral Complications in Total Knee Arthroplasty. Instr Course Lect, 50:403–407, 2001.
5. Mont MA, Booth RE Jr, Laskin RS, et al. The Spectrum of Prosthesis Design for Primary Total Knee Arthroplasty. Instr Course Lect, 52:397–407, 2003.
6. Lotke PA, Lonner JH (eds): Master Techniques in Orthopaedic Surgery: Knee Arthroplasty, 2nd. ed. Baltimore, Lippincott-Williams, Wilkins, 2002.

83. ALTERNATIVES TO TOTAL KNEE ARTHROPLASTY: OSTEOTOMY AND FUSION

Daniel P. Hoeffel, M.D., and Randall D. Neumann, M.D.

OSTEOTOMY

1. Describe the mechanical axis of the lower limb.
The mechanical axis is a straight line originating from the center of the femoral head to the center of the tibiotalar (ankle) joint.

2. Define the tibiofemoral angle.
This angle is created by the intersection of lines along the long axes of the femur and tibia.

3. What are normal values for the mechanical axis and tibiofemoral angle?
The normal mechanical axis is zero because it is a straight line. The normal tibiofemoral angle is ~ 5–7° of valgus angulation.

4. What is the load distribution across the normal knee?
Approximately 60% of the load is borne by the medial compartment, and 40% is borne by the lateral compartment.

5. Describe the load distribution across a varus knee and a valgus knee.
A **varus deformity** often results from medial compartment degenerative changes with collapse of the medial tibial plateau. As the knee progresses into varus, the mechanical axis crosses the knee joint as a point more medial than normal, which results in greater relative loading of the medial compartment.

A **valgus deformity** results from lateral compartment degenerative changes with collapse of the lateral femoral condyle. The mechanical axis moves laterally. Relatively more weight is transmitted through the lateral compartment.

6. What are the goals of knee osteotomy?
1. To transfer load from the degenerative compartment to the less diseased compartment, thus preserving articular surface and relieving pain.
2. To alter the bony alignment at the point at which the mechanical axis crosses the knee joint, thereby altering load distribution across the knee.

7. What is the usual osteotomy for medial compartment degeneration?
A proximal tibial valgus osteotomy to correct the accompanying varus deformity is usually performed.

8. Which type of osteotomy is done for lateral compartment degeneration?
A distal femoral varus osteotomy corrects the accompanying valgus deformity.

9. List the indications for proximal tibial valgus osteotomy about the knee.
1. Absence of lateral compartment and patellofemoral degenerative arthritis
2. Younger patient (< 60–65 years)
3. Good bone stock (minimal osteoporotic change)
4. Minimum flexion arc (> 90°)
5. < 15° of fixed varus

10. What are the contraindications for proximal tibial valgus osteotomy?
- Lateral subluxation of the tibia on the femur > 1 cm
- Tibial subchondral bone loss
- Flexion contracture > 15°
- < 90° range of motion
- Peripheral vascular disease
- Lateral thrust of the knee during gait
- Rheumatoid or other systemic arthritides

11. List the indications for varus osteotomies of the femur.
1. Valgus deformities > 12° and > 10° deviation of the knee joint from the horizontal
2. No flexion contracture > 15°
3. ≥ 90° range of motion
4. No knee instability

12. 12. What preoperative planning is necessary when considering a tibial osteotomy?
Full-length, weight-bearing radiographs are used to determine the desired amount of correction and the size of the bone wedge to be removed. To unload the arthritic medial compartment, the angle between the tibia and the femur should be 8–10° of valgus. Slight overcorrection provides the best long-term results.

13. What types of fixation have been used to stabilize tibial valgus osteotomy?
- Plates and screws
- Staples
- External fixators

14. What are the long-term results of proximal tibial valgus osteotomy?
At 5-year follow-up 88% of patients have satisfactory results; at 10-year follow-up the number drops to 63%. Adequate angular correction has a strong correlation with good outcome.

15. List the complications associated with proximal tibial osteotomies.
- Inadequate correction (most common)
- Overcorrection
- Violation of tibial articular surface
- Avascular necrosis of the tibial plateau
- Patella baja (low-riding patella)
- Anterior compartment syndrome
- Peroneal nerve syndrome
- Delayed union/nonunion (3–5%)
- Infection
- Vascular injuries to the popliteal vessels

16. How successful is total knee arthroplasty (TKA) after tibial osteotomy?
Results are less satisfactory than for primary TKA. Patella baja is not uncommon after tibial osteotomy, which makes adequate exposure for TKA more difficult. One study showed 81% good-to-excellent results for TKA after tibial osteotomy, whereas primary TKA had 100% good-to-excellent results.

17. Describe the usual bony deformity in the valgus arthritic knee.
Lateral compartment arthritis is usually associated with lateral femoral condyle bone deficiency. Thus, a medial closing wedge osteotomy of the tibia may cause significant obliquity of the knee joint and subluxation of the femur on the tibia. A femoral osteotomy avoids this complication.

18. What preoperative planning should be done before distal femoral varus osteotomy?
Full-length, weight-bearing radiographs are used to determine the desired amount of correction and the size of the bone wedge to be removed. The tibiofemoral angle should be corrected to 0°.

19. What types of fixation are used to stabilize femoral osteotomies?
The standard device is a 95 degree-blade plate with screws.

20. What are the follow-up results of distal femoral osteotomy?

Five to 10-year follow-up shows 70–80% good-to-excellent results that do not appear to decrease over time.

KNEE ARTHRODESIS

21. What is knee arthrodesis?

A knee arthrodesis is a surgical procedure designed to produce a bony ankylosis (fusion) of the knee joint.

22. What are the goals of a knee arthrodesis?

To create a stable, pain-free platform on which to ambulate or transfer.

23. List the disadvantages of a knee fusion.

1. Joints above and below the knee will transmit greater loads and may become stiff or undergo degenerative changes.

2. Loss of knee range of motion, which decreases gait efficiency (20% increased energy requirement)

3. Activities of daily living may be more difficult (e.g., rising from a seated position, dressing)

24. What are the indications for knee arthrodesis?

- A salvage procedure for severe unilateral knee afflictions
- Infected TKA that makes revision surgery unsuitable
- Posttraumatic arthritis in high-demand patients (i.e., manual laborers)
- Tumors requiring significant bony resection
- Severe infectious arthritis (resistant bacteria, fungal, TB)
- Paralytic conditions (especially with genu recurvatum)
- Congenital knee anomalies

25. What types of techniques are available for arthrodesis?

- Intramedullary (IM) rodding
- Compression plating
- External fixation

26. List the disadvantages of plating, IM rodding, and external fixation.

Plating

May require placing metal in previously or currently infected site

Large bulk of components

IM rodding

Rod migration

Difficult to obtain correct alignment

Difficult to remove

External fixation

Pin tract drainage/infection

Muscle and soft tissue scarring at pin sites

Long treatment course (6 months)

27. What is the ideal position for a knee fusion?

0–5° of valgus

10–15° of flexion

Slight external rotation

28. What is the reported success rate of arthrodesis with an IM nail?
Eighty-five percent of patients gain functional stability and overall union.

29. Does the type of knee arthroplasty originally performed affect the rate of fusion?
Yes. A hinged prosthesis adversely affects the fusion rate (56%). Nonhinged prostheses have a fusion rate of approximately 90%.

30. What are the potential complications of knee fusion?
- Pseudarthrosis (failure to fuse)
- Recurrent infection
- Knee pain
- Back pain
- Pin tract infection
- Fracture of bone at pin site (external fixation)
- Nail breakage
- Tibia fracture (IM rod)

BIBLIOGRAPHY

1. Arroyo JS, Garvin KL, Neff JR: Arthrodesis of the knee with a modular titanium intramedullary nail. J Bone Joint Surg Am 79:26–35, 1997.
2. Christian CA, Donley BG: Arthrodesis of the ankle, knee, and hip. In Canale ST (ed): Campbell's Operative Orthopaedics, 9th ed. St. Louis, Mosby, 1998, pp 145–187.
3. Coventry MB, Ilstrup DM, Wallrichs SL: Proximal tibial osteotomy: A critical long-term study of 87 cases. J Bone Joint Surg 75A:196–201, 1993.
4. Edgerton BC. Mariani EM, Morrey BF: Distal femoral varus osteotomy for painful genu valgum. A five-to-11-year follow-up study. Clin Orthop 288:263–269, 1993.
5. Insall JN: Osteotomy. In Insall JN (ed): Surgery of the Knee, 2nd ed. New York, Churchill Livingstone, 1993, pp 635–677.
6. Jakob RP, Murphy SB: Tibial osteotomy for varus arthrosis: Indication, planning, and operative technique. Instr Course Lect 41:87–93, 1992.
7. Kelly MA: Nonprosthetic management of the arthritic knee. In Callaghan JJ (ed): Orthopaedic Knowledge Update Hip and Knee Reconstruction. Rosemont, IL, American Academy of Orthopaedic Surgeons, 1995, pp 245–251.
8. Mont MA, Alexander N, Krackow KA, Hungerford DS: Total knee arthroplasty after failed high tibial osteotomy. Orthop Clin North Am 25:515–525, 1994.
9. Pritchett JW, Mall BA: Knee arthrodesis with a tension band plate. J Bone Joint Surg 70A:285–288, 1988.

84. UNICONDYLAR KNEE ARTHROPLASTY

Randall D. Neumann, M.D.

1. What is a unicondylar knee arthroplasty (UKA)?
UKA was developed in the 1950s to treat medial or lateral compartment osteoarthritis of the knee. The device replaces the medial or lateral articular surface of the femur with a metal component, maintaining the femoral condylar contour. The medial or lateral tibial plateau is replaced with a flat polyethylene articulating component. Both components are fixed to the bone using polymethylmethacrylate bone cement. A total knee arthroplasty uses a femoral component that completely replaces the distal femoral articulating surface including the patellofemoral articulation. The tibial component replaces the entire surface of the proximal tibia.

2. Discuss the development of the UKA.
The UKA was first designed in the 1950s by McKeever. Significant modifications were made by MacIntosh, Marmor, and Insall. Its popularity diminished in the United States after reported complications of subsidence of the tibial component led to failures. UKAs remained popular in

the 1980s and 1990s mainly in Europe, and continued to be used successfully. Excellent 10-year results reported by Repicci and Berger in the late 1990s have renewed surgeons' enthusiasm.

3. What are the indications for the UKA?

- Disabling pain in the medial or lateral compartment of the knee
- Failure of conservative care, such as injections, activity modification, nonsteroidal anti-inflammatory drugs, brace treatment
- Relatively young, less than 60–65 years of age
- Isolated medial or lateral compartment disease
- Active patient

4. What symptoms and physical guidelines should be used to determine whether a patient is a candidate for a UKA?

- Pain should be limited to one compartment, not all compartments of the knee
- Tenderness found in only one compartment
- Flexion contracture less than 10°
- Flexion greater than 110°
- Varus or valgus of 10° or less
- No translation of the tibia laterally
- No varus thrust with ambulation
- Caution in patients with a knee deficient in the anterior or posterior cruciate ligament

5. What are the contraindications to UKA?

- History of knee infection, septic arthritis, or osteomyelitis.
- Varus or valgus greater than 15°
- Flexion contracture greater than 15°
- Flexion less than 90°
- Rheumatoid arthritis and any inflammatory arthritis
- Tricompartmental disease
- Obesity
- Neuropathic arthropathy
- Severe bone deficiency
- Arthrodesis
- Extensor loss
- Ligamentous instability

6. Which compartment is affected most often, necessitating replacement?

In the author's experience, the medial compartment is much more common than the lateral. Eighty to 90% of some series involve the medial compartment.

7. What is the minimally invasive technique?

In a normal total knee arthroplasty, the skin incision is approximately 8–10 inches. The quadriceps tendon is split, and the medial capsule along the patella and patellar tendon is cut. The patella is everted and dislocated. With the minimally invasive technique, a 4-inch incision is made through the skin and along the patella and patellar tendon. The patella is subluxed, not dislocated, and the quadriceps tendon is left intact. Less tissue damage means faster recovery.

8. Describe the operative procedure.

General or spinal anesthetic is used. A leg-holder may be used, along with a thigh tourniquet. The incision is made along the medial border of the patellar tendon and the patella. The capsule is cut to enter the joint. Osteophytes are removed. The femoral guides are placed using in-tramedullary guides to align the knee components. Femoral cuts are made with a saw, and typically drill holes are made to accommodate the femoral lugs. Most prostheses have 4–6 sizes; the femur is sized accordingly. The medial tibial plateau is cut at 90° to the long axis of the tibia. Lugs or slots are drilled to accommodate the lugs and fins of the tibial component. Varying sizes are available for coverage of the tibia, and also for the thickness of the polyethylene. Sizing, range of motion, alignment, and stability are checked. The components are cemented into place. A drain may be placed and the capsule and skin are closed.

9. Describe the postoperative course.

The surgical procedure typically takes one hour. The patient is started on exercises within 6–8 hours. Patients begin ambulation within 12–24 hours. Most patients are discharged from the hospital in 24–48 hours. Aspirin is taken for prophylaxis of deep vein thrombosis. Antibiotics are given preoperatively and for two doses after surgery. Patients are allowed off crutches at 2 weeks. Excellent range of motion can be expected in 2–4 weeks. Unrestricted activity is allowed at 6 weeks. Patients are allowed to golf, play tennis, and resume other recreational activities at 6 weeks. No jogging, impact aerobics, contact sports, or heavy lifting are allowed.

10. What complications are associated with UKA?
- Infection, superficial and deep
- Deep venous thrombosis and pulmonary embolism
- Fracture
- Patellar impingement
- Tibial component subsidence
- Osteolysis
- Polyethylene wear
- Motion loss

11. What alternatives to UKA are presently popular?
- Arthroscopic debridement
- High tibial osteotomy
- Mosaicplasty
- Unicompartmental allograft
- Chondrocyte implantation (Carticel, Genzyme Corp.)
- Metal spacer (Unispacer, Sulzer Corp.)
- Total knee arthroplasty

CONTROVERSIES

12. What are mobile bearing devices?

Mobile bearing tibial components, compared with the fixed type used in the U.S., are currently used in Europe. The polyethylene articulates with the femoral component as with all other models, but the tibial base is polished and the polyethylene is free to move on this component also. One of the most popular designs, the Oxford knee, has been used extensively and has good clinical success. Reported problems include dislocation of the mobile bearing. Currently, the Food and Drug Administration does not allow its use in the United States.

13. Is the UKA indicated in 80-year-old patients?

Some surgeons believe that the older patient may benefit from a UKA, described as "the first and last" arthroplasty. It is intended to give unicompartmental pain relief. Patients are not enthused about the lengthy recovery with a traditional TKA. They respond quickly when minimally invasive techniques are used, with less morbity.

BIBLIOGRAPHY

1. Berger RA, Nedeff DD, Barden RN, et al: Unicompartmental knee arthroplasty. Clin Orthop 367:50–60, 1999.
2. Goodfellow JW, Kershaw CJ, Benson MKD'A, O'Connor JJ: The Oxford knee for unicompartmental osteoarthritis. J Bone Joint Surg 70B:692–701, 1988.

3. Insall J, Walker P: Unicondylar knee replacement. Clin Orthop 120:83–85, 1976.
4. Marmor L: Marmor modular knee in unicompartmental disease. Minimum four-year follow-up. Clinical Orthop 184:236–240, 1984.
5. Repicci JA, Eberle RW: Minimally invasive surgical technique for unicondylar knee arthroplasty. J South Orthop Assoc 8(1):20–27, 1999.
6. Scott RD: Unicompartmental total knee arthroplasty. In Insall J, Scott NW (eds): Surgery of the Knee, 3rd ed. New York, Churchill Livingstone, 2001.

85. FRACTURES ABOUT THE KNEE

Steven G. Kumagai, M.D.

1. What is a tibial plateau fracture?

A tibial plateau fracture involves the proximal 10–12 cm of the tibia, which consist largely of cancellous bone.

2. Describe the types of tibial plateau fractures.

Numerous classifications have been introduced over the years. The categories encompass many fracture configurations but are so broad that comparisons of treatment results are meaningless. Fractures can be described as minor or major and undisplaced or displaced. Compression may occur in either the medial or lateral compartment. Fractures may involve compression of one small fragment or a major fragment. The Schatzker classification is a common classification of tibial plateau fractures.

3. Describe the mechanism of injury in a tibial plateau fracture.

Strong forces directed medially or laterally at the knee joint, combined with axial loading, cause the majority of proximal tibial plateau fractures. Automobile accidents account for 40–60% of all tibial plateau fractures. Other mechanisms include falls from heights, slipping and twisting, sport injuries, and motorcycle and bicycle accidents. About 15–45% of fractures include a ligamentous rupture, commonly of the medial or lateral collateral ligaments. Meniscal lesions occur in approximately 20% of all tibial plateau fractures. Some tibial plateau fractures are quite minor and are caused by falls or minor missteps among the elderly.

4. Describe the symptoms of the patient with a tibial plateau fracture.

Most patients have had high-energy trauma and complain of severe pain and swelling of the knee. Instability may be noted when the patient attempts to bear weight. The patient also may complain of tense hemarthrosis.

5. Describe the radiographic findings in a patient with a tibial plateau fracture.

Anteroposterior and lateral radiographs of the knee usually reveal the fracture. If a fracture is suspected but not seen, oblique views or a tunnel view may be taken. Tomograms in the anteroposterior and lateral planes show evidence of plateau fractures Computed tomography (CT) produces excellent images from which to assess depressions and displacements. Magnetic resonance imaging (MRI) is often helpful because of the high incidence of meniscal and ligament injuries associated with tibial plateau fractures.

6. What are the findings of knee aspiration in patients with a tibial plateau fracture?

Some patients may have a tense hemarthrosis. Aspiration reveals blood in the joint but also may reveal fat. If fat is present in the aspirate, a fracture is surely present.

7. What complications are seen in patients with fractures of the tibial plateau?

Some patients with tibial plateau fractures have a fractured dislocation of the knee. The popliteal artery is usually injured in a knee dislocation. Prompt attention to the arterial pulses and angiography are needed for assessment of the popliteal artery.

8. Describe the indications for conservative treatment in a patient with a tibial plateau fracture.

The major indication is a minimally displaced fracture that shows depression or displacement of < 5 mm. Minimally displaced fractures may involve one or both plateaus. Instability is an important factor to consider in choosing the treatment for minimally displaced fractures. If the knee is stable to abduction and adduction stress testing, the fracture is considered stable. Stable fractures may be treated with a knee immobilizer, partial weightbearing, or cast bracing. Conservative treatments are maintained until the fracture is united and weightbearing begins.

9. Describe the operative treatment of articular depression fractures (types II and III).

Most tibial plateau fractures with > 5 mm of depression should be treated operatively, with restoration of the depressed articular surfaces. Either screw fixation or plate fixation is used. Bone graft should be used to support the elevated surface. A bone tamp may be placed through a window or through the split to elevate the depressed articular surface. Arthroscopy may be helpful for isolated or split depression fractures. Care must be taken when arthroscopy is used due to the risk of compartment syndormes in the leg. Low-pressure pumps or gravity inflow should be used with arthroscopy.

10. Describe the treatment of condylar split fractures (types I, II, IV, and V).

Open treatment is almost always indicated for displaced fragments with instability. Open reduction of the fragments are performed under direct vision. Transverse submeniscal arthrotomy is often utilized to restore the alignment of the articular surface. The reduced condyle is internally fixated with screws with or without butress plating depending on stability.

11. Describe the complications associated with bicondylar tibial plateau fractures (types V and VI).

Bicondylar fractures are generally high-energy fractures associated with a high incidence of vascular and nerve injuries. Soft-tissue damage is likely in the pre or post-operative period. Bicondylar tibial plateau fractures have the poorest prognosis for functional improvement. Treatment may consist of non-operative skeletal traction followed by percutaneous pinning and/or cast bracing. Open reduction is used when significant improvement in fracture position is likely and rigid internal fixation is possible. All tibial plateau fractures are susceptable to complications, including skin loss, compartment syndrome, wound infection, popliteal artery laceration, peroneal nerve palsy, nonunion, malunion, and degenerative arthritis.

12. Describe the surgical options for bicondylar split fratcures and bicondylar split fractures with separation from the tibial shaft (types V and VI).

If the soft tissues are amenable to operative intervention, the condyles should be reduced under direct visualiztion. Mid-line surgical approaches make salvage procedures such as total knee arthroplasty easier. The lateral condyle is secured to the generally more stable medial condyle with screws and a butress plating. Plating both sides of the tibia may be associated with more skin complications. The addition of medial-sided external fixators or fine wire-ringed fixators may be useful to limit the need for wide surgical exposures in skin which is frequently tenuous to begin with.

13. Describe the etiology of patellar fracture.

The majority of patellar fractures occur in patients between 20 and 50 years of age. The incidence is nearly twice as high in men as in women. They usually result from a direct blow to the knee sustained in a fall or a motor vehicle or pedestrian accident. Fractures also may occur from indirect forces, as in the act of stumbling or partially falling.

14. Describe the classification of patellar fractures.

Transverse fractures in the central or lower third of the patella are the most common type. Vertical fractures may occur but are generally associated with a more comminuted fracture that began as a transverse fracture. Patellar fractures may be displaced or undisplaced.

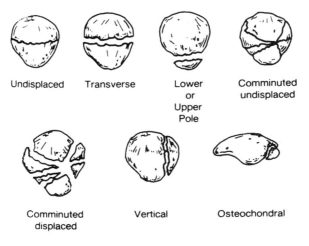

Classification of patellar fractures. (From Wiss DA, Watson JT, Johnson EE: Fractures of the knee. In Rockwood CA, Green DP, Bucholz RW, Heckman JD (eds): Rockwood and Green's Fractures in Adults, 4th ed. Philadelphia, Lippincott-Raven, 1996, with permission.)

15. What treatments are available for patellar fractures?

- Nonoperative treatment with casting or immobilization
- Operative treatment with open reduction and internal fixation
- Partial patellectomy
- Total patellectomy

16. Describe the indications for nonoperative treatment.

Patients who are able to extend the knee fully have intact retinaculum. Such fractures are usually displaced or have 2–3 mm of acceptable separation. A long leg cast is recommended for 3–4 weeks, followed by quadriceps exercises, straight leg raising, and range-of motion exercises. Partial weightbearing is easily tolerated.

17. Describe the indications for open reduction and internal fixation.

Open reduction and internal fixation are used to reconstruct the patella in patients with displacement and loss of extension. Generally the retinaculum medially and laterally to the patella is torn along with the fracture. The extensor mechanism is no longer in continuity and must be repaired. Operative treatment includes the use of K-wire and tension band or screws.

18. Describe the indication for partial patellectomy.

Partial patellectomy and repair of the extensor mechanism are indicated when there is a small remaining fragment of the patella or quadriceps tendon—usually in an avulsion fracture of the patellar ligament. The lower pole is excised, and the patella tendon is sutured into the remaining patella.

19. What is the indication for total patellectomy?

Total patellectomy is recommended for highly comminuted fractures that have no possibility of repair or reconstruction.

20. Describe the complications from patellar fractures and their treatment.
An occasional patient has an extensor lag. Quadriceps wasting may occur. Fracture fragment separation and loss of fixation occur in as many as 7% of patients. Nonunion may occur postoperatively. Other common problems include patellofemoral pain or osteoarthritic symptoms as a long-term consequence of patellar fracture.

21. What are fractures in the distal one-third of the femur called?
Supracondylar fractures.

22. Describe the classification for supracondylar fractures of the femur.
No classification for supracondylar fractures of the femur is universally accepted, but the AO classification is commonly used (see figure). Type A fractures involve the distal shaft, with varying degrees of comminution. Type B fractures are condylar fractures. Type C fractures are T and Y condylar fractures with varying degrees of comminution.

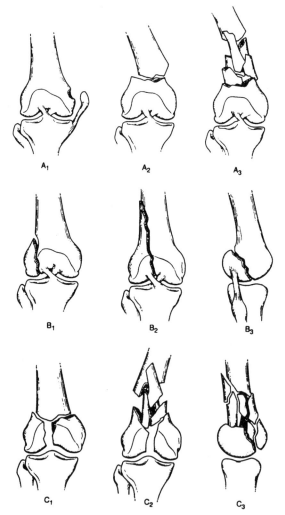

AO/ASIF classification of supracondylar femur fractures. (From Wiss DA: Supracondylar and intracondylar fractures of the femur. In Rockwood CA, Green DP, Bucholz RW (eds): Rockwood and Green's Fractures in Adults, 4th ed. Philadelphia, J.B. Lippincott, 1996, with permission.)

23. What is the mechanism of injury in supracondylar fractures?

The mechanism of injury is axial loading with varus, valgus, or rotational forces. Supracondylar fractures are typically seen after high-energy trauma related to motor vehicle or motorcycle accidents or falls from a height. In the elderly, a slip or fall on a flexed knee frequently leads to comminuted fractures through compromised osteoporotic bone.

24. Describe the initial management for supracondylar fractures.

Obtain anteroposterior, lateral, and oblique radiographs of the entire femur. CT is usually needed for all intra-articular fractures. Patients with supracondylar fractures should be treated with closed skeletal traction with a tibial traction pin. Immediate debridement is necessary for open injuries. Traction is then maintained if nonoperative treatment is elected. If operative treatment is elected, distraction of the fragments may enhance fracture mobility at the time of surgical intervention.

25. What immediate complications are associated with supracondylar fractures of the femur?

A vascular injury is found in 2–3% of patients. Vessel injury may result directly from laceration or contusion by the fracture fragments or indirectly from stretching that leads to intimal damage. Clinical examination of the leg for signs of ischemia and evaluation of pulses and motor and sensory function are mandatory. If the integrity of the vessels is in doubt, it is wise to proceed with an arteriogram to rule out vascular injury.

26. What are the indications for nonoperative therapy in supracondylar fractures?

- Nondisplaced or incomplete fractures
- Impacted stable fractures in elderly osteoporotic patients
- Significant underlying medical diseases, such as cardiovascular, pulmonary, or neurologic problems
- Severe osteoporosis
- Severely contaminated open fractures
- Infected fractures
- Fractures without joint involvement

27. What are the goals of nonsurgical treatment?

The goals of nonsurgical treatment include a stable, healed fracture with near-normal range of motion of the knee and hip. No more than 7° of malalignment in the mediolateral plane should be accepted. Anterior or posterior angulation should not exceed 7–10°. Limb shortening of 1–1.5 cm is generally well tolerated.

28. Describe the surgical management of supracondylar fractures.

Minimally comminuted fractures involving the medial or lateral condyle are best treated with open reduction, restoration of the articular surface, and internal fixation with AO screws. Severely comminuted fractures should be treated with near-anatomic restoration of the joint using K-wires and screws, followed by a medial and lateral dynamic compression plate. When comminution or defects in the cortex are present, supplemental cortical cancellous bone grafting is necessary. Alternatives are the condylar blade plate, buttress plate, intramedullary nails and flexible intramedullary nails. External fixation is frequently used in open fractures with significant soft-tissue wounds or vascular injury.

29. What is a Hoffa fragment?

A Hoffa fragment is a coronal shear of the distal femoral condyle seen best on CT axial views. If present, internal fixation requires a condylar buttress plate (broad clover-leaf plate contoured to the lateral femoral cortex) to connect the displaced condyle and Hoffa fragment to the metaphysis and shaft of the femur.

30. What are the indications for intramedullary nailing?
Extra-articular supracondylar femur fractures can be treated with retrograde intramedullary nailing. Some selected intra-articular fractures which are amenable to stable internal fixation of the condyles (such as non-displaced condylar splits) can be treated with retrograde nailing as well. (See indications for retrograde nailing in femoral shaft fracture section)

31. List the long-term complications of supracondylar fractures.

Malunion	Infection	Deep venous thrombosis
Nonunion	Implant breakage	Vascular injury
Loss of knee motion		

BIBLIOGRAPHY

1. Connolly JF, Dehne E, LaFollette B: Closed reduction and early cast-brace ambulation in the treatment of femoral fractures: Results in one hundred and forty-three fractures. J Bone Joint Surg 55A:1581–1599, 1973.
2. Connolly JF, King P: Closed reduction and early cast-brace ambulation in the treatment of femoral fractures: I. an in vivo quantitative analysis of immobilization in skeletal traction and a cast-brace. J Bone Joint Surg 55A:1559–1580, 1973.
3. Duwelius P, Connelly J: Closed reduction of tibial plateau fractures: A comparison of functional and roentgenographic end results. Clin Orthop 230:116–126, 1988.
4. Koval JK: Helfet DL: Tibial plateau fractures: Evaluation and treatment. J Am Acad Orthop Surg 3:86–94, 1995.
5. Mize RD: Supracondylar and articular fractures in the distal femur. In Chapman M (ed): Operative Orthopedics. Philadelphia, J.B. Lippincott, 1988, pp 401–412.
6. Muller ME, Allgower M, Willinegger H: Manual of Internal Fixation: Technique Recommended by the AO Group. New York, Springer-Verlag, 1979, pp 249–250.
7. Whittle AP: Fractures of lower extremity. In Canale ST (ed): Campbell's Operative Orthopaedics, 9th ed. St. Louis, Mosby, 1998, pp 2042–2179.
8. Wiss DA: Supracondylar and intercondylar fractures of the femur. In Rockwood CA, Green DP, Bucholz RW (eds): Rockwood and Green's Fractures in Adults, 4th ed. Philadelphia, J.B. Lippincott, 1996.

IX. The Lower Leg

86. EXERTIONAL LEG PAIN

David E. Brown, M.D.

1. What is the differential diagnosis of chronic exertional leg pain?
- Medial tibial stress syndrome
- Chronic exertional compartment syndrome
- Stress fracture
- Vascular claudication
- Referred discogenic leg pain
- True shin splints (myositis or tendinitis of the anterior or lateral compartment muscles)

SHIN SPLINTS AND MEDIAL TIBIAL STRESS SYNDROME

2. What are shin splints?
A shin splint is an inflammatory condition of one or more of the musculotendinous units of the leg. It is most common in the anterior compartment muscles. Repetitive loading of the anterior compartment results in overloading and fatigue, which is often the result of early season conditioning and training errors such as running on hard surfaces, overly rapid increase in training intensity, weak ankle dorsiflexors (anterior compartment), poor shoes, or poor running technique.

3. How are common shin splints treated?
Treatment involves relative rest, icing, antiinflammatory medication, stretching of the antagonist muscle groups, and strengthening of the involved muscle group. Such measures are followed by a gradual return to athletics and activity. Cross-training activities are advised during the initial treatment phase. Immobilization is not recommended. All training errors, biomechanical abnormalities, and improper equipment should be evaluated and corrected.

4. Define medial tibial stress syndrome (MTSS). What are the physical findings? How is it treated?
MTSS is an inflammatory condition involving the periosteal attachment of the deep posterior compartment. Pain usually starts after exercise and is relieved by rest. However, symptoms may persist for hours or days after cessation of exercise.

On examination, a localized area of tenderness is found over the posterior medial edge of the distal third of the tibia. Evaluation of the foot may reveal either excessive valgus or varus. The rest of the examination is usually normal. Radiographs are usually normal.

Rest is the primary treatment for MTSS. Cross-training is required, often for an extended period until the stress periostitis resolves. Strength and flexibility of the deep posterior compartment should be emphasized. Abnormal hindfoot and forefoot alignment should be corrected. Recurrences are common.

5. Explain the role of orthotics in the management of MTSS.
One of the primary causes of MTSS is overpronation, which results in excessive motion and tension on the posterior tibialis and soleus muscle attachments. Orthotics may be used to prevent this overpronation. A semirigid orthotic with a medial post that maintains the hindfoot in neutral

position is most useful. A recent study in Canada found that hindfoot-forefoot varus may actually be more prevalent. Thus, it appears that any biomechanical foot malalignment may cause MTSS.

6. Explain the role of surgery in the treatment of MTSS.

Surgical treatment of MTSS is controversial. Fascial stripping and cauterization of the posterior medial ridge of the tibia have been advocated. However, controlled clinical studies have not been performed. Release of the superficial posterior compartment may be of benefit in resistant cases.

EXERTIONAL COMPARTMENT SYNDROME

7. Name the various leg compartments and the muscles within each compartment.

The four compartments include the anterior, lateral, superficial posterior, and deep posterior. The anterior compartment consists of the tibialis anterior, extensor digitorum longus, extensor hallucis longus, and peroneus tertius. The lateral compartment includes the peroneus longus and brevis. The superficial posterior has the gastrocsoleus complex, whereas the deep posterior compartment includes the posterior tibialis, flexor hallucis longus, and flexor digitorum longus. Some include the plantaris muscle in the deep posterior compartment.

8. What is *chronic* exertional compartment syndrome?

It is intermittent excessive pressure within an enclosed fascial compartment that occurs only during exercise. Pressures then slowly fall to normal following cessation of exercise, but the pressure falls much more slowly than normal. Recent studies have shown a relative deoxygenation during exercise as well as delayed reoxygenation after exercise. This hypoxia occurs in response to the increased intracompartmental pressure. Although not yet available clinically, near-infrared spectroscopy can measure the deoxygenation in exercising muscle leading to the possibility of a noninvasive measurement tool for chronic compartment syndrome.

9. How does chronic exertional compartment syndrome present?

Athletes typically have pain in the involved compartment that begins at a consistent time in their exercise sessions. Symptoms may then slowly subside after cessation of exercise. They may note numbness in the top of the foot and weakness of ankle dorsiflexion.

10. How is chronic exertional compartment syndrome diagnosed by pressure criteria?

In the presence of appropriate clinical findings, the diagnosis of chronic compartment syndrome exists if: (1) preexercise pressure is $\geq$ 15 mmHg; (2) 1-minute postexercise pressure is $\geq$ 30 mmHg; or (3) 5-minute postexercise pressure is $\geq$ 20 mmHg.

11. What is the incidence of bilaterality in chronic exertional compartment syndrome?

Fifty to 60%.

12. What is the incidence of muscle hernia in patients with chronic exertional compartment syndrome? Which nerve can be compressed by these muscle hernias?

The incidence of muscle hernia is 45%. It usually occurs in the distal third of the lateral compartment where the superficial peroneal nerve exits the compartment and becomes subcutaneous.

13. Which compartment is most commonly involved when a leg muscle hernia is present?

The lateral compartment. On some occasions, the superficial peroneal nerve passes through the anterior compartment, making it susceptible to hernia.

14. What are the treatment options for symptomatic leg muscle fascia hernia?
- Primary repair
- Fascial graft reconstruction
- Fasciotomy

Primary repair has been identified as a causative factor in acute compartment syndrome and is therefore not advised. Fascial graft reconstruction is an acceptable technique, although it is more extensive than fasciotomy. Complete fasciotomy affords relief of symptoms and has not been associated with leg muscle weakness or other significant morbidity, and therefore is the most commonly recommended treatment.

STRESS FRACTURES

15. Where is the most common location for stress fractures in the leg?
Stress fractures of the tibia are most common in the proximal third or at the junction of the middle and distal thirds along the posterior medial margin. Fibular stress fractures are most common in the supramalleolar region.

16. Do athletes and military recruits demonstrate different patterns of stress fracture?
Yes. Military recruits most commonly sustain stress fractures of the metatarsals (40%), whereas in athletes, metatarsal stress fractures constitute only 20% of the total number of stress fractures. Of all stress fractures in athletes, 45% affect the tibia and fibula.

17. What are anatomic risk factors for lower leg stress fractures?
- Genu varum
- Tibia varum
- Subtalar varus
- Forefoot varus
- Q angle greater than 15°
- Cavus foot
- Tarsal coalations

18. Why is a stress fracture of the anterior tibial cortex a cause for concern?
An uncommon tibial stress fracture occurs in the anterior tibial cortex, usually in the middle third of the tibia. Because this fracture occurs on the OtensionO side of the tibia, it is much more likely to progress to delayed union or nonunion. Prolonged immobilization and relative rest are required. In some cases, bone grafting of the anterior tibial stress fracture is required to obtain union.

19. When are x-rays positive in the presence of a tibial stress fracture?
At least 14 days must elapse following the onset of symptoms before the characteristic findings of stress fracture are evident. Initially, a single periosteal line may occur along the posterior aspect of the tibia. Later, the subperiosteal region calcifies, resulting in a localized area of sclerosis that is most characteristic of a stress fracture.

20. What is the role of MRI in the evaluation of stress fractures?
MRI is nearly as sensitive as bone scan in detecting stress syndrome. MRI is more accurate in localizing fracture location, does not expose the patient to ionizing radiation, and requires less imaging time. It is preferred over bone scan in the evaluation of femur stress fractures.

21. What is the role of the bone scan in the evaluation of stress fractures?
Technetium bone scan allows for earlier confirmation of a stress fracture. It may become positive within 48 hours of the onset of symptoms. It also is useful in the evaluation of persistent leg pain in which the diagnosis is unclear or if the possibility of multiple stress fractures exists.

22. Discuss the treatment of stress fractures.
The athlete must perform only painfree activities. That may initially require crutches for ambulation assistance. Tibial stress fractures should be treated with a long leg Air-Cast splint. This

will allow return to play in 3–4 weeks instead of 2–3 months. The athlete should begin a walking program once painfree, progressively increasing to short jog intervals, longer jog intervals and eventually running.

23. What is the best predictive test for return to sports after tibial stress fracture?
Pain free single leg hop test (10 hops on the affected leg).

BIBLIOGRAPHY

1. Andrish JT, Bergfeld JH, Walheim J: A prospective study on the management of shin splints. J Bone Joint Surg 56A:1697, 1974.
2. AAOS Symposium on the Foot and Leg in Running Sports. St. Louis, Mosby, 1982.
3. Boden BP, Speer KP: Femoral stress fractures. Clin Sports Med 16:307–317, 1997.
4. Detmer DE, Sharpe K, Sufit RL, et al: Chronic compartment syndrome: Diagnosis, management and outcome. Am J Sports Med 13:163, 1985.
5. Fredericson M, Bergman AG, Hoffman KL, et al: Tibial stress reaction in runners. Correlation of clinical symptoms and scintigraphy with a new magnetic resonance imaging grading system. Am J Sports Med 23:472–481, 1995.
6. Holen KJ, Engebretsen L, Grontuendt T, et al: Surgical treatment of medial tibial stress syndrome (shin splint) by fasciotomy of the superficial posterior compartment of the leg. Scand J Med Sci Sports 5:40–43, 1995.
7. Korpelianen R. Orava S, Karpakka J, et al: Risk factors for recurrent stress fractures in athletes. Am J Sports Med 29:304–310, 2001
8. Lidor C, Ferris LR, Hall R, et al: Stress fracture of the tibia after arthrodesis of the ankle or the hindfoot. J Bone Joint Surg 79A:558–564, 1997.
9. Mohler LR, Styf JR, Pedowitz RA, et al: Intramuscular deoxygenation during exercise in patients who have chronic anterior compartment syndrome of the leg. J Bone Joint Surg 79A:844–849, 1997.
10. Mubarak SJ, et al: The medial tibial stress syndrome: A cause of shin splints. Am J Sports Med 10:201, 1992.
11. Pedowitz RA, Hargens AR, Mubarak SJ, et al: Modified criteria for the objective diagnosis of chronic compartment syndrome of the leg. Am J Sports Med 18:35, 1990.
12. Rorabeck CH, Fowler PJ, Nott L: The results of fasciotomy in the management of chronic compartment syndrome. Am J Sports Med 16:224–227, 1988.
13. Siddiqui AR: Bone scans for the early detection of stress fractures. N Engl J Med 298:1033, 1978.
14. Singerman R, White C, Davy DT: Reduction of patellofemoral contact forces following anterior displacement of the tibial tubercle. J Orthop Res 13:279–285, 1995.
15. Sommer HM, Valentine SW: Effect of foot posture on the incidence of medial tibial stress syndrome. Med Sci Sports Exerc 27:800–804, 1995.
16. Swenson EJ, DeHaven KE, Sebastianelli WJ, et.al.: The effect of a pneumatic leg brace on return to play in athletes with tibial stress fractures. Am J Sports Med 25:322–328, 1997.
17. Styf JR, Korner LM: Chronic anterior-compartment syndrome of the leg: Results of treatment by fasciotomy. J Bone Joint Surg 68A:1338, 1986.

87. ACUTE COMPARTMENT SYNDROME

David E. Brown, M.D., and Kristoffer M. Breien, M.D.

1. What is acute compartment syndrome?
An acute compartment syndrome is the result of increased tissue pressure within an enclosed anatomic space surrounded by semi-rigid fascia. The increase in tissue pressure leads to venous obstruction and collapse of the low-pressure arteriolar plexus, thereby reducing blood flow through the capillary network.

2. What are the primary causes of acute compartment syndrome?

Eighty-five percent of cases of acute compartment syndrome are caused by severe trauma associated with fractures or dislocations of the leg. The remainder are generally caused by marked and prolonged increase in exercise intensity, such as a forced, prolonged run by a military recruit. A small number are caused by muscle rupture, vascular injury, or prolonged externally applied pressure such as a tight cast or wound dressing.

3. How is the diagnosis of acute compartment syndrome made?

The diagnosis is made entirely based on the physical exam in an awake, cooperative patient. The three major clinical findings are:
- Palpation of firm tender compartments
- Unrelenting pain out of proportion to the injury which is not relieved by increasing levels of pain medication
- Increased pain in the extremity with passive muscle stretch.

In the case of an obtunded, intubated, or uncooperative patient, frequent mechanical measurement of compartment pressures is necessary.

4. What is a normal intramuscular compartment pressure measurement at rest?

Zero to 10 mmHg.

5. At what pressure does acute compartment syndrome exist?

Experts differ on the exact pressure at which a compartment should be released. Some advocate fasciotomy for any compartment pressure measurement greater than 30 mmHg, while others will observe and monitor pressures closely up to 45 mmHg before performing a fasciotomy. In conjunction with the above pressure measurement thresholds, many advocate fasciotomy once the compartment pressure rises to within <30 mmHg of the diastolic blood pressure of the patient.

6. Name the various leg compartments and the muscles within each compartment.

The four compartments are the anterior, lateral, superficial posterior, and deep posterior. The **anterior** compartment consists of the tibialis anterior, extensor digitorum longus, extensor hallucis longus, and peroneus tertius. The **lateral** compartment includes the peroneus longus and brevis. The **superficial posterior** has the gastrocsoleus complex, whereas the **deep posterior** compartment includes the posterior tibialis, flexor hallucis longus, and flexor digitorum longus.

7. Which compartment is most commonly involved in an acute compartment syndrome?

The anterior compartment is by far the most commonly involved. The lateral compartment is the next most frequent.

8. How are compartment pressures measured?

Compartment pressures may be measured using a variety of techniques, including needle manometer, wick catheter, slit catheter, and microcapillary infusion. The needle manometer pressure measurements are the easiest to obtain and require the least expensive equipment. An advantage of the wick and slit catheters is that they may be left in place, allowing serial or continuous pressure measurements without the necessity of repeated needle insertion into the leg. It is important to obtain measurements close to the zone of injury because pressure tends to decrease as the distance from the injury increases.

9. Is a compartment syndrome more likely to occur with a closed or open tibia fracture?

A closed tibia fracture. In open tibia fractures, the muscle fascia has frequently been effectively released due to the tissue disruption at the time of injury. However, grade III open fractures are associated with increased risk of compartment syndrome, perhaps because of the severity of the injury.

10. What is the risk of compartment syndrome in the presence of popliteal artery injury?

Compartment syndrome does not occur in the presence of popliteal artery occlusion. Rather, it is the reperfusion that follows appropriate surgical repair of a popliteal artery injury that places the leg at risk for compartment syndrome. Reperfusion following the repair often leads to marked swelling and increase in intracompartment pressures. Four-compartment release is generally advised following surgical repair of complete popliteal artery injuries.

11. What is the treatment of acute compartment syndrome?

Once the diagnosis of acute compartment syndrome is established, the only treatment is emergent surgical decompression through single- or double-incision fasciotomy. In rare instances where the compartment syndrome is the result of a constrictive dressing or tight cast, simple removal of the cast or bandage may be sufficient to relieve symptoms. Note that elevation of the affected extremity is *never* appropriate as this only serves to increase the arterial pressure required to perfuse the extremity.

12. How is surgical decompression performed?

Fasciotomy is generally accomplished by one of two different methods. The first method is performed through a single lateral incision. This lateral perifibular approach allows access to all four compartments. This technique is somewhat more technically demanding, especially in cases of trauma because normal anatomy may be distorted.

The second method employs both a medial and lateral incision. The lateral incision allows access to the anterior and lateral compartments, whereas the medial incision allows access to both posterior compartments.

Regardless of technique, the wounds must be left open. If the compartment syndrome has resulted in muscle ischemia and death, all necrotic muscle must be debrided surgically. Wounds should be reevaluated at 48–72 hours and undergo repeat irrigation and debridement. Final wound closure and possible split-thickness skin grafting is accomplished 5–7 days after the initial fasciotomy.

13. Why should the urine be monitored following treatment of acute compartment syndrome?

If muscle ischemia and death has occurred, myoglobinuria may result. The patient should be well hydrated. Renal function must be monitored closely.

14. What clinical problems are most likely to be confused with acute compartment syndrome? How are they differentiated from compartment syndrome?

The most common diagnoses confused with acute compartment syndrome are acute traumatic nerve contusion (neurapraxia), arterial injury, and traumatic hematoma.

Neurapraxia most commonly involves the peroneal nerve. The compartments are not tense; there is no increased pain with passive stretch; and pain is generally not a substantial symptom.

In arterial injury, pulses are absent, and the limb is ischemic. Arterial studies are abnormal. Conversely, in an acute compartment syndrome, pulses are present barring a concomittant arterial injury.

A large intramuscular hematoma may result in significant pain, swelling, and tightness of the compartment and occasionally may cause a compartment syndrome. In this case, vigilance and frequent examinations are crucial.

15. What are the complications of an untreated acute compartment syndrome?

An unrecognized or untreated acute compartment syndrome will ultimately lead to the death and loss of function of the neuromuscular structures within the affected compartment. Volkmann's contractures, paralysis, and sensory loss are the end result once the necrotic tissue is replaced by scar.

Surgical release of an acute compartment syndrome must be accomplished emergently once the diagnosis is made. A fasciotomy which is delayed 6–8 hours after the onset of symptoms may necessitate the debridement of large amounts of necrotic muscle. Ultimately, this may result in deep tissue infection and amputation.

16. How much time does a clinician have from the onset of acute compartment syndrome until the occurrence of tissue death and necrosis?
Muscle cell death and subsequent necrosis may occur as early as 4 hours following the onset of compartment syndrome. Muscle tissue rarely remains viable if 8 hours have elapsed prior to restoration of perfusion.

BIBLIOGRAPHY

1. Azar FM, Pickering RM: Traumatic disorders. In Canale ST (ed): Campbell's Operative Orthopaedics, 9th ed. St. Louis, Mosby, 1998, pp 1405–1416.
2. Blick SS, Brumback RJ, Poka A, et al: Compartment syndrome in open tibial fractures. J Bone Joint Surg 68A:1348–1353, 1986.
3. Cohen MS, Garfin SR, Hargens AR, Mubarak SJ: Acute compartment syndrome: Effect of dermotomy on fascial decompression in the leg. J Bone Joint Surg 73A:287–290, 1991.
4. Gershuni DH, Mubarak SJ, Yaru NC, Lee YF: Fracture of the tibia complicated by acute compartment syndrome. Clin Orthop 217:221–227, 1987.
5. Gwynne Jones DP, Theis JC: Acute compartment syndrome due to closed muscle rupture. Aust N Z J Surg 67:227–228, 1997.
6. Heckman MM, Whitesides TE Jr, Grewe SR, et al: Histologic determination of the ischemic threshold of muscle in the canine compartment syndrome model. J Orthop Trauma 7:199–210, 1993.
7. Heppenstall RB, Scott R, Sapega A, et al: A comparative study of the tolerance of skeletal muscle to ischemia: Tourniquet application compared with acute compartment syndrome. J Bone Joint Surg 68A:820–828, 1986.
8. Matsen FA III, Winquist RA, Krugmire RB Jr: Diagnosis and management of compartmental syndromes. J Bone Joint Surg 62A:286–291, 1980.
9. McQueen MM, Christie J, Court-Brown CM: Acute compartment syndrome in tibial diaphyseal fractures. J Bone Joint Surg 78B:95–98, 1996.
10. McQueen MM, Court-Brown CM: Compartment monitoring in tibial fractures. The pressure threshold for decompression. J Bone Joint Surg 78B:99–104, 1996.
11. Papalambros EL, Panayiotopoulos YP, Bastounis E, et al: Prophylactic fasciotomy of the legs following acute arterial occlusion procedures. Int Angiol 8:120–124, 1989.
12. Rorabeck CH: The treatment of compartment syndromes of the leg. J Bone Joint Surg 66A:93–97, 1984.
13. Whitesides TE, Haney TC, Morimoto K, Harada H: Tissue pressure measurements as a determinant for the need of fasciotomy. Clin Orthop 113:43–51, 1975.

88. ACHILLES TENDON

David E. Brown, M.D.

1. What are the causes of Achilles tendinitis?
- Inflexibility of the tendo Achillis
- Overpronation
- Recent change in shoe wear
- Recent increase in training, especially if it includes hill running

2. What are the signs and symptoms of acute Achilles tendinitis?
- Pain over the distal Achilles tendon
- Swelling
- Painful push-off phase of running or jumping

3. How is acute Achilles tendinitis treated?
- Relative rest (avoid painful, aggravating activities)
- Ice and/or contrast treatments
- Antiinflammatory medication
- Orthotics/heel lift
- Stretching
- If symptoms are severe and recalcitrant to the above measures, a short period of cast immobilization may be necessary.

4. Describe the treatment of chronic Achilles tendinitis.
The initial treatment of chronic Achilles tendinitis is the same as for acute injuries. Persistent symptoms, especially in individuals who have a discrete area of thickening in the tendon on physical examination, may be because of a partial tear. The tear may be evaluated by magnetic resonance imaging (MRI).

5. How should I treat the patient with chronic Achilles tendinitis who is unresponsive to conservative management?
If the patient has had symptoms for at least 6 months, has been engaged in a defined physical therapy program, and has symptoms that prevent him or her from participating in athletics or work, surgical treatment may be offered. Preoperative evaluation with MRI is usually involved. The tendon is explored, partial tears of the tendon are surgically debrided, and remaining tissue is repaired as necessary. A thickening of the peritenon should be incised or excised. Satisfactory results are obtained in two-thirds of patients. Proximal tears ($>$ 3 cm above the calcaneus) do better than distal tears.

6. Why isn't cortisone injected into the Achilles tendon when it is either acutely or chronically inflamed?
Injection of the Achilles tendon or its sheath has been implicated as the cause of subsequent Achilles tendon rupture. Corticosteroids markedly decrease the metabolic rate of chondrocytes and fibrocytes, thereby weakening the structural integrity of tendon and articular cartilage.

7. Who is most at risk for sustaining an Achilles tendon tear?
Tears are most commonly seen in males between the ages of 30 and 50 years who are generally recreational athletes or nonathletes engaged in white-collar occupations. During participation in a jumping sport, a sudden forceful contraction of the Achilles causes a rupture. At least 50% of patients who sustain complete tears have had preexisting symptoms of chronic tendinitis.

8. Describe the physical findings in an acute complete Achilles tendon rupture.
A palpable defect in the tendon is present as the proximal tendon retracts following rupture. The gap is usually 2–3 cm long. Within 24–48 hours, marked swelling and ecchymosis usually occur. The patient is able to weakly plantarflex the foot. The Thompson test is positive.

9. What is the Thompson test?
With the patient supine and the affected foot over the end of the table, squeeze the calf and observe for ankle motion. A positive Thompson test occurs when *no* plantar flexion of the ankle occurs when the calf is squeezed. The test is positive in acute complete Achilles tendon tears. In a gastrocnemius muscle tear, no defect in the tendon is present, and the foot plantarflexes as the calf is squeezed during the Thompson test.

10. What is important about the vascular supply to the Achilles tendon?
An area of relative hypovascularity is found 2–5 cm proximal to the Achilles tendon insertion, which is where most Achilles tendon ruptures occur.

11. How are tears of the Achilles tendon treated?

Surgical repair is generally indicated. Older or sedentary individuals may choose to have the Achilles tear immobilized in an equinus cast for 4–6 weeks, followed by a short-leg walking cast for another 2 weeks.

Repair of the Achilles tendon rupture results in improvement in maximum ankle plantar flexion strength, particularly in the aggressive athlete. The risk of re-rupture is much less (2% re-rupture rate in the surgically treated group compared with 8% re-rupture rate in the nonoperative group). However, surgical treatment carries the risk of anesthetic complication, skin and soft tissue breakdown, and neuroma of the sural nerve.

12. How should the patient be rehabilitated after repair of an Achilles tendon rupture?

Rehabilitation is controversial. The conservative approach places the repaired tendon in a cast for up to 3 months. Initially the cast is in an equinus cast so that theoretically the tension is taken off the repair site. The more aggressive approach places the leg in a splint for as little as 1–3 weeks after surgery, followed by a dorsiflexion stop splint, which allows the patient to plantarflex the foot from the neutral position but prevents dorsiflexion past neutral, thereby eliminating excessive tension on the repair site. Animal studies have indicated that early mild tension coupled with motion at tendon repair sites enhances healing by hastening the alignment of collagen fibrils at the repair site. Patients who are allowed early motion return to activities sooner, miss less work and have similar clinical results.

13. How much strain is there on the Achilles tendon repair during weightbearing/walking?

Minimal. Animal studies demonstrate that the strain is not statistically greater than ambulation in a non–weight-bearing cast. Thus, postoperative or postinjury weightbearing is not detrimaental to the Achilles tendon.

14. Does the plantaris muscle really rupture?

Years ago it was thought that patients with a sudden pop and pain in the medial calf had sustained a rupture of the plantaris muscle, commonly called "tennis leg." However, the plantaris muscle has never been shown to be torn in this setting. On the contrary, plantaris muscle is noted to be present and not ruptured in individuals who have sustained an acute Achilles tendon rupture and is frequently used as a tissue donor source to reinforce the Achilles repair. The injury sustained in this clinical situation is more likely a partial disruption of the medial head of the gastrocnemius muscle belly.

15. What is the treatment of a partial tear of the medial head of the gastrocnemius muscle?

- Heel lift and calf sleeve
- Avoidance of running, jumping, and push-off activities for approximately 4–6 weeks
- Ice massage
- Gentle stretching as tolerated

BIBLIOGRAPHY

1. Incavo SJ, Alvarez RG, Trevino SG: Occurrence of the plantaris tendon in patients sustaining subcutaneous rupture of the Achilles tendon. Foot Ankle 8:110, 1987.
2. James SL, Bates BT, Osterning LR: Injuries to runners. Am J Sports Med 6:40, 1978.
3. Maagard NH, Skov O, Jensen PE: Early motion of the ankle after operative treatment of a rupture of the Achilles tendon. Am J Sports Med 7:983, 1999.
4. Mafulli N: Rupture of the Achilles tendon. Am J Sports Med 7:1019, 1999.
5. Morberg P, Jerre R, Sward L, et al: Long-term results after surgical management of partial Achilles tendon ruptures. Scand J Med Sci Sports 7:299–303, 1997.
6. Motta P, Errichiello C, Pontini I: Achilles tendon rupture. A new technique for easy surgical repair and immediate movement of the ankle and foot. Am J Sports Med 25:172–176, 1997.
7. Nelen G, Martens M, Burssens A: Surgical treatment of chronic Achilles tendinitis. Am J Sports Med 17:754, 1989.

8. Nistor L: Surgical and non-surgical treatment of Achilles tendon ruptures. J Bone Joint Surg 63A:394, 1981.
9. Pritchett JW: C-reactive protein levels determine the severity of soft-tissue injuries. Am J Orthop 25: 759–761, 1996.
10. Richardson EG: Disorders of tendons and fascia. In Canale ST (ed): Campbell's Operative Orthopaedics, 9th ed. St. Louis, Mosby, 1998, pp 1889–1925.
11. Roberts JM, Goldstrom GL, Brown TD, et al: Comparison of unrepaired, primarily repaired, and poly-galactin mesh-reinforced Achilles tendon lacerations in rabbits. Clin Orthop 181:244, 1993.
12. Rupp S, Tempelhof S, Fritsch E: Ultrasound of the Achilles tendon after surgical repair: Morphology and function. Br J Radiol 68:454–458, 1995.
13. Shields CL, Redix L, Brewster CE: Acute tears of the medial head of the gastrocnemius. Foot Ankle 5:186, 1985.
14. Thompson TC, Doherty JH: Spontaneous rupture of the tendon of the Achilles: A new clinical diagnostic test. J Trauma 2:126, 1962.
15. Watson TW, Jurist UA, Yang UH, Shen UL: The strength of Achilles tendon repair: An in vitro study of the biomechanical behavior in human cadaver tendons. Foot Ankle Int 16:191–195, 1995.

89. TIBIAL FRACTURES

Matthew A. Mormino, M.D.

1. Describe the appropriate evaluation of a patient with a tibial fracture.

The evaluation of all trauma victims should follow advanced trauma life support (ATLS) protocol. The extremity should be inspected for deformity, tenderness, and crepitus. A baseline neurologic exam should document the status of motor function and sensory response to pinprick and light touch. A vascular exam should include palpation and Doppler evaluation of the dorsalis pedis and posterior tibial pulses. If pulses are absent, the extremity should be gently realigned and the exam repeated. The presence of soft-tissue injuries should be noted. Compartment syndrome may appear early after a tibia fracture and should be looked for. An anteroposterior and lateral x-ray that includes the knee and ankle should be obtained.

2. What are the signs and symptoms of acute compartment syndrome in the leg?

Pain out of proportion to the injury is the hallmark finding. Pain with passive stretch of the toes and ankle and palpably tense compartments are the other important findings. Pulselessness, pallor, paresthesias, and paralysis are findings associated with established or late compartment syndrome. In an awake patient this clinical diagnosis should be treated emergently. Compartment pressure measurements may be relied on to confirm a diagnosis of acute compartment syndrome only in obtunded or anesthetized patients (epidural and spinal anesthesia also may mask the symptoms).

3. How is acute compartment syndrome treated?

Emergent release of all four compartments of the leg (anterior, lateral, superficial posterior, deep posterior) should be performed in all cases of acute compartment syndrome via a lateral incision or medial and lateral incisions.

4. Describe Gustilo's open fracture classification.

Type I: < 1-cm wound, low-energy fracture
Type II: 1–10-cm wound, higher energy fracture
Type III: > 10-cm wound, high-energy fracture
Type IIIA: Moderate periosteal stripping, wound closure not requiring soft tissue flap
Type IIIB: Marked periosteal stripping, wound closure requires soft tissue flap
Type IIIC: Any open fracture with a vascular injury that requires repair

This classification system is the source of endless arguments among orthopaedists; do not feel bad if you cannot accurately classify a fracture. Chances are, neither can your attending.

5. How should an open tibial fracture be treated in the emergency room?

Evaluate and treat all life-threatening injuries according to ATLS protocol. Document the soft-tissue injury and neurovascular exam. Remove gross debris, apply a sterile dressing, and splint the extremity. Probing, irrigating, and culturing of the wound should be done in the operating room as part of a formal irrigation and debridement. Start appropriate antibiotics.

6. Which antibiotics are appropriate for an open fracture?

A first-generation cephalosporin (Ancef) should be given for all open fractures. Add an aminoglycoside (gentamicin) for type III injuries, and add penicillin for barnyard or heavily contaminated wounds. Tetanus status should be assessed and updated or treated appropriately.

7. What are the indications for casting a tibial fracture?

Closed reduction and casting is an option only in closed low-energy fractures in young patients. After an acceptable reduction, the fracture is placed in a long leg cast for 6–8 weeks and then replaced with a short-leg cast or fracture brace until the fracture heals. Healing rates of 90% may be expected. However, recent studies suggest that long-term knee and ankle function is improved in patients treated with operative stabilization.

8. What is an acceptable reduction?

Less than 1 cm shortening, $< 5°$ angulation in any plane, $< 10°$ of malrotation, and $> 50\%$ cortical apposition.

9. What are the indications for operative fixation?

Failure to achieve an adequate reduction, multiple trauma, ipsilateral femoral fracture, bilateral tibial fractures, fractures with compartment syndrome, fractures with vascular injury, and pathologic fractures.

10. When is external fixation recommended?

External fixation is considered the gold standard for treatment of type III open tibial fractures. Recent studies that show similar infection rates and union rates with lower rates of malalignment challenge this practice.

11. When is intramedullary nailing recommended?

Failed closed treatment and unstable fractures are the main indications for intramedullary (IM) nailing. Some authors recommend IM nailing for all open fractures.

12. What are the main differences between reamed and unreamed tibial nailing?

Reamed nailing involves machining the medullary canal to allow intimate endosteal cortical contact and passage of a large diameter nail. The use of a smaller diameter nail without reaming is indicated primarily for open fractures. The main advantage of unreamed tibial nailing is that the medullary blood supply reconstitutes faster (however, it is disrupted by the passage of the nail). The primary disadvantage is that the smaller diameter nail has a less intimate fit and is thus a less stable construct.

13. What is the infection rate for open tibial fractures?

Type I and II: 1–2%; type IIIA: 3–5%; type IIIB and C: 10–50%.

14. How are infections managed?

Irrigation and debridement of all necrotic tissue is mandatory. Removal of hardware is indicated if the fracture is healed or if the hardware is loose. The hardware is retained if the fracture is not healed and the hardware is stable. Antibiotics are used to suppress the infection until the fracture is healed and the hardware is removed.

15. What are the soft tissue coverage options for open tibial fractures?

Exposed bone should be covered in 5 days with muscle or fasciocutaneous flaps. In proximal third fractures, use a gastrocnemius flap; in middle third fractures use a soleus flap (however, the soleus is often damaged by the trauma); and in distal third fractures use a free muscle flap.

16. Describe a tibial plateau fracture.

Fractures involving the articular surface of the proximal tibia are termed tibial plateau fractures. They are usually the result of an axial loading mechanism and may involve one or both condyles and often have both split and depressed fractures. Knee ligament injury occurs in 10–20% of such fractures.

17. What are the operative indications for tibial plateau fractures?

This is controversial. Fracture type, patient age, and the patient's functional demands all influence treatment choices. In general, articular stepoff of > 3 mm, depression of > 5 mm, varus or valgus laxity $> 10°$, and fractures involving the medial plateau are operative indications.

18. What is a Segond fracture?

A Segond fracture is an avulsion fracture of the lateral tibial plateau and usually signifies an anterior cruciate ligament injury.

19. What is a tibial pilon fracture?

Fractures that involve the articular surface of the tibia are termed pilon fractures. They usually result from an axial load impacting the talus into the distal tibia. Comminution and massive soft tissue injury reflect the high-energy trauma resulting in such injuries. Surgery is aimed at restoration of the joint surface and preservation of the tenuous soft tissue envelope.

BIBLIOGRAPHY

1. Blachut PA, et al : Interlocking intramedullary nailing with and without reaming for the treatment of closed fractures of the tibial shaft. J Bone Joint Surg 79A: 640–646, 1997.
2. Gustilo RB, Anderson JT: Prevention of infection in the treatment of one thousand and twenty-five open fractures of long bones. J Bone Joint Surg 58A:453–458, 1976.
3. Hansen ST Jr, Swiontkowski MF (eds): Orthopaedic Trauma Protocols. New York, Raven Press, 1993.
4. Mast JW, et al: Fractures of the tibial pilon. Clin Orthop 230:68–82, 1988.
5. Rockwood CA Jr, Green DP, Bucholz RW, Heckman JD (eds): Rockwood and Green's Fractures in Adults, vols. 1 and 2, 4th ed. Philadelphia, J.B. Lippincott, 1996.
6. Schemitsch EH, et al: Comparison of the effects of reamed and unreamed locked intramedullary nailing on blood flow in the callus and strength of union following fracture of the sheep tibia. J Orthop Res 13:382–389, 1995.
7. Whittle AP: Fractures of lower extremity. In Canale ST (ed): Campbell's Operative Orthopaedics, 9th ed. St. Louis, Mosby, 1998, pp 2067–2111.

X. Foot and Ankle

90. ANKLE SPRAINS AND INSTABILITY

Michael P. Clare, M.D.

1. In a patient with acute ankle pain, what important historical points need to be covered?
- Mechanism of injury—position the foot was in both before and after the traumatic event
- Location of pain—medial or lateral, proximal or distal
- Weight-bearing ability
- Patient age
- Time of injury
- History of prior injury

2. What are the important physical findings?
Swelling, ecchymoses, tenderness, neurovascular status, range of motion, crepitus, stability, and deformity.

3. Which radiographic views are necessary during the initial work-up?
Ankle radiographs include an anteroposterior (AP), lateral, and mortise view. If a foot injury is suspected, an AP, lateral, and oblique view of the foot should each be obtained as well.

4. What injuries are included in the differential diagnosis?
Fracture of the lateral malleolus, medial malleolus, or both; fracture of the lateral process of the talus; osteochondral lesion of the talar dome; inversion (lateral ligamentous) sprain; eversion (deltoid) sprain; syndesmotic injury; and other muscular or tendinous injury, such as an Achilles tendon rupture, posterior tibial tendon dysfunction or rupture, or peroneal tendon rupture, instability, or tear. Additionally, foot injuries with similar mechanisms must be excluded, including fractures of the base of the fifth metatarsal or midfoot (LisFranc joint).

5. Describe the findings consistent with an inversion sprain.
The most obvious finding is the mechanism of rolling over the foot onto the lateral ankle. A previous history of similar sprains is also common. On physical exam anterolateral tenderness and swelling with a positive anterior drawer test should be present (see question 6). Pain is typically not severe enough to inhibit weightbearing, and no bony crepitus should be present.

6. How is the anterior drawer test administered, and what constitutes a positive anterior drawer test?
The test is performed by stabilizing the distal tibia with one hand and grasping the posterior heel with the other. Then, an anterior force is applied to the posterior heel in an effort to displace the talus anteriorly. A large shift anteriorly, or even a palpable clunk in severe cases, indicates a positive anterior drawer test. The uninjured ankle should be examined for comparison.

7. Which lateral ligament is most commonly injured?
The lateral ligament most commonly injured is the anterior talofibular ligament, which is the primary lateral stabilizer of the ankle in plantar flexion. The calcaneofibular ligament is a secondary stabilizer and resists inversion of the talus and calcaneus; thus it plays a major role in sta-

bility of the subtalar joint. The calcaneofibular ligament is usually disrupted in association with a tear of the anterior talofibular ligament. The posterior talofibular ligament resists dorsiflexion–external rotation forces in the ankle and is rarely sprained. Of the lateral ankle ligaments, the calcaneofibular ligament is by far the strongest, followed by the posterior talofibular ligament, and lastly the anterior talofibular ligament.

8. Describe the findings consistent with an eversion sprain.

An eversion sprain occurs when the foot is caught in a pronated, everted position with concomitant internal rotation of the upper body. Swelling and tenderness is present medially and possibly higher up the leg, indicating a syndesmosis injury. Such patients have pain with an eversion stress to their ankles but have a negative anterior drawer test.

9. Which structure is primarily injured in an eversion sprain?

The deltoid ligament is primarily injured in an eversion sprain. It originates from the inferior portion of the medial malleolus and attaches to the medial talar neck and body. It functions to stabilize the ankle during eversion and prevents subluxation of the talus.

10. How do you classify ankle sprains?

Grade I   Negative anterior drawer and talar tilt test
Grade II Positive anterior drawer/negative talar tilt test
Grade III Positive anterior drawer and talar tilt test

11. What is the talar tilt test?

The talar tilt test examines the integrity of the calcaneofibular ligament and the anterior talofibular ligament. It is performed by grasping the foot and heel while attempting to invert the talus on the tibia.

12. What is a normal talar tilt test?

Normal individuals rarely have a talar tilt test $> 5°$. A marked difference when compared with the opposite uninjured ankle usually represents insufficiency of the anterior talofibular and calcaneofibular ligaments. Clinically, this is hard to interpret. Stress x-rays are often helpful.

13. When are talar tilt stress x-rays positive?

Compared with the contralateral normal extremity, a difference of $10°$ is considered a positive test.

14. What is the initial treatment for a mild (grade I) ankle sprain?

Rest, ice, compression, and elevation (RICE). Protected weight-bearing with early mobilization and range-of-motion and isometric exercises are also involved. If the patient is improving, after 2–3 weeks advance to ankle group muscle strengthening, proprioceptive training, and functional activities with protective bracing.

15. What is the treatment for more severe ankle sprains (grade II or III) and for patients with mild sprains that do not improve?

Patients with severe sprains or sprains recalcitrant to initial home rehabilitation benefit from a supervised rehabilitation program that progressively advances weightbearing in a protected manner using isometrics or closed kinetic chain exercises. Such patients also often benefit from proprioceptive training. More severe sprains may require supportive bracing for up to 6 months during sports.

16. What is proprioception?

Proprioception involves specialized sets of mechanoreceptors within muscles, tendons, and ligaments that sense joint movement and joint position. These receptors contribute to complex motor processes for neuromuscular control and precision movements of the joint as well as to muscle reflexes that provide dynamic stability to the joint. In essence, proprioception helps determine where the joint is in three-dimensional space and thus provide protective reflexes accordingly. These receptors are present in the anterior talofibular ligament and the cervical ligament of the subtalar joint, and, to a lesser degree, in the deltoid and calcaneofibular ligaments.

17. What is the purpose of proprioceptive rehabilitation?

Proprioceptive rehabilitation includes joint positioning activities to convert conscious motor programming to unconscious in order to regain joint sense awareness and initiate reflex stabilization to prevent reinjury.

18. What structures make up the syndesmotic ligaments? What is their function?

Four ligaments form the syndesmotic ligament complex: (1) the anterior inferior tibiofibular ligament, (2) the posterior inferior tibiofibular ligament, (3) the transverse tibiofibular ligament, and (4) the interosseous ligament. The four ligaments maintain the integrity between the distal tibia and the fibula and resist the axial, rotational, and translational forces that would otherwise separate the two bones.

19. In a patient with a suspected eversion ankle sprain (see question 8), how is a syndesmosis sprain diagnosed? How is it treated?

Patients have extreme tenderness over the syndesmosis, a positive squeeze test, pain with abduction or external rotation of the ankle, pain with weightbearing, and normal x-rays. Treatment should be supervised, consisting of RICE, toe-touch weight-bearing until pain-free, gradual mobilization and range-of-motion exercises, progressive strengthening exercises, and proprioceptive training.

20. Describe the squeeze test.

The squeeze test is performed by squeezing the distal fibular and tibia together. A positive test is indicated by tenderness over the syndesmosis and is consistent with an injury to this area.

21. How is a complete syndesmosis injury (tibiofibular diastasis) diagnosed? How is it treated?

In this injury, the ligaments holding the tibia and fibula have ruptured completely; thus the ankle mortise is unstable. Pateints have similar exam findings as those with a syndesmosis sprain (see question 19). Radiographs typically show widening of the medial clear space (between the medial malleolus and medial talar dome) relative to the lateral clear space (between the lateral malleolus and lateral talar dome). The mortise needs to be reduced and held together with syndesmosis screws. The distance between the tibia and fibula is fixed and stable after reduction and screw fixation.

22. What are the findings in a patient with a muscle or tendon injury to the ankle?

The patient has swelling or bruising over the injured muscle or tendon. A palpable defect in the injured area may be found along with tenderness. The specific function of the injured muscle should be tested to determine its integrity. No crepitus or significant bony tenderness should be present.

23. What are the hallmark findings in Achilles tendon rupture?

Patients have a history of a sudden, severe pop. They have pain and swelling over the Achilles tendon or calf and may have a palpable defect in the tendon in addition to weak plantar flexion strength and a positive Thompson test.

24. How is the Thompson test conducted?

The patient is placed prone with the affected knee bent at 90°. The calf is squeezed and the foot is examined for plantarflexion. No plantarflexion with squeezing indicates a division in the Achilles tendon complex and and a positive Thompson test.

25. Describe the hallmark findings in posterior tibial tendon dysfunction or rupture.

A preexisting or increased flat foot (pes planus) deformity, swelling or tenderness medially and posterior to the medial malleolus, abduction deformity of the midfoot, decreased heel inversion on heel rise test, or inability to do heel rise, depending on the degree of severity.

26. Describe the hallmark findings in peroneal tendon instability, rupture, or tear.

A history of a plantarflexion-inversion injury, pain in the lateral ankle and posterior to the lateral malleolus, tenderness along the muscle/tendon unit, and, occasionally, dislocatable tendons with resisted eversion/plantarflexion. The peroneus brevis tendon is most commonly torn, typically from a wedging effect between the peroneus longus and the lateral malleolus.

27. Despite the correct treatment, what percentage of patients who suffer a grade III ankle sprain have persistent pain or instability that limits their activities?

Approximately 20–40% of such patients are reported to have residual pain necessitating an alteration in activities. Often the pain can be localized to the anterior or anterolateral ankle.

28. What is the differential diagnosis for a patient who presents with persistent pain after an ankle sprain?

Inadequate or incomplete rehabilitation; osteochondral lesions of the talar dome; chronic ankle ligamentous instability; peroneal tendinitis or tear; ankle impingement; a meniscoid lesion; sinus tarsi syndrome; or a stress fracture.

29. When does impingement occur? How is it treated?

Impingement occurs when the anterior capsule of the ankle is repeatedly traumatized during dorsi and plantar flexion. The trauma may eventually lead to scarring or calcifications that form off the anterior edge of the distal tibia. It may be treated nonoperatively with ice and antiinflammatory medications. If the process is recalcitrant to the initial therapy, the lesions can be resected arthroscopically.

30. What is sinus tarsi syndrome?

Pain and tenderness over the opening of the sinus tarsi characterize sinus tarsi syndrome. It is accompanied by a sensation of instability that in most cases occurs after trauma. Injecting anesthetic and steroid into the sinus tarsi usually relieves pain; however, some chronic cases may require tissue excision or even subtalar arthrodesis.

31. What is a meniscoid lesion?

A meniscoid lesion is a localized fibrotic synovitis in the lateral compartment of the ankle caused by repetitive sprains. Treatment consists of arthroscopic excision of scar tissue.

32. In the acute setting, when is surgery indicated for an ankle sprain?

Never. Studies have shown no advantage in surgical repair for ankle sprains when compared with nonoperative treatment.

33. What are the indications for surgical repair of a chronic ankle sprain?

Failure of nonoperative treatment, including proprioceptive rehabilitation, with residual mechanical symptoms of instability, episodes of giving way, and chronic pain are the most commonly reported indications for surgical repair of a chronic ankle sprain. Less than 1% of patients with ankle sprains require surgery.

34. What are the different operations that may manage chronic ankle instability?

Approximately 50 procedures are designed to stabilize the chronically sprained ankle and may be classified into two groups: (1) anatomic reconstructions and (2) nonanatomic reconstructions. At present, anatomic reconstructions are preferred and have generally been associated with more favorable results. Associated conditions include osteochondral lesions of the talus and peroneal instability, tendinitis or tears. Peroneal tendon tears may be present in up to 30% of patients with chronic ankle instability. These conditions may need to be addressed surgically at the time of ankle ligamentous reconstruction.

35. Describe an anatomic ankle reconstruction.

An anatomic ankle reconstruction repairs the injured ligament secondarily with or without augmentation. Examples are the Brostrom repair and the Gould modification of the Brostrom repair. Brostrom originally found it possible to repair chronic ankle ligament injuries by direct suture. Later techniques involving shortening of the ligaments and directly reimplanting them into bone have been highly successful. Gould later reinforced the anterior talofibular ligament with the extensor retinaculum and reinforced the calcaneofibular ligament with the lateral talocalcaneal ligament.

36. Describe a nonanatomic ankle reconstruction.

A nonanatomic reconstruction substitutes another structure or material to take the place of a damaged ligament. An example of this is the Chrisman-Snook modification of the Elmslie procedure, which uses half of the peroneus brevis tendon to reconstruct both the anterior talofibular ligament and the calcaneofibular ligament.

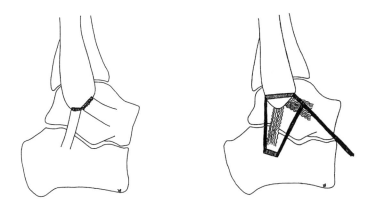

Left, Brostrom repair. The anterior talofibular and calcaneofibular ligaments are reimplanted into bone, achieving an anatomic reconstruction. *Right,* Crisman-Snook repair. One-half of the peroneus brevis tendon is used to reconstruct both the anterior talofibular ligament and the calcaneofibular ligament.

BIBLIOGRAPHY

1. Adamson C, Cymet T: Ankle sprains: Evaluation, treatment, rehabilitation. Md Med J 46(10):530–537, 1997.
2. Brown DE: Ankle and leg injuries. In Mellion MB, Walsh M, Shelton GL (eds): The Team Physician's Handbook, 2nd ed. Philadelphia, Hanley & Belfus, 1997, pp 579–592.
3. Clanton TO: Athletic injuries to the soft tissues of the foot and ankle. In Mann RA, Coughlin MJ (eds): Surgery of the Foot and Ankle, 7th ed. St. Louis, Mosby, 1999, pp 1090–1209.
4. DiGiovanni BF, Fraga CJ, Cohen BE, et al: Asscoiated injuries found in chronic lateral ankle instability. Foot Ankle 21:809–815, 2000.
5. Larkin J, Brage M: Ankle, hindfoot, and midfoot injuries. In Reider B: Sports Medicine: The School Aged Athlete. Philadelphia, W.B. Saunders, 1991, p 366.
6. Lephart SM, Pincivero DM, Giraldo JL, et al: The role of proprioception in the management and rehabilitation of athletic injuries. Am J Sports Med 25:130–137, 1997.
7. McBryde A: Disorders of ankle and foot. In Grana WA, Kalenak A (eds): Clinical Sports Medicine. Philadelphia, W.B. Saunders, 1991, p 466.

8. Povacz P, Salzberg FU, Wels KM, et al: A randomized, prospective study of operative and non-operative treatment of injuries of the fibular collateral ligaments of the ankle. J Bone Joint Surg 80A:345–351, 1998.
9. Renstrom PA: Persistently painful sprained ankle. J Am Acad Orthop Surg 2:270–280, 1994.
10. Wexler RK: The injured ankle. Am Fam Physician 57(3):474–480, 1998.

91. FOOT AND ANKLE TRAUMA

Scott T. McMullen, M.D.

1. What is a Jones fracture?

It is a fracture of the proximal fifth metatarsal diaphysis approximately 1.5 cm from the tip of the tuberosity. This term is occasionally incorrectly used to refer to all fifth metatarsal fractures. A proximal fifth metatarsal fracture is divided into three types. Type I or tuberosity fracture enters the fifth tarsometatarsal junction. Type II or Jones fracture enters the 4–5 intermetatarsal articulation. The type III fracture occurs in the proximal diaphysis of the fifth metatarsal.

2. What are the main principles in dealing with fractures and dislocations of the ankle?

1. Reduction of the injury should be performed as soon as possible.

2. The reduction should be maintained during the healing either with external immobilization or with open reduction and internal fixation (ORIF).

3. The joint surfaces must be reduced anatomically to help diminish the risk of posttraumatic arthritis.

3. What is the ankle syndesmosis?

It is the relationship or articulation between the distal tibia and fibula and is maintained by the interosseous membrane, the anterior/inferior tibiofibular ligament, posterior/inferior tibiofibular ligament, posterior talofibular ligament, and inferior transverse ligament.

4. What complications may occur following ankle fractures or dislocations?

Posttraumatic arthritis	Nonunion
Reflex sympathetic dystrophy (RSD)	Malunion
Neurovascular injury	Infection (open fractures, after ORIF)

5. What complication may develop following displaced fracture of the talar neck?

Avascular necrosis (AVN) of the talar body, which may lead to painful posttraumatic arthritis of the ankle and/or subtalar joint.

6. What is the radiographic appearance of AVN of the talus?

Increased density of the avascular body is seen compared with the surrounding bone, which is vascular and undergoing disuse resorption. Hawkin's sign is the presence of subchondral osteopenia and excludes the diagnosis of AVN. Bone scanning or magnetic resonance imaging also may be helpful in the diagnosis of AVN.

7. Which x-ray views are necessary when evaluating an injured ankle?

Anteroposterior, lateral, and mortise views. The mortise view is taken with the leg internally rotated approximately 15–20°, which aligns the beam perpendicular to the intermalleolar line.

8. What is a pilon fracture?

A pilon fracture is a fracture of the distal tibial metaphysis with extension into the joint surface. It may also be referred to as a tibial plafond fracture. Often there is extensive comminution with this injury.

9. Describe an ideal treatment protocol for dealing with a comminuted fracture of the tibial plafond.

There may be severe soft tissue injury as well, even in closed fractures. The initial treatment should include skeletal immobilization with an external fixation device and plans for delayed reconstructions after soft tissue swelling and injury have improved. Final reconstruction options include the use of a fine wire or hybrid external fixator, limited ORIF, and maintenance of the external fixation device or formal ORIF.

10. When evaluating a person with a calcaneus fracture, you must consider injuries to what other areas?

It is important not to overlook potential spinal injuries. A typical mechanism in both fractures is axial loading. Other associated fractures include femoral neck fractures and tibial plateau fractures.

11. What is the most commonly fractured tarsal bone?

The tarsal bones include the talus, calcaneus, cuboid and cuneiform bones. The calcaneus is the most commonly fractured tarsal bone. The typical mechanism for injury of the calcaneus is axial loading.

12. Name two complications of calcaneal fractures.

- Posttraumatic arthritis involving the subtalar joint and possibly the calcaneal cuboid joint
- Impingement of the peroneal tendons laterally secondary to calcaneal widening

13. Can a compartment syndrome develop in the foot?

Yes. One must consider surgical decompression if this is diagnosed.

14. What are the compartments of the foot?

There are nine separate fascial compartments of the foot:

- The medial compartment contains the adductor hallucis and flexor hallucis brevis muscles.
- The lateral compartment contains the abductor digiti minimi and flexor digiti minimi brevis.
- The deep central compartment or calcaneal compartment contains the quadratus plantae muscle, and the superficial central compartment contains the flexor digitorum brevis muscle.
- A separate fascial compartment in each intermetatarsal space contains the plantar interosseous muscles.
- In the distal medial plantar forefoot the oblique head of the abductor hallucis muscle has its own fascial compartment.

15. What are the common mechanisms of ankle fractures?

- Adduction
- Abduction
- External rotation
- Vertical loading

16. How are ankle fractures classified?

The two most common are the Lauge-Hansen and the Danis-Weber AO classification systems.

17. Describe the Lauge-Hansen classification.

The Lauge-Hansen classification is based on the suspected mechanism of injury. In each category, the injury begins in a specific anatomic location and progresses sequentially about the ankle, creating the injury patterns described.

Supination adduction (SA)
    I.   Transverse avulsion type fracture of the fibula below the level of the tibial plafond
    II. Vertical fracture of the medial malleolus
Supination external rotation (SER)
    I.   Disruption of anterior tibiofibular ligament
    II. Spiral oblique fracture of the distal fibula originating near the level of the tibial plafond
    III. Disruption of the posterior tibiofibular ligament or fracture of posterior malleolus
    IV. Oblique fracture of medial malleolus or rupture of deltoid ligament
Pronation adduction (PA)
    I.   Transverse fracture of medial malleolus or rupture of deltoid ligament
    II. Rupture of syndesmotic ligaments
    III. Short horizontal or oblique fracture of the fibula above the level of the ankle joint
Pronation external rotation (PER)
    I.   Transverse fracture of the medial malleolus or disruption of the deltoid ligament
    II. Disruption of anterior tibiofibular ligament
    III. Oblique fracture of the fibula approximately 4–5 cm above the level of the tibial plafond
    IV. Rupture of the posterior tibiofibular ligament or avulsion fracture of the posterior lateral tibia
Pronation dorsiflexion (PD)
    I.   Fracture of medial malleolus
    II. Fracture of anterior margin of tibia
    III. Supramalleolar fracture of fibula
    IV. Transverse fracture of posterior tibial surface

18. Describe the Danis-Weber AO classification system.
It is based on the level of the fibula fracture.
Type A, fibular fracture below syndesmosis
    1. Isolated fracture
    2. With associated fracture of medial malleolus
    3. With associated posterior medial tibia fracture
Type B, fibular fracture at level of syndesmosis
    1. Isolated
    2. With associated medial malleolus or deltoid ligament injury
    3. With associated medial lesion and fracture of posterior lateral tibia
Type C, fibular fracture above syndemosis
    1. Isolated fibular fracture
    2. Comminuted fibular fracture
    3. Proximal fracture of the fibula

19. What is an injury to the tarsal metatarsal joint area called?
This joint is known as Lisfranc's joint. Injuries may include disruption of the ligaments supporting the joints and associated fractures. For subtle injuries, displacement may be seen only on a weight-bearing oblique view of this region. Anatomic reduction is mandatory.

20. How are talus fractures classified?
The Hawkins classification system is used:
Type I: Nondisplaced vertical fracture of the talar neck
Type II: Displaced fracture of the talar neck with subluxation or dislocation of the subtalar joint with the ankle joint remaining intact
Type III: Displaced fracture of the talar neck with dislocation of the body of the talus from both the subtalar and ankle joints
A rare **type IV** variant is a fracture pattern that includes dislocation of the talar head. The risk of AVN increases as the amount of displacement increases.

21. What is unique about the blood supply to the talus?

Approximately 60% of the talus is covered by articular surface. Thus, only limited areas are available for vascular perforation. Most of the vascularity of the body of the talus is supplied in retrograde fashion. Displaced fractures of the neck pose the risk of AVN.

22. On the mortise view, the distance between the medial malleolus and medial border of the talus is known as the medial clear space. What is its typical distance?

Normally, this space is symmetric with the superior clear space between the talus and distal tibia. A space > 4 mm is considered abnormal, indicating lateral talar shift and a need for either closed or open reduction.

BIBLIOGRAPHY

1. Damer NT: Fractures of the proximal fifth metatarsal: Selecting the best treatment options. J Orthop Surg 3:110–114, 1995.
2. Hawkins LG: Fractures of the neck of the talus. J Bone Joint Surg 52A:991–1002, 1970.
3. Jones R: Fracture of the base of the fifth metatarsal by indirect violence. Ann Surg 35:697–700, 1902.
4. Lauge-Hansen N: Fractures of the ankle combined experimental-surgical and experimental-roentgenologic investigations. Arch Surg 60:967–985, 1950.
5. Manoli A II: Compartment syndromes of the foot: Current concepts. Foot Ankle 10:340–344, 1990.
6. Myerson MS: Experimental decompression of fascial compartments of the foot with a basis for fasciotomy in acute compartment syndrome. Foot Ankle 8:308–314, 1988.
7. Rockwood CA Jr, Greene DP, Bucholz RW, Heckman JD (eds): Fractures in Adults, vols. 1 and 2, 4th ed. Philadelphia, Lippincott-Raven, 2001.
8. Whittle AP: Fractures of lower extremity. In Canale ST (ed): Campbell's Operative Orthopaedics, 9th ed. St. Louis, Mosby, 1998, pp 2043–2066.

92. FOREFOOT SYNDROMES

Scott T. McMullen, M.D.

HALLUX VALGUS

1. What is a bunion?

The term bunion is used to describe a deformity of the great toe metatarsophalangeal (MTP) joint that is characterized by a medial prominence and lateral deviation of the great toe. Bunion is derived from the Latin word *bunio,* which means turnip. Bunion deformity is more correctly called hallux valgus.

2. What is hallux valgus?

Hallux valgus is the term used to describe the lateral deviation of the great toe. It may be due to lateral subluxation of the great toe MTP joint and/or an intrinsic deformity within the great toe proximal phalanx or at the interphalangeal joint. It may be associated with medial deviation of the first ray known as metatarsus primus varus. Pronation of the hallux may also be present with a hallux valgus deformity.

3. Are narrow shoes the only cause of the hallux valgus deformity?

No. Shoewear may play a large role in its development, particularly in feet that are symptomatic. The deformity does occur, however, in societies and cultures where shoewear is limited.

4. What are possible factors affecting the development of hallux valgus?
- Heredity
- Flat feet (pes planus)
- Metatarsus primus varus
- Hypermobile first metatarsal cuneiform joints
- Abnormal length of first metatarsal
- Joint hyperlaxity

5. What is the normal first MTP joint angle (HV angle)?
The normal first MTP joint angle is $\leq 15°$.

6. What is the normal intermetatarsal angle (the angle between the first and second metatarsals)?
The normal intermetatarsal angle is $\leq 9°$.

7. Can a painful hallux valgus deformity be treated without operative intervention?
Yes. Shoewear modification to increase the width of the toe box, which relieves direct pressure, may be helpful

8. What is hallux interphalangeus?
It is lateral deviation of the great toe secondary to deformity within the proximal phalanx or at the interphalangeal (IP) joint. It may be seen with a hallux valgus deformity.

9. What is the primary goal of surgery in the hallux valgus deformity?
The primary goal is to improve pain and function, which is achieved by restoring the normal anatomic relationship of the great toe metatarsal MTP joint and may include work on the first metatarsal as well as the great toe proximal phalanx and the surrounding soft tissue structures.

10. List the surgical options for hallux valgus deformity.
- Medial eminence resection (simple bunionectomy)
- Resection of base of proximal phalanx of great toe (Keller procedure)
- Bunionectomy with soft tissue correction at MTP joint
- Bunionectomy with soft tissue procedure and proximal 1st metatarsal osteotomy (modified McBride bunionectomy)
- Bunionectomy with distal 1st metatarsal osteotomy (Chevron osteotomy)
- Bunionectomy with distal soft tissue procedure and first metatarsal cuneiform joint arthrodesis (modified Lapidus procedure)
- Fusion of first metatarsal phalangeal joint

11. What are the main indications for performing various hallux valgus surgeries?
Isolated distal soft-tissue procedures may be used if the joint is mildly incongruent and the intermetatarsal angle is normal with a hallux valgus angle of $< 30°$.

A Chevron osteotomy is indicated when there is a mild increase of the intermetatarsal angle up to approximately $14°$ and no associated joint incongruity or mild first MTP joint incongruity.

Proximal first metatarsal osteotomy with distal soft tissue realignment is indicated when the intermetatarsal angle is $> 14–15°$ and when there is moderate to severe joint valgus subluxation at the first MTP joint. Typically the hallux valgus angle is $> 30°$ in this instance.

1st metatarsal cuneiform joint arthrodesis is indicated with an intermetatarsal angle of $> 14–15°$ and when hypermobility is present.

The main indications for fusion of the first MTP joint include the presence of degenerative arthritis or deformity following neurologic injury and also with rheumatoid arthritis. Fusion may also be a salvage procedure for failed past hallux valgus surgery. The Keller resection arthroplasty has a very limited role but may be of benefit in a very low physical demand patient.

12. What are common complications associated with metatarsal osteotomy?
- Nonunion
- Dorsiflexion at the osteotomy

- Plantar flexion at the osteotomy
- Shortening of the metatarsal
- Avascular necrosis of the metatarsal head (with distal osteotomy)

13. What results can be expected from hallux valgus surgery?

If careful preoperative planning is performed and indications for operative procedures are followed closely, one can expect 90% of patients to have good results.

14. Is pes planus related to the development of juvenile hallux valgus?

Pes planus has been believed to be related to development of juvenile hallux valgus; however, a recent study found no relationship between pes planus and juvenile hallux valgus.

15. What deformity can result if too much of the MTP head of the medial eminence is removed?

Instability develops and the MTP joint may deviate into a varus position. Correction of this deformity is treated with a transfer of the extensor hallucis longus tendon.

16. Is the hallux valgus deformity seen only in adults?

No. The deformity may develop during the teen or preteen years and is known as a juvenile hallux valgus.

17. What is hallux rigidus?

Hallux rigidus is a degenerative process that occurs with the MTP joint of the great toe. Typically, bony proliferation is present on the dorsal aspect of the metatarsal head, which limits dorsiflexion. Surgical treatment (cheilectomy) consists of generous resection of dorsal osteophytes.

LESSER TOE DEFORMITIES

18. What is a hammer toe?

A hammer toe is a deformity in which flexion of the proximal interphalangeal (PIP) and distal interphalangeal (DIP) joints exists, creating a prominence over the dorsal aspect of the PIP joint. Subluxation or dislocation of the MTP joint dorsally also may occur.

19. What is a claw toe?

A claw toe is hyperextension at the MTP joint, flexion of the PIP joint, and either flexion or extension at the DIP joint.

20. What is a mallet toe?

A mallet toe is hyperflexion at the DIP joint. Typically it is a fixed deformity.

21. With what regional or systemic processes are claw toes often associated?

They are often associated with neurologic dysfunction with weakness or loss of the intrinsic muscles of the foot. This dysfunction may be secondary to central nervous system disorders (e.g., stroke or traumatic head injury), peripheral nerve injuries, or peripheral neuropathy (e.g., Charcot-Marie-Tooth syndrome). Compartment syndrome of the foot may also lead to development of lesser toe deformity.

22. What is a flexible flexed toe?

Essentially, it is a flexible hammer toe deformity. If the deformity is truly flexible, pushing up on the metatarsal head will straighten the toes.

23. What is a bunionette?

This prominent, painful area on the lateral aspect of the fifth metatarsal head is also referred to as a tailor's bunion.

24. List the treatment options for hammer toe deformity.
- Relief of local irritation by increasing the height of the shoe toe box and direct padding
- Transfer of the flexor digitorum longus to the extensor mechanism (effective only in the flexible flexed toe variety)
- Resection arthroplasty of the PIP joint or PIP joint fusion

25. What is metatarsalgia?
Metatarsalgia is pain in the region of the MTP joints. Palpation in the involved metatarsal heads typically elicits extreme point tenderness.

26. What painful joint process in the forefoot area may contribute to deformity at the MTP joint level?
MTP joint synovitis. This has been reported both as a traumatic and a nontraumatic entity. The nontraumatic entity may lead to attenuation of the capsule ligamentous structures and resultant instability and deformity at the MTP joint.

27. What symptoms and findings are associated with MTP joint synovitis?
Metatarsal phalangeal joint synovitis. Pain may be sharp in nature. There may be a sense of fullness in the forefoot area, and its symptoms often mimic interdigital neuritis, an important diagnosis from which to distinguish it. Palpation elicits tenderness over the MTP joint, and subluxation stress testing causes pain. There may be evidence of instability.

BIBLIOGRAPHY

1. Jahss MH: Disorders of the Foot and Ankle: Medical and Surgical Management, 2nd ed. Philadelphia, W.B. Saunders, 1991.
2. Johnson KA: Surgery of the Foot and Ankle. New York, Raven Press, 1989.
3. Kilmartin TE, Wallace WA: The significance of pes planus in juvenile hallux valgus. Foot Ankle 13: 53–56, 1992.
4. Lapidus PW: Operative correction of metatarsus varus primus in hallux valgus. Surg Gynecol Obstet 58:183, 1934.
5. Mann RA, Coughlin MJ (eds): Surgery of the Foot and Ankle, 6th ed. St. Louis, Mosby, 1993.
6. McBride ED: Hallux valgus, bunion deformity: Its treatment in mild, moderate, and severe stages. J Int Coll Surg 21:99, 1954.
7. Mizel MS, Michelson JD: Nonsurgical treatment of monarticular, nontraumatic synovitis of the second metatarsophalangeal joint. Foot Ankle Int 18:424–426, 1997.
8. Morrey, BF (ed): Reconstructive Surgery of the Joints. New York, Churchill Livingstone, 1996.
9. Myerson, MS (ed): Foot and Ankle Disorders. Philadelphia, WB Saunders, 2000.
10. Rossie WR, Ferreira JC: Chevron osteotomy for hallux valgus. Foot Ankle 13:378–381, 1992.
11. Thordarson DB, Leventen EO: Hallux valgus correction with proximal metatarsal osteotomy: Two-year follow-up. Foot Ankle 13:321–326, 1992.
12. Trepman E, Yeo SJ: Nonoperative treatment of metatarsophalangeal joint synovitis. Foot Ankle Int 16: 771–777, 1995.

93. ANKLE ARTHROSCOPY

David E. Brown, M.D.

1. When was the first ankle arthroscopy performed?
It was performed in 1939 in Japan by Dr. K. Takagi.

2. What are the chief indications for ankle arthroscopy?

- Loose bodies
- Osteochondritis dissecans/osteochondral fractures
- Osseous impingement/osteophytes
- Lateral soft tissue impingement lesions/chronic synovitis
- To facilitate ankle arthrodesis
- Unexplained pain, swelling, or mechanical symptoms

3. What are the contraindications for ankle arthroscopy?

- Abnormal neurovascular status
- Severe swelling or edema
- Severe arthrofibrosis or degenerative arthritis with restricted joint volume that cannot be overcome with mechanical joint distraction

4. What are the complications of ankle arthroscopy?

- Nerve injury (usually neurapraxia), most commonly involving the superficial peroneal nerve, which is at risk from the anterolateral portal. The sural nerve is at risk from the posterolateral portal, whereas the saphenous nerve is at risk from the anteromedial portal.
- Vascular injury. The dorsalis pedis is at risk from the anterocentral portal. Posterior tibial artery injury may occur from the posteromedial portal.
- Infection
- Thrombophlebitis
- Iatrogenic joint scuffing usually related to inadequate distraction or improper portal placement

5. Describe the common portals used in ankle arthroscopy.

Anteromedial—just medial to the anterior tibialis tendon at the level of the joint line.

Anterolateral—immediately lateral to the peroneus tertius tendon at the level of the joint line.

Anterocentral—through or immediately medial to the common extensor tendons at the level of the joint line.

Accessory anterolateral—1 cm distal and 0.5 cm medial to the anterolateral portal (usually used only for small inflow cannula)

Medial midline—-between the tibialis anterior and extensor hallucis longus. This portal is 10–11 mm further from the neurovascular structures than the anterolateral portal

Posterolateral—lateral to the Achilles tendon at the level of the posterior joint space. This portal should enter the joint just medial to the transverse tibia-fibula ligament. Placement may be obtained through the use of a switching stick from the anterolateral portal.

Posteromedial—immediately medial to the Achilles tendon at the level of the posterior joint line (an uncommon high-risk portal).

6. Is distraction necessary for ankle arthroscopy? What types of distraction are available?

Mechanical joint distraction is often necessary to achieve satisfactory joint visualization and allow safe instrumentation within the joint. Operative techniques limited to the anterior aspect of the joint generally do not require distraction. Distraction may be achieved *noninvasively* with the use of a clove/hitch device that wraps around the foot and ankle. A weight is then attached to this device to provide distraction. Alternatively *invasive* distraction, using tibial and calcaneal pins with a mechanical distraction device, may be used.

7. Which arthroscopes should be used for ankle arthroscopy?

A standard 4-mm, 30° arthroscope is typically used. Especially when mechanical distraction is used, the standard 4.0-mm scope provides good illumination and the widest field of view.

Occasionally a 2.7-mm or 1.9-mm scope is needed in a tight joint with posterior pathology. Various miniprobes, graspers, curettes, rongeurs, power shavers, and burs are available.

8. Describe and discuss anterolateral soft tissue impingement lesions.

The anterolateral impingement lesions generally are a localized area of fibrosis or synovitis that occurs after an ankle injury. Symptoms include persistent anterolateral ankle pain, swelling, and catching. If these symptoms do not respond to a prolonged period of conservative treatment including rest, immobilization, and antiinflammatory medication, then arthroscopic surgical resection of the impingement lesion may be required.

9. What is the posterolateral impingement lesion?

This lesion occurs after severe ankle inverson injuries. The deep posterior fibers of the deltoid may become crushed between the medial talus and medial malleolus. Thick fibrous scar tissue may persist and impinge between the talus and malleolus. Persistant activity-related pain and tenderness posterior to the medial malleolus responds to arthroscopic resection.

10. Are ankle joint spurs amenable to arthroscopic resection?

Anterior tibiotalar impingement spurs are amenable to arthroscopic diagnosis and resection. Commonly, associated loose bodies or degenerative lesions also are amenable to arthroscopic care.

Scranton and McDermott compared open resection with arthroscopic resection. All but the most severe spurs are amenable to arthroscopic resection. Those managed arthroscopically recovered in half the time of those treated by arthrotomy and resection.

11. What is the etiology and treatment of osteochondral lesions of the talus?

Osteochondral lesions of the talus may occur from trauma or idiopathic osteonecrosis. Many terms have been used to describe these lesions, including osteochrondritis dissecans, transchondral talar dome fracture, osteochondral fracture, and talar dome fracture. Treatment includes cast immobilization, resection, drilling, internal fixation, osteochondral mosaicplasty, and bone grafting. Nearly all lesions are amenable to arthroscopic treatment.

12. Describe the Berndt and Hardy classification of osteochondral lesions of the talus.

Type I: Compression fracture
Type II: Partially detached osteochondral fragment
Type III: Completely detached fragment but nondisplaced
Type IV: Completely detached fragment, displaced

BIBLIOGRAPHY

1. Acevedo JI, Busch MT, Ganey TM, et. al.: Coaxial portals for posterior ankle arthroscopy: An anatomic study with clinical correlation in 29 patients. Arthroscopy 16(8): 836–842, 2000.
2. Alexander AH, Lichtman DM: Surgical treatment of transchondral talar-dome fractures (osteochondritis dissecans): Long-term follow-up. J Bone Joint Surg 62A:646–652, 1980.
3. Berndt AL, Harty M: Transchondral fractures (osteochondritis dissecans) of the talus. J Bone Joint Surg 41A:988–1020, 1959.
4. Buckingham RA, Winson IG, Kelly AJ: An anatomical study fo a new portal for ankle arthroscopy. J Bone Joint Surg 79B:650–652, 1997.
5. Ferkel RD, Guhl J, Van Buecken K, et al: Complications in ankle arthroscopy: Analysis of the first 518 cases. Orthop Trans 16:726–727, 1992–1993.
6. Ferkel RD, Karzel RP, Del Pizzo, et al: Arthroscopic treatment of anterolateral impingement of the ankle. Am J Sports Med 19:440–446, 1991.
7. Ferkel RD, Scranton PE: Current Concepts Review: Arthroscopy of the Ankle and Foot. J Bone Joint Surg 75A:1233–1241, 1993.
8. Hangody L, Kish G, Karpati Z, et al: Treatment of osteochondritis dissecans of the talus: Use of mosaicplasty technique—A preliminary report. Foot Ankle Int 18:628–634, 1997.

9. Kumai T, Takakura Y, Higashiyamaa I, et. al.: Arthroscopic drilling for the treatment of osteochondral lesions of the talus. J bone Joint Surg 81A: 1229–1235, 1999.
10. McGinty JB: Operative Arthroscopy, 2nd ed. New York, Lippincott-Raven, 1996.
11. Paterson RS, Brown JN and Roberts SNJ: The posterolateral impingement lesion of the ankle. Am J Sports Med 29:550–557, 2001.
12. Phillips BB: Arthroscopy of lower extremity. In Canale ST (ed): Campbell's Operative Orthopaedics, 9th ed. St. Louis, Mosby, 1998, pp 1542–1550.
13. Scranton PE, McDermott JE: Anterior tibiotalar spurs: A comparison of open versus arthroscopic debridement. Foot Ankle 13:125–129, 1992.

94. RHEUMATOID FOOT DISEASE

Todd A. Kile, M.D. and Jeffrey A. Senall, M.D.

The incidence of rheumatoid arthritis (RA) in the general population is 2 to 3 per 1000, 90% of whom eventually develop foot involvement. The ravages of RA, when left unchecked, deprive patients of the ability to ambulate effectively.

1. RA begins in the feet in what percentage of cases?

Seventeen percent. Pedal involvement with RA tends to be progressive and bilateral. Cash found that 21% of patients had involvement of the feet within the first year of disease. This rose to 53% after 3 years. In patients with longstanding RA, approximately 90% had involvement of the feet.

2. Which region of the foot is most often involved?

The forefoot is affected in up to 89% of RA patients with a predilection for the synovium of the metatarsophalangeal (MTP) joints.

3. What other areas are typically involved?

The midfoot and hindfoot are more commonly affected than the forefoot (up to 67% of adults). The sites most often involved are the talonavicular joint (39%), the subtalar joint (29%), and the calcaneocuboid joint (25%).

4. What is the most common deformity associated with rheumatoid foot disease?

Hallux valgus develops in 70–80% of patients. Hammer toes are also common, occurring in 50–80% of patients.

5. List some of the nonarticular manifestations of RA and their effects on foot function.

Extraosseous involvement often is present before other evidence of systemic disease.

Inflammation of soft tissues leads to attenuation of ligaments and tendons, which leads to flatfoot deformity (46% of patients). Posterior tibialis and peroneal tendons are most commonly involved. Rupture is caused by eroded bone surfaces, tendon degradation, or previous corticosteroid injection.

Rheumatoid nodules (immune complex-mediated vasculitis) occur in 20–30% of patients, and may develop over extensor surfaces of joints or areas of bony prominence. They usually herald a more malignant form of arthritis.

Vasculitis (inflammatory destruction of blood vessels by immune-complex deposition) results in digital infarcts, cutaneous ulcers, and diffuse rashes about the foot and ankle (rashes are rare in seronegative patients, and should alert clinicians to other systemic effects).

Neurologic involvement (evident in 46% of patients) due to nerve compression or neuropathy may be present.

6. Is hindfoot varus or valgus more common in RA?

In patients who continue weightbearing, **hindfoot valgus** is more common. The combined loss of subtalar cartilage and bone, ligamentous laxity, and posterior tibial tendon dysfunction or rupture contribute to this deformity. **Hindfoot varus** is more common in patients with severe knee flexion contractures who have experienced long periods of recumbency and in patients with juvenile rheumatoid arthritis.

7. Give a differential diagnosis for pain and swelling in the foot.
- Fracture
- Infection
- Tumor
- Sarcoidosis
- Hemophilia
- RA
- Spondyloarthropathies (Reiter's) are commonly found at the insertion of the Achilles tendon or the origin of the plantar fascia
- Psoriatic arthritis should be considered when the interphalangeal joints are affected more than other joints or if ankylosis is present.

8. Why do calluses develop beneath the metatarsal head?

The combination of dorsal dislocation of the MTP joints, causing downward pressure on the metatarsal heads, and distal retraction or atrophy of the plantar fat pad results in painful metatarsalgia and eventually callosity.

9. What is the most specific radiographic finding in RA?

Periarticular osteoporosis. Other common findings include soft-tissue swelling, loss of joint space, and juxtaarticular erosions at the insertion of the ligaments. Late findings include subluxation and dislocation.

10. Radiographs of which part of the body are more likely to provide information than radiographs of any other region?

Standing radiographs of the feet. One study of 200 patients found radiographic changes in 19% of feet and 9% of hands during the first 6 months of disease. In another study of 105 patients with definite or classic RA, 26% had foot changes without hand changes. No patients had positive hand films with negative foot films.

11. What are the nonoperative options for management of the rheumatoid foot?

Consultation with rheumatologic specialists to optimize pharmacotherapy is key. Acute phases are relieved with rest, splinting, and periods of brief immobilization, followed later by directed mobilization to preserve joint motion. Judicious use of injectable glucocorticoids is sometimes helpful. As progression is inevitable, physical therapy becomes more important to maintain range of motion and strength. Hot soaks and contrast baths may be beneficial.

12. Why do shoewear modifications make a difference in the patient with a rheumatoid foot?

By controlling instability and relieving pressure, many of the more disabling hindfoot and forefoot deformities may be delayed or alleviated, thereby allowing the patient to continue effective ambulation.

13. Of all operations done for RA, what percentage involve the foot and ankle?

Twenty-five to 35% of all operations done for RA involve the foot and ankle.

14. Does surgical treatment cure the rheumatoid foot?

No. With continued weightbearing and progression of the disease, all treatment, operative and nonoperative, should be considered palliative.

15. Preoperative evaluation of the rheumatoid patient should include radiographic assessment of the foot and what other area?

The cervical spine also should undergo radiographic assessment for C1–C2 instability.

16. Name the three surgical options for severe RA in the ankle.

1. Synovectomy may be beneficial in patients with significant ankle symptoms unresponsive to conservative therapy early in the course of the disease. Indications include patients with persistent synovitis for 4–6 months who are unresponsive to immobilization and intraarticular steroid injection with articular cartilage of 3–4 mm in width remaining on a standing ankle mortise radiograph.

2. Arthrodesis may be the procedure of choice for the rheumatoid patient with high functional demands and joint involvement limited primarily to the ankle.

3. Total ankle arthroplasty should be reserved for patients with low functional demands and involvement primarily of the ankle without deformity or instability in other joints. Bone density must be sufficient to support the arthroplasty components.

17. When hindfoot fusion becomes necessary, should a triple arthrodesis of the talocalcaneal, talonavicular, and calcaneocuboid joints be performed routinely to provide stability?

No. Only the affected joints should be fused.

18. When is an isolated talonavicular joint arthrodesis indicated?

When it is painful, the only joint destroyed, and when the hindfoot is still flexible or in neutral. This procedure has been shown to prevent later hindfoot deformity.

19. What is the only indication for surgical intervention in the rheumatoid forefoot?

Pain. Deformity or difficulties with fashionable shoewear in the absence of pain are not sufficient reasons for surgery.

20. What is the procedure of choice for painful hallux valgus in the rheumatoid forefoot?

Arthrodesis of the MTP joint. Resection arthroplasty (Keller procedure) is usually reserved for the elderly patient with fragile connective tissues and the need for immediate weightbearing.

21. What is the most important aspect of surgical treatment for the lesser toe deformities in the rheumatoid foot?

Adequate bone resection.

CONTROVERSY

22. In a patient who presents with both ankle and subtalar disease, which joint should be fused?

Occasionally, ankle pain may be referred from other sites (e.g., subtalar joint, peroneal or posterior tibial tendons). Thus it is imperative that the origin of the pain be identified, usually by careful physical examination, selective diagnostic injections, and imaging studies. If indeed both the subtalar and ankle joints are involved, both should be included in the arthrodesis. Some authors advocate a "pantalar" (tibiotalar, talonavicular, and talocalcaneal) arthrodesis. A relatively recent and innovative method stabilizes the arthrodesis with an intramedullary nail inserted retrograde through the calcaneus and talus and into the tibia to achieve rigid internal fixation. Early results are encouraging.

BIBLIOGRAPHY

Please see Bibliography of Chapter 96.

95. THE DIABETIC FOOT

Timothy C. Fitzgibbons, M.D.

1. Why all the fuss about the foot in diabetes? Certainly the other involved organ systems are more important?

There is no question that the various system failures associated with diabetes are more life-threatening; no problem, however, is more emotional, or, in one sense, more disabling than development of a diabetic foot ulcer.

2. Why not amputate the foot and ankle once they become infected?

The obvious answer, of course, is the patient's emotional attachment to his or her extremity. Some patients resist amputation at almost any cost. Of more importance, however, are the costs involved. The cost of a below-the-knee amputation, in terms of prosthetic fitting and loss of productiveness, has been shown on average to be more expensive than limb salvage. Certainly there is a point at which limb salvage is not feasible, but each patient has to be assessed individually.

3. What are the two most common complications of diabetes that affect the foot?

The two most common complications of diabetes that affect the foot are peripheral neuropathy and peripheral vascular disease.

4. What is peripheral neuropathy in diabetics?

Peripheral neuropathy in diabetics may have many different patterns, but the primary problem is the progressive loss of protective sensation in the foot and ankle. The term *neuropathic* refers to any ulceration or joint change that occurs because of this lack of protective sensation.

5. What is the incidence of peripheral neuropathy affecting the foot in diabetics?

Some signs of neuropathy occur in 10–15% of diabetics; 8–14% of patients have neuropathy at the time of diagnosis. Studies have shown a 20–50% incidence of neuropathy in patients who have had diabetes at least 25 years.

6. What is neuropathic ulceration?

Neuropathic ulceration is an erosion of the skin and subcutaneous tissue that occurs in diabetic patients because they lack protective sensation. Whereas the normal individual with a foreign object or pressure point in the shoe has discomfort and takes the shoe off, the diabetic is unable to feel the pressure and continues walking to the point that erosion occurs through the skin and subcutaneous tissue, leading to ulceration.

7. Why are diabetic ulcerations difficult to heal?

The combination of the inability to protect the foot, the high incidence of peripheral vascular disease, and the patient's inability or lack of desire to comply with treatment recommendations makes ulceration an especially difficult problem.

8. What is the incidence of peripheral vascular disease in diabetic patients?

The literature supports an increased incidence of peripheral vascular disease in diabetic patients. In one study of patients who had diabetes for less than 1 year, 22% had some vascular calcification on plain radiographs.

9. What is the concept of "small vessel disease"? How does it affect treatment recommendations?

Diabetes tends to cause occlusion and dysfunction at the capillary and arteriole level. The common teaching is that diabetics are not candidates for peripheral revascularization because the disease affects the smallest vessels. All diabetics, however, should be evaluated for possible revascularization of larger vessels to improve general perfusion to the extremity, which aids in healing of ulcers. Newer techniques of small vessel revascularization are being perfected and may be even more helpful.

10. What is the recommended treatment for diabetic foot problems?
The most important treatment recommendation for diabetic foot problems is prevention. Once diabetic ulceration occurs, it is extremely hard to heal, and the patient is committed to long-term treatment, non–weight-bearing status, and sometimes multiple surgeries.

11. How does one prevent diabetic ulcers?
The first stage of treatment is always the same. The patient must be taught to understand the disease, including the subtle progressive neuropathic changes and the risks of ulcerations. This can be extremely difficult, especially in a young diabetic male. Once the patient accepts and understands the disease, instruction in the do's and don'ts of foot care (see table below) and fitting the patient with special shoes with inlays can begin.

Instructions for Diabetic Patients: Do's and Don'ts

Do
- Use your eyes to check for problems when feeling is lost in the feet. If your vision is impaired, have your family help you.
- Check your feet every day for blisters, cuts, scratches, and nail problems. Use a mirror to see the bottom of your feet.
- Check your shoes every day for foreign objects and rough spots that could cause sores.
- Wash your feet every day. If you have dry skin, use a small amount of lotion containing lanolin on the surfaces of your feet. Keep the skin dry between the toes.
- Make sure your shoes and socks are not tight on your feet. Shoes should have extra room in the toe box and a soft upper material that can "breathe." Rotate your shoes, and do not wear new shoes more than a few hours at a time. If you have fitting problems, ask about accommodative or prescription shoes.
- Make sure your physician checks your feet at every visit. Tell the shoe salesperson that you are a diabetic.

Don't
- Don't walk barefoot. You could injure your foot on sharp objects or rough surfaces without knowing it.
- Don't use heat on your feet, which may cause a burn. Don't soak in hot water. Don't use a heating pad. Wear socks to keep your feet warm at night.
- Don't use chemicals or sharp instruments to trim calluses. Small cuts and blisters will become infected.
- Don't cut into the corners when trimming nails. Cut nails straight across. Use cotton to pack skin away from nails.
- Don't use tobacco. It impairs circulation in the foot.

12. What about diabetic shoes? Are they expensive?
In the mid-1990s medicare performed a study to assess the cost effectiveness of protective diabetic shoes. Ultimately it was clearly shown that they are cost effective and Medicare has now agreed to reimburse for one pair of diabetic shoes and two inlays per year. Private insurance carriers have followed suit and so essentially all diabetic patients now are entitled to protective shoes and should be informed of this.

13. How do you treat a diabetic ulcer?
All patients with diabetic ulcers should be evaluated in the same fashion. Radiographs must be obtained to rule out infection. A peripheral vascular examination must be done to quantify the amount of perfusion to the foot. Referral to a vascular surgeon with vascular studies should be considered for all patients to determine whether perfusion can be increased. All ulcers must be debrided of any necrotic or infected tissue. Proper antibiotics should be used when necessary. If plantar ulcers are present, the patient must be off-loaded.

14. What is off-loading?

Off-loading is the process by which the patient is prevented from putting pressure on the bony prominence that caused the ulcer. Off-loading can be done with crutches or a walker and sometimes is facilitated by special temporary shoes.

15. Describe the proper technique of wound care.

Most authorities believe that wound dressings should be moist. Various types of alternating saline and antibiotic solutions can be used. It is best to avoid the use of cytotoxic agents, such as hydrogen peroxide and Betadine, because they kill cells that aid in healing as well as bacteria.

16. Are there any newer treatments for diabetic ulcerations?

Many new treatment techniques have been advocated in recent years in the literature. The use of platelet-derived growth factors, newer occlusive dressing techniques, vacuum-negative pressure techniques, small vessel bypasses, custom neuropathic walking boots, and multiple other techniques have been advocated for the treatment of diabetic ulcers.

17. What about growth factor and its use in diabetic ulcers?

Platelet derived growth factors, which are proteins normally produced by the host to heal wounds, may be absent in the wounds of patients with diabetes. The evidence continues to mount that such growth factors are important in wound healing. The most common source of growth factor is from the platelets of the patient's own blood. The theory is that the patients cannot get such growth factor proteins to their ulcers because of circulation problems; therefore, by extracting it from their platelets and applying it to the wounds directly they may benefit. The process is complicated and expensive but appears effective. It is important, however, that patients' ulcers are properly debrided, free of infection, and that any possible revascularization to ensure growth factor's effectiveness has been performed. Recently, growth factor solutions that are not processed from patients' own blood have been introduced. Use of such prescription growth factors is encouraging.

18. Define Charcot arthropathy.

Charcot arthropathy refers to the destructive and inflammatory changes that occur usually in the ankle or tarsometatarsal joints in patients with diabetic peripheral neuropathies. Such changes can be caused by a trivial injury that is not protected or occur spontaneously. Patients present with a warm swollen foot or ankle that is often misdiagnosed as an infection. Radiographs eventually depict extensive bone and soft tissue destruction. Treatment involves immobilization and off-loading, to minimize the eventual deformity and to treat the inflammatory swelling. Long-term treatment involves custom shoes and/or bracing.

19. What are the surgical options for the diabetic foot ulcer?

The goal of all surgery in diabetic foot ulcers is to close the wound and maintain as much function as possible. Standard treatments have included extensive debridement of the ulcer with off-loading and eventual granulation by secondary intention; primary amputations of toes or portions of the foot are indicated in certain patients. Recently, a two-stage approach with eventual secondary closure has been described and has been quite successful.

BIBLIOGRAPHY

1. Clare MP, Fitzgibbons TC, McMullen ST, et al: Experience with the vacuum-assisted closure negative-pressure technique in the treatment of non-healing diabetic and dysvascular wounds. Foot Ankle Int 23:896–901, 2002.
2. Jahss MH (ed): Disorders of the Foot and Ankle: Medical and Surgical Management, 2nd ed. Philadelphia, W.B. Saunders, 1997.
3. Kumagai SG, Mahoney CR, Fitzgibbons TC, McMullen ST: Treatment of diabetic (neuropathic) foot ulcers with two-stage debridement and closure. Foot Ankle Int 19:160–165, 1998.
4. Mann RA, Coughlin MJ (eds): Surgery of the Foot and Ankle, 7th ed. St. Louis, Mosby, 1999.
5. Myerson MS (ed): Diabetes and Circulatory Insufficiency in Foot and Ankle Disorders. Vol 1. Philadelphia, WB Saunders, 2000.

96. ARTHRITIS AND ARTHROPLASTY OF THE FOOT AND ANKLE

Todd A. Kile, M.D., Jeffrey A. Senall, M.D., and Marc Bouchard, M.D.

1. What radiologic views are needed for proper evaluation of a patient with a foot or ankle disorder?
- Standing, anteroposterior (AP), lateral, and mortise radiographs of the ankle.
- Standing, AP, lateral, and oblique radiographs of the foot.

2. What serologic tests are useful in patients suspected of having an inflammatory arthritis?
Complete blood cell count (CBC), blood chemistry, rheumatoid factor (RF), antinuclear antibody (ANA), erythrocyte sedimentation rate (ESR), and the histocompatibility antigen HLA-B27.

3. List the major categories of arthritides that affect primarily the foot and ankle.
1. Crystal-induced arthritis
2. Seronegative spondyloarthropathies
3. Degenerative joint disease or osteoarthritis
4. Seropositive or rheumatoid arthritis (RA)

4. What type of crystal causes arthritis in gout?
Arthritis in gout is caused by the needle-like sodium urate crystals, which are strongly negatively birefringent under polarized light.

5. Where does gout present in the foot and ankle?
Of initial gouty attacks, 50–75% involve the metatarsophalangeal (MTP) joint of the great toe, clinically termed acute podagra. Of all gout patients, 90% experience one or more attacks in their toes. Involvement of the ankle and medial midpart of the foot is also common.

6. In what other mammal does gout occur?
None. Humans are the only mammal that lacks the enzyme uricase, which is needed to oxidize uric acid to the more soluble allantoin. Thus, purine metabolism in humans produces the relatively insoluble uric acid, which must be cleared by the kidney.

7. How is acute gouty arthritis diagnosed?
The classic history consists of abrupt onset of excruciating pain with erythema and swelling, usually at night, over the first MTP joint. The attack may be precipitated by minor trauma, binge drinking, or consumption of purine-rich foods. Most commonly it occurs without provocation. It also may occur without hyperuricemia. Diagnosis is confirmed by aspirating synovial fluid and demonstrating the presence of uric acid crystals within the polymorphonuclear leukocytes.

8. What is the proper medical management for acute gouty arthritis?
Symptomatic treatment consisting of elevation and rest of the foot and nonsteroidal antiinflammatory drugs (NSAIDs) at maximum doses (e.g., 75 mg indomethacin followed by 50 mg orally 4 times/day with food) usually provides the most rapid relief. Intravenous colchicine is reserved for patients who cannot tolerate NSAIDs or steroids.

9. What radiologic feature distinguishes gouty arthritis?
Destructive bony lesions remote from the articular surface and periarticular destruction (rat-bite lesions) are often seen in chronic disease.

10. What is pseudogout?

Pseudogout is the most frequently recognized form of calcium pyrophosphate deposition disease (CPPD). Deposits of the weakly positively birefringment, polygonal calcium pyrophosphate dihydrate crystals in synovial joints can mimic acute gout. The knee is the most commonly affected joint, but the ankle, talonavicular, subtalar, and first MTP joints also may be affected.

11. What is chondrocalcinosis?

The term chondrocalcinosis should be used as a radiographic or pathologic description for calcium pyrophosphate noted in articular cartilage or menisci and should not be confused with an actual clinical diagnosis. Chondrocalcinosis also may be noted on radiographs of patients with advanced degenerative joint disease.

12. Name the serologic spondyloarthropathies that affect the foot and ankle.
- Ankylosing spondylitis
- Reiter's syndrome (most common)
- Psoriatic arthritis
- Arthropathy of inflammatory bowel disease

13. What are the radiologic differences between the spondyloarthropathies and the inflammatory arthropathies?
- Intraarticular ankylosis
- Calcification within the adventitia
- Lack of osteopenia

14. List some clinical features of the spondyloarthropathies and the inflammatory arthropathies.
- Inflammation of the site of ligamentous or tendinous insertions (enthesopathy)
- Axial skeleton involvement, such as sacroiliitis or spondylitis
- Sites of extraarticular inflammatory disease such as skin, mucous membranes, genitourinary tract, and gut
- Increase prevalence of HLA-B27 haplotype in Caucasian patients
- Associated with peripheral arthritis
- Asymmetric involvement of distal joints (commonly the MTP joint), and inflammation of soft tissues of entire toe (sausage digits)
- Often present with heel pain (Achilles tendinitis, calcaneal bursitis, plantar fasciitis)

15. What are the most common causes of arthrosis of the ankle?

Previous trauma or malalignment secondary to lower extremity trauma or other causes are most common. Examples include: Pilon fractures, trimalleolar fractures with large posterior fragment, tibial fracture malunions (especially varus or extension), calcaneal fracture malunions, posterior tibial tendon rupture (hindfoot valgus), and subtalar coalitions or fusions.

16. List some conservative treatment options for patients with ankle arthrosis.

Change in activities, NSAIDs, cane, ankle braces, intraarticular injections, shoes with rocker bottom soles or solid ankle cushion heel (SACH), physical therapy, custom ankle-foot orthotics, and casting.

17. What are surgical treatment options for patients with ankle arthrosis?

Debridement (either open or arthroscopic), ligament reconstruction for lateral ankle instability as a cause of mild arthrosis, joint distraction arthroplasty (controversial), corrective tibial osteotomy for malalignment of the distal tibia, ankle reconstruction for fracture malunion, or arthrodesis.

18. What can be done to repair isolated ankle arthrosis (impingement)?

Anterior cheilectomy or removal of the osteophytes from the anterior aspect of the distal tibia and talus via a standard arthrotomy or arthroscopically.

19. What is the standard treatment for advanced arthrosis and failed medical and other nonsurgical treatment?

Ankle arthrodesis.

20. What is the optimum position of ankle arthrodesis?

- Neutral dorsiflexion–plantar flexion
- Hindfoot valgus 5–10°
- Neutral mediolateral displacement
- Posterior translation of the talus ≤ 1 cm (to decrease the anterior lever arm of the foot and decrease overloading of the midfoot joints)

21. How much tibiopedal motion is retained after ankle arthrodesis?

Approximately 30–40% of normal motion is retained through Chopart's (talonavicular) and Lisfranc's (tarsometatarsal and calcaneocuboid) joints.

22. Describe the various methods for achieving ankle arthrodesis.

The most important aspect of arthrodesis is rigid fixation. The numerous variations used include internal compression screws, external fixation devices, internal fixation with plates, and screws or staples and percutaneous pins. The trend is toward internal fixation with large cancellous screws (6.5 or 7.0 mm), which has high success rates. At least two screws are necessary for adequate fixation. Supplemental fibular onlay grafting has been shown to add stability. Joint debridement prior to fixation may be done using open methods or arthroscopically in selected patients.

23. What are the advantages of arthroscopic ankle arthrodesis?

- Minimal bone resection preserves anatomy and overall appearance and size of the foot and ankle.
- Patients are more likely to be able to wear normal shoes
- A statistically shorter time to fusion

24. Who is *not* a suitable candidate for arthroscopic arthrodesis?

Patients with significant malalignment or poor bone quality are not candidates for arthroscopic arthrodesis.

25. Why is total ankle arthroplasty not as common as total knee or total hip arthroplasty?

The increased force per unit area across the ankle joint, coupled with higher shear stresses, poor bone stock (particularly in the talus), and a tenuous blood supply, produce significantly higher rates of complications compared with total knee arthroplasty. Sepsis, loosening, and fractures are common complications.

26. Who is a good candidate for total ankle arthroplasty?

A patient with RA with a painful ankle having little or no deformity and adequate bone stock.

27. List the contraindications of total ankle arthroplasty.

Patient	Ankle
Youth (< 60 years old)	Hindfoot malalignment
Osteoarthrosis (primary or post-traumatic)	Avascular necrosis of the talus
Peripheral neuropathy	Painful arthrodesis

Patient (*cont.*)	**Ankle** (*cont.*)
Corticosteroid use	Pseudoarthrosis
Vascular insufficiency	Distorted anatomy
Paralysis of muscles around the ankle	Sepsis
Poor bone stock	
Neuropathic arthropathy	

28. What variables are associated with a higher rate of failure of a total ankle arthroplasty?
- Previous operative procedure on the ipsilateral foot or ankle
- ≤ 57 years of age

29. How does a total ankle arthroplasty fail?
The most common mode of failure is loosening and subsidence of the talar component.

30. What is the treatment for failed total ankle arthroplasty?
Treatment combines repeated arthrodesis of the ankle with interposition of an intercalary bone graft to minimize shortening.

31. Define triple arthrodesis.
Arthrodesis of the talonavicular, calcaneocuboid, and subtalar joints.

32. What are the indications?
- Significant arthrosis in 2 or 3 hindfoot joints
- Rigid hindfoot valgus deformity
- Certain neuromuscular foot deformities

33. Which of the three hindfoot joints has the highest incidence of nonunion following a triple arthrodesis?
The talonavicular joint.

34. What are the common causes of subtalar joint arthrosis?
Intraarticular calcaneus or talus fractures and subtalar instability are common causes of subtalar joint arthrosis.

35. List the symptoms of patients with subtalar joint arthrosis.
Symptoms include lateral ankle and hindfoot pain, pain with weightbearing, difficulty ambulating on uneven terrain, painful and restricted hindfoot motion, and tenderness over the sinus tarsi.

36. Define hallux rigidus.
Hallus rigidus is a painful degenerative affliction of the first metatarsophalangeal (MTP) joint associated with painful dorsiflexion, increased bony bulk about the joint, and loss of dorsiflexion. Radiographic features include joint space narrowing and a large dorsal osteophyte.

37. What is the treatment of hallux rigidus?
Cheilectomy—removal of the dorsal 20–30% of the first metatarsal head—relieves the dorsal impingement and increases MTP dorsiflexion in adults with pain and large dorsal osteophytes. It has the advantage of being a simple procedure with low morbidity. Cheilectomy is indicated in a patient with painful hallux rigidus and > 50% of the articular cartilage remaining.

38. What is a Moberg procedure and when is it indicated?
A Moberg procedure (dorsiflexion osteotomy of the proximal phalanx) is indicated in a younger patient with limited dorsiflexion of the hallux metatarsophalangeal joint and no dorsal prominence.

39. What are the indications for first MTP joint arthrodesis?
- A painful or damaged joint
- Unstable joint
- Degenerative arthrosis, especially with hallux valgus or failed cheilectomy
- Rheumatoid arthritis (often combined with resection of metatarsal heads 2–5)
- Salvage for total joint arthroplasty, hallux valgus surgery, or other MTP joint operations

40. What are the contraindications for a first MTP joint arthrodesis?
Acute infection and patients who find a stiff joint undesirable.

41. What is the desired position for a first MTP joint arthrodesis?
Ten to 20° valgus of the MTP joint and 10–15° dorsiflexion of the MTP joint, which provides neutral alignment of the hallux with the toe just touching the ground when standing with the ankle dorsiflexed to 90°.

42. What are the indications for resection arthroplasty (Keller procedure)?
A Keller resection arthroplasty (resection of the base of the proximal phalanx) is indicated only in elderly, low-demand patients with painful hallux rigidus, plantar ulceration, or painful hallux valgus, patients with failed silicone arthroplasty, septic arthritis, or in patients where an arthrodesis is not indicated.

43. Why is a Keller arthroplasty not recommended?
A Keller arthroplasty is not recommended because of its complications, which include: recurrence of deformity (hallux valgus), cock-up toe deformity, shortening of the first ray, loss of flexion power of the hallux, transfer metatarsalgia, and stress fractures of the lateral metatarsals.

44. When was the first MTP joint replacement performed and by whom?
The first procedure was performed in 1952 by Al Swanson. The implant—a metal head with an intermedullary stem—failed because of resorption and bone loss about the stem.

45. What is the most widely used and studied implant for MTP joint arthroplasty?
Silicone elastomer (Silastic) implants.

46. What are the indications for MTP joint arthroplasty?
- Osteoarthritis of the first MTP joint with or without hallux valgus
- Failure of other procedures resulting in damage to the joint or bone loss
- Reasonable expectations and an understanding of possible long-term problems
- A cooperative patient

Note that the surgery must be within the surgeon's ability.

47. List the complications of MTP joint arthroplasty.

1. Infection
2. Breakage of the implant
3. Implant particulation and medullary lysis
4. Cortical osteophyte proliferation
5. Synovitis
6. Possible lymphadenopathy
7. Recurrence of hallux valgus
8. Stress fractures of lateral metatarsals due to transfer
9. Hallux extensus deformity (cock-up toe)

48. What can be done for failed MTP joint arthroplasty?
- Removal of the device (resection arthroplasty)
- Replacement of the device if broken
- Arthrodesis of the MTP joint with or without interpositional bone graft

CONTROVERSIES

49. What is the current value of total ankle arthroplasty as a treatment option for degenerative joint disease of the ankle?

In 1994, Kitaoka et al published the Mayo Clinic's experience with cemented ankle replacement. The high proportion of failures and disappointing results with the first generation of implants led many surgeons to abandon this procedure. However, development of a second generation of implants over more than a decade has renewed interest in this type of procedure. Total ankle arthroplasty is currently considered a viable treatment option in appropriately selected patients.

The most widely used designs rely on the biologic fixation of semi-constrained implants with a metal-on-polyethylene interface. Surgical techniques vary, but may include fusion of the distal tibiofubular syndesmosis.

The clinical results of this second generation of implants are presently under evaluation. Current medium-term follow-up studies show promising results and encouraging prosthesis survival rates. Alvine reported 85–90% implant survivorship at 8 and 9 years. Long-term results will help to clarify the optimal indications for this treatment option; risks and benefits associated with ankle arthroplasty versus ankle arthrodesis can then be more effectively put into perspective.

50. Is metatarsophalangeal joint arthroplasty safe?

The effects that implantable silicone devices have on the body have been seen, and the media has made many Americans and lawyers aware of complications associated with their use. Cases of silicone synovitis and lymphadenopathy have been reported using such devices in the foot. Until independent clinical studies (studies not associated with the manufacturer) supporting silicone devices are done, caution should be exercised in using them. Many authors do not recommend using silicone implants.

BIBLIOGRAPHY

1. Beaman DN, Saltzman CL: Arthritis of the midfoot. In Mizel MS, Miller RA, Scioli MW (eds): Orthopaedic Knowledge Update: Foot and Ankle 2. Rosemont IL, American Academy of Orthopaedic Surgeons, 1998, pp 293–303.
2. Campbell DC, Papagelopoulos PJ: Reconstruction of the great toe: Implant and nonimplant options. In Morrey BF (ed): Reconstructive Surgery of the Joints. New York, Churchill Livingstone, 1996, pp 1811–1830.
3. Clayton ML, Winter WG (eds): The Rheumatoid Foot. Clin Orthop 340:7–94, 1997.
4. Coughlin MJ: Arthritides. In Coughlin MJ, Mann RA (eds): Surgery of the Foot and Ankle, 7th ed. St. Louis, Mosby, 1999, pp 559–699.
5. Ferris LR, Pinzur MS, Weinfield S: Ankle and foot reconstruction. In Koval KJ (ed): Orthopaedic Knowledge Update 7. Rosemont IL, American Academy of Orthopaedic Surgeons, 2002, pp 565–572.
6. Hansen ST: The ankle and foot. In Kelley WN, Ruddy S, Harris ED, Sledge CB (eds): Textbook of Rheumatology, 5th ed. Philadelphia, W.B. Saunders, 1997, pp 1759–1772.
7. Kile TA, Alford DW: Arthritis and deformities of the hindfoot and ankle. In Mizel MS, Miller RA, Scioli MW (eds): Orthopaedic Knowledge Update: Foot and Ankle 2. Rosemont IL, American Academy of Orthopaedic Surgeons, 1998, pp 279–292.
8. Kitaoka H, Johnson KA: Ankle replacement arthroplasty. In Morrey BF (ed): Reconstructive Surgery of the Joints. New York, Churchill Livingstone, 1996, pp 1757–1769.
9. Lachiewicz PF: Rehumatoid arthritis of the ankle: The role of total ankle arthroplasty. Semin Arthroplasty 6(3):187–192, 1995.
10. Mizel MS, Sobel M: Disorders of the Foot and Ankle. In Miller MD (ed): Review of Orthopaedics, 2nd ed. Philadelphia, W.B. Saunders, 1996, pp 223–243.
11. Saltzman CL, Johnson KA: The ankle and foot. In Kelley WN, Harris ED Jr, Ruddy S, Sledge CB (eds): Textbook of Rheumatology, 4th ed. Philadelphia, W.B. Saunders, 1993, pp 1855–1872.
12. Strauss E, Missirian J (eds): Arthritis, foot and ankle. Clin Orthop Research 349:9–138, 1998.
13. Toolan BC, Hansen ST: Surgery of the rheumatoid foot and ankle. Curr Opin Rheumatol 10:116–119, 1998.

97. LESIONS OF NERVES IN THE FOOT

David J. Inda, M.D., and John A. Schneider, M.D.

1. Name the five major nerves entering the foot at the level of the ankle.

Medially, the **posterior tibial nerve** divides into the medial and lateral plantar nerve branches. Anteromedially, the **saphenous nerve** parallels the saphenous vein. The **deep peroneal nerve** courses with the anterior tibial artery deep to and between the extensor hallucis longus and the extensor digitorum longus tendons. Anterolaterally, the **superficial peroneal nerve** branches into the medial and intermediate cutaneous nerves. The **sural nerve** runs with the short saphenous vein just distal to the tip of the lateral malleolus to supply the lateral aspect of the foot.

2. List the common causes of foot pain.

Interdigital neuroma	Peripheral vascular disease
Lumbar spine disorders	Diabetic neuropathy
Plantar fasciitis	Tenosynovitis
Plantar fibromatosis	Tarsal coalition
Peripheral neuritis	Reflex sympathetic dystrophy
Tarsal tunnel syndrome	

3. What is Morton's neuroma (interdigital neuritis)?

Morton's neuroma is a perineural thickening of the common digital nerve of the second or third interspace of the foot. It is most commonly seen in women (female-to-male ratio 4:1). The etiology is uncertain; possibilities include anatomic factors, direct trauma, and extrinsic pressure.

4. Describe the symptoms of Morton's neuroma.

Morton's neuroma usually presents as pain on the plantar aspect of the foot between the metatarsal heads, which is often associated with burning or tingling of the involved toes. Pain increases with activity and when wearing shoes with a narrow toe box. Typically the pain is resolved with removal of the shoe and massage of the foot.

5. What diagnostic and/or radiographic tests are helpful in diagnosing Morton's neuroma?

The diagnosis of a Morton's neuroma is based on history and physical examination. In one-third of patients the nerve and its neuroma can be palpated. It is important to differentiate metatarsal phalangeal joint tenderness from interdigital tenderness. Rarely, radiographic studies are required for the diagnosis.

6. What diagnostic approach can help differentiate metatarsophalangeal (MTP) joint synovitis from interdigital neuroma?

Differential injections can help in this difficult diagnosis. An injection of local anesthetic into the web space between the metatarsal heads causing resolution of the patient's symptoms favors a diagnosis of Morton's neuroma. If no relief is obtained, a second injection can be administered to the MTP joint, with a repeat exam noting any improvement in the patient's symptoms.

7. What is Mulder's sign?

Manual pressure applied to the forefoot results in a "click," most frequently felt in the third web space, and reproduction of the patient's pain. The presence of Mulder's sign suggests a Morton's neuroma.

8. What is the nonsurgical management of Morton's neuroma?

Always try nonsurgical treatment first, because approximately 20% of patients will have complete resolution of symptoms. The goals are to alleviate pressure on the nerve by decreasing tension on the intermetatarsal ligament and to reduce compression of the forefoot, which may be accomplished through the use of shoes with a wide toe box, firm sole, and a more rigid arch support. Metatarsal pads also may help to relieve pressure on the nerve. Anti-inflammatory medication rarely offers any benefit. Local corticosteroid injection may be helpful in relieving symptoms, but repeated injections are contraindicated.

9. Do all patients improve after excision of a Morton's neuroma?

No. In a recent large review, 20% of patients considered the operation to be either a failure or only marginally beneficial. Therefore, it is important to inform the patient that surgical excision does not always provide relief.

10. What is the tarsal tunnel? What structures lie within it?

The tarsal tunnel is a fibro-osseous tunnel formed by the flexor retinaculum or laciniate ligament, the medial wall of the calcaneus and talus, and the medial malleolus. The tunnel contains (from anterior to posterior) the tibialis posterior tendon, flexor digitorum longus tendon, posterior tibial artery and vein, tibial nerve, and flexor hallucis longus tendon. The mnemonic "Tom, Dick, And Very Nervous Harry" may be helpful in remembering the order of the structures:

T = tibialis posterior
D = flexor digitorum longus
A = posterior tibial artery
V = posterior tibial vein
N = tibial nerve
H = flexor hallucis longus

11. Define tarsal tunnel syndrome.

Tarsal tunnel syndrome is analogous to carpal tunnel syndrome and involves compression of the posterior tibial nerve or its branches (the calcaneal branch, lateral plantar nerve, and medial plantar nerve). It was first described in 1962 by Keck. The cause of the syndrome can be identified in only 50% of cases. Etiologies include fracture callus, ganglion of the tendon sheath, lipoma, exostosis, engorged venous plexus, and excessive pronation of the hind foot.

12. What are the most common symptoms of tarsal tunnel syndrome?

Patients with tarsal tunnel syndrome complain of plantar numbness, diffuse plantar burning, and tingling pain that increases with activity and decreases with rest. Occasionally, the pain radiates along a branch of the posterior tibial nerve or proximally along the posterior tibial nerve.

13. How is tarsal tunnel syndrome diagnosed?

Three criteria have been proposed by Mann:
• Characteristic pain (see Question 12)
• Positive Tinel's sign over the tarsal tunnel
• Positive electromyelogram documenting entrapment of the posterior tibial nerve or one of its branches.

14. How is tarsal tunnel syndrome treated?

Conservative treatment consisting of nonsteroidal anti-inflammatory medications and local corticosteroid injection may provide relief of symptoms. Orthotics may help to reduce tension on the nerves by limiting pronation in the patient with a hindfoot deformity. When conservative modalities fail, surgical treatment consisting of tarsal tunnel release is indicated.

15. What is reflex sympathetic dystrophy?

Reflex sympathetic dystrophy (RSD) presents with symptoms of burning pain, swelling, and vasomotor dysfunction. The cause is poorly understood, although RSD is thought to represent an abnormal autonomic response to trauma. The severity of the syndrome ranges from minor causalgia after injury to a major mixed nerve. Major causalgia results in marked vasomotor changes indicated by cool, moist skin; edema of the foot and ankle; and severe dystrophic changes, including demineralization of the bones of the foot.

16. How is RSD treated?

The mainstay of treatment for RSD involves early clinical recognition and vigorous physical therapy. If the condition is severe, lumbar sympathetic blocks are both diagnostic and therapeutic. If sympathetic blocks have been successful and symptoms continue to recur, sympathectomy may be considered.

17. What is the most common cause of peripheral nerve injury about the foot?

The most common cause of peripheral nerve injury about the foot is surgical incision. The sural nerve and superficial peroneal nerves over the dorsum of the foot are most frequently affected.

18. What other nerve entrapment syndromes have been described?

Several other less common nerve entrapment syndromes have been described. **Sural nerve entrapment** presents as pain and/or numbness over the lateral aspect of the foot. Pain and numbness over the anterolateral lower leg extending across the ankle joint to the dorsum of the foot is seen in **superficial peroneal nerve entrapment.** The area of pathology typically exists where the superficial peroneal nerve exits through a short, fibrous tunnel through the deep fascia of the lateral compartment. In **anterior tarsal tunnel syndrome,** the deep peroneal nerve may be entrapped by the inferior or superior extensor retinaculum or the extensor digitorum brevis. Trauma is the most common precipitating factor. Symptoms include neuritic pain over the dorsum of the foot.

19. What is Baxter's nerve?

It is the motor branch of the abductor digiti quinti which runs deep to the fascia of the abductor hallucis muscle and can be the cause of intractable heel pain.

BIBLIOGRAPHY

1. Baxter DE: Functional Nerve Disorder in the Athlete's Foot, Ankle and Leg. Rosemont, IL, American Academy of Orthopaedic Surgeons, Instructional Course Lectures 42:185–194, 1993.
2. Baskin JL: Nerve entrapment syndromes of the foot and ankle. J Am Acad Orthop Surg 5:261–269, 1997.
3. Mann RA: Diseases of the nerves of the foot. In Mann RA, Coughlin MJ (eds): Surgery of the Foot and Ankle, 6th ed., St. Louis, Mosby, 1993.
4. Mann RA, Reynolds JD: Interdigital neuroma: A critical clinical analysis. Foot Ankle 3:238, 1983.
5. Miller SD: Forefoot pain: Diagnosing metatarsophalangeal joint synovitis from interdigital neuroma. Foot Ankle Int 11:914, 2001.
6. Mulder JD: The causative mechanism of in Morton's metatarsalgia. J Bone Joint Surg 33:94–95, 1951.
7. Weinfeld SB, Myerson MS: Interdigital neuritis: Diagnosis and treatment. J Am Acad Orthop Surg 4:328–335, 1996.

98. TENDINITIS AND FASCIITIS OF THE FOOT AND ANKLE

David J. Inda, M.D., and Brian E. Brigman, M.D.

1. Which tendons cross the ankle joint? What do they do?
- Achilles tendon (gastrocnemius and soleus) and plantaris tendon: ankle plantar flexors
- Flexor hallucis longus (FHL): flexes the great toe and plantarflexes the foot
- Flexor digitorum longus (FDL): flexes the lesser toes and plantarflexes the foot
- Tibialis anterior: dorsiflexes the ankle and inverts the foot
- Extensor hallucis longus (EHL): extends the great toe and dorsiflexes the ankle
- Extensor digitorum longus (EDL): extends the lesser toes and dorsiflexes the ankle
- Tibialis posterior: plantarflexes and inverts the foot
- Peroneus brevis, peroneus longus, and peroneus tertius: evert and plantarflex the foot

2. How is the vascular supply of the above tendons different from that in the the hand? How does this difference affect them?
The large, extrinsic tendons of the foot have a segmental blood supply. Vessels at the musculotendinous junction and insertion supply each end of the tendon. In areas of low friction, mesotendinous vessels supply the tendon. These tendons rely relatively more on perfusion than diffusion, which may account for increased intratendinous degeneration seen in the foot compared to the hand.

3. What is posterior tibial tendon dysfunction (PTTD)?
PTTD is a spectrum of degenerative changes of the posterior tibial tendon that often occurs at the site of relative hypovascularity just distal to the medial malleolus. Obesity, diabetes, hypertension, seronegative spondyloarthropathies, steroid exposure, and previous trauma may be predisposing factors.

4. List the stages of PTTD.
Stage I: Medial ankle pain and swelling with mild posterior tibial tendon weakness
Stage II: Posterior tibial tendon disruption with a flexible flatfoot deformity
Stage III: Posterior tibial tendon disruption with a rigid flatfoot deformity

5. What is the "too many toes" sign?
In advanced cases of PTTD, the flatfooted patient will stand with hindfoot valgus and forefoot abduction. When viewed from behind, the foot appears to have too many toes.

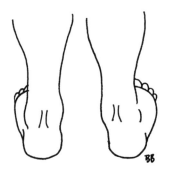

6. What else is notable on physical exam of a patient with PTTD?

Weakness of inversion may be noted. The patient may have difficulty with single heel raise (heel remains in valgus; arch is unchanged).

7. What is the treatment for PTTD?

Stage I: Anti-inflammatory medications and a trial of immobilization
Stage II: Controversial—orthotics vs. surgical reconstruction (synovectomy, tendon transfer)
Stage III: Hindfoot arthrodesis, if symptoms warrant

8. Define dancer's tendinitis.

Stenosing tenosynovitis, or tendinitis, of the flexor hallucis longus (FHL) may be a result of direct blunt trauma, previous laceration, repetitive impact, or excessive plantarflexion, as in the ballet dancer's en pointe position.

9. Where does stenosing tenosynovitis of the FHL usually occur?

It usually occurs in one of three sites: within the sheath behind the medial malleolus, at the start of the fibroosseous tunnel between the medial and lateral talar tubercles, or between the hallux sesamoids.

10. Describe the symptoms of FHL tendinitis.

The symptoms are pain, swelling, and crepitance posterior to the medial malleolus, exacerbated with active or passive motion of the hallux interphalangeal joint.

11. What is the treatment for FHL tendinitis?

Conservative treatment, including NSAIDs, stretching exercises, training modifications, and/or short-term immobilization, usually is sufficient.

12. What is the difference between Achilles tendinitis and Achilles tendonosis?

Achilles tendinitis refers to dysfunction of the tendon secondary to *inflammation* of the peritenon. This *precedes tendonosis,* which refers to the degeneration of the tendon manifested by discoloration and thickening without active signs of inflammation. Tendonosis in turn can lead to rupture of the tendon.

13. What physical exam findings are helpful in diagnosing a rupture of the achilles tendon?

Pain and palpable defects are sometimes noted in the area of the achilles tendon. Perhaps most helpful is to place the patient prone and squeeze the ipsilateral calf, noting absence of plantarflexion of the foot. This is known as the Thompson test and is considered positive because of the discontinuity between the gastrocsoleus complex and its insertion into the calcaneus.

14. Where and when is plantar fasciitis most symptomatic?

Most patients describe pain and tenderness near the medial aspect of the calcaneal tuberosity at the insertion site of the plantar aponeurosis. The pain is typically most severe with the first few steps in the morning, then subsides, only to return after prolonged activity.

15. What nerve entrapment syndromes may mimic plantar fasciitis?

Tarsal tunnel syndrome (entrapment of the tibial nerve beneath the flexor retinaculum) or entrapment of branches of the tibial nerve (the lateral plantar nerve specifically) can cause heel pain similar to plantar fasciitis.

16. What is the significance of an associated heel spur?

Up to 50% of patients with plantar fasciitis have an associated spur. The spur actually lies in the origin of the flexor digitorum brevis on the tuberosity. The pain is usually not directly associated with the spur, and spur removal usually is not necessary.

17. What is the treatment for plantar fasciitis?
Nonoperative management, including orthotics, NSAIDs, and stretching, improves symptoms in the vast majority of patients. Local steroid injections also may be considered. Recalcitrant cases may benefit from plantar fascia release.

18. What is lederhosen syndrome?
Plantar fibromatosis is a proliferative fibroplasia of the plantar aponeurosis similar to Dupuytren's contracture. Patients present with nodularity of the aponeurosis, frequently in the medial, non–weight-bearing region.

19. What is the treatment for plantar fibromatosis?
Nonoperative treatment, including modification of footwear, is the first line of treatment. For large, painful lesions, surgical resection of the lesion should include wide margins. Recurrence rates are high.

BIBLIOGRAPHY

1. Almekinders LC: Tendinitis and other chronic tendinopathies. J Am Acad Orthop Surg 6:157–164, 1998.
2. Canale ST (ed): Campbell's Operative Orthopaedics, 9th ed. St. Louis, Mosby, 1998.
3. Coughlin MJ: Disorders of tendons. In Coughlin MJ, Mann RA (eds): Surgery of the Foot and Ankle, 7th ed. St. Louis, Mosby, 1999, pp 828–829.
4. Netter FH: Atlas of Human Anatomy. Summit, NJ, Ciba-Geigy, 1989.
5. Saltzman C, Bonar S: Tendon problems of the foot and ankle. In Lutter LD, Mizel MS, Pfeffer GB (eds): Orthopaedic Knowledge Update: Foot and Ankle. Rosemont, IL, American Academy of Orthopaedic Surgeons, 1994, pp 269–283.

99. THE CHILD'S FOOT

Paul W. Esposito, M.D., FAAP, FAAOS

1. How is a congenital vertical talus (CVT) identified clinically at birth?
CVT is a rigid deformity that is more accurately defined as a convex pes valgus. It also has been described as a Persian slipper foot. CVT is characterized by a rigid equinus contracture of the hindfoot with an everted or valgus heel, marked dorsiflexion, and abduction of the mid and forefoot, creating a "rockerbottom" foot. This deformity is almost always associated with other congenital neuromuscular abnormalities, such as myelomeningocele, arthrogryposis multiplex congenita, or other syndromes.

2. How is CVT differentiated from a postural or positional deformity such as calcaneovalgus?
The calcaneovalgus foot has an extremely supple heel in a calcaneus posture (i.e., the exact opposite of an equinus contracture). Although the forefoot may be dorsiflexed to the point that it abuts the anterior tibial crest, it easily stretches downward into forefoot equinus. The lack of rigidity and contracture of the tendoachilles clearly differentiates calcaneovalgus from CVT.

3. Is it possible to document radiographically that a deformity is a CVT as opposed to a more benign deformity?

Lateral radiographs obtained in a neutral weight-bearing and plantarflexed position are the key in CVT. These x-rays usually demonstrate the inability of the talus to rotate upward into a more horizontal position with plantarflexion (one of the primary problems in CVT is that the navicular is in a flexed, dislocated position on the neck of the talus). Thus, in the neutral weight-bearing position, the talus is vertical and the calcaneus is in equinus, producing an increased talocalcaneal angle. In flexible or oblique talus foot, plantarflexion returns the talocalcaneal angle to normal (approximately 35°). Other findings include concavity on the dorsal aspect of the neck of the talus in the older toddler and subluxation or dislocation of the calcaneocuboid joint.

4. Besides the rigid equinus and dislocation of the talonavicular joint, what other pathologic findings are present in CVT?

The extensor tendons and the tibialis anterior are contracted to varying degrees. Anterior subluxation of the peroneals and posterior tibialis may be present, which in effect makes them dorsiflexors of the foot. Contractures of the dorsal talonavicular, calcaneocuboid, posterior capsule, and calcaneofibular ligaments also may be present.

5. What is the initial treatment of CVT?

The initial treatment is casting to bring the forefoot out of dorsiflexion. Almost all patients eventually require an extensive operative release with a variety of different procedures available if their associated health problems allow. These operative procedures may be done as one global procedure or in two different surgical stages.

CLUBFOOT

6. What is the inheritance pattern for idiopathic clubfoot?

Research by Dietz strongly suggests a single major gene defect rather than Mendelian inheritance pattern. Many patients, however, have no family history of clubfoot and the exact combination of hereditary and environmental factors to cause clubfeet has not been determined. There are, however, some families with a significant history of severe clubfeet who actually are manifesting a diagnosis of distal arthrogryposis.

7. What is the incidence of idiopathic clubfoot?

Approximately 1 in 1000, with a male-to-female ratio of approximately 2:1.

8. What other conditions may be associated with clubfoot?

• Myelodysplasia
• Sacral agenesis
• Arthrogryposis multiplex congenita
• Amniotic band syndrome (congenital constriction bands)

9. Are teratologic clubfeet in patients with myelomeningocele treated differently than isolated club feet?

The rigid, teratologic clubfeet seen in association with myelomeningocele, rarely, if ever respond to conservative treatment. The operative treatment of the severe form is more aggressive, requiring excision of all the tendons of the foot to leave the foot flail but balanced. Residual, unopposed muscle function always will lead to recurrent deformity.

10. Describe the clinical and pathologic findings in clubfoot.

The hindfoot is in equinus and varus. The talus also is in equinus and is medially rotated, with a short, deformed head and neck. The navicular is markedly displaced medially and may be palpated as it abuts against the medial malleolus. The cuboid also may be medially displaced on the calcaneus. The midfoot and forefoot are adducted and plantarflexed with contractures of the plantar fascia, abductor hallucis, and short plantarflexors. The gastrocsoleus and posterior tibialis muscles, as well as the ligaments and joint capsules of the ankle, subtalar joint, and midfoot, are shortened and contracted.

11. What is the initial treatment of clubfoot?
Almost all surgeons agree that casting or strapping should begin as soon after birth as possible. Serial casting allows rapid resolution of postural deformities that may mimic clubfoot. A true clubfoot may worsen with time despite casting.

12. List the principles of casting for clubfoot.
- The forefoot cavus component is corrected by molding the forefoot while stabilizing the calcaneocuboid joint.
- The forefoot adductus and dislocation of the navicular on the talus are corrected.
- The hindfoot varus is treated by externally rotating the anterior aspect of the calcaneus by placing a valgus mold on the heel.
- If correction is proceeding satisfactorily, the equinus is finally corrected.
- No forceful dorsiflexion is ever applied because deformity of the dome of the talus can occur.

13. Is casting always effective?
The success rate with casting alone varies from center to center, based on the experience of the orthopedist and the severity of the clubfoot. Most surgeons use casting as long as improvement is occurring. There is a growing interest in treating children with a highly specific program of manipulative treatment, coupled with a percutaneous Achilles tenotomy and further casting, that was pioneered by Ponsetti. Surgery is reserved for those with residual deformity. Complete partial or surgical releases are still the accepted mode of treatment at many centers between 4 and 12 months of age. The perfect treatment for club feet, however, has yet to be demonstrated. Persistent manipulation in resistant feet may lead to a rigid rockerbottom foot.

14. Is there any way to document whether casting alone is correcting the clubfoot?
A dorsiflexion lateral radiograph with a normal talocalcaneal angle indicates correction of the clubfoot. The first metatarsal should always line up with the talus and the cuboid should line up with the calcaneus on both AP and lateral x-rays.

15. What are some of the most common persistent static deformities after a primary clubfoot release?
Persistent forefoot adduction and dynamic supination are believed to result from inadequate release of the calcaneocuboid joint and plantar fascia. Intraoperative radiographs may help in recognition and prevention of this problem. A more extensive medial and plantar release, including the navicular medial cuneiform joint, may be required.

16. What causes residual dynamic adductovarus deformity in a child with a completely corrected clubfoot on static examination?
Peroneal weakness with relative overactivity of the anterior tibialis in midswing phase may cause dynamic adductovarus. If no fixed deformity such as hindfoot varus or equinus is present, a split anterior tibial tendon transfer may remedy the problem. Transfer of the entire anterior tibialis (Garceau procedure) is also done but involves the risk of an overcorrected (abducted) forefoot if the tendon is transferred too far laterally.

17. What deformity may result from the loss of function in the peroneus longus tendon after surgery for clubfoot?
Dorsal bunion may occur because the peroneus longus functions as a depressor of the first metatarsal head.

18. What deformity results from overzealous release of a clubfoot?

Soft tissue overcorrection may cause a severe flat foot. Occasionally, the calcaneus may dislocate laterally from the talus.

MISCELLANEOUS CONDITIONS

19. How does a metatarsus adductus differ from a clubfoot?

In metatarsus adductus, which may be familial or positional, only the forefoot is involved. The hindfoot is in a neutral or even mildly valgus posture.

20. What radiographic classification is used for metatarsus adductus?

Berg's classification is as follows:

Simple—isolated forefoot adductus

Complex—forefoot adductus and lateral translation midfoot

Skewfoot—forefoot adductus and hindfoot valgus

Complex skewfoot—adductus, hindfoot valgus, and lateral translation midfoot

21. Should children with metatarsus adductus be treated at birth?

Rarely is a metatarsus adductus rigid enough to require treatment at birth. Approximately 85% of cases resolve with manipulation and/or without treatment. Some controversy exists as to the time of treatment, but if the child has a stiff residual adductus that does not respond to stretching or if a crease in the mid arch is present, treatment with serial casting, special shoes, or orthoses may be effective at age 3–4 months. After 1–2 years of age, medial capsulotomy may be performed coupled with a fractional lengthening of the abductor hallucis. After the age of approximately 5 years, osteotomies may be necessary.

22. What functional problems do children with residual metatarsus adductus have?

Impingement pressure on the first metatarsal head and the base of the fifth metatarsal can occur. The impingement is caused by shoes; thus, in cultures in which shoes are not worn, it is not a functional problem.

23. What kind of shoes should be recommended for normal toddlers with flat feet (asymptomatic flexible pes planus)?

Shoes have been shown to have no effect on the development of arches. The normal developmental pattern is gradual improvement in the arch until about 5–6 years of age, regardless of shoe wear. Shoe wedges or orthotics also have been shown to be ineffective in changing torsional alignment.

24. What are the requirements of a good shoe for normal children?

Shoes should be quadrangular in shape, flexible, flat with no heel elevation, porous to prevent skin maceration, and attractive. They should be lightweight, extended above the ankle in young children (to prevent the shoe from falling off), and acceptable in appearance. Expense has little to do with the quality of the shoe. Shoes with a firm heel counter may provide some support for balance but the sole of the shoe should be flexible to allow for proprioceptive feedback.

25. Are there any indications for treatment of pes planovalgus?

Yes. Pes planovalgus should be treated if pain in the arch or the shin is present. Children with painful arches should be evaluated for underlying neurologic disease, Kohler's disease, os naviculare, or tarsal coalition. Custom-molded medially posted orthotics may be helpful. It is extremely rare for any child with flexible flat foot to require surgery.

26. Is toe walking (intermittent equinus) normal in toddlers?

Intermittent toe walking is common in normal children. However, close neurologic examination, an in-depth history, and serial follow-up examinations should be done, especially if other signs of developmental delay are evident. Toe walking may be one of the first signs of subtle spastic diplegic cerebral palsy. Unilateral toe walking may be seen in mild spastic hemiplegia, spinal cord anomalies, or tumors of the central nervous system. Idiopathic toe walking is therefore a diagnosis of exclusion, and a positive family history is frequently present.

27. What is cleft foot?

This extremely rare deformity is also known as lobster claw foot, split foot, and ectrodactyly. A varying degree of absence of the middle portion of the foot is present, including metatarsals and phalanges. Cleft foot is an autosomal dominant disorder with varying penetrance. It is most commonly bilateral, often in association with lobster claw hands. If a large cleft is present in the feet, treatment involves complex plastic surgical flaps as well as bony procedures, depending on the nature of the abnormality.

28. What are the osteochondroses? Which bones in the child's foot are involved?

Kohler's disease involves the navicular joint and presents as arch pain in a relatively young child. It is diagnosed by radiographs that show sclerosis or fragmentation of the navicular joint. Generally it is self-limited without long-term deformity or symptoms, but may necessitate a period of casting and/or orthotics. Frieberg's disease involves the second metatarsal head and causes pain in the forefoot. It usually presents in late adolescence.

29. What is the most common cause of heel pain in the preadolescent or early adolescent?

In the past, such heel pain was known as Sever's disease (i.e., osteochondrosis of the calcaneal apophysis). However, x-rays of the asymptomatic side frequently show more fragmentation and involvement than on the radiographs of the affected side. The heel pain is now believed to be secondary to inflexibility of the Achilles tendon and plantar fascia in a rapidly growing child. It responds to stretching, gel heel pads, and occasional casting. Other causes of heel pain may include stress fractures, bone cysts, tumors, and osteomyelitis of the calcaneus.

30. What is the likely pathology in an adolescent child with a symptomatic flat foot and a painful bump on the medial arch?

An os naviculare (accessory navicular) may cause a progressive and painful flat foot. The insertion of the posterior tibialis is superior to its normal insertion and thus does not elevate the arch adequately. This may be treated with a simple excision of the ossicle if the child does not respond to orthotic and or cast treatment.

31. What is a common cause of a stiff, painful flat foot in an adolescent?

A common cause is tarsal coalition, which frequently presents as recurrent sprains and pain in the medial subtalar joint or sinus tarsi. The most common sites of a coalition (fibrous or bony bridge) are in the middle facet of the talocalcaneal joint and the calcaneonavicular joint. Physical examination reveals varying degrees of stiffness. Oblique radiographs demonstrate the calcaneonavicular bridge, but computed tomography (CT) is the best method to diagnose a talocalcancal coalition. The Harris axial view of the subtalar joint may demonstrate medial talocalcaneal coalition if the medial facet is obliquely oriented and irregular or fused, but it is not as reproducible and reliable as CT. Coalitions can be excised if conservative treatment fails with results dependent on the size of the coalition and the extent of secondary changes in the involved joints.

BIBLIOGRAPHY

1. Asirvatham R, Stevens PPM: Idiopathic forefoot-adduction deformity: Medial capsulotomy and abductor hallucis lengthening for resistant and severe deformities. J Pediatr Orthop 17:496–500, 1997.
2. Cummings RJ, Davidson RS, Armstrong PF, et al: Congenital clubfoot. Rosemont IL, American Academy of Orthopaedic Surgeons, Instructional Course Lectures 51:385–400, 2002.
3. Dietz F: The genetics of idiopathic clubfoot. Clin Orthop 401:39–48, 2000.

4. Jacobsen ST, Crawford AH: Congenital vertical talus. J Pediatr Orthop 3:306–310, 1983.
5. Johnston CE II, Roach JW: Dorsal bunion following clubfoot surgery. Pediatr Orthop 8:1036–1040, 1985.
6. Kodros SA, Dias LS: Single stage surgical correction of congenital vertical talus. J Pediatr Orthop 19:42–48, 1999.
7. Kumar SJ, Cowell HR, Ramsey PL: Foot problems in children. Rosemont IL, American Academy Orthopaedic Surgeons, Instructional Course Lectures, pp 235–251, 1982.
8. Mosca VS: Calcaneal lengthening for valgus deformity of the hindfoot. J Bone Joint Surg 77A:500–512, 1995.
9. Mosca VS; Flexible flatfoot and skewfoot. Rosemont IL, AAOS, Instructional Course Lectures 45:347–354, 1996.
10. Neto J, Dias LS, Gabrieli AP: Congenital talipes equinovarus in spina bifida: Treatment and results. J Pediatr Orthop 16:782–785,1996.
11. Ponseti, IV, Becker JR: Congenital metatarsus adductus: The results of treatment. J Bone Joint Surg 78A:448–453, 1992.
12. Staheli LT: Rotational problems in children. J Bone Joint Surg 75A:939–949, 1993.
13. Staheli LT: Shoes for children: A review. Pediatrics 88:371–375, 1991.
14. Sullivan AJ: Pediatric flatfoot: evaluation and management. J Am Acad Orthop Surg 7:44–53, 1999.
15. Wood VE, Peppers TA, Shook J: Cleft-foot closure: A simplified technique and review of the literature. J Pediatr Orthop 17:501–504, 1997.

INDEX

Page numbers in **boldface type** indicate complete chapters.

Index

Tarsal bones, fractures of, 395
Tarsal coalition, 379, 424
  imaging of, 59
Tarsal metatarsal joint, injuries of, 396
Tarsal tunnel, anatomy of, 416
Tarsal tunnel syndrome, 416
  anterior, 417
  as plantar faciitis mimic, 419
  posterior tibial nerve entrapment in, 66
TDAVNH mnemonic, for tarsal tunnel anatomy, 416
Teardrop fracture, 214
Technetium-99m scan
  of osteoarthritis, 2
  of osteomyelitis, 24, 55
  of osteosarcoma, 80
  of pars interarticularis lesions, 234
Tendinitis
  Achilles', 383–384, 419
  of biceps, in athletes, 143–144
  dancer's, 419
  of flexor hallucis longus, 419
  of foot and ankle, 418–419
  of triceps, 145
Tendon injuries, of hand and wrist, **188–189**
Tendon lengthening, as spastic contracture treatment, 95
Tendonosis, of Achilles' tendon, 419
"Tennis elbow," 148, 149
Tennis elbow straps, 148
"Tennis leg," 385
Tenosynovitis
  gonococcal arthritis-related, 17
  of hand, wrist, and forearm, **207–209**
  stenosing, 208, 209, 419
Tension signs, in lumbar disc herniation, 221–222
Teres minor muscle, 66, 113
  innervation of, 103
"Terrible triad of O'Donoghue," 307–308
Terry Thomas sign, 185
Tetanus immunization, in open fracture patients, 30
Tetraplegia, cerebral palsy-related, 93
Thomas test, 243, 245
Thompson test, 384, 391
Thoracic spine, imaging of, 68
Thoracolumbar spine
  extension injury to, 241
  fractures of, 239–241
    unstable, 242
  scoliosis of, 54
Thromboembolism
  hip fracture-related, prevention of, 297
  pulmonary, 36, 37–38
Thrombolytic therapy, for pulmonary thromboembolism, 38
Thrombophlebitis
  postoperative, 291
  total hip replacement-related, 264
Thrombosis, deep venous, **33–36**
  diagnosis of, 34–35, 38
  femoral neck fracture-related, 295
  postoperative, 33

Thrombosis, deep venous (*cont.*)
  predisposing factors and conditions for, 33, 37
  prophylaxis and treatment for, 35–36
  in trauma patients, 70
Throwing injuries
  of elbow, **142–157**
  of shoulder, **112–116,** 126
Thumb
  arthrodesis in, 198
  Bennett fractures of, 180–181
  bowler's, 206
  carpometacarpal joint of
    arthritis of, 3, 193–194
    arthrodesis of, 198
  gamekeeper's, 181
  polydactyly of, 209
  Rolando's fractures of, 181
  skier's, 181
  trigger, 210
Thyroid cancer, metastatic to bone, 82
Tibia
  anteroposterior displacement measurement in, 320
  avascular necrosis of, 354
  bowing of, 100
  external rotation testing of, 333
  fractures of, **386–388**
    compartment syndromes associated with, 381
    open, 31
    pilon-type, 388
    plateau-type, 388
    stress-type, 379–380
  posterior cruciate ligament avulsion from, 325
  proximal
    in failed total knee arthroplasty, 364
    resection of, 359–360
  pseudoarthrosis of, 100
Tibial alignment jigs, extramedullary and intramedullary, 359–360
Tibial cortex, anterior, stress fracture of, 379
Tibial external rotation test, 313
Tibial inlay grafts, placement of, 327
Tibialis posterior tendon, in unilateral flatfoot deformity, 66
Tibial nerve, posterior, in tarsal tunnel syndrome, 66
Tibial plafond, comminuted fracture of, 395
Tibial plateau, fractures of, 371–372
Tibial tendon, posterior, dysfunction or rupture of, 392
Tibial transosseous tunnel preparation, 326
Tibia varum, 379
Tibiofemoral angle, 365
Tibiofibular diastasis, 391
Tinel's sign, 147, 165, 205
Tissue plasminogen activator, as pulmonary thromboembolism treatment, 38
Toes
  flexible flexed, 399
  greater, deformities of, 397–399
  lesser, deformities of, 399–400
  mallet, 399